Orthopedic Nursing

CARROLL B. LARSON
M.D., F.A.C.S.
*Professor of Orthopedic Surgery and
Chairman of the Department of Orthopedic
Surgery, The University of Iowa,
Iowa City, Iowa*

MARJORIE GOULD
R.N., B.S., M.S.
*Associate Professor, College of Nursing,
The University of Iowa, Iowa City, Iowa*

Orthopedic Nursing

EIGHTH EDITION

with 672 illustrations

THE C. V. MOSBY COMPANY

Saint Louis / 1974

EIGHTH EDITION

Copyright © 1974 by The C. V. Mosby Company

Previous editions copyrighted 1943, 1949, 1953, 1957, 1961, 1965, 1970

Printed in the United States of America

Distributed in Great Britain by Henry Kimpton, London

Library of Congress Cataloging in Publication Data

Larson, Carroll Bernard, 1909-
   Orthopedic nursing.

   [First]-2d editions by R. V. Funsten and C. Calderwood. 3d-6th editions by C. B. Larson and M. Gould published under title: Calderwood's orthopedic nursing.
   1. Orthopedic nursing. I. Gould, Marjorie, joint author. II. Calderwood, Carmelita Cameron. Calderwood's orthopedic nursing. [DNLM: 1. Orthopedics—Nursing texts. WY161 L334o 1974]
RD753.L36 1974   610.73'677   73-18221
ISBN 0-8016-2865-2

GW/CB/B   9 8 7 6 5 4 3 2

Preface

During the past decade, new scientific knowledge in the medical and related fields has resulted in many advances in patient care. Procedures and treatments have changed rapidly. As orthopedic surgery advances with new operative concepts, such as total joint replacement and new methodology in the study of bone metabolism, orthopedic nurses must understand these concepts if they are to assume responsibility for patient nursing care and assist in the management of musculoskeletal problems. But the fundamental aspects of good nursing care remain the same: the necessity to recognize and provide for the patient's physical, social, and psychological needs; the need to provide care with gentleness and a solicitous attitude; the importance of having respect for individual patients and their rights; and the necessity for teaching health maintenance and preventing disease. However, a deeper understanding of bone structure, bone physiology, and the reactions of the musculoskeletal system to stresses and strains will help the nurse to modify these established nursing skills where necessary to meet the needs of the individual patient. This revision reiterates the established fundamentals of orthopedic nursing and updates the core of basic knowledge that is the root of orthopedics and upon which the forward progress of orthopedic surgery and orthopedic nursing depends.

We are grateful for the assistance of Drs. Donald Weir, Richard Johnston, George Brown, John Albright, Merle Strottmann, and Ignacio Ponseti, and the Division of Graphic Arts of the Iowa College of Medicine, Nancy Sprague, and the secretaries and many nurses from the Department of Orthopaedic Surgery at the University of Iowa Hospitals who have each contributed their time and talent to this eighth edition to ensure its teaching value.

C. B. L.
M. G.

Contents

Orthopedic Nursing

1
Introduction to orthopedic nursing

DEFINITION OF ORTHOPEDICS

Orthopedic surgery is a medical specialty that includes investigation, preservation, restoration, and development of the form and function of the extremities, spine, and associated structures by medical, surgical, and physical methods.

HISTORY OF ORTHOPEDICS

The term orthopaedia (from the Greek, *orthos* straight, *paides* child) was coined in 1741 by Nicholas Andrey as the title for his book devoted to a discussion of the deformities of the child. Orthopedics was practiced by "strap and buckle" doctors for nearly 120 years before surgery was applied to the art. Dr. Virgil P. Gibney, Surgeon-in-Chief of the New York Hospital for the Ruptured and Crippled, advocated surgery for the correction of certain deformities, and this was looked upon by many of his contemporaries as meddlesome. His persistence produced results superior to those from other mechanical means, and in 1887 the American Orthopaedic Association was organized as a forum for orthopedic surgeons. The transactions of the Orthopaedic Association were published annually and included reports on an ever-increasing number of case studies, surgical operations, and investigations which continue today as the Journal of Bone and Joint Surgery.

World War I and the years following saw the organization of hospital orthopedic services as well as sections or departments of orthopedics in medical schools. In increasing numbers the graduates joined the general medical communities. In 1922 the Shriner's Hospitals for Crippled Children (presently 19) came into being since only 400 orthopedic surgeons were available in the entire United States, and some remote areas had none except those who worked in the Shriner's Hospitals. In 1932 the American Academy of Orthopaedic Surgeons was organized for the purpose of providing continuing education. In 1934 the American Board of Orthopaedic Surgery was formed to establish standards of training for orthopedic surgeons, and examinations have been held yearly for candidates who wish to become certified in the practice of orthopedic surgery. By 1971, over 6,000 orthopedic surgeons had been certified by the board.

Whereas the advent of orthopedic surgery as a specialty is relatively recent, medical problems that involve bones have existed for half a million years, as evidenced in the Java man. Preserved skeletons from antiquity to the present have yielded evidence by which anthropologists and archeologists have determined the state of industrial, social, and recreational activities of ancient people. Defects found in the skull rank trephining as the earliest of operations substantiated by writings in the Egyptian papyri in 1600 B.C. The translations of Hippocrates by Galen (131 to 201 A.D.) provide classic descriptions of clubfeet and congenital dislocations of the hip. In the fifteenth century Leonardo da Vinci made anatomic drawings from human dissections, but not until the seventeenth century, after the invention of the microscope by Leeuwenhoek, did Klopton Havers provide the histology of bone which is recognized to this day as the haversian system in cortical bone.

In the eighteenth century, John Hunter gave

us insight into the capability of bones to produce longitudinal and directional growth which later led Wolff to develop his famous law: "Bones in their external and internal architecture conform with the intensity and direction of the stresses to which they are habitually subjected" (1836-1902). The Wolff concept—that bone is formed through the tension of muscles and the pressure of body weight coupled with gravitational pull—constitutes the major thesis of present day authorities on skeletal development.

Normal reactions of the musculoskeletal system to the events of daily living such as standing, sitting, walking, running, and manipulative tasks of the arms and hands constitute the major concern of orthopedics. An insight into the behavior of living bone and muscle is essential if we are to relieve the handicaps to which an individual is subjected in the case of inabilities of the bones, muscles, and joints to carry out normal tasks. A clear concept of bone structure, physiologic response of bone to the stresses of gravity, and the acts of daily living is the special contribution orthopedics has to offer toward the relief of musculoskeletal abnormalities that afflict mankind.

BIOMECHANICS FOR NURSING

The application of mechanical principles to the living human body is referred to as biomechanics. The subject of mechanics deals with forces acting on bodies and the result of these forces in terms of equilibrium and movement. The human body at rest represents equilibrium, whereas the body at work represents movement. In both instances there are forces acting from within (internal) and forces acting from without (external). An understanding of the forces and how the human body translates them into rest or work is essential in orthopedics since an improper body response presents postural defects, painful strains, limps, and other impairments of the musculoskeletal system.

In biomechanics, equilibrium and motion are so closely interrelated that the principles of each will be pointed out as the occasion demands. Mechanics applied to the human body is divided into two main parts (1) statics, which is concerned with the body in balance or erect posture, and (2) dynamics, which is concerned with the body in motion.

STATICS
Posture

Standing posture is the ability of the body to remain erect, and to maintain this attitude by resisting outside forces with the least amount of energy. The anatomic variations from one individual to another are factors that account for the great differences in postural attitudes that can be observed in any queue at a box office. Postures are described as erect, good, slouchy, saggy, or tired, which raises a question: Is there a normal or proper posture? (Fig. 1-1.)

Statistically a normal posture would be the posture assumed by the majority of a healthy population. Any investigation to measure what is normal is difficult because each person may vary from day to day and in various conditions of heat, cold, sadness, and joy; thus, normal can never be a fixed value.

Physiologically posture is known to influence blood pressure, muscular effort, respiratory efficiency, and energy requirements. The rigid military posture may require 20% more energy than the at ease posture. It is known that an easy standing position requires relatively small energy costs over recumbency, hence we can say that rigid posture is not ideal.

Erect posture. In order to stand erect, the body of man must resist gravity. We learn in physics that the body has a center of gravity, that is, a point within the body around which the mass of the body is equally distributed. If the body were

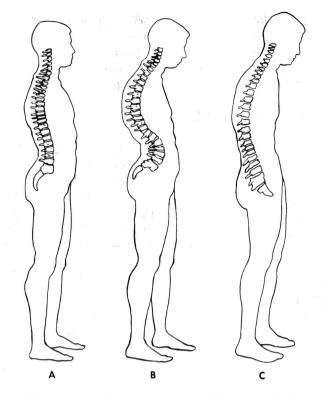

Fig. 1-1. A, Curves of the spine in good posture, **B,** curves of the spine in the slump posture, **C,** obliteration of the spinal curves as in early spondylitis.

supported at this point, it would be in equilibrium. A stable equilibrium will occur in the erect posture when a vertical line passes through the center of gravity (situated in front of the second sacral vertebra) and through the base of support (Fig. 1-2). This means an equal amount of body weight is distributed to each side of the line of gravity. If the body leans forward, an unstable equilibrium occurs since the perpendicular line of gravity through the body's center of gravity no longer passes through the base of support but is now in front of it. To prevent the body from falling, a muscle force must pull the body back to the stable position over its base of support. If the body were similar to a brick leaning forward on edge, it would continue to fall forward until it came to rest on the flat side that provides a broad base of support with the center of gravity at the lowest point. A broad base of support and the lowest center of gravity provide a stable equilibrium (Fig. 1-3).

Obviously the human body can compensate for an unstable equilibrium but it will require energy in the form of muscular effort to do so. This capability is balance, which allows the body to resist all outside forces that disturb a neutral equilibrium.

Ideal posture. Ideal posture is observed only in the trained individual. The most commonly observed posture is by no means ideal. The variations in body build and particularly the inherent inborn length of ligaments account for the marked variations of posture among humans.

Persons with relaxed ligaments stand with hyperextended knees, hyperextended hips, and very flexible exaggerated curves of the spine; hence, the individual parts of the body extend farther forward and backward from the line of gravity than those in individuals with tighter ligaments. (It must be pointed out, however, that as long as there is an equal distribution of weight of the extended parts on each side of the line of gravity, these individuals are as much on line of gravity as others and remain so with no more muscular effort than others.) The posture of these loose-ligamented persons necessarily appears slouched although it is efficient. Unfortunately the anterior longitudinal ligaments of the lumbar spine are under more continuous shear strain, which renders them more subject to low back strain. For these individuals to strive toward ideal posture would demand constant training and constant muscular energy for which very few people are suited or motivated. To attain the ideal posture would require muscular control in order to stand with knee in neutral extension and trunk control to reduce each vertebral segment toward neutral (reduce the amount of curve). Thus, a more cosmetically accepted posture would be achieved at the expense of constant muscle coordination and energy; the only physiologic gain would be relief of strain on spinal ligaments.

There are a few tricks that are easily learned to improve posture, and these can be accomplished with minimal energy expenditure. Head up, chin in, backward pelvic tilt, and standing tall practiced many times for a few seconds at a

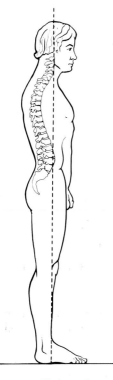

Fig. 1-2

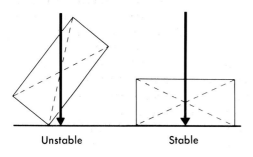

Unstable   Stable

Fig. 1-3. The large arrow is the downward force of gravity, which comes to rest outside of the narrow base of support. The brick has more weight to the right side of the base and therefore will fall to the right. The brick will fall until the center of gravity rests over a broad base as depicted in the stable position.

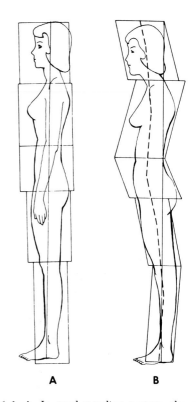

A   B

Fig. 1-4. A, In good standing posture, the weight-bearing line (line of gravity) passes just anterior to the ear, through the shoulder joint, just posterior to the hip joint, and slightly behind the patella; it strikes the floor just anterior to the external malleolus. **B,** Poor standing posture illustrating malalignment of the body segments and a distorted weight-bearing line. Note forward position of the head, round shoulders, increased lordosis, and protruding abdomen. (Courtesy M. Joan Popp; from Teaching and evaluating posture, Audiovisual Center, the University of Iowa, Iowa City.)

time will go far toward achievement of improved posture. It will eliminate the slouch that accompanies fatigue and diminish ligamentous strains. It can become a good habit to replace a bad one.

Recumbent posture. So far the discussion has related to man's ability to stand erect, which we think of as posture; however, the strict definition of posture includes other positional attitudes. If the body is lying down, this can be described as a recumbent posture; lying face down is a prone posture, and face up, a supine posture. Posture in the sense of description is synonymous with position, the word most commonly used. Gravity continues to exert its force on the body in whatever position is assumed. The effect of that force, however, is altered since the direction of the pull is no longer in the longitudinal axis of the body toward the center of the earth and the base of support is no longer the feet. The body in the supine position supported by a firm bed is pushed against the bed by the force of gravity acting at right angles or downward on each individual segment. Each segment is supported so that there is no energy requirement for balance; therefore, the body is at rest with a zero energy requirement to resist gravity.

This concept has import for the nurse who is responsible for positioning the patient's body in bed. Certain qualifications must be appreciated although the principle remains the same; namely, that wherever a force acts in one direction there must be an equal force in the opposite direction if the body is to remain at rest.

From a practical view, each body segment has its own shape and weight. A straight hard surface supporting the supine body cannot match the normal curves of the body. The consequence is that the body parts that normally protrude posteriorly must share the bulk of body weight at the midorsal spine, occiput, sacrum, and calves of the legs. Because these contact points form bridges, the segments of body in between have no base of support and, therefore, sag until the base is reached. The result of this uneven weight distribution clearly places an excessive load at the contact points and thus demands frequent change in body alignment.

An excellent example is a person who has a lordotic contracture of the lumbar spine. Lying supine on the floor would become uncomfortable as the arched lordosis flattens from the forces of gravity but never reaches the base of support. The posterior ligaments bear the strain. A supple individual, on the other hand, may be quite comfortable since the lumbar spine flattens easily to reach the floor and find support.

The ideal flexibility in the base of support (the mattress) would allow the heaviest and more

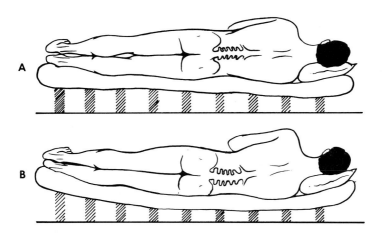

Fig. 1-5. A shows ideal mattress that allows hips and shoulder sufficient give to maintain a straight spine and an evenly distributed support throughout the body length. **B** shows sagging mattress and spring that are to maintain straight spine. This position puts a tension strain on the spinal ligaments at the convexity of the curve and a compression strain at the concavity.

rigid body segments to sink down just enough to allow the remaining segments to accept support from the mattress and maintain essentially the same body alignment as in standing. Since wide variations exist in the rigidity and weight of body segments in people, a trial and error test of spring mattress combinations would be the only way to meet the criteria of need in choosing the proper support.

In side lying, the body profile is variable; the shoulder segment is broader and heavier than the pelvis in males, and the reverse is true in females. The head requires pillow support of shoulder width to maintain a straight cervical spine. In an extended position the lower limbs lying one on the other have a very unstable equilibrium, and therefore, with relaxation tend to rotate unless flexed at the hips and knees. Even in this position the contact points at the knee and ankle provide very small surface areas of support and cannot tolerate the pressure except for short periods. A better base of support is a pillow between the knees (Fig. 1-6).

Whether the body is supine or lying on the side, there is no consistent way to relieve localized pressure points in the recumbent position. The only solution is the frequent shift of positions that occurs regularly in normal persons in sleep but must be deliberately and actively aided for the elderly, the weak, and those confined in any form of immobilization. One of the greatest responsibilities of the nurse is the recognition of the necessity of and the techniques for the implementation of bed positioning and frequent shifting of body positions for those confined to bed. These techniques are discussed in another section.

Sitting posture. In the usual sitting position, the ischial tuberosities supplant the feet as the base of support for the trunk and head. The head, trunk, and upper extremities constitute 80% of the weight of the total body. A new segmental center of gravity for the trunk, upper extremities, and head has been said to be just in front of the eleventh dorsal vertebra. The perpendicular line passing through the new center of gravity must also pass through the very narrow base of support, the ischial tuberosities (Fig. 1-7). This can

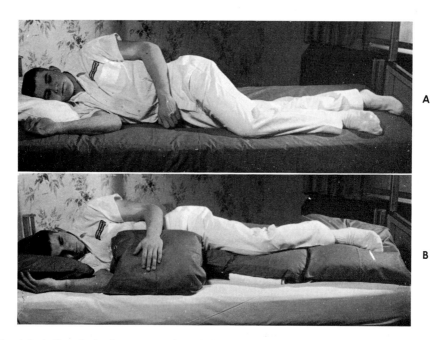

Fig. 1-6. A, Poor body alignment in the side-lying position. **B,** Good body alignment in the side-lying position. With some patients, to prevent edema of the hand, it will be necessary to maintain the hand even with or higher than the elbow.

be considered as unstable equilibrium or at least a narrow base equilibrium. If the upper thighs are added to the sitting base, the base obviously becomes more stable. Without the upper thighs, a back rest on the seat provides stability if it is inclined backward just enough to move the perpendicular back of the tuberosities.

It is common for an individual to slide forward in the chair to assure the perpendicular of gravity to be back of the tuberosities (Fig. 1-8). Such a position places the entire spine in a convex curve pointing backward, and this position, if sustained, places excessive strain on the posterior ligaments.

The ideal posture in sitting can be achieved in a chair that allows the upper thighs to add to the sitting base, while the ischial tuberosities provide the major base, the lumbar spine is in mild flexion, and the entire spine supported with the slightest backward inclination from the perpendicular. This posture is impossible in soft, deep, upholstered chairs, modern dish-shaped chairs, or bleachers without backrests. Many automobile seats are either too soft and deep or have too much backward inclination of the backrest and improper seat length for thigh rest to permit a stable equilibrium in sitting. Adjust-ments are available by proper pillow buildups or electrically driven adjusters.

DYNAMICS
Human motion

Kinesiology, the science of human motion, is studied in many fields such as anatomy, physics, mathematics, orthopedics, and engineering. A number of textbooks are geared to the specific needs of each discipline and include those for occupational and physical therapy. To be of practical value for nurses, this section is intended only to provide a new viewpoint for nurses as they deal day to day with mechanical problems in patient care. It is hoped that some insight into biomechanics as it relates to gait, traction, and the performance of mechanical tasks may aid the nurse to understand the energy costs and ways to avoid musculoskeletal strains.

Kinematics is concerned with measurement and recording of body motions and combinations of several joints to produce certain acts such as throwing a baseball. Such a series of motions constitutes a kinematic chain.

Kinetics deals with forces that produce motions and the effect of these motions on body equilibrium. The laws of forces and the classes

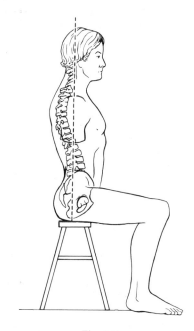

Fig. 1-7

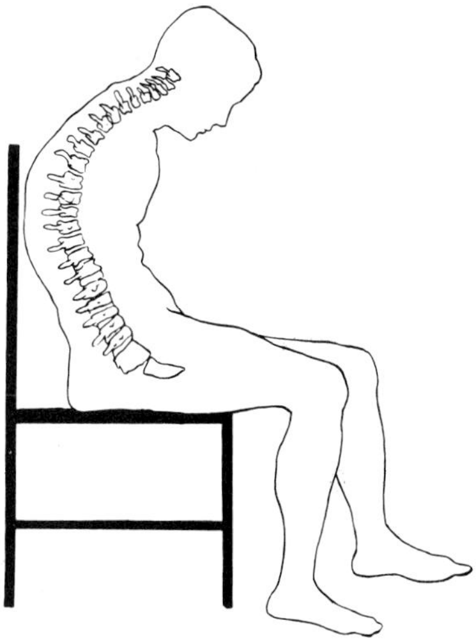

Fig. 1-8

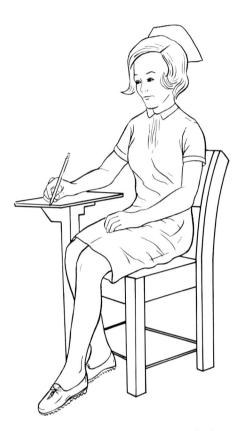

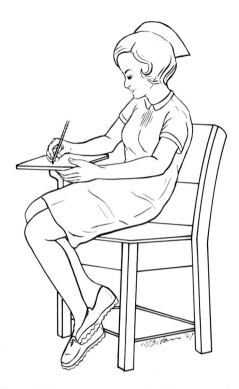

Fig. 1-10. Poor sitting posture. In this position, there is more strain on the posterior longitudinal ligaments and the interspinous ligaments of the spine than elsewhere. In addition, there is an abnormal amount of pressure placed on the anterior portion of the intervertebral disk. This compression if sustained for any length of time may be a factor in initiating the degeneration of a disk, and it certainly can perpetuate it. The depth of the seat on many overstuffed chairs does not provide for good sitting posture but tends to encourage the individual to sit with most of the weight on the lower back region.

Fig. 1-9. Good sitting posture. To provide for good sitting posture, the height and depth of the chair seat should permit the person to sit with the feet resting flat on the floor, the knees and hips flexed at right angles, and the back supported by the chair back. When sitting, the body weight should rest on the ischial tuberosities and proximal portion of the thighs.

of levers must be identified as they apply to produce bodily motions.

Laws of force

The musculoskeletal system is designed to accomplish two main objectives: (1) overcome or resist the forces of gravity, and (2) perform work. The anatomic structures of the body are arranged to achieve both with a conservation of energy, in other words, the least amount of energy needed to accomplish the job.

The same laws of force, known as Newton's laws, and the same classes of levers that apply to simple machines apply to the human body as it overcomes gravity and produces work.

Newton's Laws

Law I. A body will remain at rest or in motion in a straight line until acted upon by a force. Example: Once a heavy object, such as a bed, is put into motion, it is much easier to keep it moving than to start and stop it continually.

Law II. A force acting on a body causes the body to accelerate in the direction of the force. Example: Pushing a heavy patient in a wheelchair will require more force for a comparable acceleration than pushing a lighter patient.

Law III. For every force there is an equal and opposite reaction force. Example: A patient in bed places a force (body weight) against the mattress, and the mattress produces an equal push against the patient. Pressure sores occur on patients where heavy body parts press firmly against a mattress and receive an equal force in return. A person standing places a force (body weight) downward through the base (foot) against the floor, and the floor pushes an equal amount upward against the foot.

A knowledge of these laws of force and motion has application to every physical effort the nurse makes in the course of her work and also applies to the patient provided with nursing care. The alert nurse will think in terms of body mechanics as each act of nursing is performed in order to protect against strains that are avoidable if the proper mechanical advantage is applied to the task.

Identification of body levers

A lever is a machine, a device for transmitting energy derived from muscular contraction to move body segments which in turn transmit energy to external objects. All levers have a fulcrum, an effort arm, and a resistance arm, which are classed I, II, or III, depending upon the relative location of the fulcrum to the effort and resistance.

Class of lever

CLASS I. This is a seesaw where the weight R can be balanced by an equal force E across fulcrum F. If R is heavier than E, the seesaw is unbalanced and the lever will tilt downward. If the fulcrum is moved half the distance toward R, the lever arm for E is lengthened and E will balance R with half the effort (Fig. 1-11, *A*).

An example of Class I lever is a man using a shovel (Fig. 1-11, *B*).

CLASS II. In this lever the fulcrum is at one end, and the energy E is applied at the opposite end to lift a weight R somewhere between (Fig. 1-12, *A*). The advantage of Class II lever is obvious if the mathematics is understood. The energy in pounds times the lever arm distance to the fulcrum will lift a weight R times the lever arm distance from the fulcrum.

$$18 \text{ pounds (R)} \times 1 \text{ ft (lever arm)}$$
$$= \text{lb. E} \times 3 \text{ ft (lever arm)}$$

From this formula x equals 6 pounds. Six pounds of energy will lift 18 pounds of weight if the

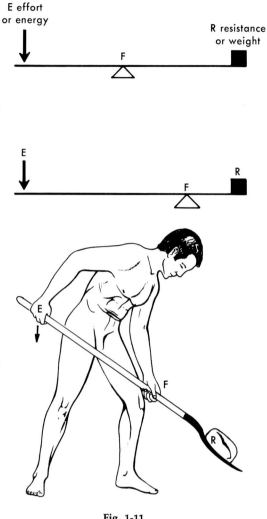

Fig. 1-11

energy is applied at the lever arm 3 times as far from the fulcrum as the weight.

An example is a man pushing a wheelbarrow (Fig. 1-12, *B*).

CLASS III. In Class III Lever the energy is applied to the lever somewhere between the fulcrum and the weight or resistance (Fig. 1-13, *A*). The energy requirement is greater than the resistance to be lifted; however, the resistance of weight can be lifted a greater distance more rapidly. The majority of single muscle levers in the body are Class III. In this example (Fig. 1-13, *B*) the fulcrum is the elbow joint, the lever is the forearm with the hand that holds the resistance. The energy is supplied by the biceps muscle inserting into the radius. Since the insertion is 2 inches forward of the fulcrum and the resistance is at least 10 inches forward of the fulcrum, it means that the biceps must pull upward with a force of 25 pounds to hold a weight of 5 pounds in the hand.

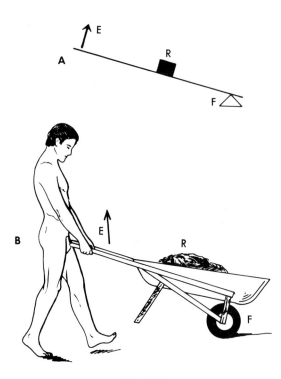

Fig. 1-12

The illustration serves to point out another important fact in body mechanics, namely the position of the fulcrum. The fulcrum can be moved to any position required to do a lifting job and must be held or stabilized in that position. Movement of the shoulder can place the elbow fulcrum and stabilize it in whatever position is required. The shoulder muscles are acting throughout the effort in exactly the same fashion as the biceps. The shoulder holds the elbow lever that holds the weight (Fig. 1-13, *C*).

The more forward the hand is held from the body, the harder the shoulder muscles must work to stabilize the position of the elbow. When the elbow is extended, the biceps muscle continues to hold the 5 pounds in the hand; however, the lever arm now is lengthened the distance from the hand to the shoulder; therefore, the shoulder muscles become the energy for a new lever system. The length of the lever from hand to shoulder is now 20 inches so the shoulder muscles must use 25 pounds of force additional to the 25 pounds of force of the biceps at the elbow to sustain the 5 pound weight in the hand.

This concept is important for nurses to understand since some positions for lifting require less energy than others for the same job. To better understand this concept requires a knowledge of torque stresses.

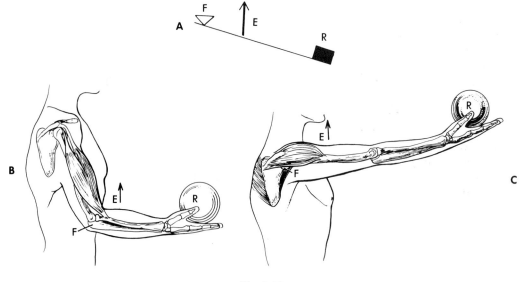

Fig. 1-13

Torque stresses

When a force acting on the body tends to rotate that body, the force is called a couple, and the moment of that couple is the torque. The direction of torque is either clockwise or counterclockwise. The moment is the distance from the center of rotation (fulcrum) to the resistance (weight). For a body to be in equilibrium and not rotate, there must be a force in the opposite direction equal to the resistance. The fulcrum in this situation is the axis of motion or center of rotation (Fig. 1-14).

The principle of torque explains why there are positions in work better than others because some require less energy and produce less strain on soft tissues. An example is lifting (Fig. 1-15). R is the weight that tends to rotate the body forward (clockwise) at the center of rotation (hip) with a force equal to the weight being lifted times the distance from the weight to the hip. To produce equilibrium and prevent the body from falling forward, the posterior muscles of the back must produce an equal force to resist the clockwise fall. The counterclockwise torque or distance from the center of rotation (hip) to the origin of the back muscles is very short compared to the clockwise torque, therefore, the muscles must generate a force of 30 pounds for the individual to hold a weight of 5 pounds.

A more efficient position for weight holding or lifting can be seen in the example of proper lifting position (Fig. 1-16, *B*). In this position the counterclockwise torque (distance from weight to hip) is reduced to one-half so that the force of the back muscles will require only 11 pounds of force to hold or lift 5 pounds in the hand.

The case of a man lifting a 5 pound ball is an excellent example of a Class III lever because it indicates the internal muscular forces at equilibrium with the weight. This is only a part of what actually happens since the arm is one segment of the total body. The 5 pound weight away from the line of gravity of the body has upset the postural (torque) equilibrium by adding weight to the front of the body's center of gravity. The body will fall forward unless a new force acting posteriorly on the body neutralizes the 5 pound weight. The center of gravity acts as a fulcrum or axis.

The rotary equilibrium of the body at the cen-

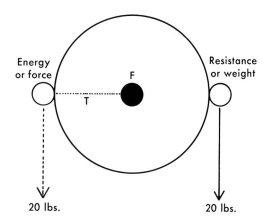

Fig. 1-14. The diagram appears as a wheel with the axis of rotation at *F* (fulcrum). If a force (weight) pulls the wheel clockwise, the wheel will rotate clockwise at the axis of motion *F*. The wheel will not rotate if an equal force (energy) pushes the wheel counterclockwise. If the wheel does not rotate, it is said to be in equilibrium.

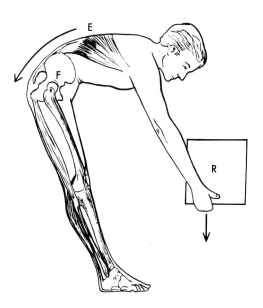

Fig. 1-15. This illustrates the torque force of *R*, which must be equalled by *E* where the fulcrum (*F*) is an unequal distance from *R* and *E*. The moment of *R* is 6 times the moment of *E* (the distance from *R* to *F* compared to the distance from *E* to *F*); therefore, the force (torque) generated by the back muscles must be 6 times the force (weight) of object *R*.

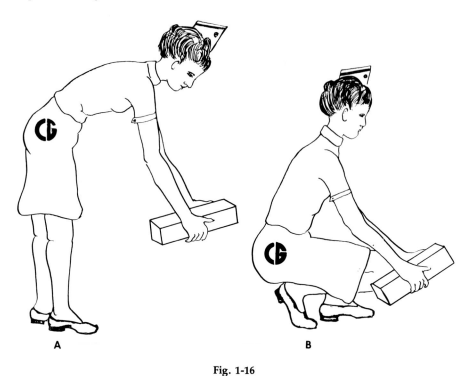

Fig. 1-16

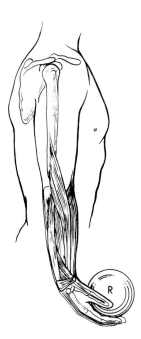

Fig. 1-17

ter of gravity axis is unstable since the 5 pound weight as an external force has added a clockwise torque. To restore equilibrium, an equal counterclockwise force must be added. Ordinarily, the contractile force of extensor muscles

of the back and pelvis will be sufficient to restore equilibrium.

If the weight is carried at the side as in Fig. 1-17, there is little or no torque and no need for a lever system. The only energy requirement will be a 5 pound finger grip to hold the weight. If the weight then must be placed at a higher level, such as a shelf, the energy requirement for the Class III elbow lever (Fig. 1-13, *B*) will suffice. If the shelf is at a higher level, much more energy is necessary for the extended lever, and body torque is increased (Fig. 1-13, *C*). It is obvious that the closer the weight is to the line of gravity of the body, the less the energy force required to do the work. The nurse can apply this principle to lifting at all times; however, there are exceptions such as when the object to be lifted cannot be brought close to the nurse's center of gravity as in the case of a patient in bed. Here a knowledge of lever systems can be helpful.

With a hand under the patient while the elbow of the same extremity rests on the bed, the fulcrum of the lifting lever has a stable base. (This is sometimes referred to as the elbow lift.) The only force required in this position will be the pull of the biceps (energy) acting on a Class III lever to lift weight. The shorter lever arm will require less energy than lifting from the shoulder, and there will be no torque of the center of gravity of the body.

In the examples of proper lifting and proper holding, there is not only conservation of muscular energy but, importantly, less *strain* on the other tissues as well.

Strain

Strains are the deformations of materials under loads, for example, the stretch of a rubber band or the bend of a wire. There are three types of strain; compression, tension, and shear.

Loads are forces or weights applied externally to a structure. Whenever a structure is loaded by a force, the structure must resist that force and the resistance becomes another force within the structure. The forces within a structure are called stresses and are intermolecular forces to resist certain loads; these are referred to as compression stress, tension stress, and shear stress. Stress forces within a structure such as bone, intervertebral disk, or ligament are not to be confused with strain.

Strain, to repeat, is another property of materials, which allows the material to respond to loads by changing shape. This is called deformation. The material elongates under tension (stretching) loads and shortens under compression loads; each material has a limit to which it can alter its shape without breaking. Solid materials have another property which is the ability to return to an original shape after the load is removed. This is called elasticity, and whereas the deformation of tension on a rubber band is easily visible as stretch, the same deformation occurs in ligaments or even bone but is too small to be visible. This is true also in compression and shear strains. As in the case of bone or ligament, each material has for its shape and size a certain measurable strain called Young's modulus of elasticity. When this is exceeded, the bone or ligament no longer returns to its original shape but rather it ruptures or breaks.

Bones and ligaments are living tissues that are capable of change in response to the load demands placed on them. The modulus of elasticity can change as the tissues grow stronger or weaker. For this reason excessive loading should be avoided if the bones or ligaments are unaccustomed to sudden excessive loading since the modulus of elasticity may be exceeded and the tissue will remain deformed. Conditioning programs can stimulate the living tissues to grow stronger to meet the demands of loads placed on them. This is just as important a part of conditioning as the development of strength in muscles by exercise. Good body mechanics will avoid excessive loading, while poor mechanics will produce excessive loading, and if the modulus of elasticity of the loaded tissues is exceeded, the tissues, particularly ligaments, will be strained and actually become painful. This type of strain can be avoided by the application of proper body mechanics to each task.

One of the most common areas of the body to be strained is the low back. This is understandable because great forces of torque are transferred to the disk and ligaments of the low back in stooping and lifting. Application of good body mechanics will lessen the torque loading on the low back throughout the working day. Good body mechanics applied to specific jobs will aid the nurse to develop good habits for herself and teach good habits to patients.

APPLICATION TO NURSING

STATICS

Practicing and establishing good posture habits, when performing nursing functions, should be an essential part of every student nurse's clinical experience. Good posture not only makes for a more pleasing appearance in contrast to poor posture, which denotes discouragement and fatigue, but also provides for correct functioning of the weight-bearing joints. It lessens the possibility of strain to joints and ligaments by preventing uneven distribution of body weight. When posture is good, muscular work to maintain balance is kept at a minimum, resulting in less muscular fatigue and strain.

Student nurses who are given the benefit of an initial posture analysis early in their careers are fortunate. They are still more fortunate if there is someone, perhaps an instructor in body mechanics, equipped to help them overcome their postural weaknesses. Corrective exercises, if prescribed, will often bring about noteworthy improvements in posture if the student understands their purpose, is adequately supervised in their performance, and is faithful in practicing them. It is indispensable that students know what they are seeking to accomplish and how to accomplish it. It would be sufficient for them to do all these things without thought—to learn good posture on what might be called a subconscious level—except that they are being educated to be health teachers as well as nurses.

We know that learning is not conceded to be effective until behavior is altered in some way because of it. Probably no nurse completes a nursing course today without being able to recite the points that the weight-bearing line should pass through for proper body stance. No doubt almost all graduates will be able to write in the state board examination, if questioned about them, some of the criteria of good posture: that the head is to be held up and the chin in, that the lower abdomen should be flat and retracted, that the curves of the spine should be maintained without exaggeration, that the knees should be in a relaxed position (not hyperextended), and that the feet should point straight ahead. However, the nurses are probably capable of writing these gems of wisdom while their own feet are wrapped tightly around the chair rungs, their chins are glued to caved-in sternums, and their backs are round as a barrel hoop.

Whether or not the students can interpret good posture to themselves in a kinesthetic sense is conjectural. Secretly they may still be convinced that slouchy posture is easier and more comfortable and that good posture is a position leading to fatigue and strain. Since they have only theoretic knowledge, with which their own experience is perhaps not in accord, it is questionable that they will be able to describe good posture in simple language for the benefit of the patient who is rising from bed after long recumbency. Even if they can do this, there is still the question of whether they will be able to confidently accompany a verbal description with a graphic example by reference to their own body alignment; unless they can, their knowledge remains academic. If they themselves do not understand the necessity for good posture and do not apply it to everyday living, they will hardly be able to transmit this knowledge to others in a vitally effective manner, nor be able to present a convincing object lesson in their own activities.

The cosmetic appeal for good posture probably does as much as any other factor to motivate the female student. Because student nurses are young and resilient, they seldom feel the result of the day's mechanical misuse of their bodies. Most female students, however, are tremendously interested in their waistlines, and their hips are a constant source of speculative consideration. Any exercises given for reduction of anatomic overloads there will usually bring about some definite display of interest and earnestness. A concept of good posture may be built upon a realization of the cosmetic benefit that results from occasional tensing of the abdominal muscles and contracting of gluteal muscles. A young woman has only to look in the mirror to observe the effects.

The nurse must remember that the laws which govern balance in the standing position also apply when the body is in motion and that maintaining correct alignment of the body segments (weight-bearing line) in relation to the base of support is important in preventing strain of supporting muscles and ligaments. Balance and motion of the human body are produced and controlled by the contraction of muscles attached to the skeletal system. Contraction of a muscle supplies the force necessary to overcome gravity and to provide for motion and work. When the nurse carries a heavy tray, the biceps muscle inserted in the radius contracts and supplies the effort needed to support the resistance offered by the tray. Carrying the tray close to the body enables the nurse to maintain correct alignment of the body segments and requires less muscular effort than holding the tray farther from the body.

When working at the bedside, if the nurse bends forward by flexing the hips and spinal column (with knees extended), the work placed on the spinal ligaments and low back muscles is very great. Lifting or working in such a position (Fig. 1-18) may result in backache due to strain of the low back muscles and spinal ligaments and may also be a factor in causing rupture of a disk. In this position there is increased pressure placed on the anterior aspect of the vertebral bodies and on the intervening nucleus pulposus. However, if the nurse, when positioning a bed patient, flexes the hips and knees, faces the work, and assumes the foot-forward position, correct alignment of the shoulders and pelvis in relation to the line of gravity and base of support will be maintained. In this position (Fig. 1-19) the nurse is able to use the strong muscles of the thighs and arms for moving the patient. Stabilization of the pelvis is accomplished by tightening the abdominal and gluteal muscles. In some instances, moving the bed patient may be accomplished with less effort by using a lifting sheet. The amount of friction between the patient's body and the bed surface is lessened. If the nurse wishes to move the mattress or the patient up in bed, the head of the bed is lowered, unless the patient's condition contraindicates the change of position. Sliding an object on a level surface requires less effort than moving it on an inclined plane. The nurse soon learns, when caring for the helpless individual, that the patient's position can be changed with less exertion by turning or sliding his body than by lifting him and that it is easier and safer for both the patient and the nurse to slide or turn the patient toward rather than away from the nurse.

Practice of nursing procedures can easily include concurrent practice in correct body mechanics (Fig. 1-20). Once the student has learned to carry out procedures while using correct body mechanics, it becomes a conditioned skill likely to be carried into similar situa-

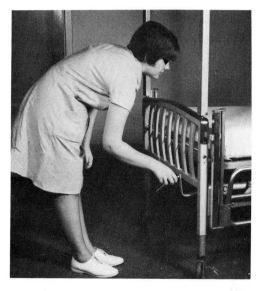

Fig. 1-18. When the kind of bed shown here is used, nursing personnel raise and lower the headrest many times a day, and in addition to changing the headrest position, it is frequently necessary to raise and lower the bed. When these activities are done with the body in the position illustrated (feet parallel and knees in extension), strain is placed on the muscles and ligaments of the lumbosacral area.

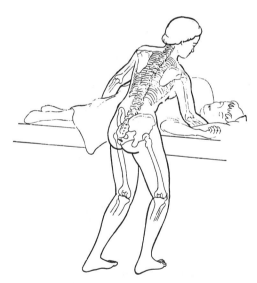

Fig. 1-19. When working at the bedside, assume the foot-forward position, face your work, flex knees and hips slightly, and maintain the shoulders in same plane as the pelvis. Protect the small muscles of the back while making the large muscles of the thigh work. (Courtesy National Advisory Service for Orthopedics and Poliomyelitis, and Alfred Feinberg, artist, College of Physicians and Surgeons, Columbia University, New York.)

tions on the ward. The carry-over to the patient will not be automatic. The situation facing the beginning student is very complex, and there are many things to remember in the early days on the ward. Guided instruction will be needed. The material on body mechanics cannot be given in one gigantic dose; it must be offered in suitable small doses and repeated often. That is why it is so important for all teaching personnel and nurse clinicians who will come in contact with the student to be well grounded in the subject and convinced of its importance.

The following reminders will help the nurse who is working at the bedside to use the body's many lever systems in an efficient manner, thus minimizing fatigue and the possibility of ligamentous strain.

1. Carry or lift heavy burdens close to the body. Since the object carried becomes a part of the body's weight, there occurs less displacement of the body's center of gravity.

2. To attain a lower work level, flex the knees and keep the back straight. If the shoulder and pelvic girdles are maintained in the same plane, the body's center of gravity is kept over the base of support. Rounding the back and reaching forward or downward to lift with the arms displaces the weight of the trunk forward. To maintain body balance in this position, excessive strain is placed on the hip and back extensors, and in addition, the strain of any lifting is placed on the small back muscles rather than on the stronger, more massive muscles of the thighs and buttocks.

3. Increase the body's base of support toward the object to be lifted or moved. A broader base of support increases stability.

4. When lifting, face the work situation and avoid rotatory movements of the spine.

5. Stand close to the object being moved or lifted. This helps to maintain the body's center of gravity over the base of support and increases stability.

6. More efficient use of muscular force occurs when the object is turned or moved toward the worker's body. To move an object toward oneself, the flexors of the elbows supply the force. These muscles

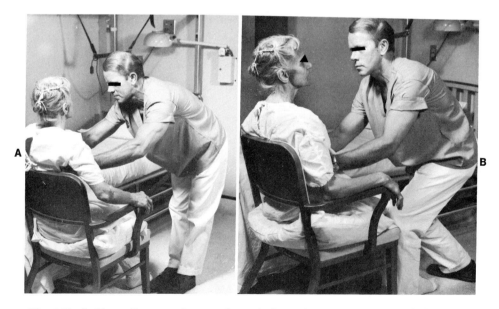

Fig. 1-20. A, Nurse illustrates the use of poor body mechanics preparatory to helping a patient assume the standing position. **B,** The nurse demonstrates correct body mechanics and in this position is able to lift and support the unsteady patient without strain to his own back muscles.

are stronger than the elbow extensors which are used when pushing or turning an object away from oneself. It should also be remembered that this is a safer procedure since the nurse has greater control over the patient's body, when the turning is done toward herself.

7. When possible, move a patient by sliding or turning, as opposed to lifting. If an object is lifted, additional effort must be used to overcome the force of gravity.

8. Move a patient on a level surface as opposed to an inclined plane. Lower the head rest (unless contraindicated) when sliding a patient toward the head of the bed.

9. Utilize smooth continuous movements as opposed to jerky start and stop movements. Less effort is needed to keep an object moving than to start its movement.

10. Use of a lifting or turning sheet decreases the amount of contact surface, and by so doing, lessens the friction between the patient and the supporting surface. When using a lifting sheet, it is helpful (when possible) to have the patient flex his knees and hips and to raise his head off the mattress.

11. When feasible, support a patient's body or extremity by utilizing the elbow lift.

12. When strenuous activity is required, prepare for it by setting the pelvis; that is, retract the abdominal muscles and contract the gluteal muscles. Sometimes this is referred to as pelvic tilt. "Up in front, down in back" and "pull and pinch" are instructions sometimes used to give this concept to the student.

13. Never lift an excessive load in an attempt to keep from asking for help.

Body alignment for the bed patient

Prolonged poor bed posture can contribute to the development of joint contractures. A sagging mattress encourages the development of hip flexion contractures (Fig. 1-21). Improperly placed pillows beneath the head and shoulders provide for a position of round shoulders. Knees continuously supported with pillows will cause an adaptive shortening of the hamstring tendons and a knee flexion contracture. To help prevent contractures, the mattress supporting the body weight must be firm enough to maintain good body alignment. Increased firmness may be obtained by placing a bedboard beneath the standard innerspring or felt mattress. To permit elevation of the backrest, a hinged board is necessary.

The footboard may or may not be considered a part of the bed, but for the patient with muscular weakness it is essential if a normal position of the feet is to be maintained. The footboard should be several inches higher than the patient's toes, supporting the foot at a right angle to the tibia, maintaining the toes in extension, and holding the bed covers off the feet. If the

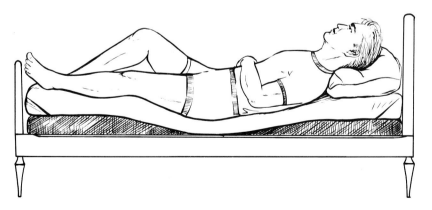

Fig. 1-21. The sagging mattress contributes to poor body alignment and to the development of hip flexion contractures.

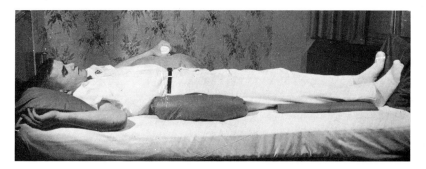

Fig. 1-22. Good body alignment in the supine position.

toes of a paralyzed extremity are permitted to curl over the top edge of a footboard, a toe drop will develop. When the patient is in the supine position, it is desirable that the footboard provide space for the patient's heels between the end of the mattress and the footboard. This position protects the heels from pressure. A footboard that is adjustable may be shifted to provide support when the patient is moved up in bed and placed in a sitting position.

For a bedfast patient, the addition of a trapeze to the bed is desirable, since it enables him to shift his position and to assist with his care, without the leverage of his elbow lift from the bed. However, in some instances it is thought that the rehabilitee will become more independent if he learns to function without this aid. The bed equipped with an electric control that enables the patient to modify his position is also helpful. In addition to maintaining good body alignment, frequent and regular changes of position are essential.

When studying the accompanying illustrations of body positions, it should be remembered that an alignment of the body segments that provides good posture for the vertical person will also provide good posture for the bedfast or horizontal person.

Supine position. Fig. 1-22 illustrates a good back-lying position. The footboard holds the covers off the toes and maintains the feet in a functional position, midway between dorsiflexion and plantar flexion. The folded bath blanket placed under the calf of the leg lessens the pressure on the heel. This arrangement also provides for a relaxed position of the knee joint and avoids pressure on the popliteal space. A bilateral

trochanter roll may be made by folding one bath blanket or two lengthwise, in thirds. This is placed crosswise of the bed beneath the patient's buttocks. The outer end of each side is rolled (under) firmly against the hip and thigh. The roll supports and maintains the limb in a neutral position, preventing external rotation. A small pillow or pad placed under the lower portion of the back gives support to the normal lumbar curve. This nursing measure will provide considerable comfort for the patient with lordosis who must remain on his back for an indefinite period of time.

The patient who has paralysis or weakness of the upper extremity muscles needs frequent and careful positioning of the arm and hand. The involved arm may be placed on the bed with the elbow and wrist in extension and the forearm pronated or supinated. At other times, the arm should be abducted with the elbow flexed and the forearm supported on a pillow with the hand maintained in a functional position. Another position for the arm is found by placing the abducted arm in external rotation (Fig. 1-23).

Prone position. When the patient is turned onto his abdomen with no support beneath the ankles, the feet are forced to remain in an equinus position (plantar flexion). To prevent plantar flexion, a pillow may be used to support the ankles (Fig. 1-24), or the patient may be positioned so that his feet extend over the end of the mattress. When one is in the face-lying position, use of a head pillow may cause hyperextension of the cervical spine. Some individuals in the prone position have better body alignment and are more comfortable with a thin pillow placed

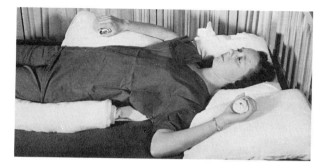

Fig. 1-23. Positions of rest for the arms. The right arm illustrates a position of abduction with internal rotation. The left arm illustrates a position of abduction with external rotation. Note the position of the wrist and fingers.

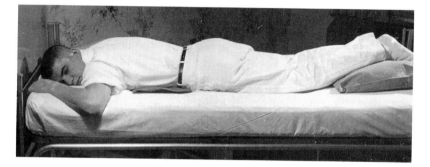

Fig. 1-24. Good body alignment in the prone position.

beneath the abdomen. Other patients, however, can be made comfortable without this pillow and still maintain good body alignment. The abducted and externally rotated (spreadeagle) position of the arms is a restful one for many patients (Fig. 1-24).

Side-lying position. When the patient is turned to this position, the entire length of the uppermost limb should be supported with pillows to prevent an adducted position. Maintaining the hip and knee in the same plane lessens strain on the hip joint and is of particular importance for the patient who has had hip or back surgery. Also it is desirable that the uppermost limb be positioned to avoid pressure on the underneath limb. When the patient is placed in the side-lying position, the underneath arm and shoulder must be made comfortable, and pillows may be used to support the uppermost arm and back as needed. (See Fig. 1-6.) Variations of this position may be utilized to change pressure points on the hip and shoulder areas

and to provide different positions for the joints of the uppermost arm.

Patient care problems associated with inactivity and bed rest

Muscle atrophy and joint contracture. Inactivity or prolonged bed rest can contribute to a number of complications by interfering with the physiologic processes of the body. Prolonged inactivity results in atrophy of muscle tissue. The muscle becomes smaller, and with disuse, circulation to the muscle diminishes. This results in decreased endurance and increased fatigability. Consequently the individual is less active, and further muscle atrophy occurs. Muscle atrophy caused by disuse may be readily observed after removal of a plaster cast that has been worn for several weeks. The circumference of the involved leg is less than that of the normal limb, and the muscles appear flabby. A period of extended bed rest will cause similar atrophy. The antigravity muscles of the lower limb (glutei, quadriceps femoris, and gastrocnemius) are the muscles most affected. Muscular inactivity and the resulting atrophy may be due to causes other than prescribed bed rest or the application of an external means of immobilization. Paralysis caused by injury or disease of the central nervous system also results in disuse atrophy. In some instances, diminished activity and loss of muscle strength and endurance seem to be a part of the aging process.

From the study of physiology the student will remember that, in order to move joints, muscles must contract or relax. For maintaining the upright posture, however, they must have a constant slight contraction. This constant slight contraction is called muscle tonus or tone. To maintain the body in a standing position, a higher degree of muscle tonus is required than is required for lying in bed. After a day of bed rest one often feels a weakness out of all proportion to the minor illness he has experienced. From this common observation the student can easily understand that when bed rest is continued over a considerable period of time muscle tone may be greatly depleted. Lack of muscle tone, even in healthy subjects, produces wasting of the muscles, often referred to as disuse atrophy. Muscles with diminished tone may become permanently stretched from being held in a lengthened position, or they can become contracted by being held in a shortened position, thus producing so-called myostatic contractures. In terms of the patient's well-being these things may mean a longer convalescence, discomfort on assuming the upright position, and possibly a persistent joint deformity.

Even 2 weeks of bed rest in faulty positions may be sufficient to bring about contractures of important muscle groups.

If joint mobility is impaired by beginning contractures, more muscular energy is required to produce motion, and thus more energy is required to perform the same act in the face of contracture. This situation may be encountered when ambulation is attempted by the patient who has developed a hip flexion contracture. Inability to fully extend the hip joint when standing interferes with easy balance of the body weight; therefore, increased muscle activity and strength are necessary to maintain the upright position and to ambulate.

The nurse also realizes that after a period of bed rest, even though there are no contractures, the patient will tire more quickly and his endurance for sitting in a chair or for walking will be markedly decreased. Walking short distances or sitting in a chair for short periods several times daily is more beneficial than extended periods of activity, which result in physical exhaustion.

A patient who is gravely ill sometimes receives less attention to body mechanics than do others on the ward. It is said, and with some reason, that the problem of keeping such a patient alive takes all the nurse's strength and energy and that effort should not be dissipated on minor details, but it is a mistake to forget that the desperately ill patient may recover. Indeed, one of the primary purposes of nursing is to help the patient get well if it is at all possible. No nurse wants a patient to recover from his original illness only to find that he has another handicap as a result of his stay in bed. Our concern for the horizontal man must not allow us to forget the vertical one.

Many deformities develop in patients with debilitating illnesses because they lie in bed in positions of adduction and flexion. The student should understand that use of flexion is one of the ways the patient learns to relieve discomfort in his back, his hips, and his knees. Sometimes he assumes these positions to keep warm when he has insufficient circulation or covers. Proper nursing care should overcome at least some of these discomforts. Sometimes making the patient comfortable may be as simple as giving support to the lower portion of the back, a little gentle massage perhaps, or an extra blanket.

Change of position is also important. Any position, however adequate it may be as far as posture is concerned, will need frequent alteration. Human beings are not static, nor were they ever intended to be; movement is the very sine qua non of life itself. Sometimes these necessary alterations—from one type of good bed posture to another one equally good—will require all the ingenuity of which the nurse is capable.

In all these considerations, as in all treatment,

we must face the irreducible and stubborn fact that patients are human beings; they do not stay where you put them. They have their likes and dislikes about these things. We may know that positions of good alignment usually produce more lasting comfort for the patient; nevertheless, if he has been so long in poor alignment that he has become accustomed to it, a little teaching and persuasion may be necessary. The student must understand that deformity cannot be corrected in a day and that zealousness should be tempered with patience and understanding. The patient's confidence and courage cannot be sacrificed in the attempt to overcome the results of neglect. Overdetermination, nagging, or sharpness demonstrates a fractional approach to the patient's total problem.

Drop-foot deformity. Of particular significance in nursing is the fact that the tendon of the muscles of the calf tends to shorten if the foot is allowed to rest in an unsupported position, whereas the muscles in the anterior portion of the leg become stretched. Even a mild degree of this muscular imbalance can cause the patient many long weeks of painful concern with his feet. A drop-foot deformity (equinus position) means that the individual in the standing position will be unable to place his heel on the floor, and walking becomes more difficult and tiring. With severe deformity of the foot, wearing of shoes is impossible and the patient must resort to a soft knit slipper. The cosmetic value of maintaining the foot in a functional position should not be overlooked.

Conscientious nursing care can do much to eliminate this unnecessary sequela of illness. Adequate support which maintains the feet in a functional position (including the toes) should be furnished during confinement in bed and exercises to maintain muscle strength and to prevent joint contractures should be utilized.

The patient should wear shoes rather than nonsupporting bedroom slippers when weight bearing is started after a period of bed rest. As previously stated, with inactivity there is generalized weakening of the muscles and attritional thinning of the ligaments. With weight bearing, the weakened ligaments and muscles, which support the arches of the feet, need the support of a well-fitted shoe. Arch strain caused by dis-

use atrophy of ligaments can be quite painful and disturbing to the patient.

Knee flexion contractures. Another set of muscles that tend to contract quickly is the hamstring group of the posterior thigh, whose tendons pass under the knee. Flexion of the knees continuously supported by pillows may bring about contractures in that area in a surprisingly short time. The nursing measures to counteract this are quite simple and obvious. Pillows under the knees must be used with caution and with constant awareness that the position of the knees must be altered from flexion to extension at frequent periods.

Preventing flexion contracture of the knee is of special significance for the arthritic patient, since paintful joints are more comfortable in the flexed position. The ability to fully extend the knee joint is also important for the below-knee amputee. A slight flexion contracture makes the fitting of a prosthesis very difficult, if not impossible. To prevent flexion contracture of the knee, a posterior splint or traction, which holds the joint in extension, may be prescribed. With some patients, instruction in active exercise is needed. This includes quadriceps setting and straight leg raising, as well as flexion and extension of the knee joint. Long periods of sitting with the knees flexed should be avoided. When flexion contracture is present at the knee joint, increased muscular strength is needed for walking, and consequently the act of walking is very tiring and frequently results in discouragement and decreased activity.

Hip deformities (flexion, adduction, and external rotation). Let us consider the problem of the patient with an acute condition of the abdomen that requires prolonged semisitting in a Gatch bed. Such a patient may be in danger of flexion contractures of hips and knees as well as of drop foot. If he sits in a slumping position on the lumbar spine with his chest caved in and his shoulders sagging forward, pulled down by the weight of his arms, pain and muscle spasms are likely to occur in the muscles of the back, particularly those muscles which lie between the scapulae. The patient confined to bed rest is most likely to lose tone in the abdominal, the gluteal, the quadriceps, and the tibial muscles, and in those of the interscapular group—all muscles that will be of great importance to him when he becomes ambulatory again.

Even though the patient's condition is such that he must be kept in the sitting position, certain measures can be used that will afford him greater comfort and also minimize the after-effects of his illness. The nurse who understands the principles of sitting posture will know that the weight of the body should be borne on the ischia and the thighs, and therefore will make certain that the hips are back as far as possible in the angle of the bed in order to prevent the patient from slumping down and sitting on his sacrum or on his lumbar spine. Although flexion of the knees is necessary to relax the spinal extensor muscles, the knees must be extended fully several times during the day. The back should be supported in its entirety, and pillows must not be allowed to bunch up under the shoulders and head, thereby forcing the spine out of its normal curves. Recognizing the dangers of prolonged outward rotation at the hips, which so often accompanies such bed posture, the nurse will improvise a simple piece of equipment for overcoming this tendency—such as a sandbag, a pillow, or a trochanter roll made by anchoring a sheet (folded lengthwise) under the patient's hips and rolling it firmly against the thigh and knee. For the feet, if the customary type of footboard does not suffice, the nurse may be able to devise a sling made of a bath blanket or sheet folded in a huge triangle and fastened to either side of the bed so that the feet may rest against it. Pillows placed under the forearms will eliminate the pull on the shoulders. When it is finally permissible for the patient to lie flat in bed for certain periods during the day, the nurse will be alert to the necessity of restoring full extension to hips and knees to overcome the results of long-continued flexion to those joints. Turning the patient to the prone position for short periods of time is also helpful in preventing the development of a hip flexion contracture. A firm support beneath the hips is important. A sagging mattress can be the cause of insidious deformity, even though the nurse is careful to arrange the patient in positions of good body mechanics and is conscientious about teaching him his part in his own recovery. A depression in the mattress at the hip level may bring about contracture of the hip flexor muscles that may make the upright position of full extension at the hips next to impossible.

The development of a sacral decubitus always presents a grave situation, particularly in a thin, elderly patient or in one in whom dehydration and pyrexia persist over a long period. The potential danger to pressure areas is always in the mind of the nurse caring for such a patient. This is one preventive feature about which no nurse is uninformed or neglectful today. Sometimes, however, the problems involved in preventing a breakdown of the skin in the threatened area are so manifold that the nurse forgets the rest of the patient's problem entirely. Perhaps he is turned on his side and allowed to lie a great portion of the time with his legs adducted and his hips and knees flexed. The danger of decubitus is overcome, but if no one thinks to place pillows between the thighs for alignment of the extremities, by the time he is ready to sit up and walk he has a dislocation of the hip that lay adducted and unsupported for so long. A crippling condition results, which will require many months, or even years, to remedy. This outcome is no hypothetical possibility; it has happened often enough to make it essential that students be taught the important part they play in the prevention of such disasters. They should be well aware of the response of the musculoskeletal system to disease, to fever, and to disuse. The necessity for good body alignment in bed will become more reasonable and immediate as comprehension of these matters is gained.

Deformities of the upper extremity. Another group of muscles that develop contractures because of faulty or unphysiologic positions in bed are the muscles at the axillary level, particularly the pectoral group. The value of providing for active range of motion of the shoulder joint following mastectomy is well known. It should also be remembered that the individul wearing a sling to support the forearm needs range of motion exercise for the shoulder joint, if tight pectorals and an adduction contracture are to be prevented. Patients lying in bed tend to be very limited as far as activity of the upper arms and shoulders is concerned. Many ambulatory patients, too, are somewhat restricted in this respect. The muscles that bring the arms away from the side and those that rotate the arms outward are used so infrequently that considerable atrophy occurs in them. The patient with a debilitating illness is likely to lie in bed with the arms held closely to the sides of the body, elbows flexed at right angles, and wrists crossed and dropped. There is usually no reason at all why he must lie this way; he does it out of apathy or from lack of knowledge that it may be harmful to him. Skillfull nurses will find reasons for making the patient use his arms in positions of abduction and outward rotation. They will have him reaching upward toward the head of the bed, combing his hair, or fastening his gown at the back of the neck. At other times they will arrange for him to lie with his arms in a position opposite to the one he tends to assume constantly; that is, they will see that the upper arms are away from the body, the elbows extended, and the hands turned palm upward. By doing this the nurse may be able to prevent the troublesome bursitis and synovitis that have sometimes followed long-continued restriction of motion in the shoulder, and certainly will be able to prevent the tightness in the axilla that so frequently follows long illness. If, however, the patient has lain for a long time at home in a restricted position, such activity must be resumed by degrees and with caution.

With paralysis of the upper extremity, positioning and change of position of the forearm, wrist, and fingers is vital to prevent fixed deformity. The wrist and fingers of the paralyzed hand may be maintained in a functional position by means of a hand roll or a posterior splint. Functional position implies a position of use: the wrist is in extension, the fingers are semiflexed, and the thumb opposes the fingers. Change of position and passive exercise will prevent tightening of the joint structure. These are some of the mishaps of poor bed posture, but there are others that may cause the patient discomfort, if not actual disability, after a period of bed rest.

As students go through the clinical services, they will become increasingly aware of situations in which knowledge of elementary body mechanics is of importance. A baby in the obstetric nursery may be noted whose head seems habitually to rest a little to one side with the chin pointed in the opposite direction. The baby may normally lie that way part of the time, but is he lying that way all of the time? And does he resist having his head turned the other way?

Again, sometimes a patient is observed in an oxygen tent with two or three pillows under his head but with no support whatever to the back or shoulders. As a result the chest is concave and sunken. The student knows, of course, that the oxygen is being given to support a failing respiratory system. The incongruity of this in the face of such a sunken and depleted chest capacity should be apparent at once. But it will not be unless instruction is given.

Charcot, the great French neurologist, once said that it was the mind that was truly alive and saw things, but it would hardly see anything without instruction. This wise observation might well serve as a professional axiom for all teachers of student nurses. The difference between a trained observer and an untrained observer is never more important than it is in these instances. Unaided observation has but little value for the young student.

Prevention of crippling, of course, includes far more than attention to bed posture. Disease and accident are the causes of a large percentage of crippling conditions today. The nurse's function in the prevention and control of disease will be emphasized in all phases of professional education, but the nurse's role in accident prevention may not be so apparent unless it is given considerable thought and analysis both in the classroom and at the bedside.

Accidents in the home cause a high percentage of fatalities yearly. Besides the fatalities there must be considered the innumerable disabilities—temporary and permanent—and the resulting economic losses that they engender. When the situations in the home and hospital that are most likely to result in accidents are brought to the student's mind, her horizon for observation is enlarged immeasurably. A clear comprehension of what constitutes individual responsibility for community health and betterment is not the least of the lessons the nurse must learn.

Hypostatic pneumonia. Bed rest, with infrequent change of position, is a contributing factor in the development of hypostatic pneumonia. The patient's position in bed, the presence of a tight bandage around the chest or abdomen, abdominal distention, severe pain, the administration of sedatives or anesthetics (which act to depress the respiratory center in the medulla), and decreased innervation of the respiratory muscles are factors that can contribute to lung congestion and decreased rib cage expansion. Also, with inactivity, basal metabolism is lowered. This results in a decreased amount of carbon dioxide being produced, and the need for oxygen is lowered. Consequently the respiratory center does not stimulate breathing and the respirations are slower and more shallow. The horizontal position tends to permit secretions to pool, and ciliary action is inhibited. The resulting stasis of the bronchial secretions provides an ideal media for the growth of pathogenic organisms, and if dehydration occurs, the secretions are more tenacious and difficult to expectorate. When lung congestion or pneumonia is present, the patient becomes lethargic, rales are heard in the chest, dyspnea is present, respirations are rapid and noisy, chills and fever with diaphoresis may occur, blood tinged sputum may be expectorated, and blood studies reveal leukocytosis. To help prevent lung congestion, nursing care must provide that the patient's position be changed at specified times, that activity be encouraged, and that he be helped to cough and deep breathe at frequent intervals. With some patients, use of the intermittent positive pressure breathing machine is indicated to accomplish deep breathing and to stimulate coughing. The use of suction may also be necessary to help remove secretions from the respiratory tract.

Pressure necrosis. Prolonged pressure from the body weight on vulnerable areas such as the sacrum, the heels the malleoli or even the greater trochanters, frequently results in breakdown of the skin and the underlying tissues. Continuous pressure from the body weight compresses the capillaries and venulas and causes a decrease in the blood supply (ischemia) to the involved tissues. When circulatory exchange is inadequate, anoxemia of the tissue and the accumulation of catabolic waste products cause cell death. An ischemic area of skin appears white but immediately becomes red (hyperemia) when body pressure is relieved. If the redness of such an area does not disappear within a relatively short time (approximately 1 hour) following relief of the pressure, tissue damage has very likely occurred. To prevent tissue necrosis, nursing care should be directed at relieving pressure and providing good skin care. To relieve pressure, a turning schedule which includes the prone, side-lying, and supine positions, as well as variations of these positions, should be established. In addition, the use of synthetic lamb's wool or other such device beneath the involved area will provide for a more even distribution of the body weight and tends to prevent pressure points. Along with relief of pressure, nursing care should provide for such things as cleanliness, adequate protein and liquid intake, the prevention of breaks in the skin, and the maintenance of normal skin oils. Massage to normal tissue increases the circulation and is beneficial. However, vigorous massage to a reddened area may cause further injury to damaged tissue. Other health factors such as circulatory problems, nutritional status, sensory deficits, and age will greatly influence the condition of the skin and the speed with which pressure necrosis can occur.

Disuse osteoporosis. It is known that inactivity and lack of weight bearing will cause loss of calcium from the skeletal system, resulting in an osteoporotic condition of bone. The mechanism of normal bone formation and resorption is not understood; consequently, the cause of osteoporosis is not known. Resorption of bone is performed by osteoclasts, and osteoblasts lay down bone matrix; but the effect of stress and activity or the lack of stress and activity on the osteoclastic and osteoblastic cells is not clearly understood. However, it is known that weight-bearing stress will lessen loss of calcium from the skeletal system. Thus, as soon as a patient's general condition permits, it is desirable to place him on the tilt table to accomplish weight-bearing stress and thereby diminish the osteoporosis that accompanies inactivity.

Renal calculi. When disuse osteoporosis occurs, the calcium lost from the skeletal system is excreted by the kidneys. Research has shown that increased calcium excretion begins as early as the second or third day of bed rest and reaches a peak by the fourth or fifth week. This increased excretion of calcium salts may lead to the formation of kidney stones. Other factors that favor precipitation of calcium and stone formation are stasis of urine, decreased urinary output, urinary tract infection, and an alkaline urine. With decreased muscular activity, the urine becomes more alkaline, and it is known that an alkaline urine favors precipitation of calcium salts. The presence of infection in the urinary tract favors stone formation by reducing the acidity of the urine and by increasing the amount of cellular debris that acts as nuclei for stone formation. Such symptoms as hematuria, severe colic-like pain, nausea and vomiting, and backache may be indicative of renal calculi. This is a very painful and distressing complication that can accompany continued bed rest. Preventive measures should include increased fluid intake. This helps to prevent urinary stasis and to decrease the concentration of calcium in the urine. In addition, frequent change of position is essential and should include sitting and standing whenever possible. In the supine position, the hilus of the kidney is uppermost. In this position gravity does not assist in the drainage of urine from the kidney. Also, as previously stated, providing for muscle activity and for weight-bearing stress will lessen the amount of calcium lost from the skeletal system and consequently the amount of calcium to be excreted by the kidney.

Bowel and bladder problems. It is not uncommon for a patient confined to bed and the supine position to have difficulty in voiding. Lack of privacy and attempting to use a bedpan or urinal in an unnatural position may make it difficult for the individual to consciously relax the perineal muscles, including the external sphincter.

The nurse needs to recognize that the patient who asks for the urinal or bedpan often but voids only small amounts or the older patient, who is frequently incontinent, may be having bladder distention with overflow incontinence. If this condition is permitted to continue, serious urinary tract complications may follow.

In many cases constipation and fecal impactions become a problem for the immobilized or bedridden patient. Defecation is dependent upon both smooth and skeletal muscle action, plus a complex visceral reflex pattern. Lack of adequate privacy and the use of an uncomfortable position tend to encourage poor habits in the bedfast patient. Neither the supine position nor a sitting position with the knees extended promotes the normal reflexes and pelvic muscle action desirable for defecation. Fecal material remaining in the lower bowel and rectum becomes increasingly hard and dry, due to absorption of water by the gut. The patient with a fecal impaction may repeatedly ask for the bedpan and will frequently pass a small amount of liquid stool; the older patient, because of relaxation of the anal sphincters, may have continuous or repeated incontinence of liquid fecal material.

Generalized weakness, loss of muscle strength, lack of activity, and changes in the patient's dietary habits and daily routines are contributing factors to bowel problems for the bed patient. To remedy or prevent this problem, it is helpful to know the patient's toilet and dietary habits. If these can be continued in the hospital situation, bowel problems may be avoided. Provision for a high residue diet, adequate liquid intake, and the use of the bedside commode as soon as permissible, are helpful nursing measures. Frequently a stool softener may be desirable.

Thrombosis. Another complication that may accompany bed rest is the development of a thrombus. Phlebothrombosis means the formation of a clot that adheres to the intima of the vein. Thrombophlebitis indicates that, in addition to the clot formation, there is an inflammatory process involving the wall of the vein. The latter is usually accompanied by pain and tenderness in the calf region and is particularly noticeable with dorsiflexion of the foot. A slight temperature elevation may be present, and if venous return is poor, edema and mottling of the skin will be apparent. A very serious complication develops if a portion of the clot (embolus) becomes detached from the wall of the vein and is carried in the bloodstream to the lung where it causes a pulmonary infarction. The severity of the infarction depends on the location in the lung and the amount of pulmonary circulation obstructed. Sudden death may occur if a large pulmonary embolus is present. Smaller emboli will cause the patient to complain of shortness of breath and of pleurisy-like pain in the chest. Blood tinged sputum may be expectorated (hemoptysis).

Anticoagulants, bed rest, and oxygen therapy

are prescribed for these patients. Because of the danger of hemorrhage when anticoagulants are administered, it is essential that a prothrombin time be taken daily. Drugs that relax smooth muscle and allay apprehension may also be indicated. Preventive measures usually stressed are early ambulation, exercise of leg muscles, and avoidance of increased pressure in the popliteal area and against the calf muscles. Indiscriminate use of pillows, knee rolls, and the knee gatch of the bed should be avoided with the bedfast patient. Frequent change of position and prescribed exercise are important nursing measures. Special precautions should be taken when placing the patient in the side-lying position to avoid pressure on the underneath limb or injury to the calf muscles of the uppermost limb. When injury to the intima occurs, a layer of platelets is laid down over the damaged area. This may be a factor in the formation of the clot. With this in mind, the nurse who moves the extremities of a helpless patient should understand the importance of supporting joints, as opposed to grasping muscle bellies. If elevation of the involved limb is prescribed, a firm support that extends the full length of the limb and maintains the foot higher than the knee is needed. Another aspect of care is providing for adequate fluid intake to prevent dehydration.

Postural hypotension. Patients who have been confined to bed may experience dizziness (vertigo) upon assuming the vertical position. In some instances fainting will occur. This is known as postural hypotension and is caused by a pooling of the blood in the muscles and abdominal viscera. Following a period of bed rest, the ability of the peripheral vessels to constrict when the individual assumes the upright position is diminished. The reason this occurs is not completely understood. However, when it does take place, it results in a diminished circulatory blood volume with a corresponding drop in blood pressure. When ambulatory activities are prescribed after a period of extended bed rest, the nurse will realize that rolling the head of the bed up for short periods, or permitting the patient to sit on the side of the bed, can be helpful in preventing dizziness and fainting. In many instances, placing the individual on a tilt table and gradually permitting him to assume a verti-

cal position is necessary. The application of elastic bandages or hose to the lower extremities is helpful not only in preventing pooling of blood but also in preventing edema of the dependent extremities.

Gentleness, a fundamental skill

If one could be arbitrary at the beginning and point out a single attainment indispensable for the nurse in any service, selecting it as a major objective for integration into all activities performed, one might be tempted to begin with the practice of gentleness. There is little argument that this is basic and a prerequisite for every new skill the nurse will attempt to master. Gentleness, as it applies to all healing arts, is too often taken for granted. It is presupposed that we, as decent human beings, will treat the people under our care with gentleness. Certainly, it is true that no nurse worthy of the name would consciously mistreat a suffering person, but to accept this as a foregone conclusion that does not need interpretation and emphasis is a questionable procedure. True, there are so many other things to be learned with great effort—methods, techniques, and manual skills—that it seems we must take some things for granted. Gentleness, we are likely to feel, should be natural and unlearned. So it is that we seldom stress this quality, assuming that it already exists. Yet this is a habit and attitude that needs developing. Paradoxically enough, we even need to create respect for it. We know that gentleness in the use of the hands is very important; when prompted by kindness and understanding, it has no counterpart in virtue. But these are overworked words—gentleness, kindness, understanding. We become supercilious in the use of them. They are adjuncts to the nurse's skill, felicitous for the patients but not indispensable for a successful career. Little emphasis is placed on acquiring them as part of one's necessary equipment for nursing.

The practice of gentleness, however, can be a conscious habit, a habit of using one's voice and hands with gentleness consciously because it is good treatment. This is thoughtful objective gentleness, based not on compassion alone but upon the knowledge that sickness is an unremitting source of human fear. If a nurse realizes this, the emotional components of the patient's illness are as important as other common symptoms observed and recorded.

Habitual gentleness is based upon understanding, experience, and an ability to identify oneself with the human race. It is cognitive as well as conative, based on intelligence as well as emotion. It seems that this is too frequently lost sight of in our nursing. Gentleness, whether it is in the handling of a patient with an acutely inflamed joint, the patient tense with fear of an oncoming treatment, or the patient pale with apprehension over a suspected malignancy, is a priceless possession. But it cannot be taken for granted that nurses automatically have this gift because they have elected nursing as their profession.

Biographers of Sir Robert Jones, the famous British orthopedist, have written often, and with deep appreciation, of the cordial spirit with which he received and handled his patients. They describe his methods of supporting a limb during examination—gently and with great skill in avoiding movement that would cause pain. Part of this skill, the cordial spirit, certainly was from the heart, but much of the rest of it must have been painstakingly learned. Both characteristics are greatly needed by nurses, particularly by those of us working with orthopedic patients.

Care of the chronically ill patient

It has been said that ward aides and practical nurses give more satisfactory care to chronically ill patients than professionally trained nurses. If this is true, we need to examine our teaching methods rather carefully to determine what it is that we do not give our students to fit them for this type of nursing. A nurse never goes through a professional career without meeting over and over again the problem of the patient who has been ill a long time—a patient exhausted in courage, short in patience, unreasonable, fearful, and demanding.

Many of these problems will be discussed in other chapters of the book, particularly those having to do with the care of the arthritic patient and the aged patient. Nurses working with the chronically ill are urged to read again Florence Nightingale's *Notes on Nursing,* especially those passages having to do with the patient who

has been confined to a bed or chair for a long time. No one has ever written of this matter with greater feeling and common sense than Florence Nightingale.

There are certain recurring problems regarding chronically ill patients that the nurse should bear in mind whether the patients are young or old. The very act of entering a hospital, for instance, may be a source of profound apprehension and fear to the patient. Perhaps he has had prolonged care in the home, care that he himself directed, wisely or unwisely. Every innovation that hospital nurses make is viewed with disfavor and suspicion, often because of the threat it offers to his comfort, but often, too, because the patient has come to take a negative attitude regarding any suggestion of change in his care. The student should realize that many of the most characteristic reactions of such patients come from a single source—fear. Nurses must recognize that they may be the exciting cause of this reaction and accept the challenge to eliminate it.

All of us who have been in orthopedic nursing for very long have seen patients forcibly taken out of our hands after a day or two of preliminary treatment, by what we justly think of as unreasonable and shortsighted relatives. Perhaps a large number of these withdrawals are unpreventable. But let us look to ourselves and to the initial treatment we give to cherished children or sheltered individuals.

The problem is resolved by use of the golden rule; it is just that simple, commonplace, and undramatic. It means that we must teach the student nurse to understand that the habitual response to these situations must be the response to a patient who is also an individual, a human being. Nurses who do this have understood and practiced democracy as truly as though they went out on a soapbox and campaigned.

DYNAMICS
Joint motion

In orthopedic nursing, nursing care concerns the patient with involvement of the musculoskeletal system. Immobilization and inactivity are frequently present. In this specialty, as in all nursing, it is necessary to remember that prolonged inactivity, regardless of the cause, may lead to complications by interfering with the physiologic processes of the body. With disuse, changes occur in muscle and in joint structure. Maintaining normal range of joint motion and providing for active or passive exercise, functional positions, and correct body alignment are some of the essential aspects of patient care. Attention must be given to the normal extremity as well as to the involved limb. The patient who has had a cerebral vascular accident resulting in a hemiplegic condition will develop joint deformity if good positioning and passive exercise are neglected. The elderly individual may have marked inactivity because of his feeble condition. Continued loss of muscle strength and increased limitation of joint motion will occur unless attention is given to correct positioning and encouragement of activity. The arthritic patient will try to find a comfortable position for painful joints. This is usually a position of flexion, and again contractures will develop unless measures are taken to encourage and to provide for activity and alternate positions. To provide care, the nurse must have an understanding of joint motion. In addition, a vocabulary to describe position and range of motion is helpful and should be used throughout the study of nursing.

The motion that is normally present for any given joint is known as the *range of motion*. Joint motion is measured in degrees of a circle by means of a goniometer (Fig. 1-25). The "neutral zero method" of measuring joint motion (approved by the American Academy of Orthopaedic Surgeons) provides that the motion of a joint be measured from a defined starting point, known as the neutral zero position. The neutral zero position for each joint is the position of that joint in the anatomic position. When the term anatomic position is used, it refers to the body in the standing position with the palms of the hands facing forward, and the toes and kneecaps pointing forward. Thus, the neutral zero position for several of the body joints is that of extension. The following example will serve to illustrate this method of measuring and recording joint motion. The elbow joint in extension is at 0 degrees (neutral zero method). As the forearm and hand are moved toward the shoulder, degrees of motion may be estimated or measured with the goniometer. Normal range of motion for the elbow is 0 degrees to 150 degrees (approximately). If an individual is unable to extend the elbow beyond a right angle, this would be referred to as a flexion deformity of 90 degrees with further flexion to 150 degrees. The range of motion for this elbow would be 90 degrees to 150 degrees. The student interested in obtaining detailed information pertaining to joint range of motion, and the measuring and recording of joint motion, will find the following reference helpful: American Orthopaedic Association: *Manual of Orthopaedic Surgery,* Chicago, 1972, American Academy of Orthopaedic Surgeons.

Knowledge of the range of joint motion enables the nurse to detect early limitations of mo-

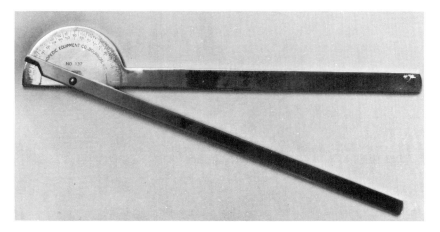

Fig. 1-25. Goniometer—instrument used for measuring joint motion.

tion. When these effects are anticipated or are recognized early, preventive measures against further restrictions can be instituted. The illustrations of joint motions in Figs. 1-26 to 1-41 are included to help the nurse gain an understanding of normal ranges. This is considered fundamental to the application of nursing care that will minimize or prevent any limitations from disuse. However, all degrees of motion given in these illustrations must be interpreted as the approximate degrees of motion possible, and not as indicating a standard or an average. Ranges of joint motion vary widely between individuals. The patient's normal extremity may better serve as a standard or a guide pertaining to his range of motion.

Normally, movements of the body parts will maintain joint motion and prevent tightness of soft tissue. When motion is present, connective tissue is reorganized and replaced in proper alignment. This permits stretching and shortening of the muscle fibers and is essential to good range of motion. When disuse of a muscle occurs, the areolar connective tissue becomes dense and fibrous, and this tends to limit motion or make it difficult. Avoidance of shortened or stretched position of a muscle for long periods of time is necessary to prevent fibrosis of the tissue and limited motion of the involved joint. With immobilization, degenerative changes also occur in the joint. The intracapsular fatty connective tissue grows excessively and forms adhesions with the non-weight-bearing surfaces of the ligaments and bones. Narrowing of the joint space occurs, and the joint cartilage becomes thin. Restriction of motion accompanies these changes. Self-care activities, passive or active exercises, and frequent change of body positions are preventive measures.

There is no active contraction of the muscle fibers with *passive motion exercise*. The extremity is moved through a range of motion by the therapist or nurse. This type of exercise is prescribed when there is paralysis or marked weakness of muscles. Passive exercise does not maintain or develop muscle strength but helps to prevent adaptive shortening or stretching of involved muscles and the tightening of the joint capsule and ligaments.

With *active motion exercise*, there is contrac-

tion of muscle fibers and movement of extremities. This type of exercise, in addition to maintaining range of motion, helps to maintain or increase muscle strength and function. Active assistive exercise may be utilized when the muscle contraction is too weak to produce motion of an extremity without assistance. Varying degrees of assistance may be provided by the therapist or some mechanical device. In some instances, relieving the pull of gravity is sufficient to make motion possible. To increase muscle strength, resistive exercise may be prescribed. As the patient moves an extremity through a range of motion, resistance to the motion is provided.

Isotonic exercise is an exercise in which the length of the entire muscle changes. It may become shorter or longer, and in so doing causes movement of the part of the body to which it is

Text continued on p. 34.

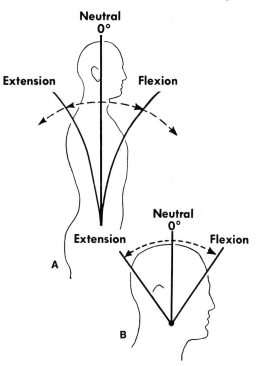

Fig. 1-26. A, Flexion and extension of the thoracic and lumbar spine. **B,** Flexion and extension of the cervical spine. Lateral bend or flexion of the cervical spine (not illustrated) consists of moving the head from the zero or neutral position laterally. The ear approximates the corresponding shoulder. Lateral bend or flexion of the thoracic and lumbar spine (not illustrated) consists of moving the trunk laterally from the zero or neutral position.

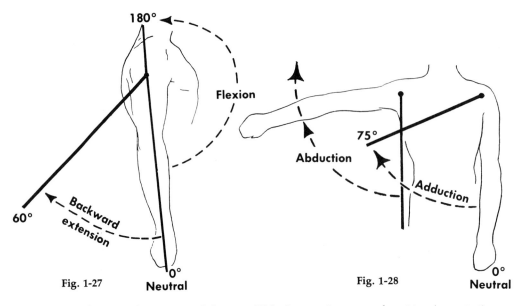

Fig. 1-27   **Neutral**   Fig. 1-28   **Neutral**

Fig. 1-27. Flexion and extension of the arm. With the arm in a neutral position (zero starting position), flexion to approximately 180 degrees is accomplished by moving the arm forward and upward. Flexion to 180 degrees includes scapular motion. Extension consists of moving the arm down and backward to the side of the body. Approximately 60 degrees of backward extension, or hyperextension, is possible—from the zero starting position.

Fig. 1-28. Abduction and adduction of the shoulder. With the arm in a neutral position (zero starting position) abduction to approximately 180 degrees may be accomplished by moving the arm outward and upward from the side of the body. Abduction to 180 degrees includes scapulothoracic motion as well as glenohumeral motion. Adduction consists of returning the arm toward the midline of the body. This motion may be continued in an upward direction beyond the midline of the body to approximately 75 degrees.

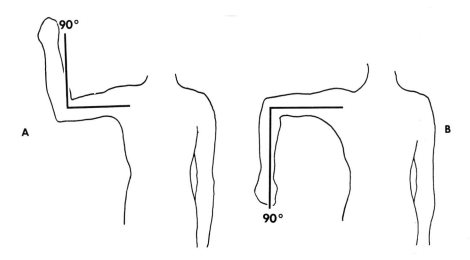

Fig. 1-29. Rotations at the shoulder joint are measured in two positions: (1) with the elbow at the side and flexed 90 degrees from the anatomic position; (2) with the arm abducted 90 degrees and elbow flexed. The diagrams indicate the second method—the more common measurement. **A,** External rotation of the shoulder to approximately 90 degrees. This is accomplished by raising the forearm and hand from the zero starting position. **B,** Internal rotation of the shoulder to approximately 90 degrees. The forearm and hand are lowered from the zero starting position.

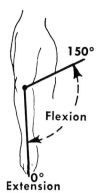

Fig. 1-30. Flexion and extension of the elbow.

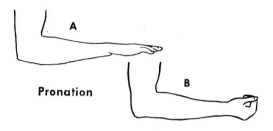

Fig. 1-31. Pronation and supination of the forearm. In the zero starting position, the forearm is supported so that the thumb and index finger are uppermost, weight of the forearm rests on the little finger or ulnar side, and elbow is flexed 90 degrees—not illustrated. **A,** Pronation is accomplished by turning the forearm 80 to 90 degrees so that the palm side of the hand is facing downward. **B,** Supination consists of turning the forearm from the zero starting position, 80 to 90 degrees, so that the palm side of the hand is facing upward.

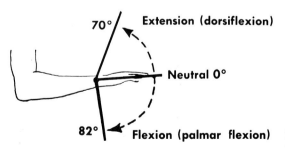

Fig. 1-32. Wrist flexion and extension. Ulnar deviation and radial deviation not illustrated here. Ulnar deviation consists of moving the hand from the neutral or zero position toward the ulnar or little finger side of the hand. With radial deviation the hand is moved toward the radial or thumb side of the hand. (See Fig. 1-47, *D* and *E*.)

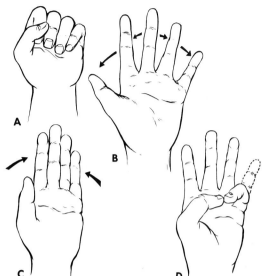

Fig. 1-33. A, Finger flexion. **B,** Finger extension and abduction. **C,** Finger extension and adduction. **D,** Thumb opposition—thumb is moved in a circling motion (outward and around) to the little finger.

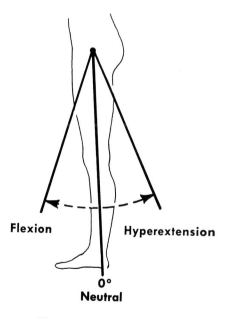

Fig. 1-34. Flexion and extension of the hip. With the limb initially in a neutral position (zero starting position), flexion is accomplished by bringing the limb forward. To measure true extent of hip flexion, the knee must be simultaneously flexed to relax hamstring restraint. Extension consists of lowering the limb to the neutral or zero starting position. Further extension (hyperextension) may be produced by moving the limb backward.

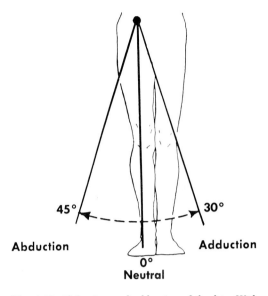

Fig. 1-35. Abduction and adduction of the hip. With the limb in a neutral position (zero starting position), abduction of the hip to approximately 45 degrees is accomplished by moving the limb outward from the body's midline. Adduction to approximately 30 degrees is accomplished by moving the limb toward and across the body's midline.

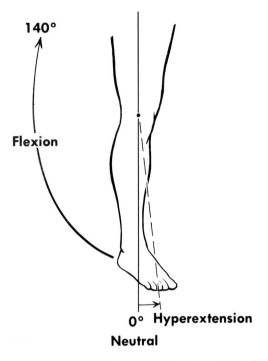

Fig. 1-37. Flexion and extension of the knee. With the knee in the neutral position (zero starting position) flexion to approximately 140 degrees is accomplished by bending the knee. Extension to the neutral position is the motion opposite to flexion. A small amount of motion beyond the neutral position is possible. This is an unnatural position known as hyperextension.

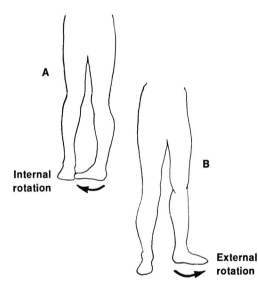

Fig. 1-36. Internal and external rotation of the hip. (In the zero starting position the limb is in a position of extension with the kneecap and foot pointing forward—not illustrated.) **A,** Internal rotation is accomplished by turning the limb toward the midline of the body. **B,** External rotation is accomplished by turning the limb away from the midline.

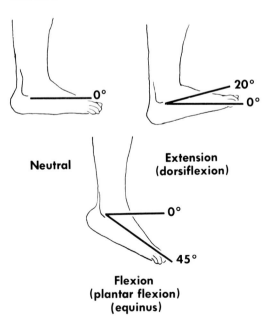

Fig. 1-38. Dorsiflexion and plantar flexion of the ankle.

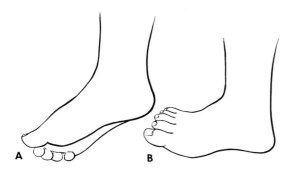

Fig. 1-39. A, Inversion—sole of the foot turned toward medial aspect of the body. **B,** Eversion—sole of the foot turned toward lateral aspect of the body.

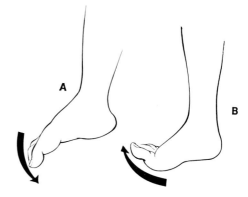

Fig. 1-40. A, Flexion of the toes. **B,** Hyperextension of the toes.

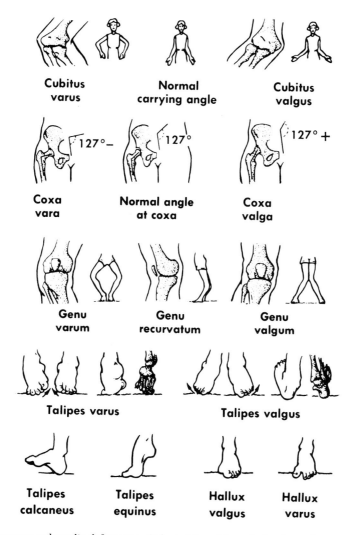

Cubitus varus   Normal carrying angle   Cubitus valgus

Coxa vara   127°−   Normal angle at coxa   127°   Coxa valga   127° +

Genu varum   Genu recurvatum   Genu valgum

Talipes varus   Talipes valgus

Talipes calcaneus   Talipes equinus   Hallux valgus   Hallux varus

Fig. 1-41. Common orthopedic deformities. (Adapted from Manual of orthopaedic surgery, Chicago, 1972, American Academy of Orthopaedic Surgeons.)

attached. Concentric contraction means a shortening of the muscle, and eccentric contraction a lengthening. When an *isometric exercise* is performed, the length of the total muscle does not change and there is no movement of body parts. This type of exercise may be used to maintain the strength of a particular group of muscles when movement of the involved joint is undesirable. The quadriceps setting exercise is an example of an isometric (static) exercise. With the knee in extension, maximum tensing of the muscle can be produced without movement of the knee joint. This may be an important exercise for the traction patient, or for the patient wearing a cast. Isometric or muscle setting exercises of the abdominal, gluteal, and quadriceps muscles may be very beneficial to the patient confined to bedrest. These exercises help to strengthen the antigravity or postural muscles of the body.

Many self-care activities provide for some degree of active exercise and range of motion. The patient who brushes his own hair or ties the neck strings of his hospital gown abducts and externally rotates his arms. Active use of the uninvolved extremities and joints is not considered corrective therapy but is aimed at preventing disuse problems related to the musculoskeletal system. However, when planning range of motion exercises and self-care activities, care and judgement must be used to make certain that the activity utilized is in keeping with the patient's general physical condition. With some patients, the nurse needs specific orders for an exercise program, and she must also be aware that any exercise regime for the involved extremity or joint is prescribed by the physician.

When caring for a helpless patient, the nurse may provide for motion of the patient's joints as part of the bath procedure. When bathing the

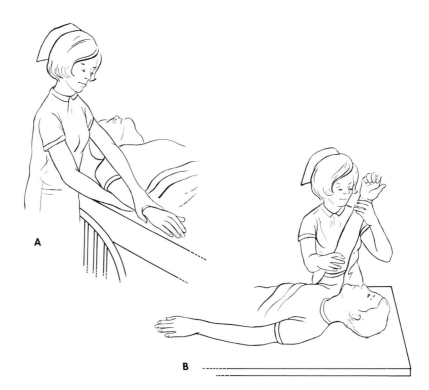

Fig. 1-42. Flexion and extension of the shoulder joint. **A,** With patient in the supine position and his arm lying at his side (thumb side uppermost), support patient's elbow and hand as illustrated. **B,** Lift arm straight up and toward head of the bed (flexion). Return arm to patient's side (extension). Do not abduct shoulder. Note that patient's elbow may need to be flexed as his hand nears head of the bed.

axillary region, the nurse moves the arm away (abduction) from the patient's side. Bending and straightening the elbow provides for flexion and extension. The movements of the wrist, plus closing and opening the hand for finger flexion and extension, can be accomplished nicely as the extremity is bathed and dried. Raising and lowering the leg and bending the knee provides for flexion and extension of the hip and knee joints. Moving the leg toward the edge of the bed helps maintain the motion of abduction, and rolling the limb in provides for internal rotation. Simple dorsiflexion of the foot during the bath procedure will help prevent tightening of the heel cord (Achilles tendon). These joint motions carried out by a nurse who knows how to support and move a paralyzed extremity can be most helpful in preventing joint contractures.

When performing passive range of motion, care must be taken that all movements are done slowly and smoothly. The patient should be relaxed and in a comfortable position. Movements should be pain-free, and the existing range of motion should not be exceeded unless the attending physician has prescribed passive exercise to provide for stretching of tight muscles. The person performing passive exercises sup-

ports the patient's extremity by cupping his hands beneath the joints or by cradling the extremity in his arm. Grasping of muscle bellies is uncomfortable to the patient and should be avoided. Figs. 1-42 to 1-53 will be helpful to the nurse who is responsible for providing passive range of motion for the joints of a patient who is paralyzed or for some other reason is inactive. This type of nursing activity should be supervised by the attending physician.

Mechanics of human gait

Gait is man's self-powered means of travel from one place to another, to reach a position to see, to hear, or to perform a task. There is no means of transportation as versatile as man's bipedal locomotion to adapt to diverse terrain and simultaneously protect the brain and vital organs against sudden impacts.

Normal gait is accomplished by a series of intricate and coordinated muscle and joint actions of the legs and trunk. The coordinated actions require energy (or force) and direction to carry the body forward in a smooth gliding fashion. A normal person tends to walk at a fairly well defined velocity of 2.5 miles per hour, at a cadence of 90 to 110 steps per minute, and an

Text continued on p. 42.

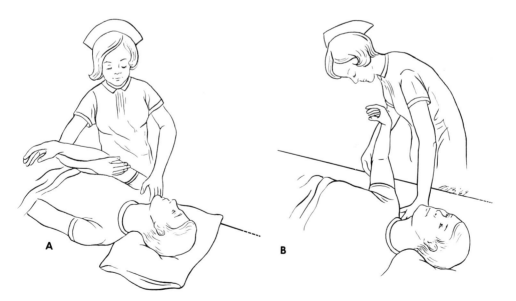

Fig. 1-43. Abduction of the shoulder joint. **A,** With patient in the supine position, "cradle" his arm as illustrated. Use other hand to hold shoulder in a fixed position. **B,** Move patient's arm away from his side (maintain arm at bed level).

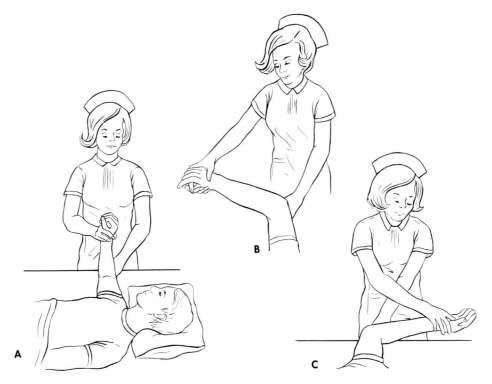

Fig. 1-44. Internal and external rotation of the shoulder joint. With patient in the supine position, the upper arm is supported on the bed in a position of abduction (90 degrees) and the elbow is flexed (90 degrees). **A,** Grasp patient's hand, supporting his thumb with your fingers. Your thumb is on the dorsal aspect of his hand. **B,** Patient's forearm is moved toward the bed, palm downward (internal or medial rotation). **C,** The forearm is returned to the starting position and moved backward toward bed with palm upward (external or lateral rotation).

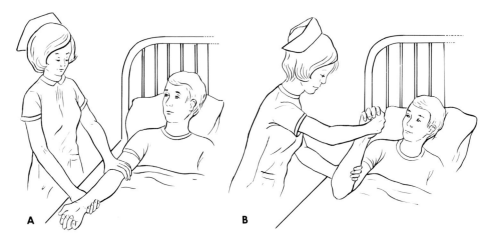

Fig. 1-45. Flexion of the elbow. Place patient in the supine position, with arm resting at his side, palm side uppermost. **A,** Support patient's hand and wrist as illustrated. **B,** Flex elbow, moving hand toward patient's shoulder. Straighten elbow by returning patient's hand to the bed (extension).

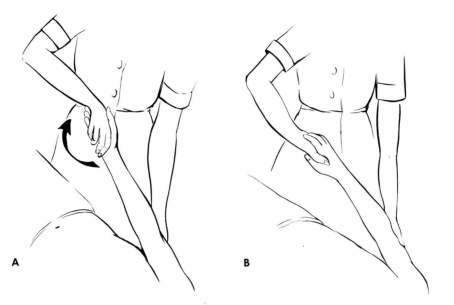

Fig. 1-46. Supination and pronation of the forearm. With patient in the supine position, support his hand in a hand-shaking position. Support his bent elbow with other hand. **A,** Turn palm of his hand upward (supination). **B,** Turn palm of patient's hand downward (pronation).

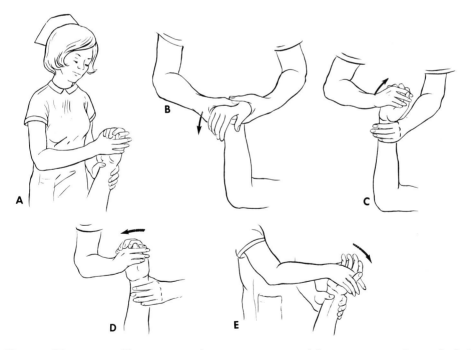

Fig. 1-47. Wrist motion. Place patient in the supine position, with his upper arm resting on the bed and elbow flexed. **A,** Support his forearm with one hand, and with the other hand grasp the patient's hand, supporting his thumb with your fingers. **B,** Flex patient's wrist by moving the palm of his hand toward his forearm. **C,** Move hand backward, palm of patient's hand turned upward (dorsiflexion or extension). **D,** Supporting his wrist in the neutral position, move patient's hand toward the "little finger" side of his hand (ulnar flexion). **E,** Move patient's hand toward "thumb side" of his hand (radial flexion).

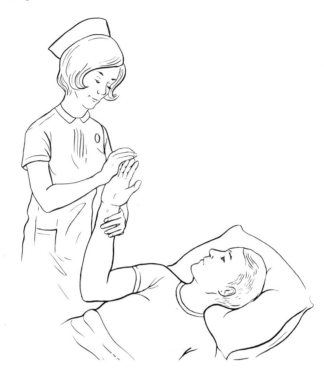

Fig. 1-48. Finger flexion. With patient's elbow flexed and resting on the bed, support his extended wrist with one hand. Place your other hand and fingers (palm side) over dorsum of the patient's hand and fingers. Flex patient's fingers to make a fist. Fingers are then straightened. Thumb opposition (not illustrated)—with the elbow resting on the bed and the fingers held in extension, the thumb is moved in a circling motion (outward and around) toward the little finger.

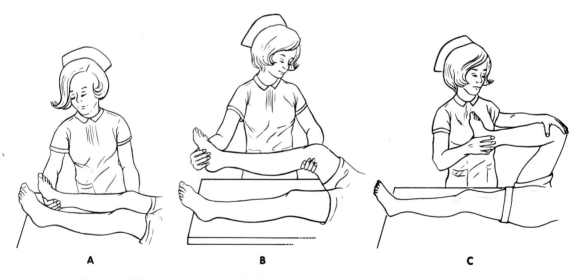

A B C

Fig. 1-49. Flexion and extension of the hip and knee. **A,** With patient in the supine position, the nurse places one hand beneath his knee and uses other hand to support his heel. **B,** Patient's knee and hip are flexed as the limb is lifted off the bed. Limb is maintained in a neutral position (without external rotation or abduction). **C,** As the knee is moved and guided toward patient's chest, the nurse's hand is moved from beneath the knee to the patella region. As the limb is slowly returned to the bed, the nurse's hand must again support the knee as in **B.**

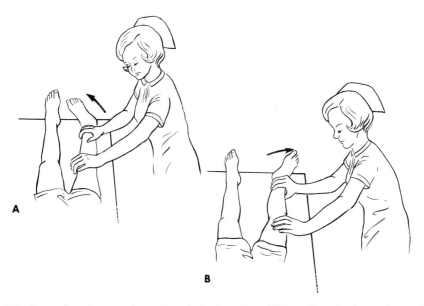

Fig. 1-50. Internal and external rotation of the hip joint. With patient in the supine position, the nurse places one hand above patient's ankle and her other hand above his knee. **A,** The thigh and lower leg are rolled gently toward the midline of the patient's body, then returned to a neutral position. **B,** Entire leg is rolled outward, away from the midline.

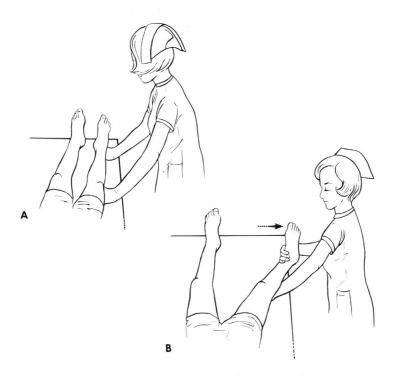

Fig. 1-51. Abduction and adduction of the hip joint, with patient in the supine position. **A,** One hand of the nurse is placed beneath patient's ankle and heel, and her other hand beneath his knee. **B,** Limb is moved slowly and gently toward the edge of the bed, while being kept at bed level and in a neutral position (no external rotation). Limb is then moved back toward midline of the body as in **A.**

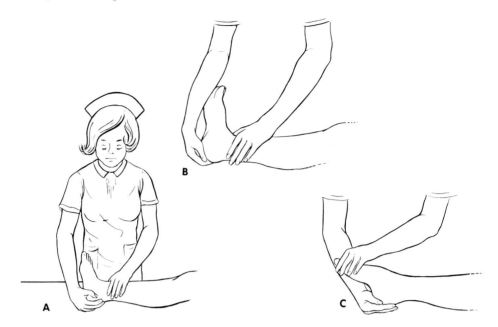

Fig. 1-52. Dorsiflexion and plantar flexion of the foot, with patient in the supine position. **A,** Nurse grasps patient's heel with one hand, permitting the sole of the foot to rest against forearm. Her other hand supports the limb just above the ankle. **B,** The forearm is used to dorsiflex the foot. **C,** The hand on the ankle is moved to the forefoot and the foot is plantar flexed.

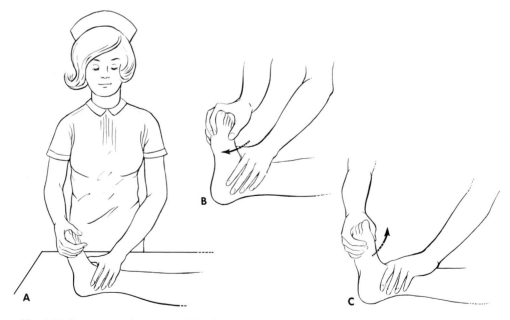

Fig. 1-53. Inversion and eversion of the foot. Patient is placed in the supine position. **A,** With one hand the nurse grasps patient's forefoot (fingers on the plantar surface of the foot). Her other hand holds the limb at the ankle region. **B,** Moving foot toward "little" toe side of the foot (eversion). **C,** Moving foot toward the midline of the body (inversion).

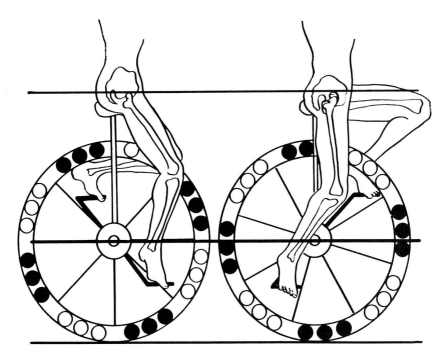

Fig. 1-54

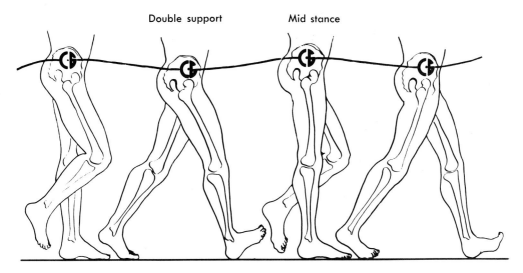

Double support   Mid stance

Fig. 1-55. The heavy line follows the pathway of the body's center of gravity. The low point is at the moment of double support; the high point at mid stance. The small rise and fall throughout the cycle of walking conserve energy.

average step length of 30 to 40 inches. Energy consumption at this velocity seems to be optimal. Whenever a person lacks the required range of motion in the joints or muscle strength and central nervous system balance and coordination, he will limp or have to exaggerate other actions to compensate for the deficiencies.

Children up to age 3 or 4, whose early walking patterns are evolving from the stage of support to no support, have less uniform gait patterns than older children and adults. From step to step they show variability in speed, stride length, cadence, and knee and ankle motion patterns which become more uniform in adults. A limp in young children must have a consistency before it can be qualified as a gait abnormality. Not infrequently a show-off tendency, mimicry, or attention-getting will show itself in gait peculiarities in young children so that again the consistent presence and a consistent pattern should be observed to ascribe a pathological cause to the abnormality.

If the human body operated or moved like a wheel, the hub of the wheel (its center of gravity) would not oscillate up and down on smooth ground but follow a straight line (Fig. 1-54). The center of gravity of the human body in walking follows a pathway which shifts up and down as well as from side to side in a smooth undulating fashion (Figs. 1-55 to 1-56). These shifts of body weight are kept to a minimum since energy is required for each shift of lowering and raising the body weight in each cycle of gait. The shift, although minimal, is necessary

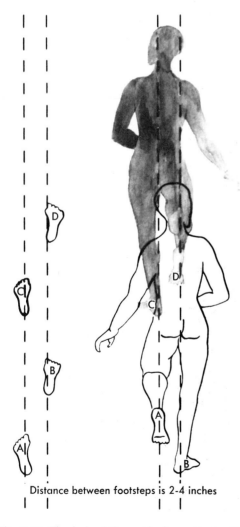

Distance between footsteps is 2-4 inches

Fig. 1-56. The body shifts gently from side to side to assure that the center of gravity is supported on a single leg alternately.

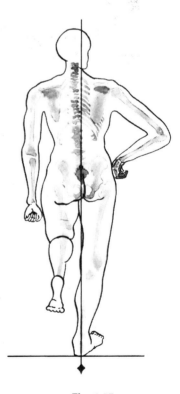

Fig. 1-57

since two requirements of bipedal gait must be met:

1. Single leg stance means that one leg must support body weight while the other leg swings (Fig. 1-57) forward to take a step.

2. The swinging leg cannot reach the ground unless the pelvis on the swing side is lowered and rotated forward to make heel contact with the ground.

The pelvic dip and rotation are insufficient to allow the forward-swinging leg to contact the ground unless the knee of the weight-bearing limb is flexed simultaneously. The knee flexion lowers the center of gravity. As the weight-bearing leg with the bent knee prepares to push the body forward at toe-off, the knee goes into extension at the same time that the foot pushes off from a position of equinus. The knee extension plus ankle extension in effect lengthens the trailing leg to prevent a rapid fall of the center of gravity. The center of gravity is at the low

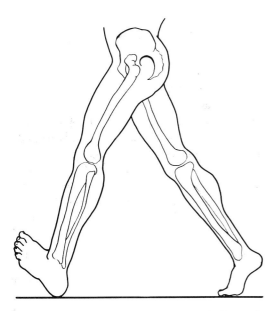

Fig. 1-58. When the leading foot receives body weight (heel strike) and the trailing foot pushes the body forward (push-off), double support takes only a fraction of the walking cycle time. This is the low point for the center of gravity of the body. The forward progression would be a sudden surge from the push-off energy unless the surge is modified by the heel strike, which receives the momentum and slows it to a steady progression by lowering the foot to the floor gradually.

point when both feet are on the ground (double support) (Fig. 1-58) and at the high point at mid stance. The walking base controls the horizontal side to side shift.

The muscle effort of push-off, which comes mainly from the gastronemius, is the force that accelerates the body forward. In order that each push does not appear as a forward surge, other muscles decelerate the body to keep the momentum smooth and uniform. The greatest acceleration of the forward progression of the body occurs as the heel of the reaching foot strikes the floor. The anterior tibial muscle is holding the foot in dorsiflexion at heel strike. The muscle lowers the foot slowly into a flat foot position, and this serves to lessen the impact to the body at heel strike as well as to decelerate the forward momentum of the body.

In summary, the functional tasks of walking are forward progression, single leg balance, and limb length adjustment. When these are accomplished by proper body mechanics, normal walking becomes a smooth, minimal rise and fall of the center of gravity and a fairly uniform forward acceleration with an optimal expenditure of energy.

A limp occurs whenever any individual component of joint motion or muscle force is abnormal. If the abnormality is known, it is possible to predict the type of limp to be expected. This approach may serve to focus the viewpoint of the observer on that portion of gait which is abnormal.

Classes of limp. The commonplace limps encountered may be more meaningfully reviewed if illustrated by specific abnormalities such as those related to hip pathology, knee problems, muscular diseases, and so on.

HIP LIMPS. The hip joint is the major weight-bearing joint in the body and must function properly to produce a normal gait. Body weight is balanced over a single ball-and-socket joint in stance phase. The hip joint is the fulcrum over which muscle force must provide balance. If the pelvis is to remain level when body weight is balanced on one hip, the mechanical arrangement resembles a seesaw (Fig. 1-59). The force of the abductor muscle on the outer end of the lever must equal the weight of the body at the inner end of the seesaw. The Trendelenburg

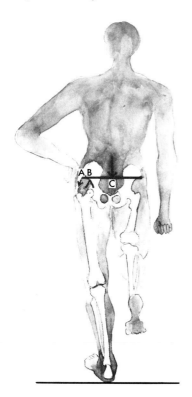

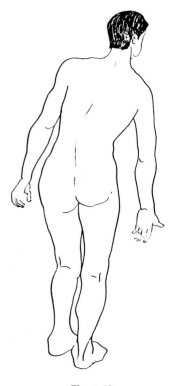

Fig. 1-59. The abductor mechanism of the hip allows single leg stance to support the entire body weight. The pelvis is balanced on fulcrum *B*, the hip joint. The body weight at *C* must be balanced by an equal force at *A*, the abductor muscle. Ability to balance body weight and maintain a level pelvis in single leg stance is known as a negative Trendelenburg test. If the abductor mechanism fails and the pelvis drops on the nonsupport side, the Trendelenburg is positive.

Fig. 1-60

test is negative if the pelvis remains level during single leg stance. The test is positive if the pelvis drops on the non–weight-bearing side (Fig. 1-60). A positive test indicates an abnormality in the abductor mechanism and will show an associated limp. In normal gait the pelvis must be tilted and rotated during stance phase, as previously described. Also, the pelvis must be shifted laterally to receive body weight and keep the center of gravity over the base of support.

Limp in congenital dislocation of hip. The pelvic fulcrum at the hip joint is lacking, which will affect single leg balance. As the body center of gravity shifts laterally to provide single leg balance, the hip abductor cannot regulate pelvic

tilt, which becomes excessive. The body would fall sideways away from the dislocated side unless it compensated by bending the spine toward the dislocated side. This can be observed in gait as a body lurch to the dislocated side each time body weight is transferred to the dislocated limb. This has been called an abductor lurch or Trendelenburg gait (Fig. 1-60). It is indistinguishable from the gait of a paralyzed abductor muscle as often seen in polio. In bilateral dislocations the gait has beeen described as waddling.

Paralysis of the hip abductors. If paralysis of the hip abductors is present, the limp will be similar to that in congenital dislocation of the hip; however, the lurch is apt to be of greater magnitude since the loss of all control of one end of the lever requires a greater compensatory shift of the body.

Stiff hip gait. The word limp has deliberately not been applied since a hip that is stiff in a position of slight adduction, mild external rotation and 30 degrees of flexion will show very little abnormality in gait. If the hip is stiff in a position of 50 degrees flexion, the gait will be altered in two components: First, the pelvis cannot rotate forward or tilt downward when the stiff hip is in stance phase; thus the length of stride of the opposite limb is diminished. Second, at push-off the hip cannot be extended; therefore, to compensate the lack of hip extension, the lumbar spine extends to allow an upright posture for the trunk.

Limp in slipped capital femoral epiphysis. In this condition the range of motion in the hip joint has been altered, and a resultant limp occurs. The hip lacks internal rotation; therefore, pelvic rotation to extend the length of stride for the opposite limb will be shortened; however, the pathway of the center of gravity will remain quite normal. As the gait is observed, two deviants of gait are likely: first the involved limb will be externally rotated throughout the walking cycle, and second, the step length will be slightly shortened on the opposite side (Fig. 1-62). An antalgic component may be present if the hip is also painful.

KNEE LIMPS. Keep in mind that flexion and extension motion is needed in the knee to provide the center of gravity a smooth ride, to clear the floor for the swing-through limb, and to extend the leg to reach the floor at heel strike.

Knee flexion deformity limp. Fixed flexion of 40 degrees at the knee shortens the length of the limb; therefore, as the limb reaches forward for heel strike, the opposite knee must bend to lower the center of gravity more than usual. This has three observable effects on gait: first, the rise and fall of the center of gravity will be more abrupt and greater from the midstance of the good limb to midstance of the flexed limb; second, there will be a shorter step on the flexed limb, and third, often the flexed limb will walk on tiptoe to gain length. If the deformity at the knee is 20 degrees, the compensatory mechanisms will allow a gait that seems almost normal to the casual observer.

Stiff knee gait. If the leg length is normal and the knee is stiff in the extended position, there are two main problems. Heel strike will be quite normal, but the knee flexion that occurs immediately after will be absent. This will mean that the center of gravity, starting low at heel

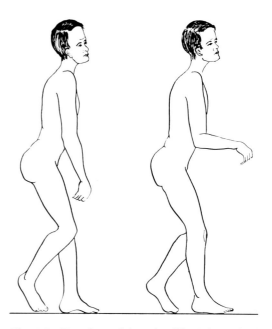

Fig. 1-61. Note that in bilateral stiff hips the angle of flexion remains constant and there is no swing phase of gait. The entire propulsion and leg length adjustment occur at the knee and ankle.

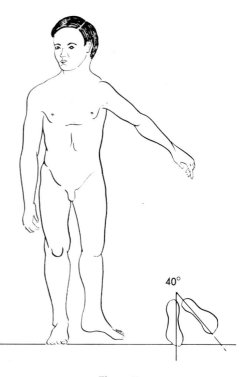

40°

Fig. 1-62

strike, will rise to the normal height of mid-stance but in a more abrupt rather than gradual curve.

In swing phase of the stiff knee limb, the foot will have difficulty clearing the ground; thus, in order to assure clearance, the limb will circumduct (swing out in an abduction circle) as the foot swings over the ground. To the observer this gait can best be described as vaulting when the body is carried forward over the stiff-kneed limb and a sweep of the leg laterally in the swing phase. Chester in "Gunsmoke" typified this gait.

OTHER COMMON LIMPS

Short leg limp. A short leg will affect the limb length adjustment and require the center of gravity to be lowered more than usual for the short limb to reach the floor at heel strike. This can best be observed by watching the entire body drop more at heel strike on the short leg than body drop at heel strike of the normal leg.

Intoeing. The most common gait problem in children under five is that of intoeing (pigeon toe). Recognition of intoeing is simple; however, the cause is not so clearly discernible. Three primary defects produce intoeing, and the gait appears the same in each. To differentiate the primary defect—whether it be hip, knee or foot—the observer must have knowledge of normal leg alignment. Normally in two-legged standing, the feet are separated 2 to 4 inches, slightly toed out, tibias parallel to each other and perpendicular to the ground. The femoras angle outward from the knee the distance required to place the femoral heads into the acetabular sockets. The kneecaps face straight ahead. The normal alignment just described will show 3 variants to account for intoeing:

1. Metatarsus adductus. In this condition the feet appear toed in because of the adducted position of the forefoot, which appears exaggerated in walking (Fig. 1-63).

2. Internal torsion of the tibia. The entire foot appears toed in while the kneecap points or faces straight ahead (Fig. 1-64).

3. Anteversion of the neck of the femur. In this condition the foot and kneecap are in proper alignment, but both appear internally rotated. The internal rotation of the entire limb is an accomodation at the hip to rotate the tronchan-

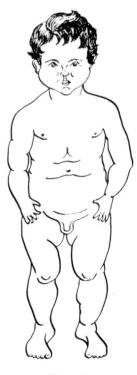

Fig. 1-63

ter forward for better mechanics of the abductor mechanism. This is a compensation to relieve the posterior position of the trochanter caused by anteversion (Figs. 1-65 and 1-66).

Antalgic gait. The word antalgic means relieving pain and is often used to refer to a limp. This term does not describe the limp, nor does it imply a specific mechanical component of gait; thus it is the same as saying the limp relieves pain. Although the condition may appear in a variety of forms, there is one common denominator of all antalgic limps, namely that the less time weight rests on the painful joint, the less pain; hence, the average antalgic limp is a "quick step" gait, which is obvious to the observer. Other abnormalities of gait may be associated in the same individual; however, the associated limps are usually explainable by known associated deformities, limited motions, or muscle deficiencies. An antalgic limp would relieve pain in any joint, the hip, knee, or ankle, or even pain caused by a nail in the shoe.

Slap-foot (drop-foot) gait. In the beginning of stance phase of gait at the time of heel strike, the limb is suddenly loaded by body weight

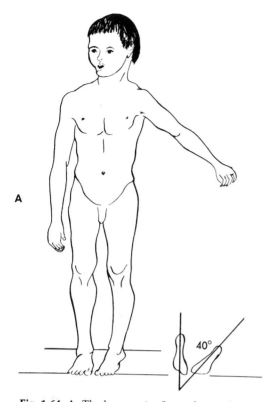

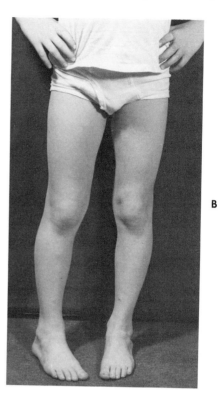

Fig. 1-64. A, The knees point forward properly, yet the left foot is toed in because of internal torsion of the tibia. **B,** Internal torsion of right tibia.

which has just been propelled forward by the push off limb. At the next instant, the dorsiflexed foot would be forced rapidly to the ground with a slap sound unless the foot were lowered more gradually. The gradual lowering is accomplished by the anterior tibial and toe extensor muscles whose forces hold the foot dorsiflexed. A weakness of these muscles, as in peroneal palsy, allows the foot to slap to the ground. Likewise, if these muscles are absent the foot is never dorsiflexed, and instead of heel strike the entire foot slaps flatly to the ground. In this instance, the observer will note two things—first, the knee is raised higher in swing phase to keep the dropped foot from scraping the ground, and, second as the foot strikes the ground, there will be an audible slap.

Miscellaneous limps. Cerebral palsy, polio, and neuromuscular defects provide an array of limps and gait abnormalities that defy accurate description. Often the compensatory mechanisms alter the anticipated limp in the case of known muscle deficits. Inability of reciprocal

muscle relaxation may restrict a joint movement in an otherwise normal joint. Cerebral balance from brain damage may produce a drunken gait. Lack of proprioceptive positional feedback will exaggerate the movements of an otherwise normal gait. Such persons may be unable to walk in darkness since eyesight gives the only positional feedback.

Extensive spasticity is most commonly displayed by the scissor gait in which the extended legs become crossed from persistent overwhelming adductor muscle spasm. A jerky, slow deliberate effort manages to swing one leg past the other in each step (Fig. 1-67).

If the knees are simultaneously held in flexion by quadriceps and hamstrings in unrelenting spasticity, neither of which will relax to allow alternating motion, each leg will suddenly spring forward as though released from a spring trap at each step. The body center of gravity, usually riding with the smooth even undulations, is now moved by a series of jerks (Fig. 1-68).

Add permanent spastic equinus to the flexed

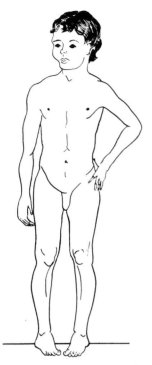

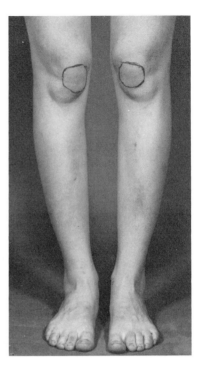

Fig. 1-65. Kneecaps point inward as do the feet, which indicates that the entire extremity is rotated inward at the hip joint. The usual cause is excessive anteversion of the femoral neck, which is normally 12 degrees at growth completion. The anteversion in this intoeing could well be 35 degrees.

Fig. 1-66. Actual case of a 17-year-old girl with anteversion of 35 degrees by roentgenographic measurement. Note the knees pointed inward and the feet straight ahead. Frequently the tibias show a compensatory external torsion.

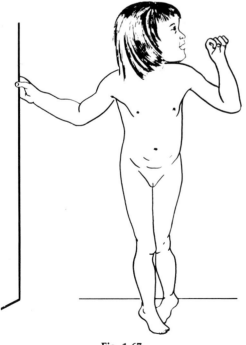

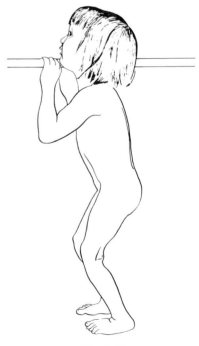

Fig. 1-67

Fig. 1-68

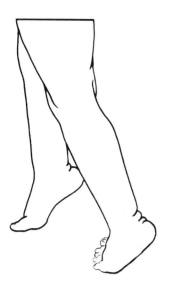

Fig. 1-69

knees and scissored legs, and the commonly described jump gait is produced (Fig. 1-69).

Take away the gastrocnemius, as in myelomeningocele, and the individual shows a calcaneus gait.

STUDY QUESTIONS

1. List criteria for evaluating:
   (a) Standing posture
   (b) Sitting posture
2. Demonstrate use of correct body mechanics when:
   (a) Moving a patient to the side of the bed
   (b) Assisting patient from bed to chair
   (c) Giving back care to a bed patient
3. Describe or demonstrate the normal range of motion at each of the following joints:
   (a) Shoulder
   (b) Elbow
   (c) Wrist
   (d) Metacarpophalangeal
   (e) Hip
   (f) Knee
   (g) Ankle
4. Be prepared to demonstrate good posture for the bed patient in:
   (a) Supine position
   (b) Prone position
   (c) Side-lying position
5. What nursing care would you suggest to prevent?
   (a) Foot drop
   (b) Knee flexion contracture
   (c) Hip flexion contracture
6. Bed rest or inactivity may contribute to a number of complications by interfering with the physiologic processes of the body. Explain.

REFERENCES

Abramson, A. S., and Delagi, E. F.: Influence of weight-bearing and muscle contraction on disuse osteoporosis, Arch. Phys. Med. **42:**147-151, 1961.

Anderson, T. M.: Human kinetics ang good movement, Physiotherapy **57:**169-176, 1971.

Basmajian, J. V.: Man's posture, Arch. Phys. Med. **46:**26-36, 1965.

Brower, P., and Hicks, D.: Maintaining muscle function in patients on bed rest, Am. J. Nurs. **72:**1250-1253, 1972.

Browse, N. L.: Physiology and pathology of bed rest, Springfield, Ill, 1965, Charles C Thomas, Publisher.

Brunnstrom, S.: Clinical kinesiology, ed. 3, Philadelphia, 1972, F. A. Davis Company.

Cadogan, D. R.: Handling the handicapped, Physiotherapy **57:**467-470, 1971.

Carnevali, D., and Brueckner, S.: Immobilization—reassessment of a concept, Am. J. Nurs. **70:**1502-1507, 1970.

Civca, R., Bradish, J., and Trombly, S.: Range of motion exercises, active and passive: a handbook, Nursing, '73 **3:**25-37, Dec. 1973.

Coles, C., Grendahl, B., Hannan, V., Plass, J., and Ulrich, P.: Rehabilitative nursing techniques. 3. A procedure for passive range of motion and self-assistive exercises, Minneapolis, 1964, Kenny Rehabilitation.

Cooper, J., and Glassow, R.: Kinesiology, ed. 3, St. Louis, 1972, The C. V. Mosby Co.

Covalt, N. K.: Bed exercises for convalescent patients, Springfield, Ill., 1968, Charles C Thomas, Publisher.

Daeso, M.: Prevention of secondary deterioration of the chronically ill patient, Postgrad. Med. **38:**90-96, 1965.

Daniels, L., and Worthingham, C.: Muscle testing: techniques of manual examination, ed. 3, Philadelphia, 1972, W. B. Saunders Co.

Evans, F. G., editor: Biomechanical studies of the musculo-skeletal system, Springfield, Ill., 1961, Charles C Thomas, Publisher.

Fixsen, J. A.: Common postural deformities in children, Nurs. Times **68:**1086-1088, 1972.

Foss, G.: Body mechanics, Nursing '73 **3:**25-32, 1973.

Foss, G.: The "how to's" of bed positioning, Nursing '72, **2:**14-16, 1972.

Fronst, H. M.: Laws of bone structure, Springfield, Ill., 1964, Charles C Thomas, Publisher.

Gough, J. V., and Ladley, G.: An investigation into the effectiveness of various forms of quadriceps exercises, Physiotherapy **57:**356-361, 1971.

Greenwood, M. W.: An illustrated approch to medical physics, ed. 2, Philadelphia, 1966, F. A. Davis Company.

Griffin, W., Anderson, S. J., and Passos, J. Y.: Group exercise for patients with limited motion, Am. J. Nurs. **71:**1742-1743, 1971.

Hopkins, J.: Surrender to gravity, Phys. Ther. **48:**862-865, 1968.

Human locomotion, Washington D. C., Fall, 1969, V. A. Administration Department of Medicine and Surgery Bulletin of Prosthetics B.P.R.

Joint motion—method of measuring and recording, Chicago, 1965, American Academy of Orthopaedic Surgeons.

Jordan, H. S., and Kavchak, M. A.: Transfer techniques, Nursing '73 **3**:19-22, 1973.

Kamenetz, H. L.: Exercises for the elderly, Am. J. Nurs. **72**:1401, 1972.

Karpovich, P. V.: Exercise in medicine: a review, Arch. Phys. Med. **49**:66-76, 1968.

Kelly, M. M.: Exercises for bedfast patients, Am. J. Nurs. **66**:2209-2213, 1966.

Kendall, H., and Kendall, F.: Developing and maintaining good posture, Phys. Ther. **48**:319-336, 1968.

Kern, C. C., and Poole, L.: Transfer techniques, Nursing '72, **2**:25-28, 1972.

Kottke, F.: The effects of limitation of activity upon the human body, J.A.M.A. **196**:825-830, 1966.

Kottke, F., and Anderson, E.: Deterioration of the bedfast patient—causes and effects and nursing care, Public Health Rep. **80**:437-451, 1965.

Kottke, F. J., and Blanchard, R. S.: Bedrest begets bedrest, Nurs. Forum **3**:57-73, March 1964.

Krusen, F., Kottke, F., and Ellwood, P.: Handbook of physical medicine and rehabilitation, ed. 2, Philadelphia, 1971, W. B. Saunders Co.

Larson, C. B.: Low back pain, Postgrad. Med. **26**:142-149, 1959.

Madden, B. W., and Affeldt, J. E.: To prevent helplessness and deformities, Am. J. Nurs. **62**:59-61, 1962.

Manual of orthopaedic surgery, Chicago, 1972, American Orthopaedic Association.

Millen, H. M.: Physically fit for nursing, Am. J. Nurs. **70**:520-523, 1970.

Muller, E. A.: Influence of training and of inactivity on muscle strength, Arch. Phys. Med. Rehab. **51**:449-462, 1970.

Olson, E. V., Johnson, B., Thompson, McCarthy, J., Edmonds, R., Schroeder, L., and Wade, M.: The hazards of immobility, Am. J. Nurs. **67**:779-797, 1967.

Perry, J.: The mechanics of walking, Phys. Ther. **47**:778, 1967.

Rehabilitative aspects of nursing, a programmed instruction series, Part I. Physical therapeutic nursing measures: unit 1, Concepts and goals (1966); unit 2, Range of joint motion (1967), New York, National League for Nursing.

Saunders, J. B., Inman, V. and Eberhart, H.: The major determinants in normal and pathological gait, J. Bone Joint Surg. **35-A**:543-558, 1953.

Stillwell, D., McLarren, G., and Gersten, J.: Atrophy of quadriceps muscle due to immobilization of the lower extremity, Arch. Phys. Med. **48**:289-295, 1967.

Works, R. F.: Hints on lifting and pulling, Am. J. Nurs. **72**:260-261, 1972.

2

General features of orthopedic nursing

NURSING CARE OF PATIENTS IN CASTS

To preserve the efficiency of a cast and, at the same time, to maintain the patient in cleanliness and comfort taxes the ingenuity of the best nurse. This skill is one of the most essential of orthopedic nursing, and doctors frequently judge the competency of the nursing staff by the care given to patients in casts. No one way of caring for these patients can be arbitrarily defined, and the nurses are learning new and better methods daily. The directions given here are offered solely to the perplexed nurse who has not had sufficient experience in these matters to assume the care of patients in casts satisfactorily.

Safeguarding the efficiency of the cast (that is, its ability to maintain the position for which it has been applied, over the period of time necessary for the accomplishment of the doctor's purpose) is the nurse's responsibility. Yet one must be constantly aware that the patient inside the cast is the first concern. One thing to understand clearly from the outset is that the patient's every complaint must have prompt attention, even though his complaint seems trifling and the nurse may privately consider him a chronic complainer. The patient who seldom complains is given solicitous attention when he reports a burning sensation over common points of pressure, such as the heel, the malleoli, or the sacrum. It is the constantly complaining patient who may be overlooked, so that when the cast is finally removed a sloughing sore appears over an area he told the nurse about at one time. It is the old "wolf-wolf" story in an orthopedic version.

OBSERVATION OF CIRCULATION

Nurses have been warned repeatedly about the dangers of impaired circulation in an extremity upon which a new cast has been applied, and it seems as though the subject could be passed over with little more than a word. However, it must be remembered that inspecting fingers or toes when the extremity has been recently encased in plaster is as important as taking a pulse after an operation. Circulatory impairment is important to watch for as well as signs of hemorrhage. The rapidity with which it may progress from bad to worse is difficult for the inexperienced nurse to comprehend. A paralysis of such seriousness that the patient may never again be able to use his hand or foot may be produced within a 24-hour period.

Nurses should be familiar with the blanching sign. This is particularly important in caring for patients who have casts applied to the leg or arm. The nail of the thumb or great toe is momentarily compressed, and the return flow of blood to the nail is observed. The compressed area should refill with blood immediately upon the release of pressure; that is, the nail should turn from white to pink at once. It must be emphasized, however, that some blood often remains in the fingers or toes even after circula-

51

tion is impaired, and the nurse may be misled to believe that the circulation is satisfactory because blood does return, although somewhat sluggishly. The anemic area must flush rapidly with blood, and the fingers or toes should be warm and of good color. Inspection should be made every 10 to 15 minutes if there is any sign of impaired circulation.

Often the physician will cut a hole in an arm cast near the radial artery, so that the nurse can take the pulse of the patient frequently through this opening to ascertain whether the circulation to the hand is normal. This does not mean that the nurse is to take his pulse to be assured of the patient's general condition, as with other patients postoperatively, but rather to keep an accurate check of the circulation in the extremity in the cast. Failure to feel the pulse is warrant for notifying the physician at once. Symptoms of coldness, pallor, blueness, edema, loss of motion, numbness, pain, and a slow return of blood to the part on blanching are cardinal. In addition, it is important to be able to see all the fingers and toes. Nor should the nurse be satisfied with 12 or 24 hours of close watching. The extremity must be watched during many succeeding days. A feeling of security is not justified merely because the patient is conscious and in apparently good condition after the operation.

CARE OF THE CAST

Supporting the wet cast. The care of the patient as an individual is primary, but the cast is also important. The doctor has spent considerable time and thought on the cast. It has cost both time and money, and its importance in the patient's recovery is considerable.

The care of the cast begins before the patient returns to the ward from the plaster room. It begins with the preparation of the bed. A firm mattress is a necessity. Boards spread, preferably lengthwise, under the mattress are essential when the cast is the body type or a hip spica, enclosing the legs and the body. Pillows should be ready to support the wet cast (Fig. 2-1). These pillows need rubber or plastic covers to prevent dampness and mustiness that would result from absorption of moisture from the plaster. They also need to be pliable and easily adjusted to the coutour of the patient's body. If the patient is to have a body cast, three pillows laid crosswise on the bed are usually satisfactory. For a hip spica cast it is best to arrange one pillow crosswise at the level of the waist with two laid lengthwise for the single leg in the cast. If both legs are to be encased, two more pillows are needed for the second leg of the adult patient. A pillow for the head and shoulders is necessary if the patient has not had an anes-

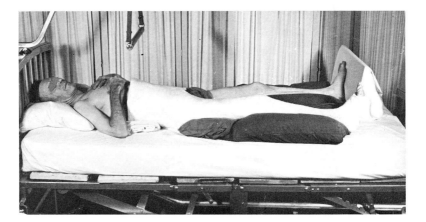

Fig. 2-1. Correct support for the patient in a hip spica cast in the supine position. The pillows beneath the limb enclosed in plaster provide support for the thigh and avoid pressure on the heel. The small pad that supports the lumbar region prevents the anterior portion of the cast from pressing on the abdomen, and the pillow for the head, placed well down under the shoulders, maintains good alignment of the cervical spine. Boards beneath the mattress provide a firm surface for the cast. Note the trapeze, which facilitates nursing care of the patient in a hip spica cast.

thetic. Under no circumstances is the damp cast to be lifted directly onto the hard bed when the patient is returned from the plaster room. If this occurs, the cast will become flattened over the bony prominences, particularly the back of the heel and the sacrum, and damage to the underlying soft tissues will be unavoidable.

Some doctors prefer to have one sandbag placed under the groin on the affected side and another under the heel. These are used to prevent excessive weight on the damp cast. It is essential that no sharp break in the pillow alignment under the cast be allowed that might cause the cast to sag at some strategic point, particularly at the junction of the leg and body sections of the hip spica cast.

The patient must be lifted carefully onto the bed. The nurse helping with this procedure uses the palms of the hands, not the fingers, to lift the cast. Fingers may make indentations in the soft plaster if it is not sufficiently set. This is particularly important in handling the foot and leg section of the cast.

Drying the cast. If the patient has not been anesthetized, the cast is usually left uncovered for several hours. Many physicians prefer that casts be dried in this way—by natural evaporation. If, however, quick drying is essential, as it often is when the patient is to leave the hospital

shortly, it can be started as soon as the cast is set. After the cast has set, it is usually satisfactory to use some form of external heat for drying it. Heat lamps or a cradle on which a low-watt incandescent lamp is suspended at a safe distance from the patient and the cast may be used for this. Cages of wire encircling these lamp bulbs are desirable, and a distance of at least 15 inches from the cast to the light is usually considered safe. The cradle should not be covered with bedclothes because the moisture will go back to the cast as the confined space under the bedclothes becomes saturated. Escape for the moisture-laden air is essential.

A hand dryer, such as that used for hair drying, may be employed and is especially good for small areas of plaster that have become dampened through mishaps. Intense heat is never recommended because it tends to cause the outer layers to dry too swiftly while the underlying layers remain moist (Fig. 2-2).

It has been frequently observed that during warm weather with the early setting and drying process, the cast becomes very hot. If the cast is left entirely uncovered, the air will greatly hasten evaporation and hardening, and the heat of the cast will be transitory.

It may be wise to insert here something about the basic chemistry of plaster of paris, so that

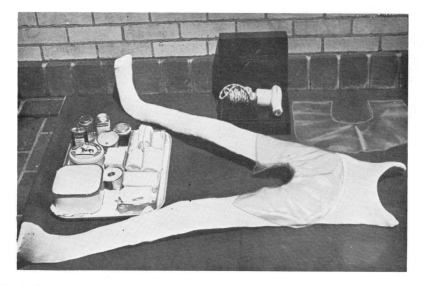

Fig. 2-2. Bedside cast tray and hair dryer for daily use on casts. Anterior shell is covered with stockinet and protected with waterproofing.

the nurse may know exactly what is happening in the cast as it sets and hardens. The plaster of paris commonly used when a cast is applied is made from gypsum (calcium sulfate, $CaSO_4 \cdot 2H_2O$). When the gympsum crystals are heated, the water of crystallization is driven off, and the remaining calcined gypsum is plaster of paris ($CaSO_4 \cdot \frac{1}{2} H_2O$). The finely powdered plaster of paris is incorporated into a mesh bandage to produce the plaster of paris roll or splint. When this plaster of paris bandage is placed in water, preparatory to use, the reverse action takes place: water is absorbed and crystals of gypsum are formed. During formation of these gypsum crystals the potential full strength of the plaster is determined according to the closeness with which the crystals interlock. The maximum strength is obtained only after all excess water has been evaporated from the cast's surface. When this is accomplished and the cast is wholly dry, it is strong and firm and able to withstand sudden stresses.

Turning the patient. The time of the first turning of a patient in a new cast frequently depends on the physician's order, but in orthopedic hospitals a standing order usually exists that all patients be turned by the evening of the day the cast is applied. This is done primarily for the comfort of the patient and so, also, that the cast may be dried on its posterior surface. The first turning of a patient in a body cast or a hip spica cast requires more help than will be needed subsequently when the cast has become rigid and firm through drying. To turn a patient with a new cast without assistance endangers the cast and should not be attempted if it can be avoided.

With a crew of three people, an adult patient in a hip spica cast can be turned without much risk either to the patient's comfort or to the integrity of the cast. The patient is gently pulled toward the side of the bed that corresponds to the leg in plaster. It is possible to effect this moving by exerting a pull on the pillows beneath the cast. When the patient is pulled to this side, two of the crew should go around the bed, where if necessary a fresh drawsheet can be started and the pillows can be arranged to receive the cast when the patient is turned (Fig. 2-3).

Dry pillowcases may be necessary if the ones in use are damp. When the pillowcases do not need changing, it is sometimes possible to pull the pillows partially through from under the cast without allowing the cast to drop from them.

Turning should always be done on the side

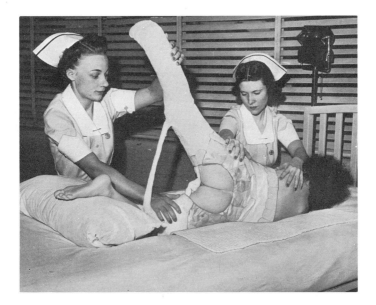

Fig. 2-3. Turning the patient in a hip spica cast. Note the pillow in place for foot support. The abduction bar should not be used as a handle when lifting or turning the patient. Strips of protective material have been applied to protect the cast in the perineal area.

not enclosed in plaster or toward the side that has not been operated upon if the cast is a double spica. The patient is thus turned on his normal leg and toward the nurses who are assisting him. One nurse remains on the side of the bed toward which the patient has been pulled in order to overcome any sense of insecurity he may have from a fear of falling. The other two nurses turn the patient toward them from the opposite side. The patient is told exactly what is to be done, and he is instructed to place the arm on which he is turning above his head. With adult patients it may be easier to have the patient keep his arms close to his sides. To avoid pressure on the arm on which he is turning a folded towel should be placed between the arm and the cast. The pillow beneath the patient's head should be removed during the turning. In this procedure, care is taken to move in unison. One nurse places her hands on the shoulder and hip of the patient, and the other supports the thigh and foot of the extremity in the cast. The nurse on the opposite side assists with the turning by pulling the shoulder through as the patient is gently eased onto his face.

Pillows along the entire length of the cast must be in readiness in order to avoid lifting the patient once he is turned. Lifting the cast is exceedingly hard on the patient and endangers the soft cast. In addition, it is an unnecessary strain to the nurse's back that can be avoided with foresight. After the patient has been turned, the nurse should observe his position to see that the toes of the leg in the cast do not jam against the bed. A pillow laid crosswise on the bed will provide support for both feet. If there is wide abduction in the cast, the toes of the foot in plaster may hang over the edge of the mattress. Another point to observe is the position of the body section of the cast. If there are too many pillows under the patient's head and shoulders, the plaster may press into the back just below the ribs. If the pillow under the abdomen is not placed correctly, the cast edges may press into the soft tissues of the chest and abdomen (Fig. 2-4).

Later, when the cast is completely hardened, one or two nurses may turn the patient with a minimum of difficulty. Patients soon learn to assist with turning—to such an extent that little help is needed from the nurse or attendant. When the cast is dry, pillows are needed only for the patient's comfort and may be dispensed with except at points of pressure. A support for the heel so that it does not rest on the bed is usually considered essential, and patients are generally more comfortable with a pillow beneath the body portion of the cast as they lie prone. When this pillow is in place, the patient's chest will be the forward portion of the body.

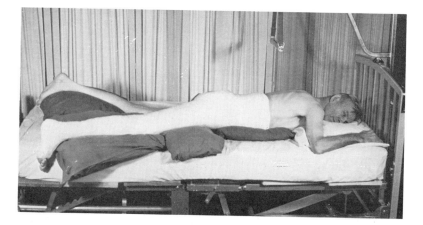

Fig. 2-4. Correct support for the patient in a hip spica cast in the prone position. The extremity enclosed in plaster is supported by pillows to prevent strain on the cast at the groin area. There is enough abduction to permit the foot enclosed in plaster to extend over the edge of the mattress. The thin pillow placed crosswise at the top edge of the cast prevents undue pressure on the abdomen, and one pillow for the head maintains good alignment of the shoulders and neck. Note the position of the normal extremity.

When the patient is turned the first time, the cast will still be damp on its posterior surface and will usually be rather compressed against the back. Some method of quick drying should be used at this time, and the patient's back should be given meticulous care. The buttocks will be blue and creased and will need particular attention. The skin around the cast edges and immediately beneath the cast can be reached with the fingers, and this area can be rubbed and gently stretched away from the cast to increase comfort and circulation. Any rough edges on the posterior surface of the cast must be cared for at this time. Insufficient room for defecation should be noted and reported.

After the cast has been trimmed, if necessary, the stockinet lining may be pulled over the cast edge and secured with a moistened plaster of paris splint or bandage.

If the patient is a child, however, some thought must be given to the protection of the buttocks region. It is never safe to expect the child to get through the night without soiling his cast. Small strips of waterproof material may be tucked under the cast, and the outer edges be secured with a plaster of paris splint.

The patient should be urged to lie prone as long as he can. Encouragement from the nurse may often prolong this period to as much as 45 minutes to an hour. When this rest period is completed, he is again turned with the precautions described.

If the surgeon has ordered a window cut over the abdomen or chest, it is usually wise to wait until the cast is dry before having this done. There is a tendency for the cast to break or buckle if the window is cut too early. The surgeon, of course, should be consulted in this matter.

Finishing the cast edges. When sheet wadding or similar material has been used to line the cast, it is impossible to pull this material over the cast edge as is done with stockinet. However, adhesive tape may be used to cover the cast edges. If tape is used (without additional plaster of paris to secure the outer edge) the cast must be thoroughly dry to prevent the tape from rolling. This usually requires 24 to 48 hours, depending on the thickness of the cast and the humidity of the air. Petals of tape, cut

round or pointed and about 1½ inches in length, are excellent to bind cast edges or to apply waterproofing. When tape is applied to the dry cast, it is important that the edges be pressed securely against the plaster to prevent the tape from rolling and sticking to the bed linen. To prevent rolling of the tape, a plaster of paris strip can be moistened and placed over the outer edge of adhesive tape; this will hold the petals in place and maintain a smooth, tape-covered cast edge. Likewise, the edges of the newly applied, damp cast can be finished with such petals, if a plaster of paris splint or bandage is used to secure their outer edges. The adhesive petals adhere nicely to the sheet wadding on the underneath side of the cast and are held in place on the outer aspect of the damp cast with a moistened plaster of paris splint. This permits finishing the edges of a cast, lined with sheet wadding, immediately following application and trimming of the cast. An easy method of cutting petals is to fold a length of 1½- or 2-inch wide adhesive tape lengthwise (sticky side out) and cut through it at a 45-degree angle (Fig. 2-5).

If stockinet has been used to line the cast, the ideal method of finishing the cast is to pull the stockinet over the edges and secure it with a moistened plaster splint. This can be done be-

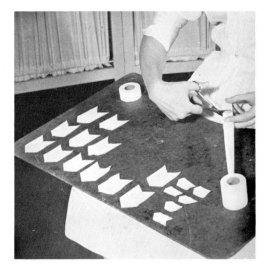

Fig. 2-5. Lapboard used in cutting petals for finishing the edges of a cast. Note the position of the tape strip. It is folded so that the sticky sides are out and then cut diagonally toward the center fold.

fore the cast is completely dry, thus sealing off the edges and eliminating plaster crumbs.

Before the cast edges are finished, all rough spots or irregularities likely to cause pressure areas or irritation of the skin must be removed. Also, before the cast is finished around the buttocks, enough room for the patient to have proper care after voidings and defecations must be ensured. If the cutout space seems unnecessarily small, the physician should be consulted before it is bound. Most doctors are eager to give nurses enough room for proper care of these patients, and usually the insufficient space cut out is an oversight rather than a design. An exception to this may occur in the case of patients in whom adductor tenotomies have been performed and whose incisions are very close to the perineum.

Protection of casts. The protection of casts from soiling and moisture is a point of considerable interest. The ingenuity of a generation of nurses has been taxed by this troublesome problem. The impossibility of properly protecting casts made such men as Dr. V. Putti and Sir Robert Jones declare that plaster of paris could be used for home treatment only with the greatest risks and danger. However, the modern nurse can devise many methods of protecting casts that are also simple enough to make home care of patients in casts not only safe but also quite satisfactory.

To protect the perineal region against body excretions, a waterproof material is used. Inexpensive plastic materials provide excellent protection when they are properly applied (Figs. 2-6 to 2-8).

Waterproof material is cut in strips from 4 to 5 inches in width and tucked under the cast around the curved area at the buttocks. It is secured on the outside of the cast with either adhesive tape, mending tape, or a single layer of plaster of paris.

Casts cannot be washed, for water will soften them. The life of the cast will be shortened and its efficiency lessened, and mold will almost inevitably appear on the surface of a frequently dampened cast. It is usually considered permissible to remove very minor stains from casts with a cloth squeezed almost dry and rubbed over a cake of Bon Ami. If the area is large, this must be followed by some form of artificial heat or sunlight to dry the cast as quickly as possible. Shellac, varnish, or lacquer must not be used to waterproof casts until they are thoroughly dried, preferably not until 48 hours have elapsed. Waterproofing the entire cast before it is dry prevents the proper evaporation of moisture beneath.

Old stockings may be used to cover casts in the home and provide excellent protection for leg casts on children. In some clinics all casts are covered completely with stockinet before the patient is discharged. Outer stockinet is sewed to that which has been used beneath

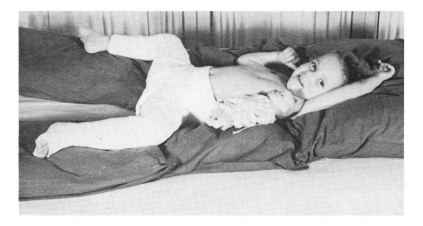

Fig. 2-6. Supine position in hip cast, illustrating Pliofilm strips tucked about the perineum. A piece of Pliofilm may be tucked over the diaper, which is being used as a perineal pad. This will help prevent wetting of the cast.

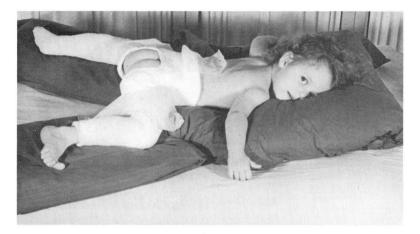

Fig. 2-7. Hip cast illustrating position of plastic material used to protect the cast. The protective material is applied in strips, with the outer end secured with tape or plaster of paris bandage. The strips have been pulled out to permit air to get to the posterior aspect of the cast. This helps to maintain a dry cast and prevents formation of mold. Before the child is turned to the supine position, the strips of plastic material will be tucked under the cast edges of the buttocks area.

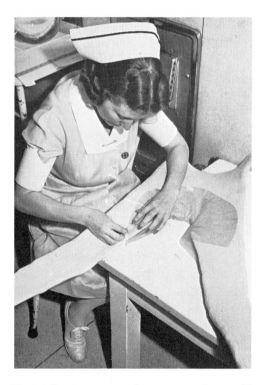

Fig. 2-8. Basting waterproof pattern around removable shell of a hip spica cast. Pattern is a double semicircle of Pilofilm cut out to fit cast opening and basted together on concave edges before it is applied to the shell.

the cast as a lining. Unquestionably, this method does preserve the cast more satisfactorily than any other, but it entails a considerable amount of time, more than is usually available in the modern hospital.

It has been suggested that the waterproof material used to protect casts be applied in strips rather than in a solid piece. The reason for this is obvious because a curving surface is to be bound. The material is tucked under the cast so that it folds back very tightly, thus forming a dam against excretions, but too much material must not be used under the cast or it will become wrinkled. The plaster of paris bandage or tape used to hold the outer edge should be applied in such a fashion that the waterproof material can be easily slipped out from under the cast without entirely detaching it.

Placing the patient in a cast on the bedpan. Even with the most artful padding and waterproofing, the nurse's worries are not over. Extreme caution must be taken when placing the bedpan so that the buttocks are not higher than the head. Inevitably, this situation will cause urine to flow backward inside the cast, and the drying of the cast afterward is no small problem. Elevating the head of the bed slightly and placing another pillow under the back while the patient is voiding will prevent this accident. Unless a patient is in shock or is hemorrhaging, it is al-

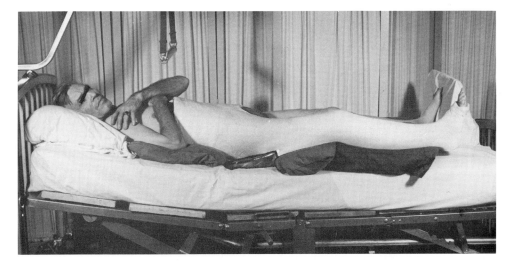

Fig. 2-9. Placement of patient with hip spica cast on the bedpan. To avoid strain on the cast at the groin area, pillows have been placed beneath the limb enclosed in plaster and beneath the lumbar and hip regions. The head of the bed has been elevated slightly to help prevent soiling or wetting the posterior aspect of the cast.

most always permissible to elevate the head and shoulders for use of the bedpan. Sharp angulation at the groin must be avoided to prevent breaking the cast. A second precaution that may be taken is that of placing a folded diaper or gauze pad on the posterior aspect of the bedpan. This padding will absorb moisture and prevent the lining of the cast from becoming wet with urine (Fig. 2-9).

To place an adult patient on the bedpan one of two methods is usually employed. The patient is turned onto his good side, the bedpan is placed so that the fleshy part of the buttocks contacts the posterior section of the pan, and pillows or blankets are arranged to support the legs and back on the same level as the buttocks. The patient is then returned to the back-lying position. By the other method, with an overhead trapeze to support himself, the patient may be placed on the pan without turning. The nurse elevates the hips with one hand while the pan is slipped under them with the other.

With the small child in the hip spica cast the problem is more complicated. A Bradford frame hung on hooks in the crib or supported on boxes with the head end slightly higher than the foot end may be used. The frame is prepared with a two-piece covering, so arranged that a space is left under the buttocks. A bedpan is kept con-

stantly under this space. However, in recent years, with better methods of protecting the cast, it has been possible to care for the small child and to maintain a clean intact cast without the use of the frame. Plastic-covered pillows are used beneath the child. These pillows are arranged to provide for a slight elevation of the head and shoulders, to help prevent urine from running backward and inside the cast. As previously described, the perineal area of the cast must be protected with waterproof material. A folded diaper is used as a perineal pad and may be held in place by a regular diaper. In addition to applying the waterproof material, it is very essential that this child be checked frequently and that diaper changes be made as needed.

CARE OF THE PATIENT'S SKIN

Good powers of observation are necessary in caring for the patient in a cast. All visible skin must be inspected daily for signs of abrasions or irritation. All areas that come in contact with cast edges must have particular attention, for cast sores are very frequently encountered at these places. Fingers moistened sparingly with alcohol should explore under the cast as far as it is possible to reach. If beginning abrasions or skin blemishes are noted, they should be inspected frequently during the day. Sometimes collodion-based or tar-based emollients are prescribed to protect the skin at these points against further irritation. Nurses should learn to inspect casts with the sense of smell as well as with the senses of sight and touch. It is not enough, however, for nurses merely to sniff at the cast while standing in an upright position. They must get down to within an inch of the plaster and learn to smell discerningly. It takes experience to learn to detect abnormal odors, but sometimes even an inexperienced nurse will be able to locate the exact position of a musty odor that may be the only evidence of a sloughing area beneath a cast. It is sometimes possible to detect an underlying pressure sore by the temperature of the cast, for the cast tends to become much hotter over an area that is beginning to discharge. Eyes, nose, and fingers are of equal importance in cast care.

Each time the patient is given nursing care, the waterproof fabric around the groin and buttocks should be pulled out from beneath the cast. The cast under this waterproofing should be inspected for soilage, dampness, and mold.

Time should be taken to dry this portion of the cast before the waterproof material is reapplied. The waterproof fabric should be washed with hot soapy water, rinsed, dried, and powdered. It is then tucked neatly and smoothly under the edges of the cast. If this is done at least once a day, the life of the material will be greatly prolonged. It will also prevent the forming of small troublesome pimples on the skin that appear around the edges of the cast when the skin and cast are neglected.

Certain other areas of the patient in a cast are commonly vulnerable to pressure sores. The heel of the normal foot may become sore because the patient habitually pushes himself up in bed with that leg. The elbows sometimes become sore because the patient braces himself on them to see what is going on around him. These places can be cared for more easily than areas covered by casts and should never be allowed to reach the stage of skin breakdown.

The importance of providing support for the uninvolved extremity cannot be overemphasized. The patient's good extremity should be in excellent condition to withstand the strain that will be put upon it when he becomes ambulatory. Provision for support should be made in the form of footboards, boxes, pillows, or sandbags. Bed exercises will do much to maintain muscle strength and joint range of motion.

CLEANING THE CAST

The orthopedic nurse should take pride in keeping casts as spotless as possible. With the best care we can give, however, accidents do occur, particularly with small children. Knowing how to repair damage is a satisfactory accomplishment and seems like nothing short of a miracle to the onlooker.

The outside of the cast may be easily repaired. Bon Ami, carefully applied with a damp cloth, will remove the most superficial stains. For the larger areas of soilage, the pattern method of repair is recommended. From a plaster bandage of suitable width a double thickness is cut to fit exactly over the soiled area. This pattern is swiftly immersed in water so that it is barely moistened through when it is lifted from the pan. The pattern is applied directly over the soiled area and is carefully rubbed into the cast. It must be well incorporated by rubbing, or it will peel off later like an onion skin. Some orthopedists advise that the cast be roughened slightly with a nail file or scissors before the pattern is applied. A generous sprinkling of baby powder rubbed into the moistened plaster will remove the odor that may accompany soilage.

A more troublesome problem is encountered when the inside of the cast becomes soiled. To remedy this, the stockinet lining of the cast may be carefully detached from the area around the buttocks or groin with either a razor blade or sharp scissors. The stockinet can then be pulled down and the soiled area trimmed off. Stockinet stretches to a considerable degree and is not at all difficult to manage. The clean edge is then brought out over the cast edges and secured to the cast either with adhesive tape or a bit of damp plaster of paris bandage. Repeated soiling of this kind would deplete the available stockinet lining.

If stockinet has not been used to line the cast, small portions of the sheet wadding must be carefully pulled out, and the inside of the cast must be cleaned with a sparingly dampened cloth.

On the adult wards, where all this elaborate precaution seldom seems necessary, protection may be managed by small disposable waterproof pads, put in place only when the patient uses the bedpan. To risk such underprotection on a child's ward is usually dangerous to the cast, however. Nor should too much confidence be placed in the adolescent girl in a spica cast. Any patient in a cast is relatively helpless in taking care of his own toilet needs, and the orthopedic nurse must understand this from the outset.

ARM AND LEG CASTS

Most of the admonitions mentioned earlier have to do with patients in the larger types of casts, but there are things that must be borne in mind about the patient in the foot or leg cast or in the arm cast reaching from the wrist to the shoulders. Paramount in importance, as has been stated, is the matter of circulation in the part.

To prevent edema following the application of an arm or leg cast, it is usually necessary that the extremity be maintained in an elevated position. To relieve edema, the doctor may request that the extremity be maintained in a position even with or higher than the heart. Application of cold (ice bags) may also be ordered to help prevent edema. To avoid pressure, these should be placed at each side of the cast. Arm casts should be supported in a sling if the patient is ambulatory, and it scarcely seems necessary to remind the nurse that a sling should support the arm and not allow it to drop forlornly at an angle of 120 degrees at the elbow. It must be remembered, too, that the hand and wrist should be supported and not permitted to hang in a wrist-drop position. The weight of an unsupported cast on the shoulder is considerable and will cause the patient discomfort that a well-applied sling can eliminate.

In this connection the nurse should be reminded of the potential danger and discomfort of a sling tied in a hard knot over the back of the neck, so that the knot constantly presses on the cervical spine. The triangle sling is more comfortable if it is pinned in two places neatly with two small safety pins dividing the stress of the weight. Various types of slings made from dur-

able material and in dark colors are available from surgical supply houses for the person who must use a sling for an extended period of time. These slings are applied in a manner to provide for maximum comfort and to provide the needed support. In addition to information pertaining to application, the patient using a sling for an extended period of time should be instructed in range of motion exercise for the shoulder joint. Failure to use this joint due to hand or lower arm injury may be followed by tightening of the soft tissue around the joint and result in limited shoulder motion.

Long leg casts should be supported on pillows when the patient is placed on a bedpan. Otherwise, the patient will be insecure and uncomfortable with his legs unsupported in space as his body is elevated to the level of the pan. The groin area of long leg casts in children needs protection with a waterproof material.

Short leg casts with an abduction bar as illustrated in Fig. 2-10 may be used to maintain the desired position of the extremities. When the patient is being turned, the abduction bar should not be used to lift or support the limb.

The bathing care of toes and fingers in casts is frequently a point of neglect. The patient may be well bathed otherwise and the toes or fingers overlooked. Applicators moistened in alcohol can be used to clean, refresh, and deodorize otherwise unreachable fingers and toes. Cast crumbs at these points are dangerous as well as annoying. They can be eliminated to a great extent by binding the edges of the cast around toes and fingers with adhesive tape if there is no stockinet to be taped over these edges.

ANTERIOR AND POSTERIOR SPLINTS

Quite frequently, hip casts are bivalved and made into removable shells so that the patient may receive the benefits of sun treatment, massage, or exercises. If these casts have been on the patient for some time, considerable cleaning may be necessary in order to renovate them. A change of stockinet lining may be easily effected without disturbing the cast's padding. The cut edges may be bound with adhesive tape or the entire cast may be covered with stockinet that can be stitched on. Straps are used to secure

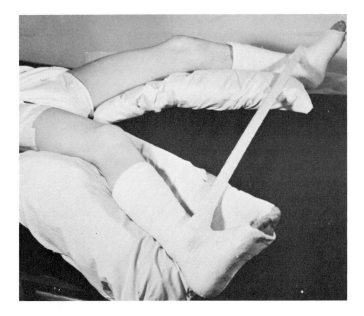

Fig. 2-10. Use of plaster to maintain the desired position of the lower extremity. The right limb is held in a position of abduction and internal rotation by means of bilateral short leg casts and an abduction bar.

the bivalved sections securely on the patient's body while he is being turned. If many such casts are in use on the wards, it is a good policy to keep circular pieces of waterproof material on hand for protection of the gluteal region. These are made in various sizes, half-circle in shape, and stitched on the sewing machine around the concave section. They may then be turned inside out and neatly fitted into the curved area of the perineal buttocks region. Simple basting stitches will secure them nicely to the stockinet-covered bivalved shell; or they may be attached with adhesive strips.

Frequently, posterior splints or bivalved casts are made to maintain the patient's extremities in good alignment. The splint illustrated in Fig. 2-11 is designed to maintain a neutral position of the foot and limb. The posterior shell provides support for the foot, preventing drop foot, and the bar placed at the ankle prevents external rotation of the limb. This type of support may also be worn to help prevent flexion contractures of the knee. It is held in place by an elastic bandage, or figure-of-eight straps placed around the ankle and knee. Nursing problems, however, are not eliminated with the application of the bivalved cast. If it is not applied correctly, the patient

may pull his foot up within the splint, and the foot is then held in a definite drop-foot position. Pressure areas at the heel also must be prevented. Although these casts are lined carefully, the heel may be a constant source of trouble. Sometimes this can be prevented by placing a small piece of padding, felt or sponge rubber, in the cast just above the heel space. This tends to relieve the pressure and helps to prevent blisters or pressure sores.

Bivalved casts may be aired daily and placed in the sunlight for drying. A rack to hold such casts is an excellent device to have on hospital sun decks. An ordinary clotheshorse will serve the purpose and will hold a number of such bivalved sections.

CARE OF THE PATIENT WHEN THE CAST IS REMOVED

Nurses who have watched orthopedic surgeons apply casts have observed the comfortable support that such casts give the joints. Although we may have a private conviction that casts are clumsy things to handle, a well-applied cast is as perfect a fixation apparatus as can be devised for the human body. The patient himself may never realize this until he

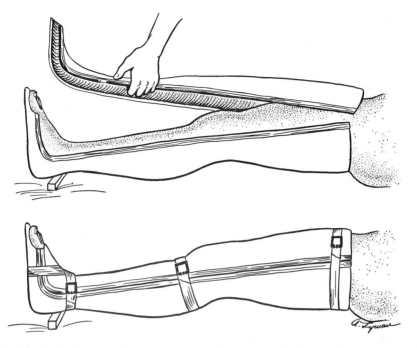

Fig. 2-11. The bivalved cast used frequently in convalescent care of patients with fractures, sprained ligaments, bursitis, poliomyelitis, arthritis, synovitis, and many other conditions, when protection is still necessary but access to the limb and joints is needed for daily treatments. Illustration also shows use of a heel bar to prevent rotation of the limb.

is removed from its support. Once out of his cast, he will become conscious of many aches and discomforts, and even minute changes in the position of the joints will cause him pain. Joint structures have become somewhat contracted, and muscles that have been immobilized are suddenly stretched. In addition circulation is sluggish, and coldness, mottling, and swelling are often present. If the primary trouble has been in the hip, the patient may be acutely alarmed because his greatest discomfort and stiffness now seem to be in the knee. This is a common occurrence and usually results from the fact that the quadriceps muscle group, which forms the bulk of the muscle at the front of the thigh, has suffered considerable disuse atrophy from the weeks spent in the cast. This muscle group is the main extensor of the knee and is absolutely essential in rising from the sitting position to the upright standing position. When attempting to rise, the patient will be much concerned with the weakness, instability, and pain he experiences in the knee. If he can be told that the cause of his discomfort is merely the result of disuse and is not a permanent

deformity, he will be able to bear it with much more fortitude.

To minimize the patient's discomfort, support to the joints is necessary immediately after the cast is removed. Slight relaxation rather than complete extension is usually the goal in applying casts, and it is important that this position of relaxation be maintained after the cast is removed. The normal curve of the lumbar spine should be supported with a firm narrow pillow or with a sheet folded to make a firm pad measuring about 6 by 20 inches. Soft wide pillows do not give the correct anatomic support that is needed in this area. The knee should be slightly relaxed by placing a rolled towel beneath the head of the tibia. A footboard or box should be used to maintain the anatomic position of the feet, a 90-degree angle leg position, with the toes pointing toward the ceiling. Frequently outward rotation of the hip will be a troublesome feature that may need attention. Sandbags placed from the hip to below the knee may be used to overcome this, or a trochanter roll may be made of a sheet or bath blanket.

The boards that have been in use under the

mattress should not be taken out because the cast has been removed. A firm bed is necessary to protect the patient from the aches that a sagging bed would cause him.

Some physicians feel that support should also be given immediately to the integumentary system after the cast is removed. If this is done, the edema that so often occurs after the removal of a cast can be somewhat lessened. All-cotton elastic bandages or elastic hose may be used and must be applied immediately after the cast is removed to be effective. Other physicians feel that elevating the limb for certain periods of the day may be sufficient to reduce the edema. If elevation is ordered, nurses should see to it that support is given along the entire limb from the buttock to the heel and that the knee is not acutely flexed.

After the cast is removed, movement in bed is usually freely permitted, but certain precautions should be observed. Nurses should remember that considerable decalcification has occurred and that the bone is more brittle and vulnerable to stresses that would not affect it under normal conditions. Fractures brought about by minor stresses sometimes occur at this time and are sometimes disguised by the patient's general discomfort. In addition, muscles that are weakened need careful handling to eliminate unnecessary pain and discomfort. Nurses should be careful to lift a limb newly out of a cast by providing adequate support at contiguous joints. Such a limb should never be lifted by grasping the muscle belly.

When plaster casts that have been on the patient a considerable period of time are removed, the skin will be noted to be caked with a yellow exudate that is partly dead skin and partly secretions from the oil sacs of the skin. It is generally conceded to be poor policy to try to soften the skin or forcibly remove the closely adhering exudate, particularly if a new cast is to be applied at once. If the patient is to remain out of the cast permanently or for a considerable period of time, the skin can be cleaned at the nurse's leisure and the patient's comfort, never forcing the caked matter off in such a way as to cause bleeding or rawness. There is plenty of time for this, and no one will be accused of neglect if this is allowed to take several days.

Zeal in this matter is misplaced. If the patient is not to be put in a cast again, the use of olive oil on the skin is an easy and safe method of cleaning the skin.

CUTTING CASTS

Cutting windows or holes in casts is usually considered a dangerous procedure, because the flesh under the opened area bulges out alarmingly after an hour or so and the patient's discomfort is only exacerbated. If the doctor in charge of the patient orders windows cut out, it is customary for him to request the nurse to apply a pad of felt over the area that has been removed and to use a snug bandage for eliminating this complicating edema. Sometimes a window is cut in the cast so that a surgical dressing may be applied, or the heel may be cut out to relieve pressure on a tender area. In any case the nurse must not discard the part of the cast that has been removed. These pieces are nearly always put back and held in place by a new roll of plaster.

Every nurse should know how to cut a cast if an emergency arises. The short, curved-bladed plaster knife is not a difficult tool to handle; and the electric cast saw provides for fast and safe cutting of a plaster cast. However, use of the saw may be a frightening experience for a small child. The saw blade, which vibrates, does not cut through the material used for padding but may feel very warm to the patient. If a cast knife or cast saw is not available, an ordinary shoe knife or a pruning knife may be used. Very heavy casts may be spread with household pliers. A spoon handle may be inserted under the cast to protect the patient's skin from the plaster knife. The spoon is advanced as the cast is cut. Vinegar or water is sometimes used to soften the cast before it is cut. The liquid is dropped on the line of cutting with a syringe of the Asepto variety.

When an arm or leg cast is to be split to relieve edema, it should be cut along its entire length. Splitting the cast only part way will often add to circulatory congestion. It is always a mistake to attempt to prevent or overcome swelling of toes or fingers by cutting the edges of the cast. Usually, the more the cast is cut or trimmed back, the greater the area that will swell. When edema and circulatory problems are present, the cast is split along its full length and spread slightly.

It is not enough to cut the plaster only, for frequently the underlying bandages or dressings may be the cause of the circulatory impairment or the pain. They should be loosened so that no constricting material binds the extremity. When a newly applied cast is split to relieve congestion, it may be taped together loosely until further instructions can be obtained from the physician.

It is never safe to postpone reporting circulatory congestion of an extremity in a cast. Night nurses sometimes feel that they can risk waiting until daylight or for the early morning rounds of the house physician. Although it is prompted by the best of motives, such a policy is dangerous. Irremediable damage may be caused by 2 or 3 hours of neglect.

INSTRUCTION OF PARENTS

What nurses have been taught or have learned through experience and the application of their ingenuity concerning the care of casts is no sacred professional secret. It must be shared with all those to whom care of casts is confided. Parents must be given adequate instruction before taking children with plaster of paris casts away from the hospital, and this includes instruction in all the details that have been mentioned: close check on circulation of the exposed body parts, attention to complaints of pressure and burning, the manner of detecting odors in casts, the care of the skin under the cast, and the cleaning and protection of the plaster itself. If possible, the parents should observe the patient's bath and cast care completely. They must be told that young children often make a game of hiding things in their casts, which may cause damage to the skin. They must understand why the patient is wearing the cast and must recognize when the cast has become inefficient for maintaining the position essential to correction of the child's deformity. They must be taught to look for signs that the child is outgrowing the cast. If the parent is manifestly slow to understand such instructions and seems confused by the number of things to watch for, instructions of this nature may be written down and sent home with the child. On the whole, patients in casts spend only a small portion of their convalescence in the hospital. It is but a short interlude, and the excellent care the child

experiences in the hospital will be absolutely negated unless a follow-up of some type is provided for him when he returns to his home.

Written instructions for parents on the care of patients in hip casts

Even though the plaster cast may seem extremely bulky and awkward, the patient has been placed in the cast for definite reasons, mainly to immobilize the hip joint and to maintain a corrected position. Consequently, if a definite position of the hip joint is to be maintained, the care of the patient must be such as to prevent softening or cracking of the cast. Equally as important, this care must provide for the general welfare of the patient and prevention of cast sores or bed sores.

Skin care

Special attention should be given the skin of the patient in a cast.
1. Daily cleansing of the skin is desirable.
2. Reach under the cast to eliminate plaster crumbs or foreign objects.
   Feel and look for skin irritations at the cast edges.
   Do not permit youngsters to poke crayons or other small objects down in the cast. Such articles may cause severe pressure areas.
3. Turn patient every 4 hours during the day and encourage him to lie on his abdomen several hours each day. Frequently, a patient will find it possible to sleep in this position.
   If reddened areas appear on the sacral area, the patient must stay on his abdomen for longer periods of time.
4. Rub the back, especially around the edges of the cast and over the sacral area, with rubbing alcohol several times daily.

Check the following closely when caring for a patient in a plaster cast

1. Is there swelling or discoloration of the toes?
2. Is the patient able to move his toes? Are they warm?
3. Does he complain of pain or numbness?
4. If the patient is a small child, does he fuss and seem unduly irritable?
   (If for any reason you are in doubt concerning any of these things, consult your doctor.)

Drying the cast

If the cast becomes damp, it can be dried by exposing the area to the air or by using an ordinary hair dryer.

Cleaning the cast

If the cast becomes soiled from stool, it may be cleaned by using a damp cloth with Bon Ami.

Finishing the edges of the cast

To eliminate plaster crumbs in the bed and to provide a smooth nonirritating cast edge, adhesive tape may be used to bind the edges of the cast. To do this one must wait until the cast has dried. This usually requires 24 to 48 hours.

Protecting the cast from urine

On the baby or small child plastic waterproof material may be used to protect the cast around the perineum and buttocks.

This material should be cut in 4 by 6 inch strips.

One end of the strip is tucked under the cast at the perineum opening and the material is folded back over the outer side of the cast.

The outer end of the material is secured with adhesive tape to the plaster cast.

Six to eight strips of the plastic material are needed to protect both the back and the front of a hip cast on a small child.

These strips may be pulled out at the perineum, washed, dried, and powdered daily. (The nurse will provide you with the plastic material and show you how to apply it.)

In addition to the plastic material a perineal diaper may be used on the child who is not toilet trained. Fold a diaper in the form of a perineal pad and place it across the perineum, tucking it under the edges of the cast in the front and in the back. The ordinary diaper may be applied over this.

It is essential that this pad or diaper be changed as soon as it becomes wet or soiled.

The small youngster or baby in a hip cast may be supported by placing plastic- or rubber-covered pillows so that the head and shoulders are slightly higher than the buttocks. This will aid in keeping the cast dry.

Placing the patient on the bedpan

Elevating the patient's head and shoulders by using pillows when he is on the bedpan will tend to keep the cast from becoming wet with urine running back from the pan.

A folded diaper, soft cloth, or gauze pad placed on the back of the bedpan will absorb any moisture and will help to keep the cast clean and dry. It must be removed with the bedpan.

Turning the cast patient

If only one leg is enclosed in the cast, turn the patient toward the normal leg (the leg not in the cast). Turn the body simultaneously to prevent undue pressure on the cast at the groin.

PLASTER ROOM TECHNIQUE

Several types of instruments are usually considered necessary for the application and removal of casts. Cast knives, cutters, and saws are needed for removing an old cast. Bandage scissors will be necessary for removing bandages under the cast, and a heavy pair of shears will be essential for cutting pieces of felt (Figs. 2-12 to 2-14).

Sheet wadding, a thin unabsorbent cotton web covered with starch to hold it together, is

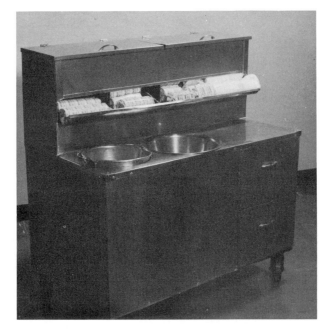

Fig. 2-12. The plaster cart may be taken to the operating room or to the bedside when plaster of paris is to be applied.

commonly used for padding. Piano felt, cut in suitable sizes, is used to provide additional protection against pressure on bony prominences. Sponge rubber may occasionally be used for this purpose. Material will be needed for reenforcing the cast at points of stress, and plaster splints, aluminum strips, yucca board, and plywood are among the most popular of these. Tubular stockinet, which comes in many different widths, from 2 to 18 inches, is used for a cast lining. A deep pail for soaking bandages, a pan of splints, and a waste water vessel, all of them lined with brown paper or old pieces of cloth to filter the waste plaster, will be necessary. Gloves

and gowns should be at hand for the surgeon and assistants who are to apply the cast.

The temperature of the water that is used to soak the bandages should be between 95° and 105° F. Warmer or cooler water will delay the setting of the plaster.

Paper-wrapped bandages retain plaster satisfactorily when they are put on edge in water until the bubbling ceases. They may then be lifted vertically from the water with the ends firmly grasped in the palms. Bandages not so wrapped are usually submerged horizontally, with the nurse or assistant keeping her palms cupped over the end of the bandage to prevent

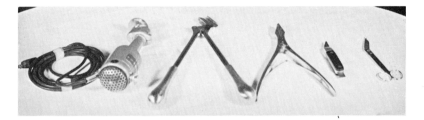

Fig. 2-13. Cast instruments: cast saw, cutter, spreader, knife, and bandage scissors.

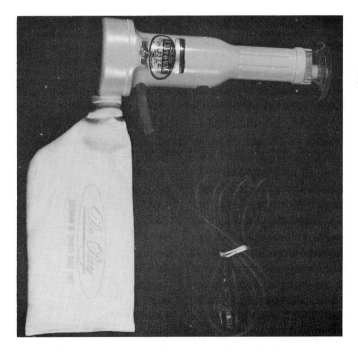

Fig. 2-14. Prevention of skin irritation caused by cast crumbs in the bed or inside the body cast is facilitated when a cast saw with a vacuum bag is used for trimming the cast.

loss of plaster. No compression of the bandage must take place at this time.

The bubbles of air in the water will rise until the bandage is completely saturated; that is, until the water has penetrated every part of the bandage. When this is completed, the bandage should be removed immediately, because the crystallization (setting) process will have begun.

The bandage is lifted from the water and held horizontally with the ends secured in the nurse's palms. Water is expelled by gently compressing the bandage in a short twist—no more than is necessary to supinate the right hand a single time, keeping the left hand in pronation. The bandage should not drip when it is handed to the surgeon; but, on the other hand, it must not be wrung so dry that the surgeon will have difficulty incorporating it into a cast. The end of the plaster bandage is unrolled about 2 to 4 inches before it is handed to the doctor. Only a few bandages should be put in the water at one time. Change of immersion water may be necessary if a large cast is being applied. A waste basin lined with paper may be used to receive the plaster that is wrung from the plaster bandage when it is removed from the water.

By the time the cast application is over the plaster in the basins used for immersion will usually have settled to the bottom. The water above this plaster is poured into the sink, with the faucet wide open to assist in washing what plaster is still present in the water through the drain. If paper has been used to line the immersion basins, this is lifted from the container and deposited in waste containers. Caution must be exercised in the care of all this equipment so that plaster is not allowed to gather in the sink and to clog plumbing fixtures.

TRACTION

MODES OF TRACTION

The following brief classification of traction has been inserted to clarify the different methods of securing traction.

1. *Skin traction* is applied to the skin and soft tissues and thus indirectly to the skeletal system. Traction tapes made of various kinds of material with provision for adherence to the skin surface are most commonly used for this type of traction.

2. *Skeletal traction* is applied directly to the skeletal system. The Steinmann pin or Kirschner wire is used in applying traction to an extremity. Skeletal traction to the skull is secured by Crutchfield tongs, Vinke tongs, or other devices.

3. *Manual traction* means the application of traction to a part of the body by the hands of the operator. The nurse, when assisting with the application of traction or a cast, may be asked to apply manual traction. This calls for a smooth firm grip on the extremity and sudden jerking movements should be avoided. Occasionally, when nursing care is being given or when traction is changed, it is necessary to apply this type of traction to the extremity. Permission to substitute manual traction for the regular traction must be secured from the attending physician.

PURPOSE OF TRACTION

Perhaps the best way to begin studying the care of the patient in traction is to consider why the patient has been placed in this apparatus. The application of traction means that a pulling force is applied to an extremity or a part of the body.

The student caring for patients on an orthopedic service will discover varied reasons for the application of traction. Frequently when the physician wishes to immobilize an extremity, traction is applied. The desired rest and immobilization for a patient with a tuberculous joint may be secured in this manner. Traction may be applied to the extremity of a patient with a fracture, first to lessen the muscle spasm and to reduce the fracture and then to immobilize and to maintain the corrected position. The patient with arthritis who has flexion contractures of the hip and the knee may have traction applied to correct or prevent the development of these deformities. The child with scoliosis may have traction as a form of treatment to lessen the deformity. Occasionally, the patient with back pain may be placed in traction to relieve muscle spasm, or traction may be applied to lessen muscle spasm around a joint.

Countertraction. Provision for countertraction must always be made if effective traction is to be maintained. Countertraction means a pull exerted in the opposite direction of the pull produced by the traction apparatus. This can be obtained when the traction pull is exerted against a fixed point (such as the pelvis when a Thomas, Hodgen, or Keller-Blake splint is used), or by elevating the bed under the part that is being placed in traction; for example, the foot of the bed is elevated for traction on the lower extremity, causing the body itself to exert countertraction in its gravitational pull away from the limb extension. Elevation of the bed should be from 8 to 12 inches. Sufficient countertraction prevents the patient from sliding toward the foot of the bed, when traction has been applied to the lower extremity. If a child or a thin adult is being subjected to many pounds of traction, this amount of countertraction may not suffice to keep the patient balanced against the traction being applied. Further elevation of the bed may be of assistance here, and of course, nurses must be most conscientious in aiding the patient to pull himself up in bed at frequent intervals during the day. The footplate or spreader must never be allowed to come in contact with the foot of the bed at any time, or traction on the extremity will become entirely useless.

Friction. Any friction created by ropes riding on the foot of the bed, ropes impinged by bedclothes, or heels digging into the mattress will lessen the efficiency of traction greatly. Orthopedic nurses must train themselves to observe these details and others that their experience and common sense tell them mitigate efficiency of the traction. A firm, thin pillow does much to eliminate bed friction when it is placed under

the limb in extension. Correct placement of the pillow also prevents pressure on the heel, a likely spot for a pressure sore.

Continuous traction. In caring for patients in traction a safe rule to follow is that traction cannot be released for any nursing procedure and that it must be continuous for 24 hours of the day. There are exceptions to this rule, but they must be given by the physician for a specific patient. Patients with arthritis who have had traction applied to prevent or correct flexion contractures of the joints are sometimes an exception to the rule and frequently are allowed to be released from traction for a few hours during the day. There may be others from time to time who have this privilege, but it is given only on the explicit order of the doctor in charge.

TRACTION EQUIPMENT

Traction cart. A traction cart, in addition to the traction room, is a useful piece of equipment for orthopedic hospitals or wards and will save

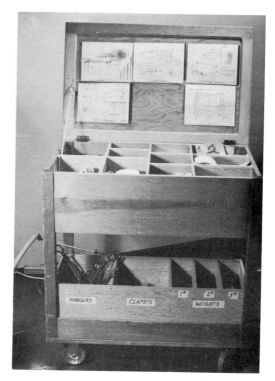

Fig. 2-15. The well-equipped traction cart is a time-saving device when traction is to be applied. Traction equipment can be taken to the bedside without delay or preparation.

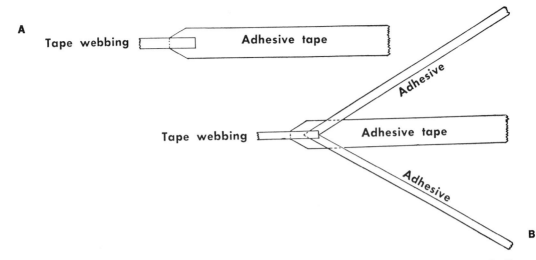

Fig. 2-16. Two types of adhesive tape patterns for skin traction. **A,** Adhesive strip is tapered off, and a 1-inch width of tape webbing is sewed or stapled onto the adhesive tape. This must be done firmly; otherwise, separation will occur if considerable weight is applied. **B,** The three-tailed design is also stitched or stapled where the strips adjoin. The tape backing is left attached until the tape is used, but it is not sewed or stapled to the tape.

much time and effort when traction is to be applied. Any kind of wheeled carriage can be used for the purpose. The cart may be stocked with various types of orthopedic equipment such as moleskin strips sewed or stapled to tape webbing, self-adhering traction strips, felt, stockinet, bandages (cotton elastic, muslin, and gauze), bandage scissors, a screwdriver, tincture of benzoin, and a razor. A lower shelf or a drawer might contain various types of pulleys, weights, carriers, ropes, footplates or spreaders, sandbags, hammocks for limb suspension, pelvic girdles, and chin halters.

Type of bed. The patient in traction must have a firm mattress that does not sag under his body. A bed that sags beneath the hips prevents the free play of the traction rope on the pulley and decreases the efficiency of the apparatus considerably. Furthermore, it may be the cause of a permanent flexion deformity at the hips of the patient who is in traction over a long period of time. The bed may be made firm by placing boards beneath the mattress. It is preferable ... s extend lengthwise and that ... the backrest level.

... esirable, but in most types of ... sary to have a bed with over- ... on, the modern hospital bed ... lowering and raising either ... lpful in positioning the pa-

tient and maintaining countertraction. If this type of bed is not available, shock blocks may be used to provide for countertraction.

The trapeze (unless contraindicated) should not be omitted from the patient's bed. It facilitates nursing care and enables the patient do many things for himself (Fig. 2-17).

Braun-Böhler inclined plane splint. The inclined plane splint (Fig. 2-18) is frequently used for patients with fractures of the lower end of the femur, either in conjunction with skin or skeletal traction. Since this type of frame and traction rests on the bed, it does not maintain immobilization as automatically as a suspension apparatus. The physician should be consulted concerning the amount of motion permissible for the patient. As a general rule, it is permissible to turn the patient toward the splint for back care. In changing linen it is more convenient to use two folded sheets for the under part of the bed. One sheet rests under the splint, and the other reaches from the head of the bed to the level of the splint. It is thus possible to change the sheet under the patient frequently without disturbing the sheet under the splint. Two or three rolls of 5-inch muslin bandage may be used to cover the splint and to provide support for the affected limb. The bandage is started around the base and wrapped smoothly and tightly over the inclined plane.

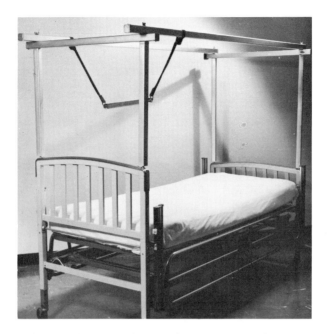

Fig. 2-17. Frame attached to bed makes application of suspension type of traction possible. Additional longitudinal and abduction bars may be clamped to this frame to provide for correct placement of pulleys.

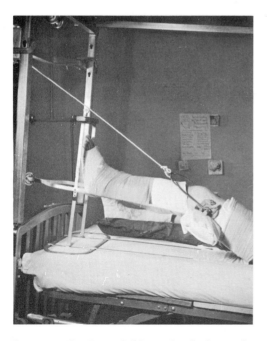

Fig. 2-18. The Braun-Böhler inclined plane splint may be used to support the limb after application of skeletal traction. Note that the splint supports the entire thigh and that the knee joint corresponds with the beginning of the inclined plane.

Other splints. Half-ring or full-ring Thomas, Hodgen, or Keller-Blake splints or the canvas hammock can be used in applying suspension traction (Figs. 2-19 and 2-20). Suspension is frequently used with traction because it will permit the patient to move himself about in bed without disturbing the line of traction. Furthermore, suspension improves circulation and allows freer motion of the suspended part than would be possible if the patient had to lift the extremity against gravity.

TYPES OF TRACTION

Buck's extension, rubber surface traction, and Bryant traction may be described as straight or running traction that exerts a pull on the affected part but does not provide a balanced support by means of a hammock or splint.

With Russell traction, suspension traction, and Dunlop traction, the extremity has traction applied and is then supported by means of a hammock or splint held in place by balanced weights attached to an overhead bar.

Head traction, pelvic traction, and ankle traction are applied with some type of fitted apparatus, such as a corset, head halter, or anklet.

Skill in the nursing care of the patient in traction is an attribute that comes with knowledge

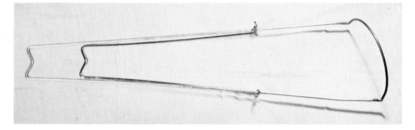

Fig. 2-19. The half-ring Thomas splint (Hodgen splint) with Pearson attachment.

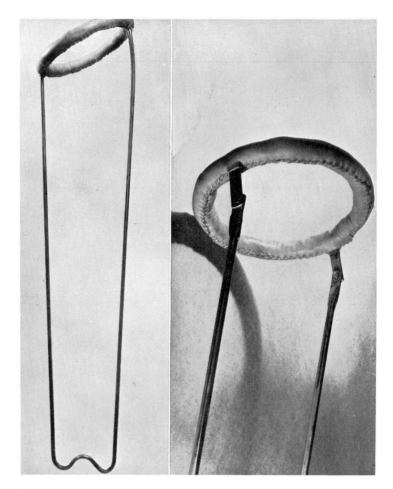

Fig. 2-20. Thomas splint for lower extremity and modified Thomas splint with hinge for upper extremity. (From Crenshaw, A. H., editor: Campbell's operative orthopaedics, ed. 5, St. Louis, 1973, The C. V. Mosby Co.)

and experience. The patients in casts present their problems, but they are much simpler than the problems of the patient in traction. The patient in a cast may be moved as frequently as is necessary for the care of his back or for his comfort. He may lie on his back, abdomen, or side without endangering the immobilization of the diseased part. Patients in traction, on the other hand, usually have but one position to lie in— the dorsal recumbent position. Good nursing care of these patients must include keeping the patient clean, comfortable, and free from pressure sores despite the handicap of his enforced and prolonged recumbency.

Buck's extension. Buck's extension (named after Gordon Buck, who described the apparatus in 1851) is perhaps one of the easiest types of traction to apply (Figs. 2-21 to 2-23). Also,

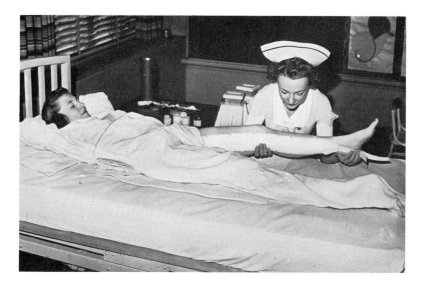

Fig. 2-21. Buck's extension. Note notching of adhesive tape to fit leg contours.

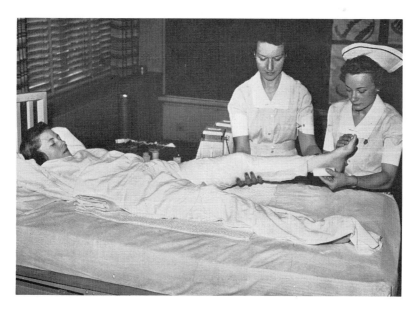

Fig. 2-22. Buck's extension is covered first with sheet wadding. Straps are retracted and sheet wadding is continued over malleoli as padding. An elastic bandage is usually applied over the sheet wadding and traction tapes.

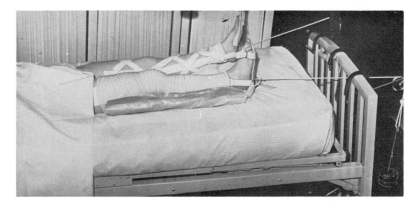

Fig. 2-23. Two types of adhesive traction for leg. Note firm pillow positioned under leg to eliminate friction and to free the heel of pressure. The left foot is supported by an adhesive strip to prevent drop foot. Aluminum footplate is used for right leg. Right leg traction is applied with a single strip and is held in place with a spiral reverse elastic bandage. The left leg has three-tailed adhesive strips wound obliquely over leg and thigh. Note bracelet of stockinet and cotton over malleoli on left ankle. Also note strips crossed high above dorsum of foot to prevent circulatory impairment. Both extremities are maintained in a neutral position. External rotation is to be avoided.

it provides the basis for most other types of skin traction, and in an emergency it can be applied with improvised equipment: two strips of 3-inch adhesive the length of the patient's limb, a block of wood to be used for a spreader below the foot, some type of pulley, and a weight that may be a window-sash weight or a canvas bag filled with salt or sand. A chair may be used to elevate the foot of the bed to provide countertraction. Hospitals usually have on hand more elaborate equipment for applying traction, but it is well for the nurse to understand how such traction can be applied and maintained satisfactorily with homemade equipment.

Some contraindications to the use of skin traction should be remembered and observed. This type of traction cannot be applied to the patient with a severely injured extremity with open wounds or to the patient who is allergic to tape. Circulatory disturbances, dermatitis, or varicose veins may prohibit the application of traction to the skin. The patient with diabetes may present a problem if skin traction must be maintained for a long period of time. Traction applied to the skin with adhesive type of tape may slip if a large amount of weight is applied.

The area to which adhesive tape is to be applied is usually shaved. However, some physicians feel that shaving the area with a razor before applying tape is not advisable in that epithelium is invariably removed and infection may occur under the tape. Clippers are frequently used instead of the razor. When a razor is used, shaving must be done very carefully, and accidental denudation or cuts of the skin should be reported before the tape is applied.

There are a few landmarks on the leg that must be given special consideration when traction tapes are applied. Strips of adhesive with tape webbing stapled or sewed to one end frequently form the basis of the equipment. However, in recent years commercially prepared traction tapes have been made available. With these, as with the adhesive or moleskin tape, some provision must be made for the traction tapes to adhere to the skin and thus provide for a "pulling force" (traction) on the extremity.

The traction tapes extend from the malleoli to the thighs, and in many instances surgeons feel that these strips alone are sufficient for the pull. However, it is the custom in some clinics to use oblique strips of narrower adhesive tape to augment the lateral strips. These pass across the tibia and obliquely encircle the leg, crossing in the back of the calf and then above the knee. Although these strips add to the staying power of the traction as a whole, they present a distinct menace to the circulation of the foot if they are applied too snugly or they are applied too near the dorsum of the foot. There is an inevitable amount of slipping of the adhesive tape when weights are applied, and oblique strips tend to be pulled down by the lateral strips and to cut into the flesh. An ischemia of the foot with resulting paralysis has been known to develop from the pressure on the dorsalis pedis artery which lies beneath.

Another landmark of which the nurse should be conscious is the upper 3 inches of the fibula—that is, the outer aspect of the calf just below the knee. It is here that the peroneal nerve lies close to the surface, and it can be easily compressed against the bone over which it passes. The result of this compression may be a peroneal paralysis. Such a paralysis is a serious thing, involving plantar flexion and inversion of the foot. This area should be well padded with felt or cotton before tape is applied. The foot should be observed daily for the tendency to turn toward the midline of the body. Any complaint of pain or of a burning sensation under the tape must be carefully checked.

Although pressure upon the Achilles tendon will not cause paralysis, it must have special consideration. No tape should at any time pass directly over this tendon or very near above it. The tendon is exceedingly superficial and tends to become sore and denuded with great rapidity. Placing an oblong piece of felt over this area before applying bandage or traction will eliminate danger to the area.

Oblique strips crossed on the tibia at any point are a threat to the underlying skin, and padding should always be applied at these points. Adhesive skin traction is not supposed to pull directly on bone. The pull is to be exerted on skin and subcutaneous tissues, and this fact should be borne in mind during application of the tape. Superficial bony points are to be guarded.

There are a few common errors in the use of apparatus that should be mentioned at this point. One of these is the use of a single pulley for more than one rope, a practice that greatly limits the efficiency of the pulley. Another is the use of a foot spreader so narrow that the traction tapes connecting it to the leg contact the bony points of the ankle, always vulnerable spots for pressure sores. A third error is the use of a foot spreader so wide that the traction tapes constantly pull

away from the skin of the leg, thus adding unnecessary discomfort to the patient.

Tincture of benzoin is frequently used for painting the skin before the application of the adhesive, with the idea that it serves as a disinfectant for the skin and gives the tape greater properties of adherence. However, the use of tincture of benzoin is not routinely accepted as having these benefits, and some authorities do not think its use is always warranted. It is not always safe to apply it to the skin of an infant because the adherence of the tape to the skin is so great that, on removing it, bleeding points are almost invariably encountered on the baby's skin.

In any case the skin should be dry and clean before tape is applied. Massaging the tape gently into the skin after its application will prevent much of the slipping that occurs when the weights are applied. Wrinkles or creases in the tape are to be avoided scrupulously since they may be the cause of pressure areas on the underlying skin.

Traction tapes should be applied with the knee in slight flexion to prevent hyperextension of the joint. The tape should cover a generous area of skin. The largest area of skin and subcutaneous tissue of the extremity is on the thigh, and the nurse should plan to utilize all of this, provided no contrary orders are received from the physician.

The tape should be started about 1 inch above the malleolus. It should never be applied directly to the malleolus but slightly above it. This is advisable, also, because space can be allowed for the tape to slip down, as it inevitably will do for the first 24 hours. If a moderately large amount of weight is used, a downward slipping of the tape for 1 or 2 inches may be expected in 24 hours. It is advisable to clip the tape obliquely every inch or so, beginning from the top. These nicks should be no more than ¼ inch in depth. They are to aid in fitting the adhesive tape more snugly and neatly to the contours of the leg.

The traction tapes are then applied to the leg on its inner and outer aspects. However, under no circumstances should the strips be allowed to pass over the patella or over the popliteal space; this may happen if the tape is hastily or carelessly applied. The tape is massaged gently into the skin and, if circumstances permit, it is advisable to allow time to elapse between the application of the tape and attaching of the weights. Slipping will be much less likely to occur if this is done.

As has been stated, the use of these two straps alone is preferred by a number of surgeons. This is particularly true in children's hospitals, where the delicate quality of the child's skin is a consideration and where only small amounts of weight are necessary to obtain traction.

With the straight longitudinal traction tapes unsupported by the transverse sections, a securely applied bandage is needed to maintain the position of the tape. In many clinics sheet wadding is applied over the adhesive in a simple spiral bandage, followed by an elastic bandage put on in an ascending spiral reverse. In these cases the sheet wadding is brought under the tape webbing at the ankle and provides effective protection of the bony points. Some orthopedists feel that the upper ends of the tape should be visible at all times in order that slipping may be detected without removing the outer bandage.

Temptation to apply the bandage very snugly to improve its appearance must be firmly resisted. Circulation in the foot should be inspected after the bandage has been in place for several minutes. Signs of mild cyanosis will be present if the bandage has been applied too tightly.

Pressure areas may form under traction straps with none but the mildest complaints on the part of the patient. Needless to say, every complaint from the patient in traction deserves prompt attention. With these patients, as well as with those in casts, the nose is of definite assistance in detecting the musty odor that may result from pus forming under the bandage.

Once traction tapes and bandage are securely applied, a footplate with buckles or a spreader is attached to the sole of the foot. The spreader must be wide enough to keep the traction tapes spread out somewhat from the malleoli. A small hook on the bottom of a footplate makes it possible to attach the rope.

The other end of the rope passes over a pulley secured at the foot of the bed. The weights attached to a carrier are suspended from this and

must be high enough from the floor so that the patient's slipping down in bed will not cause them to come in contact with it. Also, traction weights must be attached in a manner that prevents their resting on the bed frame when the patient changes his position. Canvas bags are sometimes used around traction weights to minimize noise and to prevent accidents from loosened knots. Weights must not be attached so high that if the patient alters his position in bed, the knot will rest against the pulley. Rope should be of good quality, neither frayed nor pieced together. When a large amount of weight is applied to an extremity, nylon rope should be used. The added strength prevents sudden breaking of the rope and release of the traction.

All knots should be secure. The patient's comfort demands that no sudden release of knots occur to jar the leg in traction. All nurses should know how to tie a square knot and should make use of it in their orthopedic nursing. Narrow strips of adhesive tape may be used to make such knots additionally secure.

The amount of weight to be used depends upon the physician's order. For fractures large amounts may be applied at once. A large amount of weight should be an indication to the nurse to be very solicitous in observing that patient's traction so that injury to the skin does not occur at any point.

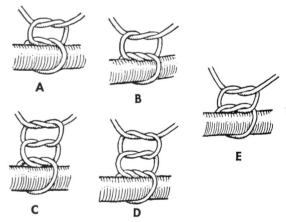

Fig. 2-24. Knots: **A,** square knot; **B,** surgeon's knot; **C,** square knot reinforced; **D,** surgeon's knot reinforced; **E,** granny knot. (From Mobley, H. E.: Synopsis of operative surgery, ed. 2, St. Louis, 1947, The C. V. Mosby Co.)

Orders regarding patients in traction are sometimes confusing to student nurses. For patients with scoliosis, for instance, it is occasionally the practice of surgeons to order a small amount of weight at the beginning with a substantial increase each day. In patients with fractures the reverse may be true. A large amount of weight is frequently used during the first 24 to 48 hours, followed by a decrease in the amount after reduction is obtained. For patients with scoliosis permission is frequently given to remove weights for short intervals during the day, but for those with fractures this would not be permitted. The maximum amount of weight for reduction of the fracture is put on immediately, and once reduction has been obtained, only such weight as is needed to maintain the bone ends in good position is used. However, this remaining amount of weight is important and should not be disturbed without specific order from the surgeon.

A word should be said about the danger of tape constriction in patients with fresh fractures to which traction has been applied. Traction for patients with fresh fractures should always be applied by the physician, but the nurse must realize that in trauma of this nature swelling inevitably occurs and an alarming degree of constriction may occur within the first 3 or 4 days. This must be watched for and reported to the surgeon immediately before any permanent damage is done to the extremity.

Rubber surface traction. Traction tapes are made from strips of synthetic sponge rubber backed with strong fabric. These are applied directly to the skin, as described for Buck's extension, and are secured to the leg by means of one or two 3-inch cotton elastic bandages. There is relatively little slipping when the weights are attached because of the suction of the rubber on the skin. The advantage of this type of traction is that the apparatus may be removed for physical therapy treatments and for hydrotherapy. Furthermore, it can be used on skin that needs more watching than would be possible if adhesive tape were applied.

There are dangers, however, that the nurse must not ignore. To prevent slipping, the elastic bandage must be wrapped securely. This in turn may cause swelling and constriction of

circulation, which is a real hazard with the older patient who has poor circulation.

Ankle traction. Ankle traction may sometimes be ordered as a temporary measure. It is obtained with a boot made of leather or canvas that is laced onto the foot and has straps extending below for rope and weight attachment (Fig. 2-25). The shoe must be thoroughly padded over the dorsum of the foot as well as over the heel cord. Otherwise skin denuding and circulatory impairment will occur after a few hours in such traction. It is not the most satisfactory type of traction, although frequently its use is a necessity. Applying considerable weight to such a meager portion of the extremity is painful and dangerous. The nurse should release the laces over the dorsum of the foot frequently and rub the area with alcohol. Ridged blue areas across the top of the foot inevitably occur after a few hours in this type of traction. Deep fissures have been known to form at this area within 24 hours.

Bryant traction. Bryant traction has its foundation in bilateral Buck's extension on the child's leg. Bryant traction is used in the treatment of a femoral shaft fracture in a child under 6 years of age. For this type of traction two overhead bars passing longitudinally over the crib or traction bed will be necessary. Two pulleys are attached to each bar. The first set of pulleys is placed overhead at the level of the child's pelvis, making it possible to suspend his legs at right angles to his body. The second set of pulleys is placed on the overhead bars near the foot of the bed, and provide for attachment of the weights distal to the child's body. When the weights have been applied, the child's buttocks must just clear the bed. This makes caring for his toilet needs much easier than when traction is applied in a horizontal direction.

Some form of restraint will be necessary to maintain this position, either a specially designed jacket or a Bradford frame with a harness restraint to keep the child in position (Figs. 2-26 and 2-27).

The position of the bandage must be checked to see that it does not slip in such a manner as to cause increased pressure over the dorsum of the foot or around the heel cord.

The child in Bryant's traction should have

his feet checked at frequent intervals for circulatory disturbances. Discoloration, pallor, loss of motion, or loss of sensation must be reported to the attending physician. Immediate loosening of the elastic bandage, reduction of the traction force, or lowering of the limbs to a less than vertical position is indicated to correct the circulatory problem.

When callus formation at the fracture site is sufficient (3 to 4 weeks), the child may be placed in a unilateral hip spica cast, which is worn for an additional 3 to 4 weeks.

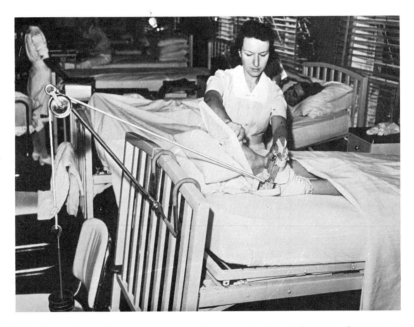

Fig. 2-25. Ankle traction with canvas boot and aluminum footplate. This type of traction is intended to be only temporary. Prolonged use results in pain and constriction over dorsum of foot and Achilles tendon.

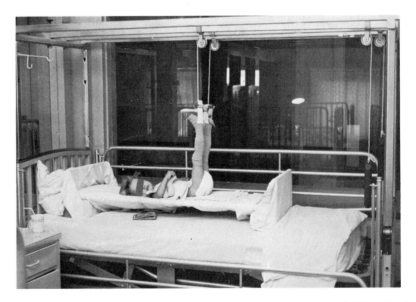

Fig. 2-26. Bryant traction for use in fracture of the shaft of the femur in young children. The frame is used to restrain child. Small blankets or divided linen must be used to keep the child warm.

Russell traction. Russell traction, when it has been properly applied and is in good mechanical working efficiency, is a comfortable device for the patient.

The equipment required is not elaborate (Fig. 5-6). A single section of the common Balkan frame can be attached to the bed, with the overhead bar directly above the injured limb. Four pulleys are used. These pulleys are arranged so that one is on the overhead bar at a level directly above the tubercle of the tibia of the fractured leg. A second is attached to the footplate or spreader. Two pulleys are attached to a crossbar at the foot of the bed and are placed at about the level of the mattress. A canvas hammock, which is used for the knee sling, and traction tapes form the basis of the traction.

In the original method these strips were applied only to the knee. Russell believed that it was best to extend the tape only from the ankle to the knee because he wanted the pull exerted at the point of insertion of the large muscles of the thigh into the tibia and fibula—namely, the hamstring and quadriceps muscles. However, many modifications to this original method have been devised.

When the traction tapes have been applied, the hammock is slipped under the knee and a rope is attached to it. This rope passes to the overhead pulley and then to the uppermost of the two pulleys on the crossbar at the foot of the bed. It is then passed over the pulley on the foot spreader and back to the remaining pulley on the end of the bed. Weight is then attached. The amount usually ordered for an adult is 8 or 10 pounds (Fig. 5-6).

Important nursing points are as follows: The angle between the bed and the hip should be approximately 20 degrees. The heel of the foot in traction should just clear the bed. Firm pillows should support the thigh and the calf along their entire length, leaving the heel free of the bed. The popliteal space must be watched for ridging and skin denudation. Back rest is usually permitted, and no difficulties are encountered in giving nursing care, because the fractured leg is not at the mercy of gravity and will not be altered in position during any type of nursing care. Provision should be made for prevention of drop foot on both feet.

Because Russell traction includes suspension of the limb in traction, nursing care of the patient is much simplified. The patient is usually allowed to sit up, to turn, and to move at will, because the line of traction is not disturbed by these movements. Care of the back, making the bed, and giving the bedpan are much simplified. Other nursing features that are important in caring for the patient in Russell traction are as follows:

1. To prevent wrinkling of the sling under the popliteal space, a piece of felt may be inserted between the sling and the patient's skin. This will assist in eliminating pressure areas that sometimes form at this spot.

2. Whatever position the patient assumes, the angle of flexion of the hip in traction should be as near 20 degrees as possible at all times. (This is the angle between the thigh and the bed, not between the thigh and the abdomen.)

3. The heel should clear the bed. The ideal position for the heels of the patient in Russell traction is that of a person standing with his heels 4 inches apart. Abduction is to be avoided.

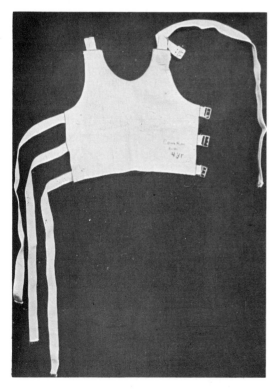

Fig. 2-27. Vest or jacket restraint for use with or without frame. (Courtesy University Hospitals, The University of Iowa, Iowa City.)

4. Two pillows are usually used under the traction: one of them is under the thigh to maintain the desired angle and the other is under the calf down to and including the Achilles tendon.

Care of patient in a Thomas splint. When a Thomas splint or any type of ring splint or suspension apparatus is used in conjunction with skin or skeletal traction, the patient is usually allowed more latitude in moving about in bed. If the leg rests on the bed, as it does in Buck's extension, any movement the patient makes with his body will alter in some degree the position of the traction. When suspension is used, however, the slack occasioned by the patient's movement is taken up at once by the suspension apparatus and the line of traction remains unchanged. Suspension allows freedom of the body as a whole while efficient traction on the limb is maintained.

We are told by Dr. McCrae Aitken—historian for Hugh Owen Thomas who invented the Thomas splint—that Thomas invented the hip splint for a certain Sara McTurk in the year 1867. He had long disliked any type of traction apparatus that rested on the bed, because he noted the sagging of the limb that occurred when a bedpan was placed beneath the patient. The invention of the Thomas splint was an attempt to allow the patient to be moved for using the bedpan and for other nursing requirements without changing the position of the limb in traction.

Since the patient may be moved more safely, the problem of the sacral decubitus is not as troublesome as it is in patients with other kinds of traction. Furthermore, the splint is usually suspended or hung, and pressure on the heel of the leg in traction can easily be avoided. There are other nursing problems to consider, however, because of the pressure of the ring on the adductor and ischial area.

The ring of the Thomas splint is usually covered with smooth, moisture-resistant basil leather. It is usually considered advisable not to pad these rings with cotton or gauze.

When the daily bath is given, the area of skin that is contacted by the ring and the leather ring itself must have special care. The patient may be turned toward the leg in the splint.

The tendency for pressure sores to form in the adductors and the ischial region can be overcome by elevating the foot of the bed from 12 to 18 inches. The patient will thus pull away from the splint somewhat. In some cases this may be considered undesirable. The surgeon should always be consulted before this is done.

A half-ring Thomas splint (Fig. 2-19) is frequently used in balance traction. The splint is placed with the half ring on the anterior aspect of the thigh. With this arrangement the patient does not sit on the ring, there is less irritation in the groin area, and the difficulty and discomfort in using the bedpan are considerably lessened. The ring is not covered with padding and leather; consequently there is not the nursing problem of keeping it dry and clean. Pressure in the groin and on the anterior aspect of the thigh is prevented by using a properly fitting splint, maintaining adequate countertraction, and placing a correct amount of weight on the rope suspending the ring. The weight lifts the ring slightly, and adequate countertraction keeps the ring from pressing in the groin area; thus need for padding of the splint is minimized (Fig. 2-28).

Position of extremity in suspension traction. The position of the extremity in traction is determined by the doctor, but the nurse should know that the limb is usually held in a neutral position or in a position of slight internal rotation. The amount of abduction may vary with the patient. However, the nurse must recognize that when only one leg is in traction, the position the patient assumes may greatly alter the amount of abduction being maintained. If the patient lies diagonally in bed, abduction is lost. Fig. 2-29 illustrates the use of a sandbag to remind the patient of the position he should maintain. Most patients with traction applied to the lower limb are encouraged to dorsiflex and plantar flex the foot at frequent intervals. Also, to maintain muscle strength, the patient may be taught to do muscle-setting exercises (quadriceps, gluteal, and abdominal). To prevent hip flexion contractures, a firm mattress is necessary and, in addition, it is desirable and usually permissible that the backrest be completely lowered for short periods, several times daily. This provides for extension of the hip

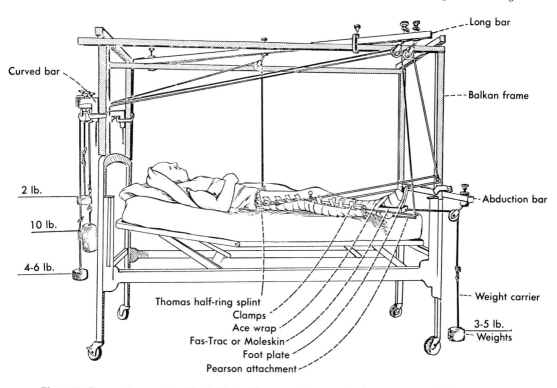

Fig. 2-28. Suspension traction. The half-ring Thomas splint provides for suspension of the extremity. Skin traction has also been applied to the limb. (From Nursing procedure manuals, University Hospitals, The University of Iowa, Iowa City.)

joints. A footboard for the uninvolved limb (Fig. 2-29) helps the patient to maintain the desired position; in addition, a bolster may be placed at the foot end of the bed to keep the mattress from sliding down.

With suspension traction, the patient's knee should correspond with the fastening of the Pearson attachment to the splint. Generally speaking, it is desirable to have the Pearson attachment (the part that supports the leg from the knee down) horizontal with the mattress and just high enough to swing clear of the bed. The position of the ring should be observed frequently. It should rest in the groin but not cause undue pressure or irritation.

Pelvic traction. The pelvic girdle customarily used to apply pelvic traction is made of canvas, darted to fit the shape of the body. It is more comfortable if it is lined with flannel, which may be quilted in several thicknesses. This girdle is not to be made to fit the waistline except in its upper border. It is a pelvic girdle and is to pull from the bony crests of the ilia, so that its lower border

will be considerably wider than the upper. It should fit snugly over the crests of the ilia and the pelvis, much as a girdle or garter belt does. On either side are tape webbing straps, usually two or three, joined together to form one strip at about the level of the midthigh. If possible this strip should contain a steel ring for securing the rope for traction. The girdle is customarily fastened in front with tape webbing straps and buckles (Fig. 2-30).

Because the girdle is exerting traction on bone, the crests of the ilia must have constant care and frequently, padding over the crests will be necessary for the thin patient. Weight in pelvic traction is usually increased gradually, and although it may be started with as little as 5 pounds on each side of the pelvis, it is usually increased considerably. The hazards of this amount of pull to thinly padded bony prominences are readily understood.

At the foot of the bed two pulleys about 2 feet apart are necessary. Ropes attached to the girdle extend through these and are attached to weight

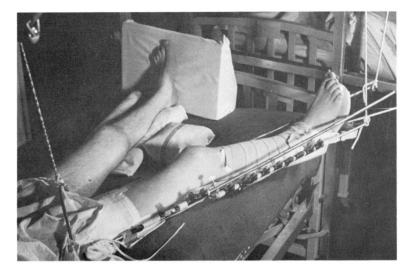

Fig. 2-29. Suspension traction applied following cup arthroplasty. Note position of the extremities and use of sandbags to maintain this position.

carriers and weights. It is the prerogative of the surgeon to order the number of weights, but when this is left to the nurse's judgment it is better to begin with too little than too much. Discouragement on the part of the patient during the first few hours may make further treatment difficult. Weights are not lessened or removed without the permission of the doctor who has given the order to apply them. Orders may occasionally be given to remove some of the weights at night to enable the patient to rest more comfortably. This type of traction may be applied to the patient with scoliosis to relieve pain and to gain some correction, or it may be applied to the patient with back pain to relieve muscle spasm.

The greatest complaint a patient in traction will have during his first 24 hours will probably have to do with pain in the lower part of the back, in the lumbar region. Usually placing a narrow firm pillow to support the lower back will provide relief from this discomfort. This pain in the lower portion of the back is the result of a spasm of the extensor muscles of the back that occurs in conjunction with the pull upon the flexor muscles of the thigh.

At all times during the period that the patient is in traction the feet must be given protection. Some kind of foot support must be placed at the foot of the bed in such a fashion that the ropes

are not contacted. Simple foot exercises carried out during morning and evening care help maintain muscle strength and range of motion. Dorsiflexion combined with toe flexion (not toe extension, which is the patient's usual tendency while dorsiflexing) is considered an adequate exercise for maintaining tone in muscles to be used for walking. When lying prone, the patient's feet must be supported or allowed to lie over the edge of the mattress.

Another point of discomfort to the patient newly in traction is a feeling of strain under the knee. A very small pad which could be made by folding a towel, placed under the head of the tibia, will relax this joint satisfactorily and contribute much to the patient's comfort.

Usually, the physician will request that the patient with acute back pain be placed in a semi-Fowler position in conjunction with pelvic traction.

Traction used in the treatment of fractures of the pelvis is discussed in Chapter 5.

Head traction. Various types of head halters may be obtained from orthopedic and surgical supply houses. These include soft disposable halters, as well as those made from leather or canvas (Figs. 2-31 to 2-33).

In addition to the halter, a spreader is needed. It should be wide enough to prevent pressure on the side of the head. The jaws and ears will

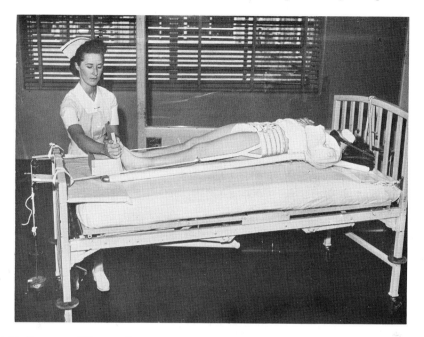

Fig. 2-30. Patient on Whitman frame with pelvic girdle and head traction in place. Note boards to prevent frame from cutting into mattress. Foot support is always necessary, but some orthopedists feel that anything more than a pillow for this will disturb efficiency of traction.

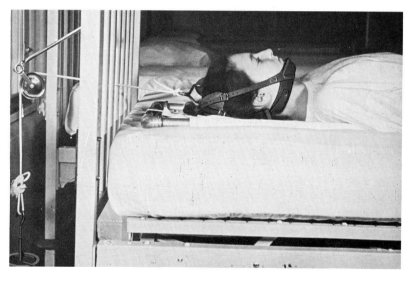

Fig. 2-31. Leather halter for exerting traction on head.

become irritated if the spreader is too narrow. These two items plus the rope, weights, and pulley attachment are needed for the application of head traction with a halter.

Too much emphasis cannot be placed on the necessity for conscientious care of the chin during the period of traction. Alcohol rubs are almost always permissible, except for patients with acute inflammation, and should be given at stated intervals during the day. Massage or oils should not be applied in the presence of acne, since inflammation is likely to follow. This

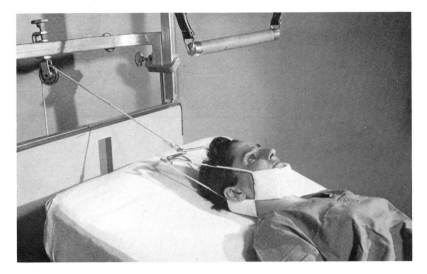

Fig. 2-32. A disposable head halter used to apply traction to the cervical region. To maintain the desired angle of pull, it is necessary to raise or lower the bar supporting the pulley, when the headrest is elevated or lowered. Traction apparatus that provides for anchoring the pulley to the headrest will maintain the desired pull regardless of the position of the bed's headrest.

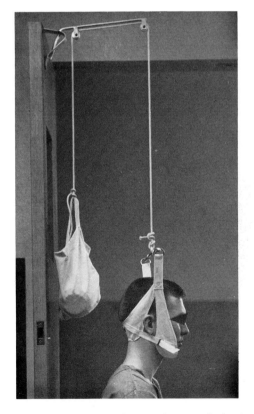

Fig. 2-33. Head traction that may be prescribed to be used intermittently in the home for the relief of cervical pain due to arthritis.

is especially true in hot weather. Soft material such as sheet wadding or silence cloth, inserted into the chin cup and changed frequently, gives the patient considerable comfort. Should the skin condition prohibit the use of the chin itself for traction, occipital traction can be substituted. In these cases the back of the head must be inspected closely each day for signs of irritation or pressure. The use of frequent shampoos with any type of head traction is indicated to improve the circulation of the scalp and to lessen the danger of decubitus ulcers.

Head traction may be applied to relieve muscle spasm and pain caused by an injured cervical disk or a "whiplash" type of injury. The patient suffering with cervical arthritis may recieve relief when this kind of traction is applied. Head traction is used to relieve pain caused by the presence of a cervical rib or a scoliotic condition. Frequently, some type of head traction is applied following surgical correction of torticollis. The traction helps to maintain a position of overcorrection. Head traction with a leather or canvas halter may be applied to provide temporary immobilization and support when fracture of the cervical vertebrae has occurred.

Intermittent head traction is sometimes used in the home for short daily periods for patients with dorsum rotundum, cervical arthritis, and other conditions requiring hyperextension of the spine (Fig. 2-33).

When constant head traction is necessary for an extended period of time, skeletal traction is nearly always applied. However, to provide for adequate care of the chin and occiput, if constant head traction is being maintained with a halter, the surgeon *may* permit the nurse to remove the chin strap, if manual traction is applied to the head. When manual traction is applied, the grip is more comfortable to the patient if the nurse's palms are placed against his cheeks with the fingers flexed under his chin. The thumbs are not used during the process, and care should be taken not to encircle the patient's neck with the hands at any time during the process. Increased flexion or hyperextension of the cervical spine must not be permitted. A second nurse bathes (shaves male patient) and gently massages the skin and subcutaneous tissues of the lower jaw and chin.

NURSING CARE OF PATIENTS IN SKELETAL TRACTION

Skeletal traction applied to an extremity. Various types of surgical apparatus for applying direct traction to bone have been used in the past, but for the most part these have been supplanted by the Steinmann rustless steel pin and the Kirschner wire of chromic steel (Fig. 2-34). The latter is perhaps the most commonly used type of skeletal traction and is preferred to the Steinmann pin because it is smaller in diameter and the disturbance to the bone occasioned by its use is almost negligible. Skeletal traction may be applied to the lower extremity through the proximal or distal end of the tibia, through the heel, and through the distal end of the femur. It may also be used in the upper extremity and in the skull.

The wire or pin may be inserted in the operating room or, if necessary, on the ward. The anesthetic used may be general or local. It is a surgical procedure and requires the most scrupulous aseptic technique in its performance. Usually, the area where the pin will be inserted is prepared surgically in advance of the procedure.

The wounds made by the introduction of the wire may be dressed with sterile gauze sponges, and the doctor usually prefers that the dressing not be disturbed after it is applied unless there is evidence of infection. Daily inspection of the wound is not necessary, and infections have been traced to overzealous dressing and cleansing of these wounds. Care should be taken not to allow the dressings to become contaminated by the patient's hands or through accidental spilling of fluids on the dressings.

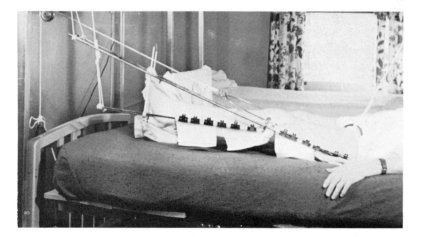

Fig. 2-34. Skeletal traction applied to the distal end of the femur. The limb is supported by means of a half-ring Thomas splint with Pearson attachment. The clips placed on the lateral aspect of the splint hold the canvas strips taut. The limb is in a neutral position and from the knee down is supported by the Pearson attachment. The position of the foot support can be adjusted to the patient's needs. Note U-shaped clamp attached to the Kirschner wire.

It is usually wise to have a Thomas splint and Pearson attachment prepared and sent to the operating room with the patient. If the wire or pin is to be inserted on the ward, the splint should be ready to be put on the patient's leg before the skin area is surgically cleansed.

Equipment to attach the weight to the U-shaped clamp that will be attached to the nail or wire should be available in the recovery room when the patient returns from the operating room if the procedure is carried out there. Much discomfort can be eliminated if the weights are attached before the patient becomes conscious or before the local anesthetic has completely worn off.

A cork or adhesive tape is usually applied over the sharp end of the wire or pin to protect the nurses and patient from injury. All handling of the U clamp, the rope, and the attached weights must be exceedingly careful to avoid causing pain and discomfort to the patient.

Skeletal traction is frequently used in fractures of the lower third of the femur, when it is essential that the fracture be treated with the knee in flexion. The Thomas splint with a Pearson attachment is generally used with this type of fracture. The splint and attachment are prepared with wide canvas strips or slings to support the thigh and lower leg. These strips should be fastened securely with large traction clips or safety pins on the lateral aspect of the splint to make tightening them more convenient. An overhead frame with pulleys is necessary for suspending the Thomas splint. The Thomas splint will usually be elevated at a 45-degree angle with the bed. The Pearson attachment is fastened to the Thomas splint at the knee joint. The knee is flexed to 45 degrees, and the lower leg lies in the Pearson attachment, which is horizontal with the mattress. Buck's extension is sometimes applied to the leg below the knee.

Equipment for preventing drop-foot deformity consists of an adhesive strip fastened along the sole of the foot and attached by rope to an overhead pulley. (Care must be taken not to exert pressure on the toes as contracture of the toe extensors will be likely to occur.) Also, commercial foot supports that clamp to the Pearson attachment are available.

Ropes are attached to the U-shaped traction clamp that holds the pin. This rope passes to a pulley at the end of the bed, where the weights are attached. The pull is in line with the Thomas splint and with the long axis of the femur.

The patient is allowed to move about rather freely in bed. He may sit up, or he may turn to his side as much as the traction will permit. The nurse must handle the apparatus with gentleness, however, for jarring movements are particularly dreaded by the patient. The rules applying to efficient skin traction also apply in skeletal traction, and nurses should be alert in their observations to see that the apparatus is mechanically correct and in good working order at all times.

When the wire or pin is to be removed, the skin is prepared as carefully as it was for the original procedure. Sometimes the surgeon will ask that the area surrounding the wire be saturated with alcohol solution for 24 hours before the removal.

The traction clamp and weights are removed from the limb, and the wire end on the outer aspect of the leg is sterilized with iodine, alcohol, and ether. The skin is then pushed inward, and the wire is cut beneath the surface of the skin. The wire is pulled through from the opposite side. Small sterile dressings are applied to the pin areas until healing takes place.

Skeletal traction applied to the head. Nursing care of the patient with skeletal traction applied to the head is included in the care of the patient with fracture of the cervical spine.

Bathing patients in traction. Patients in traction, like most other orthopedic patients, are bathed over the anterior surface of the body as the first step of their morning care. During the bath the toes are carefully cleaned and the sole of the foot is massaged with alcohol or oil. At this time the area around the traction tapes or bandage should be inspected. Particular attention is given to the back of the heel and the Achilles tendon, which so often become sore when adhesive tape and bandage have been applied too snugly. The dorsum of the foot is inspected for signs of ridging or cyanosis. If the protective bandage over the traction tapes has become loosened either at the ankle or the groin, it should be reenforced or reapplied.

Without explicit permission, weights are never

removed at any time during the nursing care given these patients. This is an axiom of such serious import that it can scarcely be emphasized too strongly. The damage that can be done in fractures of the extremity by this kind of thoughtlessness may on some occasions be almost immeasurable.

The nurse will frequently need assistance, when giving back care and changing the bed linen of the patient, newly operated on, who has been placed in suspension traction. Generally speaking, it is not permissible for the traction patient to turn for this procedure. However, with the aid of a trapeze, the patient learns to help with this aspect of his care. By grasping the trapeze and pulling, he is able to lift his shoulders off the bed, enabling the nurse to bathe and care for the upper portion of his back. To bathe the buttocks and the sacral area, the assistance of a second nurse is needed to help the patient lift his hips off the bed. The patient, by flexing his uninvolved hip and knee and pushing with his foot on the mattress as he pulls on the trapeze with his hands, is usually able with the assistance of a second nurse to lift his buttocks off the bed. This makes it possible for the first nurse to complete the back care and to change the bed linen. To change the bottom sheet, the clean linen is placed in position on the side of the bed beneath the patient's uninvolved limb. Then with the aid of the second nurse (on the opposite side of the bed) the patient's hips and shoulders are lifted as described above, and the clean linen is pushed underneath the patient, replacing the soiled linen. The soiled linen is removed and the bed-making process completed. If the patient is a child, it is sometimes more convenient to change bed linen from the bottom or from the top of the bed. Many variations of bed-making and bath-giving procedures are necessary in caring for the patient in traction, and no one way can ever be set down dogmatically as the best for all patients.

An overhead bar, or trapeze, is almost indispensable for the adult patient in traction. With this device he can support himself for back care and thus spare the nurse much unnecessary lifting.

The following observations should be made when caring for the traction patient.

1. Circulation—check skin color, joint motion, complaints of numbness, coldness, or swelling of the extremity. Avoid pressure in the popliteal space.

2. Condition of the skin—check skin areas over the Achilles tendon, dorsum of the foot, heel, and sacral region.

3. Body alignment and position of the extremity—is the purpose of the traction being accomplished?

4. Prevention of deformity—have measures been provided to prevent drop foot, hip flexion contracture? Is the backrest lowered several times daily to provide for complete extension of the hip joints?

5. Countertraction—is countertraction sufficient or does the footplate frequently rest against the foot of the bed?

6. Slipping—is there slipping of the traction tapes, and does outer bandage need rewrapping?

7. Pressure—is there pressure on the lateral aspect of the leg over the head of the fibula? Pressure in this area may result in a palsy of the peroneal nerve.

8. Patient's comfort—traction should never be a source of undue discomfort for the patient. Listen carefully and heed complaints of discomfort.

9. Complication—because of prolonged bed rest and minimal activity, hypostatic pneumonia is a constant threat, particularly to the elderly patient. Encourage coughing and deep-breathing.

In washing the patient's back, close attention should be paid to the sacral area, which is an extremely vulnerable spot that must have constant care to prevent breakdown of the skin. It should be emphasized that nurses giving care to such patients should take the trouble to inspect this area. The fact that the area is below the eye level often makes the nurse content to wash and rub the part without sufficient inspection. As sensitive as one's fingers are, they miss change of color, the purplish redness of the skin in the early stages of pressure before skin breakdown has occurred. Further damage may be prevented at this time, and it is important to detect the oncoming trouble before it progresses further. If signs of pressure are present, the area should be massaged gently and covered with a thin coating of talcum. Squares of sponge rubber or acrylic fiber pads (artifical lamb's wool) may be placed under the sacral area. Most important of all, especially for the patient who cannot be turned, is frequent massaging of the part. This can be done, of course, without raising the patient each time. The nurse may slip her hand under the area and give an acceptable massage several times a day without changing the patient's position. Even moving the skin back and forth for a short period may prevent undue pressure on any point for a dangerous period and will be valuable.

In making the top of the bed the efficiency of the traction and the warmth of the patient are the important considerations. The appearance of the bed is always secondary. Undersheets and drawsheets must be snug and tight, but the upper part of the bed may be made according to the individual case.

The nurse's well-worn ingenuity comes into play when caring for such a patient, and no set rule can be laid down except that the comfort of the patient and the efficiency of the traction come before the appearance of the bed in orthopedic wards.

Divided linen with ties may be helpful in some instances; however, this type of linen may, also, interfere with the efficiency of the traction and with prescribed exercises. Many patients prefer that the top linen not be tucked under the mattress in the conventional manner, but be tied loosely to the foot of the bed. Small blankets may be used to keep the limb and foot in traction warm.

Traction and bedpans. Because a great majority of patients in traction lie in a bed that has a foot elevated for countertraction, some difficulty in the use of the bedpan may be encountered. In most instances, however, elevating the headrest is permissible and helpful. Also, the fracture bedpan with a tapering back can be slipped under the patient's buttocks without altering the position of the hips, and with very little disturbance of the traction. With women patients, the use of a female urinal may cause less discomfort than use of the regular bedpan, plus the fact that less lifting is necessary to position the patient. The patient (unless contraindicated) should be encouraged to use the trapeze and the uninvolved limb to assist in placement of the bedpan.

Prevention and treatment of pressure sores. The problem of preventing pressure sores on patients in traction is an extremely serious matter. Traction seems to predispose patients to this condition, first, because in many instances alteration of position is not allowed, and, second, because a great number of patients in traction are elderly. It is very common for the older person in traction to have a continual 30- to 45-degree back elevation as a safeguard against pulmonary congestion. This, of course, places a considerable portion of the body weight on the sacral area, and pressure sores tend to occur at that point with great frequency. In addition, the elderly patient often has dry tender skin, and the protective fat pads are gone from over bony surfaces. Often their nutrition is inadequate, particularly regarding protein and vitamin C, both of which are exceedingly important elements for promoting tissue health.

It is important that nurses recognize these hazards before trouble begins to occur. They should consult the doctor in regard to proper diet and obtain his assistance and advice in meeting the problem. He will often be able to help them in planning for change of position. Usually, some latitude will be allowed the elderly patient who must be in traction over a considerable period.

A great deal of the problem of pressure sore prevention is the responsibility of the nurse. It must be recognized that trauma of any nature that endangers tissue integrity is a great factor in the production of skin abrasion, and the trauma need be no more than that caused by a few crumbs in the bed. Trauma can occur to the skin from wrinkles in the undersheet, the rubber sheet, or the drawsheet; it can occur from grit in talcum powder. A wet bed is a well-recognized cause of skin abrasion, and the necessity for keeping the bed dry and smooth can hardly be overemphasized. Patients who lift themselves on their elbows many times during the day may develop pressure sores at these areas. Another vulnerable site is the heel of the unaffected foot because the patient has a tendency to push himself up in bed with this foot.

Pressure areas go through certain rather well-defined stages. The first stage of redness will usually be accompanied by the patient's complaint of a hot burning pain at the site involved. After a day or so the initial reddened area may cause the patient little pain because of the paralysis of the sensory nerve endings in the skin. The redness in the area may take on a purplish cast which will not disappear upon blanching. The skin may break, because of an almost undetectable vesicle formation. Unless this progression is checked, ulceration may follow, and the denuded area may become the source of secondary infection by an endemic *Staphylococcus*. Culture of these sores and appropriate antibiotics may be indicated in selected cases. Tissue necrosis may cause deep craterlike holes in the skin and underlying soft tissues that may reach down to the bone.

Fundamental to all treatment for this condition is removal of pressure. Frequently, permission may be given to turn the patient to his side for short periods to relieve pressure on the sacral area. If this is done, the nurse should be careful to keep the legs in good alignment. The top leg should be supported with pillows to prevent sagging. A brisk rubbing to restore circulation to the threatened area can be given, but it should not be vigorous enough to endanger the skin. Alcohol may be used to toughen the skin, but it is advisable to use oil on the area once during the week to prevent excessive drying. Sponge-rubber squares or squares of unclipped sheepskin are often effective in preventing the progress of pressure areas if they are used during the early stages.

Small pressure pads placed around such points as the heel and the malleoli should not be circular but semilunar in shape. Too often the circular pad with its doughnut-like hole cuts off what little circulation is left to the part. A half moon that only partially closes the area accomplishes relief from pressure without the accompanying circulatory loss. Sponge rubber, cut into varying sizes and shapes, makes excellent pressure pads for heels, elbows and other bony prominences.

Some physicians prescribe drying powders such as boric or zinc. Tincture of benzoin is sometimes beneficial in the early stages of denudation.

Treatment for the advanced pressure sore with its craterlike hole is a more difficult problem.

If a culture taken from a decubitus ulcer grows a *Staphylococcus* organism, the patient should be isolated and precautions taken to protect other patients and personnel. Gloves and mask should be worn when dressings are changed. The physician may request that the ulcer be cleansed several times daily, depending on the amount of drainage. Because of its infection-inhibiting properties, pHisoHex solution may be the prescribed cleansing agent. Daily irrigation with sterile saline solution, Dakin's solution, or solutions containing antibiotics are commonly used. Elase ointment, because of its action on necrotic tissue, may be placed on the ulcer. Packs of gauze impregnated with penicillin ointment or other antibiotics are frequently used. A and D ointment, granulated sugar, and many other drugs may be prescribed and are used with varying degrees of success. The physician frequently requests that dressings be omitted for certain periods of the day to permit drying of the area. Sunlight or treatment by the bactericidal lamp has been helpful in many cases. Dressings should be held in place with a minimum amount of tape, because adhesive itself can be a frequent cause of skin breakdown. With some patients it is advisable to use cellophane tape or Blenderm surgical tape. These tapes are usually less irritating to the skin.

Surgical closure of a decubitus ulcer may be necessary to facilitate rehabilitation. Pressure sores treated conservatively heal slowly and, in some instances, healing is superficial. The area breaks down when activity is started, revealing a larger underlying ulcer. It is necessary, therefore, to precede surgical closure of a pressure sore with several weeks of preparation. The patient must understand the importance of assuming positions that eliminate pressure on the involved area, and thus provide for a more adequate blood supply. Frequent cleansing and irrigation of the area are prescribed to lessen infection and to promote growth of healthy tissue.

Activity to prevent atrophy and stiffness of uninvolved extremities. It is always important that the parts of the body not in traction be kept in the best condition possible. No unnecessary stiffness or atrophy should be allowed to occur because of the immobilization of the injured part. Exercises for the uninvolved portions of the body should include flexion and extension of the hip and knee of the good leg; dorsiflexion and inversion of the ankle; static exercises to strengthen the quadriceps, gluteal, and abdominal muscles; exercises to develop the extensors of the elbows and wrists to facilitate future crutch walking; and breathing exercises. The patient with only lower extremity involvement is also encouraged to use his upper arms and shoulders freely, particularly in positions of outward rotation and abduction. Activities such as combing his hair, fastening his gown at the back of the neck, or lying with his arms out at the sides with elbows flexed and palms upward are beneficial and prevent shoulder restriction that often results from long bed rest. Equipment must, of course, be supplied to encourage the patient to lie in good physiologic positions: a footboard or box, rolls for use under the knee, and a firm pad for under the lumbar region; the latter is indispensable for the comfort of the patient who has traction applied with the legs in full extension.

Diversional therapy. It is also extremely important that the patient be given something to do. A patient in traction is confined so closely to his bed for such long periods that restlessness and depression occur rather easily. If an occupational therapist is available, he will be able to suggest many crafts suitable for this type of patient. Otherwise the nurse should provide some type of activity attractive to the patient, so that he will have the satisfaction of creating something with his hands while he is bedfast. Wherever possible, schooling should not be interrupted.

Patients in traction may be moved without too much difficulty to recreational courts or porches to provide variation in their daily program. If swinging weights are attached to the bed, moving should not be done by one person. Someone should be responsible for holding the weights during the moving process so that they do not swing or become dislodged from the pulley.

BRACES

During recent years, increased interest has led to advancement in the use of braces and other aids that make functional activity possible for the handicapped individual. New materials have been made available, which are light in weight but still provide for strength and durability. Braces, splints, or other supportive devices are prescribed for many reasons. They are frequently necessary to permit the patient to walk without undue strain or fatigue. They are also used to prevent or overcome mild deformity or tendencies toward deformity. In other instances, a brace may be used to prevent motion in a joint or part of the body. The cock-up splint, which maintains the wrist and hand in a functional position, is often prescribed for the hemiplegic patient. Night splints may be worn by the arthritic patient to help prevent or correct knee flexion contractures. The child with Legg-Perthes disease may wear an ischial weight-bearing brace to protect the hip joint. A spinal brace is frequently prescribed to provide support and immobilization for the patient with back pain. Various types of back braces have, also, been devised to help correct and prevent spinal deformity for the scoliotic child. The Frejka pillow or the abduction brace may be used to maintain the congenital dislocated hip in a corrected position, and long leg braces provide the support necessary to make ambulation possible when muscle weakness or paralysis is present in the lower extremities. The purpose of using "the brace" as with other methods of treatment is to help restore the patient to normal living. Braces are a step in this direction. However, when possible, the ultimate aim is to eliminate the use of braces either by further development of the patient's own remaining powers or by some type of reconstructive surgery.

When braces are ordered a considerable outlay of expense is involved. A respect for the cost and skilled labor going into these braces is a healthy virtue for the nurse to develop in the patient. Their care is part of the teaching that the nurse does for the family. Knowledge of their purpose and the correct way to apply them, with recognition of the purpose of each part and the necessity for keeping them intact, is essential. Nurses may encounter some resistance to the use of braces. Many persons honestly believe that to walk in any manner, however hazardously, without braces is preferable to walking with them. Nurses will need to be well informed about the reason for the prescribed brace.

Short leg brace. The short leg brace serves primarily to control motion of the ankle and foot. Motion at the ankle joint (dorsiflexion and plantar flexion) may be controlled by a particular type of ankle stop. Prevention of plantar flexion (dropfoot position) can be accomplished with the posterior stop. This is frequently used when there is weakness or paralysis of the dorsiflexors of the foot. If the dorsiflexors are of normal strength and the plantar flexors weak, an anterior stop is used to prevent the patient from walking on his heel (calcaneus position). If the muscles that produce ankle motion are normal, the ankle joint in the brace is made without "stops," making free motion possible. If there is flaccid paralysis of all the muscles controlling ankle motion, the brace's ankle joint is made to provide only a few degrees of dorsal and plantar flexion. To control varus deformity of the foot, a leather T strap is attached to the lateral aspect of the shoe and buckled around the medial upright bar of the brace (Fig. 2-35). The reverse is used to control pronation (valgus deformity) of the foot.

Long leg brace. A long leg brace with knee pads or cuffs is necessary to prevent buckling of the knee and to permit weight bearing when there is paralysis or marked weakness of the knee extensor muscles (quadriceps). Knee pads worn over the anterior aspect of the knee should tell the nurse of strong hamstring or flexor muscles around the joint combined with relatively weaker extensor muscles. Such pads are placed in front of the knee to prevent the

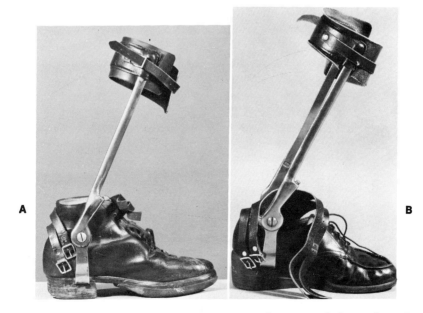

Fig. 2-35. A, Klenzak inner upright brace. **B,** With inner and outer upright bars and outside T strap. The hinge has a built-in spring stop that prevents plantar flexion and is useful in the treatment of foot drop from muscle paralysis. The T strap stabilizes the foot against varus position.

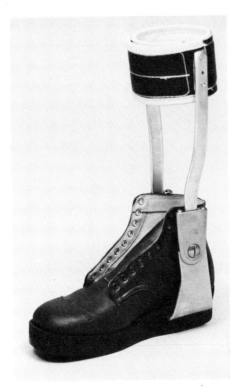

Fig. 2-36. Short leg brace with bichannel ankle. The main use for this brace is the prevention of drop foot from weakness of the dorsiflexor muscles. The anatomical ankle joint is aligned with axis of the mechanical joint in the brace. A spring can be loaded to aid dorsiflexion or plantar flexion, whichever is required.

patient's feeling insecure and fearful of jackknifing as he walks. A similar pad on the posterior aspect should indicate the presence of strong quadriceps, extensor muscles, that tend to pull the knee into a hyperextended position (genu recurvatum). Frequently these knee pads get lost because the nurse and the patient do not recognize them as an essential part of the brace. Also, to prevent hyperextension when there is paralysis of the hamstring muscles, padded metal cuffs are placed posteriorly on the long leg brace above and below the knee joint.

Various types of locks have been devised to permit flexion of the knee joint. Any such lock must function with a high degree of safety, if buckling of the knee with weight bearing is to be prevented. It must, also, be devised so that the individual wearing the brace can manipulate it without difficulty. The most common type of lock is known as the "sleeve" or "ring" lock, which is placed on the lateral upright of the brace. This sleeve or ring slides up and down over the hinge joint. The automatic lock (Fig. 2-37) is one the patient must learn to operate. The spring that controls the lock is released by pressure on the seat of the chair. The patient is then able to bend the knee.

The long leg brace constructed for a child is usually made with upright bars that overlap. This allows for frequent adjustment of the brace to meet the growth needs of the child.

When there is paralysis of the hip and trunk muscles, a pelvic band or body brace may be added to the long leg braces (Fig. 2-39). This arrangement provides for control of hip motion and for good body alignment with correct support of the body weight. Pelvic bands should fit just below the iliac crests. The trunk part of the brace must be observed to be certain that the fastening is in the midline of the body; any minute variation of this will make the fitting of the entire apparatus faulty.

Attachment of the brace to the shoe. The brace made for the lower limb may be attached directly to the shoe or may have a footplate that fits inside the patient's shoe. The attachments commonly used to fasten the brace to the shoe are known as the caliper and the stirrup. With the stirrup attachment, the shoe cannot be separated from the brace. With the caliper attachment, the brace may be removed from the shoe, enabling the individual to attach the brace to more than one pair of shoes. However, the caliper attachment has the disadvantage of producing motion at the heel. The brace with the footplate that is placed inside the shoe enables the individual to wear different shoes, but when fitting shoes it is necessary to remember that space must be allowed for the footplate.

The selection and fitting of the shoe to be worn with a brace is a significant factor. Many times adjustments such as arch supports or metatarsal pads are necessary. To provide proper weight bearing and position of the foot, the shoe may be altered with a metatarsal bar, with inner or outer wedges, or shoe lifts may be used to equalize leg lengths. The nurse must remember, when helping parents or a patient select a

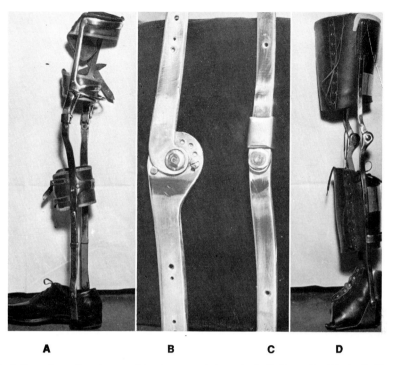

Fig. 2-37. A, Long leg caliper brace with an automatic knee lock. **B,** Set or fixed lock. **C,** Sleeve lock. **D,** Long leg brace with footplate and no knee lock.

shoe to which a brace will be attached, that the sole must be fairly thick and of a quality that will permit the brace maker to make the necessary alterations. For brace attachments a walking shoe with a low broad heel is preferable. If there is considerable spasticity of the ankle and foot muscles, it is desirable to have a shoe that opens over the toes. Care must be exercised when putting the spastic foot into the shoe, to make certain that the toes are in the correct position. With a tight heel cord, it is difficult to keep the heel of the foot down in the shoe. The high-top, laced shoe may be helpful. If the individual has no sensation in the foot, a great deal of care must be taken to prevent the development of blisters and ulcers on the heels and toes. Frequent and careful inspection of the skin for reddened areas is necessary. In some instances lining the shoe with sheep's wool has been helpful..

Arm splints. If arm splints are used, they should be inspected frequently to see if the splint is actually maintaining the arm in the position designed. Patients wearing arm splints have a tendency to lift the shoulder by con-

tracting the strong upper trapezius muscle, thereby robbing the upper arm of the support of the splint. It may be necessary to take a little time to instruct the patient to relax the trapezius muscle so that the arm may rest in the splint as prescribed. If weakened shoulder or back muscles are present and no splint is worn, the weight of the arm in the splint should not be allowed to pull the shoulders downward in undesirable postural attitudes. Some provision to eliminate this pull may need to be devised. If the patient is bedfast, canvas hammocks may be suspended from an overhead bar that will support the arms and prevent the pull on weakened shoulder muscles. If the patient spends considerable time sitting, the arms may be supported by armrests constructed of pillows, pads, or boxes, which may be placed on the desk or table top or on the arms of the chair. It is sometimes possible to improvise an upright support with an overhead bar to a wheelchair. Hammocks or cuffs may be suspended to this bar to support the hands and arms for part of the day. It is usually permissible for the patient to use his hand and elbow functionally in eating, writing,

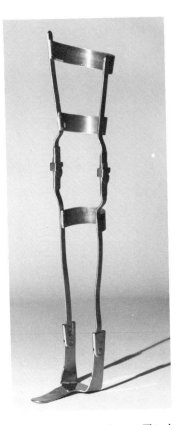

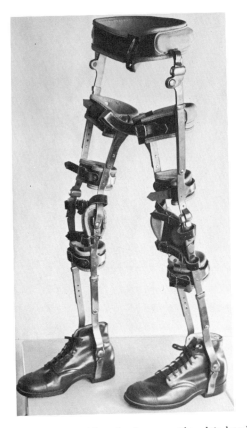

Fig. 2-38. Modular long leg brace. This brace provides support to the entire leg and is applicable to different uses. The knee joint can be locked in extension in the case of thigh muscle paralysis. It can be used with a free knee if the knee requires lateral support. The ankle portion of the brace can provide "stops" to prevent excessive dorsiflexion or plantar flexion of the foot. This can be spring loaded to aid either dorsiflexion or plantar flexion, whichever is needed. The ankle is also provided with lateral stability without interference of ankle motion since the bichannel joint produces motion anatomically through a mechanical joint in the same axis.

Fig. 2-39. Bilateral long leg braces with pelvic band.

or holding a paper if there is no involvement in these areas even though weakness is present in the shoulder muscles. Too constant use of the forearm, however, may put more strain than is desirable on the shoulder, and frequent periods of rest from activity are advisable.

Care of braces. All joints and locks on a brace should be oiled weekly with 3-in-1 oil, or a similar lubricant, and surplus oil be removed immediately so that it does not stain the surrounding leather. Lint should be removed from screws before they are oiled. Saddle soap and small amounts of water cleanse leather parts satisfactorily. Leather should be polished after the use of saddle soap. This both refurbishes and imparts a certain amount of water resistance to the leather.

For the patient's comfort and for the cleanliless and long life of the brace, a cotton shirt may be worn beneath a body brace. Oiling of the skin tends to stain leather portions of braces, and these stains are very difficult to remove. When incontinence is present, the upper portion of the leather thigh cuff sometimes may be protected with waterproofiing. Although it is desirable, it is not always possible to get the bulky diapers and rubber pants beneath the brace, and these have to be applied outside, leaving the leather portions near the groin exposed to frequent wetting.

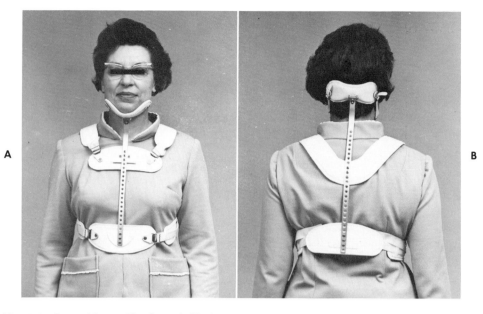

Fig. 2-40. Cervical brace. This brace holds the cervical spine immobilized and is adjustable for any degree of flexion. There is considerable freedom of flexibility for the wearer to adjust to positions of necessity from the waist down while providing support for the cervical spine.

All straps on braces should be securely fastened, but care should be taken, as the child puts on weight or grows, that constriction of circulation does not develop because of the straps. Nurses new to orthopedic services will need instruction in the application of each of the more complicated types of braces, particularly the corrective scoliosis braces, the different kinds of clubfoot braces, and the Taylor spine brace. Automatic locks should be explained and their use demonstrated. The student deserves to have this information from a clinical instructor rather than from the patient, who often gives poor instruction.

Lacings or shoestrings used on braces should be kept in good condition, without knots, and be changed as they become frayed. If the tips fall off, new ones can sometimes be constructed by applying collodion in successive layers. Frayed straps and soiled or worn felt pads should be replaced by the brace maker.

Missing parts (screws, laces, hooks, straps, pads, or felt lining) should be reported as soon as they are noticed. The patient will learn respect for his apparatus by the nurse's prompt attention to such details. The shoes attached to his braces, usually by caliper through the heel, must be inspected frequently for signs of wear and abnormal pressure. Children tend to outgrow shoes and braces with alarming rapidity. Points to be recognized as indications that the child is outgrowing the braces or shoes must be called to the attention of the parents when correct application is demonstrated to them.

If elastic straps are attached to braces or shoes, inspection of the brace should include examination of this elastic for its resilience. These straps may go from the sole of the shoe to a point just below the knee to form a sort of external dorsiflexor to relieve drop foot caused by paralysis of the anterior tibial muscle. Elastic is also used in many types of scoliosis braces.

Inspection of the skin when the brace is removed may reveal bruises, discolorations, skin abrasions, or dermatitis. Any deviation from the normal condition of the skin or underlying tissues should be reported. Suitable alterations can usually be made to overcome such friction.

In teaching parents and relatives, the nurse must constantly emphasize the necessity of periodic checkups for all patients wearing apparatus of this nature.

EQUIPMENT FREQUENTLY USED TO FACILITATE
CARE OF THE DISABLED PERSON

Alternating pressure pad or pneumatic mattress. The alternating pressure pad is made of air cells 1¼ inches in diameter, running longitudinally to the bed. Every other cell is connected to an air tube that comprises the edge of the mattress. This arrangement provides for two systems of air cells. These air cells are alternately inflated and deflated by an electrically driven air pump. The air is shifted first into one system and then into the other. This means that the patient's body is alternately resting on the odd-numbered cells and then on the even-numbered cells. The cells are inflated and deflated at intervals of 2 to 3 minutes. This interchange of air in the cells is so smooth that it is barely perceptible to the hand. It produces a massaging effect to the cutaneous tissues and provides for a continuous change of pressure points. With improved circulation to the skin and changing pressure points, the danger of decubitus ulcers is somewhat lessened. This pad not only facilitates the care of the patient in the hospital; it also may be used in the home to help prevent pressure areas (Fig. 2-41).

Nursing care of the patient on a lateral turning frame. The patient whose care necessitates immobilization of the spine and who needs to be turned at frequent intervals to prevent pressure sores is usually placed on a Foster or Stryker frame. This apparatus is similar to the Bradford frame, except that both the anterior and posterior frames have been fitted on a standard that has a pivoting device. This pivoting device makes it possible in many instances for one nurse to turn an adult patient. Not only is it easier to turn the patient but better immobilization is secured; consequently, the patient experiences less pain in turning. These frames are used primarily in the treatment and nursing care of patients with various back conditions. The patient with spinal cord damage may be placed on this type of bed. Good position can be maintained, and it is possible to turn the patient frequently, thus changing the pressure points.

Canvas covers are used with these frames. They may be fastened with buckels or with lacings but must be firm and taut continuously. Divided covers are frequently used. This can vary, however, depending on the diagnosis and the purpose for which the frame is being used. The divided cover for the upper half of the posterior frame should extend from the top of the frame to the level of the patient's buttocks (gluteal cleft). A space of approximately 4 inches is left for the perineal opening. The lower half of the posterior cover extends to the end of the frame. The upper portion of the divided cover for the anterior frame will extend from the patient's shoulders to the symphysis pubis. Again a space of 4 inches is maintained for the perineal opening, and the lower portion of the anterior cover extends to the level of the patient's malleolus. This arrangement permits the patient's feet to extend over the frame cover when he is lying in the prone position. Some type of support must be arranged for the patient's forehead or face. This usually consists of a narrow canvas strip buckled at the top of the anterior frame. When caring for a patient with incontinence on the frame, it will be necessary to protect the canvas covering around the perineal opening with waterproof material. A narrow canvas strip is buckled across the perineal opening when the bedpan is not in place. This prevents the patient's buttocks from sagging and helps to maintain a good back-lying position (Fig. 2-42).

The frame may be padded with cotton blankets folded to fit the frame, or strips of sponge rubber cut in the desired size can be used. The outer linen covering is made to fit the frame and is held in place by tying it to the underside. When the patient is being turned from the supine to the prone position, a pillow should be placed crosswise above the dorsum of the

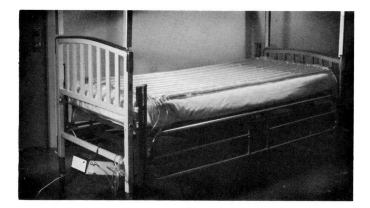

Fig. 2-41. Alternating pressure pad. The pad is placed on top of the regular mattress. Plastic material attached to each end of the pad is tucked beneath the mattress and maintains the pad in position. The smaller air cells or tubes, at the foot end of the pad, provide better protection for the patient's heels.

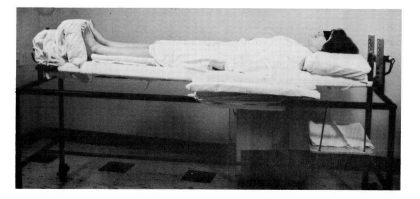

Fig. 2-42. Supine position on the Foster bed. Note the footboard maintaining neutral position of the feet and the small pad to prevent pressure on the heel.

feet. The top frame is fastened in place so that the patient is held snugly between the two frames. Two or three canvas turning straps are buckled around both frames and the patient. This gives the patient added security and will prevent the limbs from slipping during the turning process. The arm boards are removed, and the screw or spring lock that keeps the frame from turning is released. The patient is instructed as to which way he will be turned. If he is being turned by one nurse, it is best that the nurse move to the side of the frame. The turning should be done quickly and smoothly. After patient is turned, the screw or spring lock must be in place before the nurse's grasp on the frame is released. This screw or lock holds the frame firmly and prevents turning. The straps and upper frame are removed, and back care can be given. The covers and linen are changed when that half of the bed is not in use.

These frames may be used even when it is necessary for the patient to have traction applied. The frames are constructed so that traction can be applied to the patient's lower extremities or to the cervical region (Figs. 2-43 to 2-45).

The CircOlectric bed. A vertical turning frame may also be used when it is necessary to apply cervical traction (Fig. 2-46). The bed is equipped with a traction bar and pulleys, which place the traction weight at the side of the bed (outside the circle). When the bed is rotated, the weights hang free and thus provide for

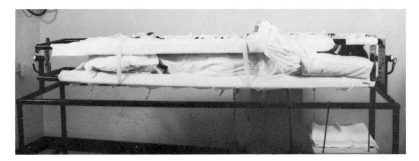

Fig. 2-43. The anterior frame has been fastened so that the patient is held snugly between the two frames. Turning straps have been applied to give added security. The adjustable arm boards have been removed in readiness for turning. Note the pulley at each end of the frame. These may be used in the application of cervical or leg traction.

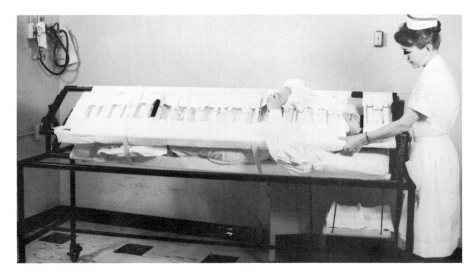

Fig. 2-44. The screw lock has been loosened and the turning process started. Note ties of muslin sheet covering the canvas frame cover. Also, note the narrow strip of canvas used to support the patient's forehead when in the prone position.

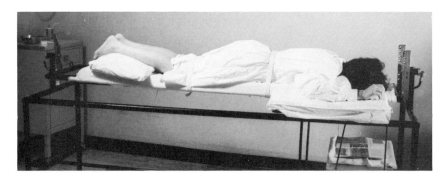

Fig. 2-45. Prone position on the Foster bed. The posterior frame has been removed and will have needed linen changes while the patient is on the anterior frame. In this position the patient can use the lower shelf for holding reading material, or the diet tray may be placed here.

continuous traction. Nursing care given to the patient in a CircOlectric bed is usually adjusted to the turning schedule. When the anterior frame is being placed, the face support is positioned carefully. Change of position in the cervical region must not be permitted. A pillow may be placed over the lower limbs to help maintain proper body alignment, the footboard is positioned prior to fastening of the frame, and straps encircling the two frames will add to the patient's feeling of security during the turning process. The control button makes it possible to turn the patient slowly and without jerky movements. At the beginning of the turning process, the head end of the bed rises vertically, while the foot end descends. The stop on the frame prevents the bed from turning too far. Adjustments in the patient's position, which facilitate feeding and diversional activities, can be made. When positioning the patient, the

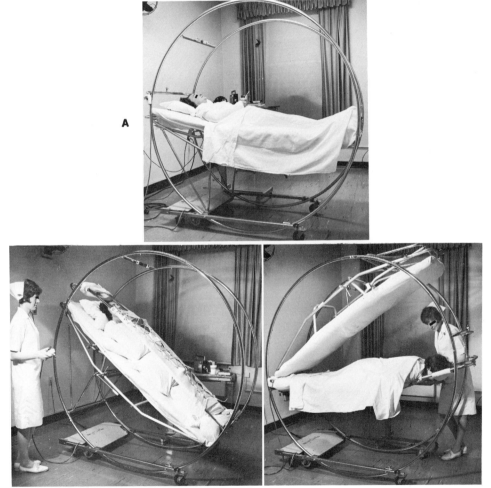

Fig. 2-46. The CircOlectric bed consists of an anterior and a posterior frame and provides for vertical turning as opposed to lateral turning of the patient. Thus, standing, Trendelenburg, and sitting positions may also be utilized. Since the bed is operated with an electric motor, even the very helpless patient may be able to adjust his position and assume a greater degree of independence. The many benefits (physiologic and psychologic) derived from frequent position changes and from self-dependence may be augmented with the use of this bed. In addition to hospital use, it has been found that the CircOlectric bed can be used advantageously in the home to facilitate care of the disabled person. **A,** Supine position. **B,** The anterior frame has been put in position and turning of the patient is started. **C,** Prone position, with the posterior frame in the elevated position.

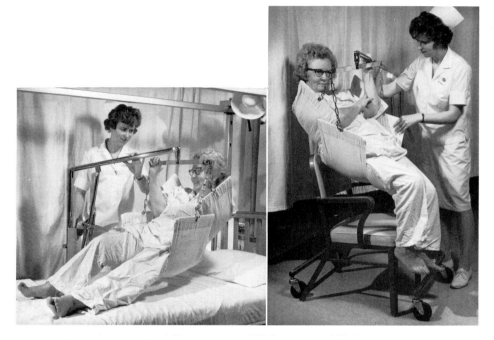

Fig. 2-47. Various types of "lifts" have become useful devices in the hospital as well as in the home for lifting and moving helpless patients. They make it possible for one person to move a patient from the bed to a wheelchair and vice versa.

nurse should remember (if cervical traction is being used) that sufficient countertraction must be maintained to prevent the cervical tongs from resting against the pulley, resulting in a decrease in the traction force. Also, careful checking prior to the turning process is essential to prevent interference with the traction apparatus, which extends laterally to the bed.

The general nursing care of the patient is the same as for other bed patients. Skin care, change of position, prevention of deformity, and maintenance of normal joint motion are essential for his rehabilitation.

Lifting devices. Lifting devices (Fig. 2-47) facilitate caring for the disabled person and make it possible for one person to safely transfer the paralyzed or helpless patient from his bed to a chair or, in some instances, to a tub. Canvas strips that are placed beneath the patient's shoulders and buttocks support the patient as the "arm" of the "lift" is raised. The "lift" is then moved so that the patient is positioned over the chair. The "arm" is lowered slowly, placing the patient in the chair. The canvas hammocks are detached from the "lift" and remain beneath the patient in readiness for his return to the bed.

CRUTCH WALKING

The orthopedic patient usually has ample time to anticipate the moment when he will be able to move about on crutches. It is a goal that he sets for himself and looks forward to with great eagerness because once again he will be able to get around and do things for himself. This is the feature that usually appeals most to him. Sometimes this same eager patient is considerably disappointed when he begins to use those crutches. He is weak; progress is slow, and many limitations of which he was previously unaware become apparent.

The nurse needs patience and foresight to manage this situation. Many institutions have physical therapy departments to teach patients to walk on crutches. This is ideal for the patient. He receives careful instruction and guidance from a physical therapist skilled in this procedure. In the smaller hospitals, however, no such assistance is available to the nurse who must assume the responsibility for this part of the patient's treatment.

MEASURING FOR CRUTCHES

The nurse must first of all have some knowledge of crutches. The most common way to measure the patient for a crutch the correct length is to have him lie on his back with arms straight at the side. When the patient lies with the arms elevated over the head, measurement is often inadequate; contracture of the muscles in the axillae is essential for correct measurement. The tape measure extends from the axilla to a point 6 to 8 inches out from the patient's heel. He should be measured in the shoes he will wear to learn to walk. When it is inconvenient to have the patient lie down, measurements can be made by subtracting 16 inches from the patient's total height.

Crutches that are more than 2 or 3 inches too long should not be cut off to fit the patient without some provision being made for altering the hand bar, which will otherwise be too low. The position of the hand bar should allow practically complete extension of the elbow. The wrists are to be held in hyperextension. The palms of the hands should bear the weight. See Fig. 2-48 for the types of ambulation aids that are most ·frequently used by disabled persons.

Crutch tips should be of good quality and should be inspected from time to time for wear. A worn crutch tip is a menace and must be recognized as such, since slipping is likely to result. Slipping may be undesirable for a normal person, but for the handicapped person it may spell disaster. The soft rubber suction crutch tip is most desirable. The entire tip has contact

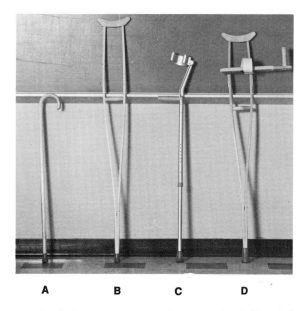

Fig. 2-48. Various types of ambulation supports. **A,** The cane with a half-circle handle is available in wood or metal. **B,** The underarm crutch illustrated is not adjustable but is lighter in weight than the adjustable crutch. This type of crutch is available in either wood or metal. **C,** Adjustable forearm crutch. **D,** An underarm crutch with a forearm adaptation platform. This type of crutch may be used for the arthritic patient who is unable to fully extend the elbow or who is unable to grasp the crutch hand bar. (Courtesy Physical Therapy Department, University Hospitals, The University of Iowa, Iowa City.)

with the floor and is less likely to slip than the hard rubber crutch tip.

Padding over the axillary bar is not necessary, but frequently it is used because the patient thinks it is more comfortable. Some authorities believe that such pads encourage the patient to lean on the crutches, thus bearing too much weight on the axillae. Since crutch paralysis is not an infrequent complication from too much pressure on the axillae, under which the radial nerves lie, it is well to discourage this attitude from the beginning.

PREPARATORY EXERCISES FOR WALKING ON CRUTCHES

In hospitals or clinics where intensive treatment of disabled persons is carried out, attention is first directed toward developing and strength-ening the muscles of the shoulders, chest, arms, and back. The patient is made to recognize the fact that he must have strong upper extremities and back muscles to support his weight when he becomes ambulatory. It is important that these things be accomplished before he begins to walk. An overhead trapeze is extremely valuable in encouraging the patient to use his arms and shoulders to lift his weight from the bed. He should begin standing exercises as soon as his general condition permits him to do so. The tilt table is frequently used to help the patient adjust to the vertical position (Fig. 2-49). Prolonged lying in bed can lead only to loss of muscle tone and incipient deformities that will make standing and walking all the more difficult when they are finally undertaken.

During the time the patient is carrying out

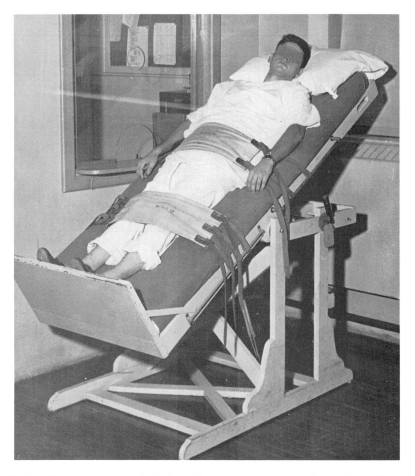

Fig. 2-49. The tilt table is used to help the patient adjust to the standing position. Several times daily he is placed on the table, and gradually the vertical position is attained. This activity has psychologic as well as physiologic values.

active and active-resistive exercises to strengthen the upper extremities, the weak legs are carried through the full range of joint motion several times during the day to prevent muscle contractures and to minimize joint stiffness.

For preparing the patient to use the parallel bars and crutches, push-up exercises from the prone position are useful in strengthening the triceps muscles. Sawed-off crutches that may be used in a sitting position in bed will help the patient to become accustomed to the sensation of having crutches under the arms and will also give him the feeling of bearing his body weight on his hands (Figs. 2-50 to 2-52). He can be taught how to hold his shoulder girdle as he practices with these sawed-off crutches, so that he will avoid hunching and will keep the shoulders at a normal or slightly depressed level. He can learn to shift his weight on the crutches while he is still sitting in bed. These sideways shifts will enable the patient to transfer himself to the wheelchair when he is ready for that experience. Exercises may also include the use of weights. Push-ups may, also, be practiced

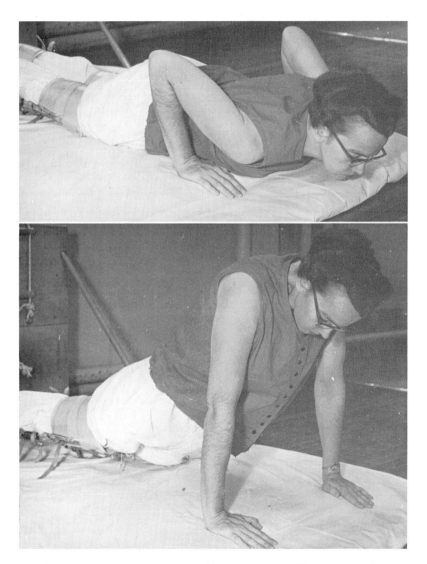

Fig. 2-50. Push-up exercises are done prior to walking on crutches. This activity is of special value in strengthening the triceps muscle (elbow extensor).

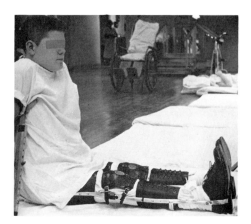

Fig. 2-51. Short crutches may be used in preparation for walking on crutches. Using the crutches to lift the body weight off the bed or mat is valuable in strengthening the shoulder depressors, elbow extensors, wrist dorsiflexors, and finger flexors.

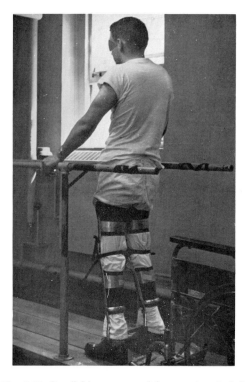

Fig. 2-52. Parallel bars are used for exercises in balancing, standing, and walking. They provide added security and safety for the disabled person.

when the patient is sitting in a wheelchair or chair with armrests. The armrests are grasped and as the patient straightens the elbows, the buttocks are lifted off the chair seat. Care should be taken to avoid "hunching" or elevating the shoulders. This type of exercise strengthens the shoulder depressors, the elbow and wrist extensors, and the finger flexors. If the lower extremities are not paralyzed, the following exercises that include development of the hip and knee extensors are helpful. Tightening the quadriceps, by lifting the heel off the bed or by straight leg–raising (SLR) will strengthen the knee extensors. (See Figs. 3-5 and 3-6.) Lying in the prone position and lifting the leg off the bed (hyperextension) will strengthen the hip extensor muscles.

GOOD CRUTCH WALKING POSTURE

The standing position is not attempted until the patient has mastered the bed exercises and has learned to transfer himself without help into a stabilized wheelchair. Standing with crutches may take a considerable time to master, for it is vitally important that the patient learn to balance himself on the crutches (Fig. 2-53) before he undertakes any further activity. Two hospital beds, placed with foot ends together and stabilized with wooden blocks, may be used as parallel bars for exercises in balancing, standing, and walking.

Nurses will not usually be required to teach the severely handicapped patient to walk on crutches. However, they must know what constitutes safe and efficient crutch walking for this type of patient if they are to supervise such activities on the wards or in the home. They should be able to recognize the patient's maximum degree of good crutch-walking posture and to encourage it at all times. The desirable stance is one in which the head is held straight and high, with the pelvis over the feet if that is possible with the muscular power the patient possesses. The crutches are placed about 4 inches in front and about 4 inches at the sides of the feet, which makes a large standing base. As in all crutch walking, the patient should extend his elbows and carry his weight largely on his hands. He must not hunch his shoulders, and very little weight should be taken by the

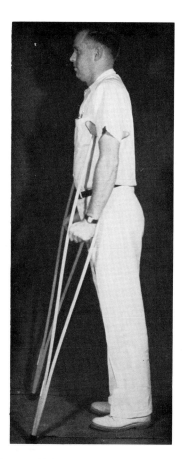

Fig. 2-53. Balancing in the tripod position.

axillae at any time. However, the crutches will lean somewhat against the rib cage and are grasped there by the adductor muscles of the arm and chest.

If involvement is such that this position is impossible—that is, when the patient has little or no use of the muscles of the hip joint, the back, or abdomen—he is usually taught to balance himself in the tripod position. In this position the weight is forward from the ankles, with the hips forward and the crutches ahead and out at each side. It is important to keep the pelvis as far in advance as possible with patients who have severe muscular involvement. They have little muscle power in the front of the body to support them if the pelvis is held too far behind the feet, and so they must depend on anterior hip joint ligaments to stop them from going too far forward.

The patient must, of course, always be as-

sured of his own safety. Usually, one attendant will stand behind him and one in front, but care is taken not to touch the patient unless it is absolutely necessary for his safety.

Attention to details of good posture is essential when the patient begins to walk. If he starts badly, he is likely to continue in the same attitude. Rounded shoulders, stooping back, slumping, flexion at knees or hips, outward rotation of hips, and eversion of the feet are postural defects particularly common to the patient walking on crutches. Fatigue, over-determination to make progress, and muscular weakness from prolonged bed rest may account for some of this. Discouragement also may play its part. If the patient is allowed to see himself in a mirror, there is sometimes amazing automatic improvement in posture.

Sitting with back and feet well supported either on the bed or in a chair should precede actual walking by several days for the patient who has been bedfast for a long time. This is followed by standing at the side of the bed in good position, hips and knees extended, back straight, chest forward, and head up. Contracting the abdominal and gluteal muscles will assist with later easy natural locomotion and good posture. As the patient stands at the bedside he can be helped to shift his weight from one foot to the other without slumping, provided his disability permits. Alternate knee flexion and extension and deep-breathing exercises may be used to prepare the patient for walking. This is the slow approach, and the patient may be impatient to start actual locomotion. The situation and reasons for the delay must be carefully pointed out to him. Getting a patient out of bed and allowing him to walk on crutches in the space of one day usually ends in tears and discouragement.

The patient should learn from the first day the proper way to balance on crutches, as a safety measure and to give him a feeling of security. The starting position is a tripod formed by the patient's body and the two crutches. The patient stands with his feet slightly apart, and the crutches are placed forward and out from the body in such fashion that a line drawn between them would form the base of a triangle whose apex would be the patient's feet. All the factors of good standing posture must be observed. In teaching the patient to walk on crutches our aim is ultimately to enable him to walk without the crutches. Faulty unnatural habits developed during this period will inhibit ultimate return to a normal gait. Hips will tend to sag backward; the chin will be low on the chest, and the eyes will be directed toward the floor. These defects should be corrected before the patient actually begins to walk.

The patient is taught to extend and stiffen his elbow and to place the weight of his body on the wrists and the palms. He is taught to avoid bearing any weight at the axillary level, because the radial nerve passes under this area superficially and pressure on it may cause paralysis of the extensor muscle of the hand and arm. It is, however, usually considered permissible to allow the patient with considerable arm and trunk involvement to lean on the axillary bar for brief periods in order to rest the hands. The patient should be aware of the danger involved in using this position too frequently.

Persons beginning to walk on crutches have a tendency to try to lift a crutch when bearing weight upon it. Nurses should be alert to this tendency and explain the fallacy to the patient. This habit of taking a longer step with the weaker leg is another common mistake made by beginners. Patients should be instructed to take rather short steps of equal length with both legs.

The Canadian crutch (Fig. 2-54), without axillary rest, is preferred in some clinics. One advantage in the use of these crutches is that there is more tendency on the part of the pa-

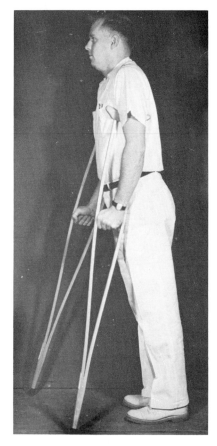

1

Fig. 2-55. Four-point crutch walking: **1,** right crutch; **2,** left foot; **3,** left crutch; **4,** right foot. Parts **2** and **4** of this group also illustrate the two-point crutch walking gait: opposite foot and crutch are advanced simultaneously; that is, right crutch and left foot are advanced together, followed by left crutch and right foot. With the four-point and two-point crutch walking gaits, weight is taken on each extremity. This pattern is frequently used by the patient with poliomyelitis, arthritis, or cerebral palsy.

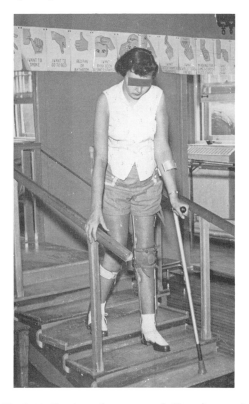

Fig. 2-54. Aluminum forearm crutch (Canadian type).

tient to make better anatomic use of the hips and pelvis in locomotion. In other words, the patient tends to depend on himself and his own muscles more than on the crutches, which are really not much more than canes. Absence of the axillary bar is considered to be advantageous also because likelihood of crutch paralysis is decreased greatly.

These crutches are particularly useful for the patient who is likely to need them only for a short period, but the longer crutch with the axillary bar gives more adequate support. It is usually considered advisable to use the standard type of crutch for patients who have involvement in the trunk, hips, and arms. When fitting the patient with the Canadian crutch, the hand-bar should be in such a position that the shoulder girdle can be relaxed comfortably when the hand is dorsiflexed on the bar with the elbow in almost complete extension.

TYPES OF CRUTCH WALKING

The type of disability that the patient has determines the type of crutch walking he should do. Where help is available through a hospital physical therapist, it should be solicited in making the choice. In general, the following will apply to the most common types of orthopedic patients:

1. When the patient may bear some weight on each limb, teach the four-point or two-point crutch gait (Fig. 2-55). This is applicable to patients with poliomyelitis, arthritis, cerebral palsy, and so forth.

2. When the patient must bear little or no weight on one extremity, teach the method of advancing both crutches and the affected limb at the same time, the three-point crutch gait (Fig. 2-56).

3. Swinging through crutches is sometimes permissible when paralysis of hips and legs is

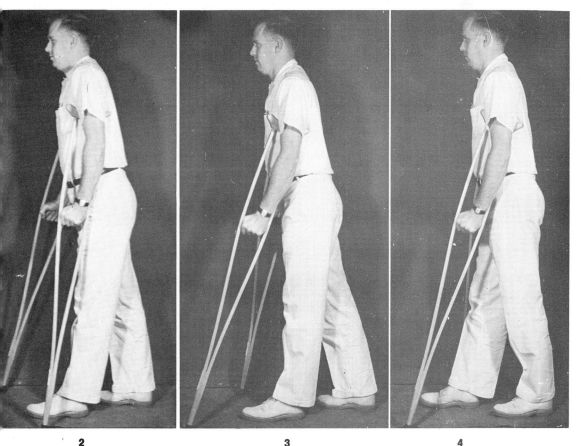

2   3   4

Fig 2-55, cont'd. For legend see opposite page.

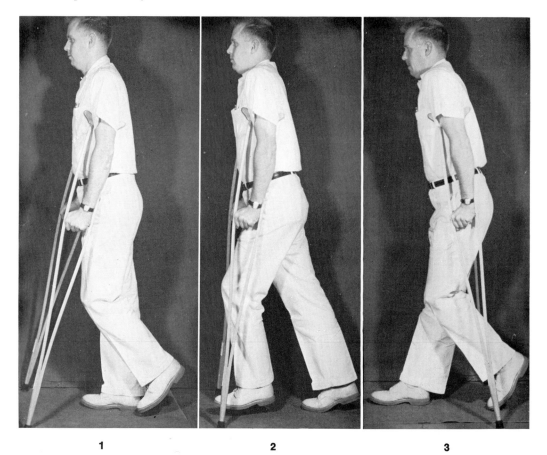

1   2   3

Fig. 2-56. Three-point crutch walking gait is used when there is involvement of one extremity. It may be used when no weight bearing has been ordered or when partial weight bearing is permitted. The affected extremity advances with the crutches, and the patient's weight is taken on the hands as the normal extremity comes forward.

complete. This is the type so frequently seen on the street. It does not simulate normal walking in any way and leads to atrophy of legs and hips.

Modifications are recognized to be essential. For instance, although swinging between crutches is not recommended as a permanent practice for patients, it may frequently be necessary when speed in walking is essential. Also, the use of one crutch or cane is an advanced procedure for the preceding method. The crutch is used on the normal side, because it is put forward at the same time as the disabled limb, thereby taking the weight off that foot.

Four-point crutch gait. The four-point gait can be performed to a count of 1-2-3-4. The pa-

tient puts one crutch forward, then the opposite foot, the other crutch, and the opposite foot. This is hard for a normal person to do, although it approximates normal walking motions of arms and legs. However, with a little practice the patient becomes automatic in its use.

Two-point crutch gait. The two-point gait is the same as the four-point gait, except faster. With this gait the patient advances the opposite crutch and limb simultaneously—left crutch and right limb, right crutch and left limb.

Three-point crutch gait. Walking on crutches is usually an ordeal for the patient who has been inactive over a period of time. Everything possible should be done to make the experience safe and comfortable. The patient will need instruction and constant encouragement if he is

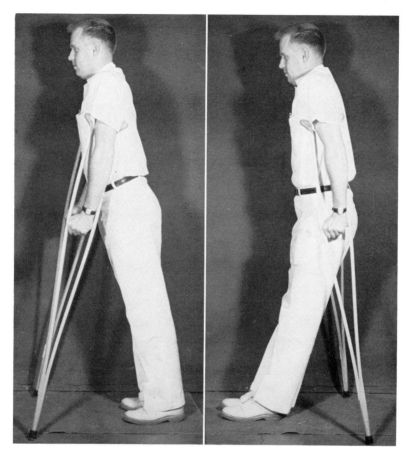

Fig. 2-57. The swing-through crutch gait is used when both lower extremities are paralyzed. The limbs are braced and swung forward together.

to learn to use crutches without undue fatigue. When no weight bearing has been ordered or when partial weight bearing is permitted on the affected extremity, the three-point gait is usually considered preferable (Fig. 2-56). The patient may be taught the mechanics of this gait by means of a diagram before he is out of bed. The affected limb and both crutches are advanced at the same time. Then, with the body weight balanced on the two crutches and the weak leg, the normal leg is advanced. The patient should be instructed to take steps of equal length; otherwise he will tend to take a long step when using the crutches and a very short one when advancing the normal extremity.

When the physician wishes the patient to begin bearing weight on the affected leg, it should be begun gradually. As the patient advances in the ability to manipulate himself on crutches, one crutch may be discarded. The single crutch should be used on the normal side because its purpose is to carry the weight of the body when the normal leg is advancing forward.

Swing-through crutch gait. The swing-through gait (Fig. 2-57) is frequently used by the patient with paralyzed lower extremities. The limbs are braced and swung forward together. This is a rapid gait but does not simulate normal walking.

Tripod crutch gait. The tripod gait is often taught to patients with severe involvement of the lower extremities. The right crutch is advanced first, then the left crutch, and the body is then

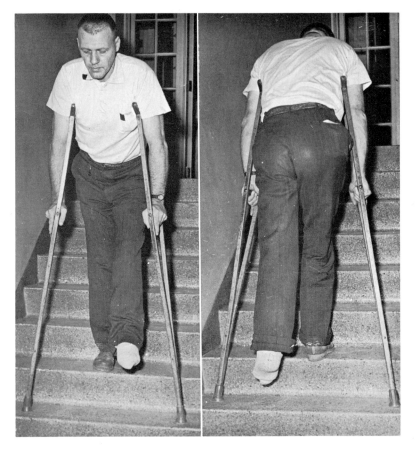

Fig. 2-58   **Fig. 2-59**

Fig. 2-58. Down the stairs with crutches. The crutch walker who is accustomed to the three-point gait will place his crutches on the lower step, take his weight on his hands, and bring the normal extremity down to the lower step with the crutches. Then with the body weight on the normal extremity, the crutches are placed on the next step and the procedure is repeated.

Fig. 2-59. Up the stairs with crutches. When going up steps, the body weight is taken on the hands and crutches and the normal extremity is advanced to the upper step. The body weight is then taken on the normal extremity, and the crutches and involved limb follow. A safe rule to remember when teaching the three-point crutch gait is that the involved limb always goes with the crutches.

Fig. 2-60. Standing with axillary crutches. **A,** This young woman keeps her crutches handy by hooking them on the back of the chair. To stand she slides forward in the chair, with the foot of her strong leg slightly under the chair. **B,** She pushes down against the armrests and leans slightly forward as she stands. **C,** She pivots on her strong right foot. **D,** Placing one hand on the armrest, she picks up both crutches with the other hand. **E,** She then places both crutches under one arm before shifting one crutch to the other arm. (Reprinted with permission of *Patient Care* magazine. Copyright, 1968, Miller & Fink Publishing Corp.)

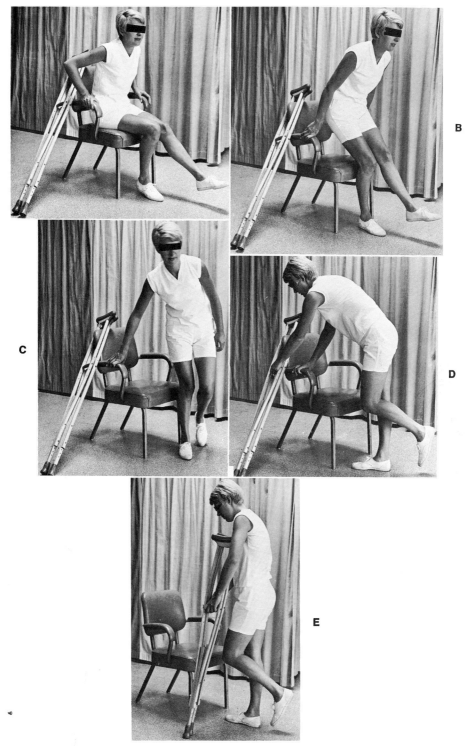

Fig. 2-60. For legend see opposite page

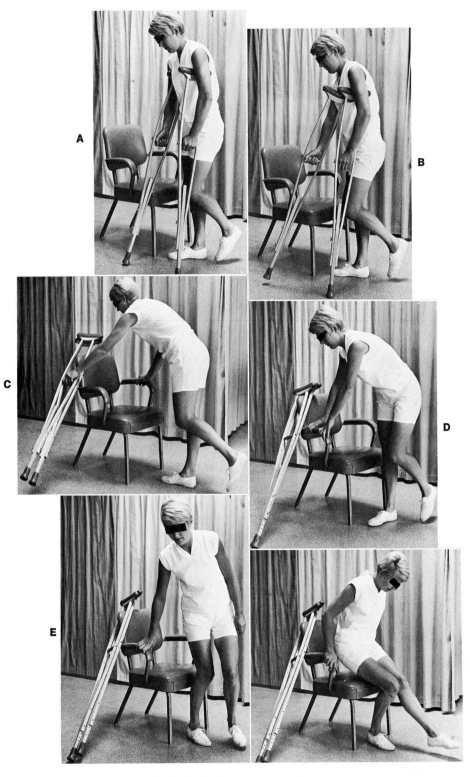

Fig. 2-61. For legend see opposite page.

dragged up to the crutches. If the upper extremities and shoulders are strong, the patient can use the swinging crutch gait. For this gait the crutches are placed together in front of the body. The patient then bears down on the crutches and lifts his body so that it is brought up to the crutches. The next step in advance of this method is the swing-through gait, when both crutches are placed ahead and the body is lifted and swung beyond the crutches. This is more involved than the first swing gait because the body is swung through the crutches and therefore comes to the floor ahead of the crutches.

Figs. 2-58 to 2-61 illustrate one method of going up and down steps, and directions for sitting and rising from a chair with the aid of crutches.

HAZARDS OF WALKING ON CRUTCHES

Everything possible should be done to ensure the patient's safety, for a fall is extremely hazardous after a long period of inactivity. Even a mild mishap may lead to a fracture. When the patient begins to walk, there should be one worker in front and one behind him. He should not be encouraged to lean on his assistants, but he should feel confidence in their presence at all times. No wet spots, loose rugs, or other obstacles to safe walking should be near the patient. Crutch tips must be intact and should be replaced when there is any sign of thinness in the rubber. Suction crutch tips, as the name implies, adhere to the floor surface and decrease the possibility of slipping.

Common errors for which the nurse should be alert are (1) walking with the knee and hip flexed, the foot everted, and the hip in outward rotation; (2) a tendency to walk with the weight on the ball of the foot and with the heel elevated; and (3) a slouching posture, with the eyes fixed on the floor, the chin on the chest, and the shoulders and back rounded.

USE OF A CANE

The cane is frequently prescribed to improve the patient's balance and to lessen the weight-bearing strain on an involved knee or hip. It probably provides the least amount of support of any of the walking appliances. However, it does widen the base of support and, by so doing, helps to maintain the patient's feeling of confidence and sense of balance. When one cane is used, it is used in the hand opposite the involved limb and is advanced with the involved limb. Thus the body weight is taken partially on the cane and the involved limb as the uninvolved limb is moved forward. The height of the cane should permit a few degrees of flexion at the elbow point. As weight is taken on the hand, the elbow is extended. A rubber tip with a wide flat surface for contact with the floor is desirable. Canes that have three or four small legs are, also, available and are helpful to the elderly person who walks slowly and has poor balance.

Fig. 2-61. Sitting down in chair with crutches. **A,** As the young woman approaches the chair, she moves her strong leg in close to the chair. **B,** She then places both crutches under her left arm. **C,** Placing her right hand on the left arm of the chair, she hooks the crutches on the back of the chair. **D,** Now she pivots on the right foot. **E,** Placing her right leg against the chair, she brings her left hand around to the left chair arm. **F,** She gently lowers herself into the chair. (Reprinted with permission of *Patient Care* magazine. Copyright, 1968, Miller & Fink Publishing Corp.)

NURSING CARE OF THE ORTHOPEDIC SURGICAL PATIENT

Nurses will remember from their surgical nursing experience that hemorrhage, wound infection, and pain are the three great obstacles to success in surgery. In orthopedic surgery, impairment to circulation caused by mechanical obstruction must be added. Nurses should be alert for symptoms that indicate the presence of any of these conditions.

GENERAL CONSIDERATIONS

A great number of reconstructive operations on bones are performed on people past middle age. Steindler states that when the constitutional background of the patient is abnormal, it will have a definite primary influence upon the surgical risk. It is for this reason that laboratory tests are done on a large scale. In addition to the routine laboratory tests done on all surgical patients, such as blood count, hemoglobin estimation, bleeding and clotting time, and urinalysis, the orthopedic surgeon often requests determinations of serum calcium, phosphorus, and phosphatase, as well as of the blood sedimentation rate. All these things are especially necessary in older persons in whom the surgeon suspects metabolic changes in the bones. Renal function tests are sometimes ordered, because certain anesthetics offer a definite threat to the patient with kidney damage. During and after surgery, parenteral fluids are given to replace body fluids lost by perspiration, vomiting, and hemorrhage.

Nurses should be able to read laboratory sheets with some degree of facility and intelligence in order to understand more satisfactorily their patients' conditions. Understanding preoperatively the risk facing the individual patient will enable the nurse to assist in his recovery more confidently. A high sedimentation rate is not a good prognostic sign. Excessively high or low blood pressure may lower the patient's vital capacity. Specific gravity of less than normal in the urine adds to the gravity of the outcome. Blood urea nitrogen of over 35 mg per 100 ml. of blood indicates a considerable degree of kidney

damage. It is a well-known fact that postoperative mortality in patients with nephritis complicated by hypertension is high. Any patient who has been confined to bed over an extended period is not considered a good surgical risk.

Dehydration, present or threatened, is an outstanding danger that may be recognized preoperatively. An increase in fluid intake is of greater value before operation than afterward. A daily intake of at least 3000 ml. containing a high percentage of glucose is advisable, and a diet predominating in carbohydrates is advised by some authorities for 48 hours preceding orthopedic surgery.

Delayed coagulation time demands special treatment. Frequently, an intravenous injection of 10 ml. of 5% sterile calcium chloride solution is given for 2 days preceding operation. Transfusion is of greater value if it is given before operation than afterward. Menstruation is not considered a contraindication to orthopedic surgery. However, it should be reported to the doctor before the patient is sent to the operating room.

The mental condition of the patient demands respect. This is particularly true with the spastic child. Severe excitability is known to bring about acidosis. When possible, the patient with cerebral palsy should be allowed to obtain some mental equilibrium before surgery is performed. Some surgeons scoff at preoperative psychic depression. Others feel quite definitely that such depression adds to the gravity of a postoperative prognosis particularly when premonition of death exists. Such mental states should be reported to the physician by the nurse as accurately as a definite physical symptom.

Excessive obesity causes the surgeon concern because of the impairment in respiration that sometimes accompanies it. Wound infection and fat embolism are possibilities to be feared, especially in these patients. A marked degree of weight loss is not considered a good indication, because a loss of glycogen reserve is likely to exist. After operation, persistence of nausea and vomiting will increase the gravity of such a patient's condition extremely because acidosis may occur very quickly.

Inhalation anesthesia is usually preferred by orthopedists, largely because it is a controllable anesthesia; that is, it can be discontinued at once if the patient's condition seems to warrant it. Spinal anesthesia is sometimes used in older persons or in those with hypertension. Danger signals in this type of anethesia are rapid fall of blood pressure and diminution of the respiratory rate. The surgeon will usually order ephedrine in these cases.

PREOPERATIVE PREPARATION OF PATIENT

Preoperatively, a general physical examination will be performed by the physician. His preoperative instructions will usually consist of orders for increased fluid and carbohydrate intake, cathartics, enemas, and preoperative sedation. Antibiotics may be administered to patients who have had osteomyelitis or some septic bone condition in former years.

Although breakfast is omitted for all surgical patients receiving general anesthesia, some orthopedists order the juice of one orange to be given 2 or 3 hours before surgery to all young children. The use of strong cathartics is not recommended by most surgeons. Enemas may or may not be given. If they are ordered, they are usually given the night before the operation, the morning of the operation, or both, depending on the surgeon's wishes. Barbiturates may be given the night before surgery to ensure proper rest. These are especially advisable for the nervous patient and are frequently given on the morning of operation also, particularly when rectal, spinal, or local anesthesia is to be used. The usual preoperative medication of morphine or a derivative combined with atropine or scopolamine is used, except in very young or elderly patients.

Attention to the physical and mechanical data should not deter the nurse from the psychologic treatment that must accompany much of the preparation of any patient for surgery. Most orthopedic conditions are not acute. The patient has perhaps anticipated this operation for some time. Probably, if he is an adult, he has debated over a long period of time the advisability of having the procedure performed. The emotions he feels are a mixture of hope and doubt—hope perhaps that he will regain the use of a long-paralyzed limb and fear that the surgery and long convalescence may be of no avail. It is an important moment in his life. The nurse should recognize this and realize that the difference between the operative procedure for the orthopedic patient and that done for the ordinary surgical patient lies in his hope that some lost function of his body will be restored. This hope often overrides the natural fear. While preparing the operative site, the nurse has an opportunity to establish rapport with the patient and to listen to his story in order to gain some knowledge of his social background. Also, it is a good time to explain to the patient his own part in his recovery and the necessity for patience and cooperation to ensure a successful outcome.

PREPARATION OF OPERATIVE SITE

Because the consequences of infection in bone surgery are so grave and may lead to crippling through stiffness of the joints or chronically infected bone, the preparation of the operative site must be carefully and conscientiously executed. The exact procedure used will vary from clinic to clinic. Recently, however, there has been a tendency to omit the long 48- or 72-hour sterile orthopedic preparation. Instead, the orthopedic patient may be given a preparation similar to that given the general surgical patient.

The antiseptic solutions used vary in different clinics. The method of preparation, however, is much the same. It is now well recognized that mild soap and water are probably the best agents available, not only for removing dirt and grease from the skin but also for eliminating bacteria safely and effectively. Some surgeons feel that no other antiseptic is necessary for cleansing the skin.

After the preliminary cleansing of the skin, shaving is the next step in the operation preparation. The area to be shaved is usually designated by the doctor in the preoperative orders, but the nurse should know what constitutes the area of preparation for all types of orthopedic surgery. Surgery performed on the toes will usually require a surgical preparation to the knee; surgery on the ankle, to the midthigh. In spinal surgery the area will depend on the site of injury or disease. If the operation is to be performed in the high cervical area, the shaving will no doubt include the back of the neck and occiput and will continue to the buttocks. Preparations for operations on lower spinal fusions will include the backs of the buttocks and the upper parts of the thighs and will extend upward to the shoulders. If a graft is to be taken, the leg will be prepared from ankle to midthigh or groin. Knee operations usually indicate preparation of the leg from the toes to the groin. For operations on the hips the preparation usually extends to well below the knee and to the lower border of the ribs, the umbilicus being the limit anteriorly and the spine posteriorly. The pubic area is always included. The nurse must remember that a preparation for operation on one joint should include preparation of the joint above. This is not always a rule, but it provides a generous enough area that little dissatisfaction will be found (Fig. 2-62).

Nurses should develop a deep respect for the importance of the skin, recognizing the fact that the intact skin serves as a mechanical barrier to keep bacteria out of the body. Indeed, some investigators feel that a clean, healthy, and intact skin may actually have a self-disinfecting power. Nothing that is done during the sterile preparation should lessen in any way the defensive powers of the skin.

The shaving must be most carefully done. The blade should be new and of good quality. It is not a procedure to be hurried. Two things can happen with a hurried shave: denuding of the skin area or omitting a small field of fine hair. Hair is not easy to disinfect and may be a source of infection. A denuded area is a grave threat and may mean postoperative infection. The surgeon may refuse to operate in the face of it. Abrasions of the skin of any sort should be reported.

Shaving is usually done in the direction opposite from which the hair lies in order not to omit fine hairs. A wet shave is usually considered more satisfactory, but in case of emergency, when it is not desirable to use water or when the electric razor is used, a dry shave may be given.

After the area is shaved, the extremity for operation must have special attention. It must be thoroughly washed and absolutely clean. If grime persists on feet or hands after this washing, it should be reported to the surgeon. The

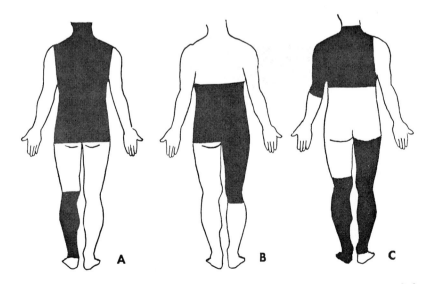

Fig. 2-62. A, Sites commonly prepared for surgery of the spine with autogenous graft from left tibia. **B,** Site prepared for bone operation on hip. **C,** Sites prepared for operations on shoulder, ankle, and knee.

toenails or fingernails must be clipped and thoroughly cleaned. Frequently, it is necessary to soak the foot or hand in warm sudsy water for 30 minutes prior to scrubbing.

After these preliminary but important details have been attended to, the procedure that follows will vary somewhat according to the wishes of the surgeon. In general, however, the area that has been shaved is well scrubbed with mild soap and water for 3 to 5 minutes. A brush may be used for this scrubbing unless the skin is sensitive and tender, and then sponges are used. The nurse must recognize that this mechanical cleansing of the skin prior to the preparation in the operating room is of the utmost importance and must be done conscientiously.

A tray or cart for these preparations should be on every orthopedic service (Fig. 2-63). It should contain an extension light, a razor with fresh blades, unsterile towels for protecting the bed from moisture, bottles containing mild liquid soap, and the antiseptic preferred by the doctor. A small cup or basin to contain water for the shave, paper sacks, cotton balls or sponges,

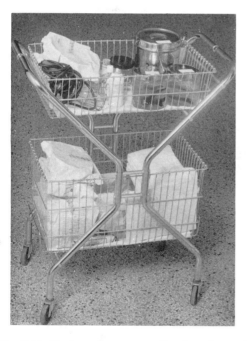

Fig. 2-63. Equipment necessary for cleansing and preparing the skin for a surgical procedure can be taken to the bedside in this lightweight cart.

gloves if they are used, and brushes will complete the tray.

BLOOD TRANSFUSIONS

The transfusion of blood has become a common procedure and is done frequently on a busy hospital service. Yet the transfusion of blood carries a death risk as great as that from an uncomplicated appendectomy. The observations made by the nurse during this procedure are a vital part of the patient's care. The alert well-informed nurse can prevent some dangerous reactions, and her prompt recognition and treatment of others can be life-saving.

When the blood is delivered to the patient area, prior to the time that it is to be given, it should be placed in a refrigerator and kept at a temperature above freezing until it is to be transfused. Blood should not be permitted to stand at room temperature for several hours.

Before the transfusion is started, both the physician and the nurse should compare the patient's name and registration number on the label of the blood container with that on the patient's identification wrist band. In addition to the patient's name the type of blood and the Rh factor appearing on the bottle label should be checked against the accompanying slip. Dangerous reactions and deaths have occurred because blood has been given to a patient for whom it was not intended.

During the entire transfusion the recipient should be watched carefully. It is essential that the drop indicator on the transfusion set be checked frequently and adjustments in the rate of flow be made when necessary. The soft tissues around the needle should be checked for swelling. A hematoma caused by blood going into the subcutaneous tissues can be very painful and may result in serious slough of tissue. The complaints of a patient receiving blood must not go unheeded. Any complaint of respiratory difficulty, such as pain or tightness in the chest, fast breathing, wheezing, coughing, pain in the abdomen or lumbar region, or the appearance of chills or hives, is an indication for the nurse to stop the transfusion and to notify the attending physician. The appearance of respiratory difficulties may necessitate the prompt application of tourniquets on all four extremities, the upper arms and the thighs. The purpose of the tourniquets is to prevent pulmonary edema by pooling the blood in the extremities away from the heart. The tourniquets should be pulled tight enough to hold back venous blood but not tight enough to occlude arterial pulses. The tourniquets should be released one at a time for 2 minutes, then replaced and another one released. No tourniquet should be in place more than 10 minutes without a respite.

Do not permit the tubing to empty completely before discontinuing the transfusion. Near the end of the transfusion watch the apparatus carefully so that the blood flow may be stopped when there is still 20 ml. or so in the container or tubing. If the transfusion has been discontinued because of a reaction, place the used equipment containing the residual blood in the refrigerator. The labels and unused blood should be available for posttransfusion tests in the investigation of transfusion reactions.

After a transfusion, take the patient's temperature at 2-hour, 4-hour, and 6-hour intervals. An elevation in the temperature should be reported to the physician.

A 24-hour collection of urine should be made for all patients receiving transfusions. Note the volume and color of each specimen as it is collected. Oliguria is the output of a dangerously small amount of urine, usually less than 600 ml. in a 24-hour period. If a single specimen, collected over a known period of time, has a volume of less than 25 ml. per hour, or if a red color is present in a urine specimen after transfusion (probable hemoglobinuria), save the specimen and notify the physician.

Immediate transfusion reactions

Transient fevers. These are often initiated by a chill. The fever may occur during or soon after transfusion. The cause may be the presence of polysaccharides called pyrogens in the blood mixture. These pyrogens are produced by the growth of nonpathogenic bacteria in the fluids or equipment used in the transfusion. These substances are not destroyed by sterilization. A second cause may be the presence of small amounts of heated plasma protein left in reused equipment. A third cause may be the onset of a hemolytic reaction in which the donor's or

recipient's erythrocytes are destroyed. Early hemolysis may be excluded by drawing a fresh specimen of the patient's blood, centrifugating it, and demonstrating the lack of pink coloration in the plasma or serum.

Urticaria. Hives occur in about 1% of the patients receiving blood transfusions. During or soon after giving the blood, patches of hives or angioneurotic edema appear on the skin. This can be promptly dealt with by an intramuscular injection of 0.3 ml. of a 1:1000 solution of epinephrine. The transfusion can then be continued.

Hemolysis. Destruction of the red blood cells may occur from (1) damage to the donor's blood by improper storage, overheating, or freezing of the blood, or the mixing of the blood with distilled water, glucose solutions, or solutions other than isotonic sodium chloride, (2) the transfusion of blood containing red blood cells that are destroyed by the recipient's antibodies, or (3) the administration of blood whose plasma contains strong antibodies against the recipient's blood cells. Some of these incompatibilities cannot be detected by the usual laboratory tests. However, some may occur from errors in blood grouping or crossmatching, errors in labeling blood containers, or errors in reading the labels by the nurse or physician. Hemolytic reactions often start with a chill and fever, accompanied by pain or a constrictive sensation in the chest and pain in the lumbar regions or thighs. These symptoms should indicate the immediate discontinuance of the transfusion, notification of the physician, examination of a fresh urine specimen for hemoglobinuria, and the collection of a fresh blood specimen from the patient for examination of plasma hemoglobin. Between 6 and 24 hours after transfusion hemolysis has occurred, the patient may develop painless jaundice that lasts a day or two. Two dangerous complications may result from hemolysis. A state of immediate shock may occur in which the patient has few symptoms except lethargy and low blood pressure. Death may occur in a few hours. More insidiously, the kidneys may be damaged so that the urinary output is less than 600 ml. in a 24-hour period. Complete cessation of urinary excretion is called transfusion anuria; when some urine, but an insufficient amount, is produced, it is termed oliguria. The prognosis is the same for both; normal urinary excretion may resume any time up to 3 or 4 weeks, or death may occur from renal failure.

Circulatory overload. This occurs when the increase in blood volume from transfusion causes acute cardiac failure and pulmonary edema. The patient suddenly becomes extremely short of breath, with wheezing respirations and cyanosis of the lips. When these signs occur, the transfusion should be discontinued at once and tourniquets (as described previously) placed on all four extremities. Preparation should also be made for a phlebotomy, which the physician may wish to perform.

Air embolism. This condition occurs rarely but it is possible whenever a leak is present in certain parts of the transfusion apparatus, or when all the blood has run out and air follows it into the vein. The patient has pain in the chest with severe dyspnea and cyanosis. The nurse can hear thumping in the heart at a distance. Prompt action may be life-saving. If this occurs, the transfusion should be discontinued and the physician notified. The patient should be placed on his left side so that the air bubbles float upward in the right ventricle away from the outlet to the lungs, and oxygen should be administered.

Delayed transfusion reactions

These need not concern the nurse directly but are mentioned for general information.

Transmission of disease. In the United States infectious hepatitis (serum type), or homologous serum jaundice, is the most common disease transmitted by transfusion. The donor is a carrier of the causative virus but usually has no clinical signs or symptoms of the disease; thus there is no method of excluding him from giving blood. The incubation period in the recipient is roughly from 60 to 120 days. The patient may become jaundiced with signs of severe liver damage, and there is considerable mortality. In some parts of the world transfusion malaria is a serious problem. With ordinary storage of blood the malarial parasites outlive the erythrocytes. The only method of preventing the disease is to reject all donors who have had untreated malaria within 5 years.

Transfusion syphilis is usually not possible to contract from blood that has been refrigerated for more than 2 days, because the causative treponemas are readily killed at low temperatures. Syphilis may be transmitted by transfusion of fresh blood when the donor has a chancre and enough time has not elapsed to confirm the diagnosis of syphilis by a positive Wassermann reaction. The disease differs from that acquired by physical contact in that when the blood of a syphilitic person is given to another person, the recipient will also acquire the disease but without the chancre. The incubation period of syphilis acquired in this manner is from 1 to 4 months.

Isosensitization of the recipient. If a patient does not possess a particular blood antigen, he or she may be sensitized when cells containing this antigen are received in transfusion. Antibodies gradually develop in the recipient over weeks and months, so that a succeeding transfusion with the same antigen results in destruction of the red blood cells. Women who are Rh-negative may also be sensitized from a fetus that received Rh-positive antigens from the father's genes. In this case the mother's antibodies may hemolyze the red blood cells of her infant to produce a disease called erythroblastosis fetalis. The red blood cells of a woman sensitized in this fashion will also hemolyze blood containing the antigen when it is received in transfusion.

Postoperative nursing care

A recovery room where intensive nursing care can be provided for the postoperative patient is almost a must in the modern hospital. Here the recovery room nurse can give undivided attention to the post-anesthetic patient. Constant observation for signs of shock and hemorrhage or for an obstructed airway is a vital part of the nurse's concern. The administration of blood or intravenous fluids started in the operating room usually continues in the immediate postoperative period. Emergency equipment and drugs are readily available and the timely use of suction and oxygen have greatly reduced postoperative hazards. Encouraging and helping the patient to cough and to breathe deeply at frequent intervals are almost routine postoperative orders. Use of a breathing tube to build up carbon dioxide is helpful when deep breathing and coughing are vital to the patient's welfare. In addition to a recovery room, many hospitals provide post-operative units or intensive care units, where the patient who has had major surgery may receive care for several days. By grouping these patients together in small units, superior and constant nursing care can be provided. Many postoperative complications can be prevented when good nursing care is provided the first few days after surgery.

In orthopedics it is absolutely essential for all patients other than those receiving surgery of the foot or hand and arm to have a firm bed. This frequently necessitates the placement of boards under the mattress. Preferably these boards are placed lengthwise, but when long boards are not available, the shorter ones may be placed across the bed. A sagging bed has no place in orthopedic nursing. Almost every type of postoperative patient will need one or more plastic-covered pillows. However, the use of large numbers of pillows never assures the safety or comfort of the patient in a cast. Care in the arrangement of pillows will frequently eliminate the need for a number of them. Body alignment should approximate the body align-ment desirable for all bed patients. The chest should be the part of the body farthest forward. All nurses know that this is true, because it applies to good posture in any position, but frequently they forget to apply it to the patient in the hip spica cast. The extremities should be supported along their entire length, not merely at one or two points such as the knee and heel. Pillows placed under the head should support the shoulders as well. If the head is to be elevated, one pillow should support the back from the lumbar spine to the shoulders and two pillows are arranged crosswise to support both shoulders and the head. A common error is to elevate head and chest without providing for this support under the back, and the result is that an actual bending of the body occurs just above the body section of the hip spica cast. This causes the edges of the cast to press against the soft portion of the abdomen and frequently results in a feeling of fullness and

pressure in the abdomen that is mistaken for distention. It will usually be found that once a pillow has been placed lengthwise under the cast to the sacrum, this troublesome feature can be eliminated.

Pillows should be arranged so that the leg portion of the spica cast is supported along its full length and no strain is imposed on the groin section, which is always vulnerable to cracking.

Following surgery on the foot or hand, it is usually necessary that the extremity be elevated to prevent edema. In some instances, the sur-geon may request that the part operated on be maintained at a higher level than the heart.

Long leg casts usually require three pillows for elevation or an overhead frame with one crossbar and a hammock that may be sus-pended from the frame. This will eliminate the use of pillows and ensure constant elevation of the limb (Figs. 2-64 and 2-65). Pillows may also be used to support the upper extremity; however, continuous elevation of the part is more likely to be maintained if the arm can be sus-pended from an overhead frame. When a cast has been applied to the forearm, muslin band-age may be used for this purpose and when a soft dressing has been applied to the hand, stockinet of the proper width and length may be slipped over the extremity. The proximal end of the stockinet is anchored to the upper arm. The distal portion extends beyond the fingers and can be used for suspending the extremity to the overhead frame. Holes will need to be cut in the stockinet to facilitate checking circu-lation in the fingers. When the forearm is sus-pended in this manner, the elbow and upper arm must be supported by the mattress or a pillow to prevent discomfort of the shoulder and undue pressure on the operative site.

When skeletal traction is being used, it is well to have the equipment for establishing traction at hand for immediate application. This will consist of pulleys for the foot of the bed, rope, footplate, and weights. An overhead frame or Braun-Böhler splint may be necessary. With all patients who are to have hip spica casts it is advisable to have the overhead frame ready with a trapeze for helping the patient to lift himself. For reconstructive operations on the hip a

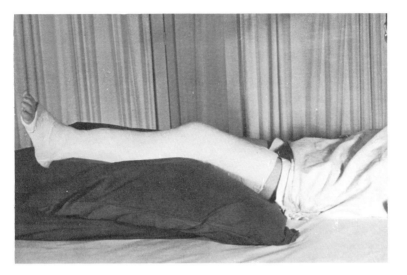

Fig. 2-64. Placement of pillows to support long leg cast. Note that the support is continued along the entire limb in order to eliminate strain on any muscle group. The patient's foot extends beyond the edge of the top pillow, thus preventing pressure or weight on the heel. With some patients it will be necessary to place a sandbag or trochanter roll along the lateral aspect of the thigh to prevent external rotation of the extremity. To prevent edema, the foot is maintained level with or higher than the knee and hip.

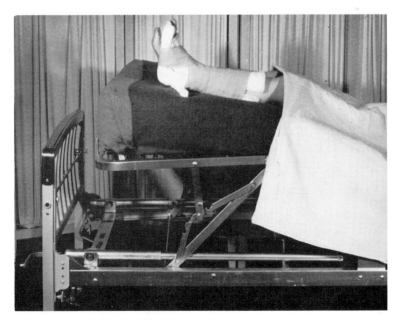

Fig. 2-65. With the type of bed illustrated, short leg casts may be elevated by raising the knee roll and the lower portion of the springs.

Thomas or Hodgen splint with a Pearson attachment or some modification of these will probably have been ordered by the doctor. The splint must be properly prepared with the Pearson attachment in place. Small towels, or preferably strips of bandage 6 inches wide, and at least 2 dozen safety pins are needed for preparing the Thomas splint. If desired, canvas strips and metal clips may be used in place of the towels and safety pins. Buck's extension equipment should be accessible if the nurse is not sure that it will be applied in the operating room.

After any type of orthopedic operation it is important that the nurse know the limitations of activity for the patient. This is essential for intelligent care, and it is as unwise to restrict the patient unnecessarily over a long period as it is to allow him more activity than the doctor wishes. Every orthopedic nurse should ascertain the limits for each patient. When and how often may he be turned? Will he be allowed to lie on his side with proper support, or is the prone position more advisable? May he have his backrest elevated at intervals? It is also advisable for the nurse to inspect the cast early. Are all the toes visible? Is the cast cut out enough around the buttocks for good care? (It is almost never necessary for the cast to come down over the gluteal crease, and if it is left in this fashion it is usually the result of oversight.)

It will be said many times in the course of this book that close observation of circulation in extremities in plaster is one of the nurse's chief responsibilities. To quote directly from Lovett and Jones, "Every plaster cast where there is any definite slowing of the return of blood in the fingers or toes or any considerable swelling of fingers or toes should be immediately bivalved, the lid removed, and all constricting soft bandages cut through. The latter point is more important."*

It must be remembered, too, that apparatus or casts applied for the remedy of acute conditions, such as fractures, osteomyelitis, or septic joints, may be followed, or rather are likely to be followed, by constriction and circulatory embarrassment as late as 3 or 4 days

afterward. The cardinal symptoms the orthopedic nurse should watch for are (1) pain, (2) color—cyanosis, anemia, or blanching, (3) swelling, (4) depressed local temperature, (5) diminished sensation, (6) loss of motion, and (7) sudden elevation of temperature that cannot be accounted for.

ORTHOPEDIC SURGICAL DRESSINGS

Dressing of orthopedic surgical wounds should be done by the most scrupulous technique. Patients with infected wounds should be segregated from those with clean ones, preferably in a different ward or room. Clean wounds are always dressed before infected ones, and there should be a separate dressing tray for each patient. Greater control of environment is, of course, possible if a special room is set aside for dressings. Wartime experiments showed conclusively that many hazards exist in wound dressings that were not formerly recognized as being important. For example, if clean and infected bone cases are housed in the same open ward, the bedclothing may be a source of contamination. Bedclothes contain great quantities of lint and dust, and if they are exposed to purulent discharges from wounds and dressings these particles may be loaded with bacteria. The gradual spread of certain strains of bacteria through an entire ward by this method was demonstrated forcefully during World War II.

For this reason some orthopedists make it a rule not to dress wounds until at least an hour after all the beds have been made, in order that dust and lint may have a chance to settle. Sweeping or dusting is never done during dressing periods. Even turning a patient in bed may be hazardous in that it will release quantities of lint and dust. Blankets and soiled linen should be carefully handled and never shaken in the ward as the beds are made. They should not be thrown on chairs or on the floor where dust and lint may be deposited. It is preferable to have containers for soiled linen in the ward, and place the linen in them immediately as it is removed from the bed. In some institutions nobody is admitted to the ward during the dressing period and windows and doors are kept closed. Doctors, nurses, and the

*From Jones, R., and Lovett, R. W.: Orthopedic surgery, Baltimore, 1929, Williams & Wilkins, Co.

patient wear masks while the dressing is being done.

Bandage scissors are sometimes a source of infection in surgical dressings. It is inexcusable to cut the outer dressings of both infected and clean wounds without disinfecting the scissors. In removing dressings it is wise to cut the bandage and remove it in one piece. Unwrapping soiled bandages may fill the surrounding air with bacteria-loaded lint that may infect other wounds. It is considered safer not to touch anything with the hands until the outer bandage is applied unless the hands have been washed in the meantime. All saturated dressings should be reenforced immediately after they are observed, and when the wound is a clean one, the reenforcement must be sterile to avoid contamination by capillary action. This means, of course, that the dressing should be applied with a sterile forceps. The practice of placing sterile dressings on a wound by hand is uniformly condemned by surgeons.

POSTOPERATIVE COMPLICATIONS

Nurses caring for patients who have had bone surgery should be familiar with the symptoms of fat embolism. This condition will usually occur within the first 24 hours but can be distinguished from symptoms of shock by the fact that it usually does not occur until 12 hours after surgery. When the pulmonary vessels are involved, symptoms are rapid breathing, increased pulse rate, and pallor followed by cyanosis. Some war surgeons have noted that the condition is often accompanied by petechiae over the chest and shoulders. If the fat embolus is in the brain, it will manifest itself in delirium, pupillary changes, twitching of the muscles, and coma. The condition is severe and frequently fatal. The patient must be kept absolutely quiet. If he is in a cast, no attempt should be made to remove it in trying to save his life. Intravenous therapy, heart stimulants, and artifical respiration may be ordered.

Thrombophlebitis may occur as the result of immobilization or enforced bed rest. The causes of this condition are a general slowing of the blood flow, collapse or compression of the veins, and endothelial damage. Complaints of pain in the calf of the leg, swelling, or heat and redness of the extremity should be reported immediately to the attending surgeon. Rest, avoidance of sudden movements, and elevation of the extremity are usually ordered as treatment. When an anticoagulant (heparin) is prescribed, frequent determination of clotting time is required. When Dicumarol is substituted for the heparin, measurements of prothrombin time daily or at other suitable periods of time are indicated. To prevent dislodgment of a clot the surgeon may desire to interrupt the involved vein or veins.

Pulmonary embolism is another grave complication that sometimes follows surgery. It comes on much later than fat embolism, usually in from 10 to 20 days, although it may occur much later. If the embolus is large, death may occur instantly. If there is a partial block, the patient will complain of sudden severe chest pain.

Gradual stretching of nerves may bring about epileptiform convulsions. These are not as grave as the convulsions that accompany fat embolism and occur later, usually from 2 to 6 days after operation. The dyspnea is slight; the pulse does not become increased; the respiratory rate is approximately normal, and recovery may be expected after 2 to 4 days. Treatment is removal of plaster and sedation.

The presence of backache after operation as a result of the complete relaxation of the muscles of the back during anesthesia is so commonly known that it seems hardly necessary to mention it. It is almost axiomatic that the lumbar spine be supported with a firm pad during anesthesia and after return to bed to prevent this disturbing postoperative complication.

Urine retention may occur in patients who have had orthopedic surgery. It is frequently necessary to catheterize adult patients who have had operations on the back or hip. This may continue to be a problem for several days postoperatively, and the utmost care must be taken to prevent cystitis or kidney infection.

It is not uncommon for the adult patient who has had a major orthopedic operation to have abdominal distention. Rectal tubes, enemas, and neostigmine methylsulfate may be ordered to relieve discomfort. In some instances relief is not obtained until gastric suction has been started.

The alert orthopedic nurse will provide measures to prevent postoperative pneumonia. This applies to any surgical patient but is of special importance for older persons. They must be encouraged to cough up mucus and to do deep-breathing exercises. Their position must be changed frequently, and as much activity as possible should be permitted.

The risk of operative intervention on spinal deformities of great extent (severe scoliosis or kyphosis) is increased by the effect these deformities have upon the rib cage, the lungs, and heart. The large vessels of the thorax, too, may be affected. Patients with severe scoliosis should be observed postoperatively for dyspnea, cyanosis, and edema of the lower extremities.

PREVENTION OF WOUND INFECTION

In surgery of bones and joints the greatest possible care is exercised to prevent infection. The outcome of most orthopedic operations depends largely on bone union, and bone will not unite in the presence of infection. Furthermore, the presence of postoperative infection of bones and joints often leads to lifelong crippling. For these reasons techniques used by nurses in preoperative skin preparation and in postoperative dressings should be as nearly faultless as possible.

The prevention of wound infection will depend to a large extent on attention to the following details:

1. Careful skin preparation preoperatively
2. Meticulous operating room techniques
3. Observation of wound site to keep dressings and cast intact and free from contamination
4. Careful wound dressing technique—masks, use of forceps rather than fingers, segregated space for dressings, and individual dressing trays
5. A clean ward for clean patients where no patients with infected bone conditions are housed simultaneously
6. Careful removal of any foreign bodies or dead tissue from wounds, since such foreign objects will increase the susceptibility to infection five-hundredfold

Postoperative drainage from clean surgical wounds should be reported by the nurse as soon as it is observed. Staining of the cast either by serum or by purulent drainage must be watched for. Immediate reenforcement of saturated dressings with a sterile pad so that capillary action will not bring about further contamination is important.

Children who have been walking barefoot are often predisposed to tetanus infection. When dirt is grimed into the soles of the feet before surgery, it is sometimes difficult to attain the surgical cleanliness desired. The physician should be informed of this circumstance. Occasionally, prophylactic antitoxin may be given to these patients before surgery is performed.

EARLY AMBULATION AFTER ORTHOPEDIC SURGERY

Although bed rest is being whittled down to very short periods in patients with surgical conditions that are not of the skeleton, a certain amount of recumbency is still indispensable for many orthopedic patients. Even in orthopedic wards the tendency is to promote as early ambulation as is compatible with the healing time of bone.

New sets of skills are necessary for the nurse who wishes to help the patient toward an early and uncomplicated convalescense; there is nothing helter-skelter about the procedure. It requires wisdom, understanding, and knowledge of new techniques. It is not merely a matter of saying "arise and walk." Equipment for preparing the patient for ambulation is seen in most hospitals today. One sees trapezes on many beds and portable overhead frames of lead piping on wheels, that make it possible for patients to exercise arms and shoulders for using crutches. Sawed-off crutches are often provided the badly affected patient for learning to manage crutches while he is still in bed. Footboards are used for support and for maintaining the standing reflex. Pulleys and ropes for resistive exercises are not uncommon. Printed lists of simple instructions for bed conditioning exercises prescribed by the physician are seen.

Present-day nurses know that standing is preferred to sitting for the patient's first out-of-bed periods, and they understand the relationship of the cough and the elimination of mucus to his welfare. Standing is almost always preferred to sitting in early rising after surgery. There are certain dangers that attend the patient who is allowed out of bed early only to sit for many hours in a chair. For patients who must sit, it is important to see that the seat is not too long, because a long seat causes pressure on the popliteal vessels, with the inevitable danger of thrombosis. A backward tilt to the seat is preferable because it serves to keep the hips from slipping forward toward the edge of the chair—a posture that encourages sagging shoulders and rounded back. The elderly thin patient must not sit with his legs crossed because of the danger of peroneal palsy from pressure on the very superficial peroneal nerve on the outer aspect of the knee.

Wheelchair restraints should provide a good sitting position for the patient. Hips should be maintained in contact with the back of the chair, and shoulders should be persuaded to an upright position so that stooping forward does not occur as the patient operates the chair.

No restraint is foolproof, and all of them need constant adjusting.

The procedure for getting a patient out of bed by having him turn to his side, flex his hips and knees as though sitting, and then swiveling him gently to the sitting position is entirely acceptable in orthopedic nursing. Unfortunately most orthopedic patients are encumbered with apparatus that makes getting up a much more complicated procedure. Nevertheless, adaptations may be made to fit the needs of each patient without too much difficulty if sufficient help is available.

STUDY QUESTIONS
Cast care

Nursing care of the patient in a cast must provide for patient comfort and safety, as well as the maintenance of a clean intact cast. Discuss the following factors as they relate to the care of the patient in a cast.

1. Circulation checks of part enclosed in the cast.
2. Preparation of the bed and proper placement of pillow to support the patient with a newly applied hip spica cast.
3. Provision for elevation of the extremity enclosed in plaster.
4. Checking of postoperative bleeding.
5. Method(s) of turning patient in a hip spica cast.
6. Placement of the patient with a hip spica cast on the bedpan.
7. Methods that may be used to finish the cast edges. Why is this necessary?
8. Provision for protecting the perineal area of the cast.
9. Methods that may be used to repair a soiled or blood-stained cast.
10. Instruction of the mother pertaining to care of the small child in a hip spica cast.
11. Skin care and positioning of the extremity following removal of a cast.

Traction

Many adaptations in the application of traction have been devised to provide proper treatment for the individual patient. However, if the nurse has an understanding of the basic modes of traction and principles involved, she will be able to meet the nursing needs of the traction patient, regardless of the variations that are necessary.

1. There are three basic modes of applying traction to a part of the body. These are referred to as manual, skin, and skeletal traction. Explain.
2. A variety of material is available, which may be used to apply traction. List and describe equipment available in your hospital for application of skin traction; skeletal traction.
3. The following types of traction usually refer to skin traction: Buck's extension, Russell traction, Bryant traction, and balance suspension traction. Review the equipment needed for each type and nursing implications.
4. Skeletal traction involves the use of head tongs, Kirschner wire, Steinmann pin, or other apparatus. Review nursing care of a specific patient pertaining to:
   (a) Application of this type of traction
   (b) Care of the patient wearing Crutchfield tongs (Chapter 5)
   (c) Care of the patient with skeletal traction applied to the femur
5. Discuss the following aspects of nursing care as they pertain to the traction patient. (Apply to a specific patient and type of traction.)
   (a) Prevention of skin irritation or development of pressure sores
   (b) Factors that may interfere with maintenance of continuous traction
   (c) Provision for correct body alignment
   (d) Prevention of secondary contractures
   (e) Patient activity that may be permitted
   (f) Maintenance of countertraction for the patient in head traction; for the patient with traction applied to the upper extremity; the lower extremity
   (g) Changing the bed linen and placement of bed covers to provide for warmth and coverage of the patient.

Crutch walking

1. Discuss several methods of measuring a patient for crutches.
2. What nerves and muscles are involved when "crutch paralysis" develops?

3. List the most important muscle groups used in crutch walking. Explain the various types of exercise that may be prescribed to strengthen these muscles.
4. Demonstrate the following crutch gaits:
   (a) Two-point
   (b) Three-point
   (c) Four-point
   (d) Swing-through
5. For what type of patient is each gait most likely to be prescribed?

REFERENCES

Alder, R. H., and Brodie, S. L.: Postoperative rebreathing aid, Am. J. Nurs. **68:**1287-1289, 1968.

Anderson, M. I.: Physiotherapeutic management of patients on continous traction, physiotherapy **58:** 51-54, 1972.

Bailey, J., Jr.: Tractions, suspensions, and a ringless splint, Am. J. Nurs. **70:**1724-1725, 1970.

Beaumont, E.: Wheelchairs, Nursing '73 **3:**48-57, Nov. 1973.

Beckwith, J.: Analysis of methods of teaching axillary crutch measurement, Phys. Ther. **45:**1060-1065, 1965.

Bonner, C., Hofkosh, J., Jebsen, R., and Neuhauser, C: Tips on choosing and using crutches, canes and walkers, Patient Care **2:**17-54, 1968.

Crenshaw, A. H., editor: Campbell's operative orthopaedics, ed. 5, St. Louis, 1971, The C. V. Mosby Co.

Dalton, A.: Using a Stryker frame, Am. J. Nurs. **64:**100-101, 1964.

DeVeber, G.: Fluid and electrolyte problems in the postoperative period, Nurs. Clin. North Am. **1:**275-284, 1966.

Dison, N. G.: An atlas of nursing techniques, ed. 2, St. Louis, 1971, The C. V. Mosby Co.

Foss, G.: Breaking the architectural barrier with crutches, wheelchairs, and walkers, Nursing '73 **3:**17-31, Oct. 1973.

Granger, C., Iannuzzi, N., Boivin, G., Yanasy, S., and Piatrowski, K.: Laminated plaster-plastic bandage splints, Arch. Phys. Med. **45:**585, 590, 1965.

Grant, W. R.: Aids to mobility: walking aids, wheelchairs, and hoists, Physiotherapy **52:**146-150, 1966.

Hicks, M. L.: Decubitus ulcers—alternating pressure pad, Am. J. Nurs. **58:**1008-1009, 1958.

Hrobsky, A.: The patient on a CircOlectric bed, Am. J. Nurs. **71:**2352-2353, 1971.

Jebsen, R. H.: Use and abuse of ambulation aids, J.A.M.A. **199:**63-68, 1967.

Jordan, H. H.: Orthopedic appliances, ed. 2, Springfield, Ill., 1963, Charles C Thomas, Publisher.

Kamenetz, H. L.: Selecting a wheelchair, Am. J. Nurs. **72:**100-101, 1972.

Kamenetz, H. L.: The wheelchair book—mobility for the disabled, Springfield, Ill., 1969, Charles C Thomas, Publisher.

Kerr, A.: Orthopedic nursing procedures, ed. 2, New York, 1969, Springer Publishing Co.

Knapp, M: Orthotics (bracing), Postgrad. Med. **43:**241-246, 1968.

Knapp, M.: Orthotics: bracing the lower extremity, Postgrad. Med. **43:**225-230, 1968.

Knapp, M.: Orthotics: bracing the upper extremity, Postgrad. Med. **43:**215-219, 1968.

Knocke, L.: Crutch walking, Am. J. Nurs. **61:**70-73, 1961.

Lane, P. A.: A mother's confession—home care of a toddler in a spica cast—what it's really like, Am. J. Nurs. **71:**2141-2143, 1971.

Latham, H. C.: Thrombophlebitis, Am. J. Nurs. **63:** 122-126, Sept., 1963.

Lehneis, H. R.: New developments in lower-limb orthotics through bioengineering, Arch. Phys. Med. Rehab. **53:**303-310, 1972.

Levenstein, B. P.: Intravenous therapy: a nursing speciality, Nurs. Clin. North Am. **1:**259-267, 1966.

Licht, S., and Kamenetz, H. L., editors: Orthotics etcetera, New Haven, 1966, Elizabeth Licht, Publisher.

Marmor, L., and Treach, J.: A new balanced suspension, Clin. Orthop. **85:**146-147, 1972.

Meyer, S.: Functional bandaging including splints and protective dressings, New York, 1967, American Elsevier Publishing Co.

Moore, F. D.: Blood transfusions: rates, routes and hazards, Nurs. Clin. North Am. **1:**285-294, 1966.

Narrow, B. W.: An hydraulic patient lifter, Am. J. Nurs. **60:**1273-1275, 1960.

Nayer, D. D.: They don't notice her wheelchair, Am. J. Nurs. **71:**1130-1133, 1971.

Owen, R.: Indication and contra-indications for limb traction, Physiotherapy **58:**44-45, 1972.

Peacock, B.: A myographic and photographic study of walking with crutches, Physiotherapy **52:**264-268, 1966.

Powell, M.: Application of limb traction and nursing management, Physiotherapy **58:**46-51, 1972.

Principles of lower extremity bracing, Phys. Ther. **47:** entire issue, Sept., 1967.

Ranalls, J.: Crutches and walkers, Nursing '72 **2:**21-24, 1972.

Raney, R. B., and Brashear, H. R.: Shad's handbook of orthopaedic surgery, ed. 8, St. Louis, 1971, The C. V. Mosby Co.

Rusk, H. A.: Rehabilitation medicine, ed. 3, St. Louis, 1971, The C. V. Mosby Co.

Sarno, J. E., and Lehneis, H. R.: Prescription considerations for plastic below-knee orthoses, Arch. of Phys. Med. **52:**503-510, 1971.

Schmeisser, G.: A clinical manual of orthopedic traction techniques, Philadelphia, 1963, W. B. Saunders Co.

Schneider, R. F.: Handbook for the orthopaedic assistant, St. Louis, 1972, The C. V. Mosby Co.

Senf, H. R.: Caring for the patient in the CircOlectric bed, Am. J. Nurs. **60:**227-230, 1960.

Shafer, K., Sawyer, J. R., McCluskey, A. M., Beck, E., and Phipps, W. J.: Medical-surgical nursing, ed. 5, St. Louis, 1971, The C. V. Mosby Co.

Smith, D. W., and Gips, C.: Care of the adult patient; medical-surgical nursing, ed. 3, Philadelphia, 1971, J. B. Lippincott Co.

Spiegler, J. H., and Goldberg, M. J.: The wheelchair as a permanent mode of mobility; a detailed guide to prescription, Part I, Am. J. Phys. Med. **47:**315-326, 1968; and Am. J. Phys. Med. **48:**25-37, 1969.

Stolov, W. C.: Progressive ambulation, Postgrad. Med. **47:**229-235, 1970.

Wiebe, A.: Orthopedics in nursing, Philadelphia, 1961, W. B. Saunders Co.

3

Rehabilitative aspects of orthopedic nursing

Rehabilitation as we know it envisions a total effort directed at restoration of the abilities of a physically handicapped person to lead a happy and useful life. Total effort means surgical correction, functional restoration through exercise, special education, vocational training, and finally, employment (Fig. 3-1). A team of doctors, nurses, physical and occupational therapists, speech therapists, social workers, educators, vocational and employment counselors combine their efforts to meet this responsibility. Rehabilitation, for the sake of discussion here, will refer to the medical segment of the total effort. Obviously, not all handicapped persons are equally capable of complete rehabilitation.

Many of the hospitals have established rehabilitation units where efforts on the purely physical elements of restoration can be concentrated. This includes medical direction of physical therapy, occupational therapy, speech therapy, brace-fitting, rehabilitative nursing, psychological evaluation, and on-the-spot work training. A pattern of treatment that will help achieve maximum rehabilitation is available for many physical defects, such as those that result from paraplegia, amputation, poliomyelitis, hemiplegia, and cerebral palsy. The Army rehabilitation centers in World War II showed how special exercises after acute trauma can hasten recovery. Graduated exercise programs, including heavy resistance exercises, are now commonplace therapy after surgical operations on bones and joints. The field is so broad that it would be impossible to outline all the details here, but discussion throughout this book will

include rehabilitation as applied to specific conditions.

DEVELOPMENT OF HEALTHY ATTITUDES TOWARD HANDICAPPED PERSONS

Irresponsible sentimentality and excessive sympathy are not conducive to rehabilitation. Nurses should avoid such shallow responses to the handicapped person. They must recognize and control their emotional reactions to physical disabilities. It is urgent that they avoid doing too much for the person. Rather they should work with the handicapped individual to encourage and help him to master doing things for himself. Threaded through orthopedic nursing is the need not only for helping the person with a handicap become capable of functioning independently but also for helping him to develop the desire and motivation to help himself. This thread must run through all nursing care for the handicapped and through teaching the patient's family. A nurse may feel a desire to protect and indulge the patient and care for his wants so solicitously that he has no need to do anything for himself. This urge is often even more potent among the family of the patient and may seem good and natural to them. To the parents, the rehabilitative procedures used for a handicapped child may seem almost cruel, and they may call the nurse heartless and unfeeling. Parents, in trying to create greater self-reliance in their crippled child by showing a little healthy neglect, may be criticized by their neighbors.

I once saw an 11-year-old boy with cerebral

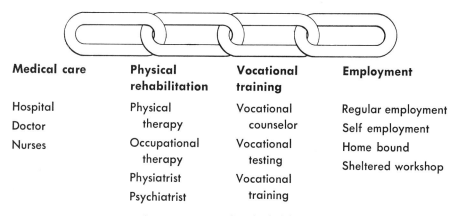

Medical care	Physical rehabilitation	Vocational training	Employment
Hospital	Physical therapy	Vocational counselor	Regular employment
Doctor	Occupational therapy	Vocational testing	Self employment
Nurses	Physiatrist	Vocational training	Home bound
	Psychiatrist		Sheltered workshop

Fig. 3-1. Concept of total rehabilitation.

palsy who was brought to a hospital by a mother who had cared for him in every detail since birth. He could neither walk nor talk beyond a few guttural noises. A year later, after an expensive course of treatment that included muscle re-education and intensive training in self-help, that boy left the hospital walking, unsteadily but still walking, on crutches. The mother had been told repeatedly by the nurses and doctors that all this expensive treatment must be continued faithfully at home. However, they had little hope. He was an only child; his father and mother were indulgent and emotional, and they adored him with what seemed excessive affection.

Two months later, across the street, I saw this boy walking on crutches, appearing as unsteady as a drunken man, his eyes fastened fiercely on the mailbox at the corner, which I guessed was his goal. Half a block away I saw his mother. She took on a sort of nobility to me that afternoon—walking slowly, no doubt conscious of every staggering unbalanced effort of her son, but walking half a block behind him. God knows what emotions of apprehension and agonized fright were in her heart. When he got to the mailbox, he stopped, turned around triumphantly, and waited for her to catch up with him. She came unhurried and, in attitude at least, calm and unperturbed.

To avoid over-protection of the handicapped person, one must teach him not only to care for his own needs insofar as he is able, but also to take responsibility for his mistakes and misdeeds equally with his more normal brothers and sisters. If the patient has had such training at home, the student nurse should recognize the importance of doing nothing to undermine it in spite of personal feelings. In many cases, the individual has not been taught these things at home. Occasionally tyrannical traits in the patient will be observed when his family visits him. The nurse should be aware that the incomparable experience in communal living that is given this overprotected person in an orthopedic ward is not the least of the benefits he may receive in the hospital. Sharing his pleasures with the other patients, in turn sharing theirs, and assuming his share of responsibility for misdemeanors will perhaps be new to him, but the nurse should recognize the opportunity to use these as first steps in his long fight for social and emotional maturity. The wise nurse points out and makes purposeful these problems in everyday living on the ward. Properly directed, the experience should be highly beneficial to the handicapped person. It should help him adjust to other disabled individuals and to normal companions. It should help to prepare him to live with greater harmony in his own family. It may serve also to help overcome a crippled attitude of mind—a more serious disability, after all, than a crippled spine.

THE REHABILITATION TEAM

In rehabilitation, the nurse always works as a member of a team. The team includes all those who are in some way contributing toward the total care of the patient, whether it be physical, psychologic, social, spiritual, or vocational. The team, always working under the leadership of the physician, may consist of the hospital nurse and assistants, the public health nurse, the psychologist, the physical and occupational therapists, the chaplain, the teacher, the social worker, the speech clinician, the vocational counselor, the parents or family, and, last but not least, the patient himself.

For everyone working with a team, it is of course extremely important that the common objectives be clearly recognized. It is equally important to learn how to work with people. It may often be necessary to subordinate one's own ego for the good of the whole group. The complete rehabilitation of a patient may require more of one group of workers than it does of another at certain stages of the program, but there are actually no stars on the team except the patient.

Rehabilitation teamwork demands that the nurse, particularly the hospital nurse, have long range perspectives. The period of time that the rehabilitation patient spends in the hospital is, as a rule, only a small episode compared with the long years that he may have been or will be disabled. The nurse should look both backward and forward. There was a time, before the disability occurred, when the patient lived as a normal member of a family and a community. Then the illness or accident happened that changed him from a normal person to one with a handicap. There may have been a period before he decided, perhaps with considerable anxiety and dread, to submit himself for treatment. Then there is a brief but intensive period of treatment in the hospital where nurses, occupational and physical therapists, and others work with the surgeon on physical restoration or on some reconstructive problem that in itself is only a beginning. He will then return to his home, his family, and his community to continue the treatment begun in the hospital. There may be a new group working with him, including perhaps the social worker, the public health nurse, and the visiting physical therapist. Other therapists in a sheltered workshop may help round out his functional recovery. It is a long road, and on it the rehabilitation patient meets many people working to help him.

The more aware hospital nurses are of the road the patient has traveled beforehand and of the distance he must go before reaching maximum recovery, the more intelligent and unselfish will be their contribution to the rehabilitation team.

It is sometimes difficult to work harmoniously with other groups when one is under pressure. Often it seems that there are endless conflicts in aims and methods and one may feel that there is a great deal of pulling in opposite directions. It is vital for the efficiency of the program that such conflicts be resolved as soon as they occur. Frequent conferences between groups with opportunities to discuss troublesome problems are bound to pay dividends in easier working relationships. The goal of all team members is the same: to assist the patient in his fight for recovery and rehabilitation (Fig. 3-2.)

What can the nurses do to promote better working relationships with other clinical groups?

First and most important, they can develop a cordial spirit for other people working in the rehabilitation area. Since nurses may feel more at home on the ward or unit, they are able to make other persons who work there feel comfortable and welcome.

Second, nurses must seek to learn as much as possible about the work of other clinical workers, including the aims of treatment of various team members, the problems, and many of the skills and therapeutic techniques that enter into the care of the patient. It will be necessary to encourage the patient to carry out correctly the instructions agreed upon by the team. Without follow-through, the relatively brief periods the patient spends with a therapist may be of little lasting value. The nurse must supervise the patient's practice of the exercises given him, or he may sometimes use slipshod methods, knowing that the therapist is not there to observe him. Also, the nurse must work with other team members and with the social worker to plan a coordinated home program to fit the needs and capabilities of the patient. Instructions given to family or patient at the time of discharge should be a joint responsibility, and conferences should be held frequently so that no overlapping or omissions will occur.

Third, the nurse should help prepare the patient to go to the occupational or physical therapy departments, to the school, or to the

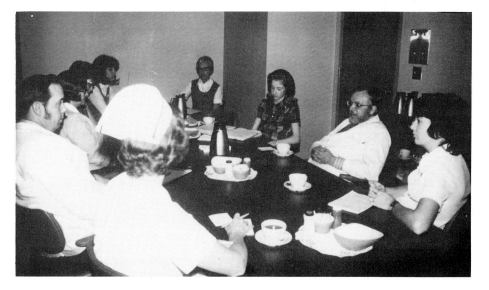

Fig. 3-2. In a rehabilitation team conference the physician, nurses, physical and occupational therapists, social worker, and speech clinician discuss the progress of a patient and plans for further care.

speech therapist by caring for his basic needs. He should be clean and dressed, and he should have had an opportunity to use the bedpan or urinal before he goes. If he is scheduled for walking exercises, his braces should be correctly applied and his crutches placed beside him. If he has had an enema that has not been fully expelled, the therapist should be notified before he is sent to the department. He should be sent there on time; if some unavoidable emergency makes this impossible, the department should be notified so that the therapist is given an opportunity to rearrange his schedule with as little time loss as possible. The attitude of ward personnel toward the therapy should be positive and cooperative.

It must be assumed that each worker on the rehabilitation team is trying sincerely to aid the patient's full recovery. However, unless one views the recovery process in its entirety, it may resemble a jigsaw puzzle with each worker concentrating on his own phase of the work to the exclusion of the others. The central theme is always the patient. He is the focal point. The pieces of the puzzle must be fitted together for his benefit with tolerance, understanding, and mutual respect. This will result in a coordinated program for the patient and in more satisfac-

tion and sense of accomplishment for the workers themselves.

The whole truth, Steindler once wrote, cannot come from a solitary voice. Similarly, planned rehabilitation does not come from a solitary pair of hands. The nurse who recognizes and wholeheartedly accepts this will occupy an important role on the rehabilitation team with great benefit to the patient and a feeling of professional satisfaction.

VARIOUS ASPECTS OF REHABILITATION NURSING

The basic principles and practices used in good nursing care are applicable and essential in rehabilitation nursing. In fact, they are the essence of rehabilitation nursing.

Good hygienic care is very important for the handicapped patient. It is not only conducive to good physical health but also has value in sustaining morale and sense of well being. The rehabilitation patient is taught and encouraged to care independently for as many of his personal needs as possible. Longer periods of time must be allowed for him to complete these activities. Considerable patience is required of the nurse who works with and encourages the disabled patient to manipulate his own toothbrush or

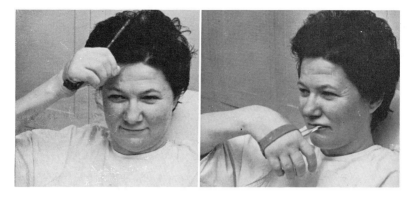

Fig. 3-3. By using the leather holder, this patient with guadriplegia is able to comb her hair and brush her teeth.

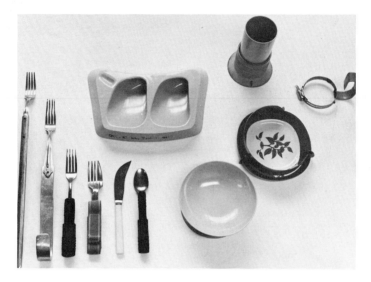

Fig. 3-4. Mechanical aids that facilitate self-feeding for the person who has weakness or paralysis of the muscles of the upper extremity. Suction-cup dishes that adhere to the table and have divided compartments make getting food onto the spoon easier. Padded or enlarged handles may make it possible for the disabled person to grasp the eating utensil.

cup or to manage his own brace. Which mechanical aids can be used? Can the patient with weakness of the upper extremities be taught to feed himself and to light his own cigarette? One no longer concentrates on doing things to or for the patient but thinks in terms of how the patient might do it for himself (Figs. 3-3 to 3-5).

Maintaining good nutrition is important in the care of the rehabilitation patient. A strenuous exercise program increases his nutritional requirements. The paralyzed patient needs adequate intake of protein to help prevent breakdown of the skin and underlying tissues. The individual with an arm or hand disability may experience fatigue when feeding himself and not consume an adequate diet unless help is offered. The problems of the overweight patient must not be forgotten. Extra pounds may make ambulation impossible. At mealtime the nurse who understands what the rehabilitee is being taught by the occupational therapist can help him practice self-feeding. If he can learn to feed himself, mealtime can become a sociable hour. This is important for the handi-

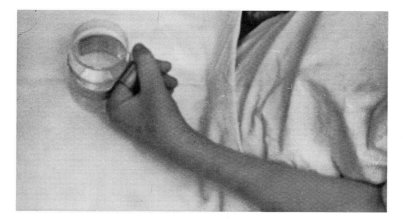

Fig. 3-5. This glass holder enables the person who is unable to grasp objects with his fingers to drink from a glass.

capped person attempting to find his place in family and community life. A dining room equipped with tables that accommodate wheelchairs provides a more normal situation for practicing the activities of daily living.

Prevention of decubitus ulcers is another important aspect of rehabilitation nursing. Many patients are paralyzed in one extremity, or more. Frequently, incontinence is a problem. One or both of these factors make the maintenance of healthy skin a real challenge to nursing personnel (Fig. 3-6). Frequent change of the patient's position (every 1 or 2 hours) is important to relieve pressure. Protection of bony areas with foam rubber, flotation pads, or a water bed and the maintenance of a clean dry bed are necessary nursing measures if pressure lesions are to be prevented. This sounds simple, but to maintain this 24 hours a day requires the vigilance of all nursing personnel, constant teaching of new personnel, and an adequate amount of nursing help.

Regardless of the cause of disability, the prevention of deformity is important from the onset. Emphasis is placed on teaching the handicapped individual and his family how joint deformity can be prevented. "An ounce of prevention is worth a pound of cure" was never more applicable than in the prevention of secondary joint deformity. Those of us who have seen patients spend weeks receiving treatment directed at the correction of contractures, to say nothing of the pain endured, can appreciate the importance of their prevention. Applying knowledge of

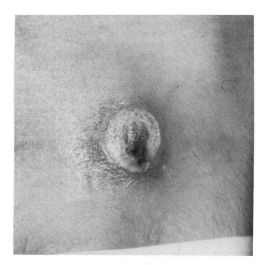

Fig. 3-6. Sacral decubitus ulcer in a quadriplegic patient. Muscle paralysis, sensory loss, leakage from a Foley catheter, and failure to turn the patient frequently were contributory factors leading to this lesion.

proper body alignment, providing for frequent change of position, and maintaining a normal range of joint motion are necessary if deformity is to be prevented.

During the bath, the nurse can easily perform simple passive exercises of the involved extremities to help maintain normal range of motion. As the axillary region is bathed, the arm is moved away (abduction) from the patient's side. Bending and straightening the elbow provides flexion and extension. The movements of the wrist, plus closing and opening the hand for finger flexion and extension, can be accomplished nicely as the extremity is bathed and dried. Raising and lowering the leg and bending the knee provide for flexion and extension of the hip and knee joints. Moving the leg toward the edge of the bed helps maintain the motion of abduction, and rolling the hip inward provides for internal rotation. Simple dorsiflexion of the foot during the bath procedure will help prevent tightening of the heel cord (Achilles tendon). These joint motions carried out by the nurse who knows how to correctly support and move a paralyzed extremity can be most helpful in preventing joint contractures.

In addition to exercises of the involved extremities by the nurse or therapist, the disabled patient is taught and encouraged to do simple exercises of the uninvolved extremities himself

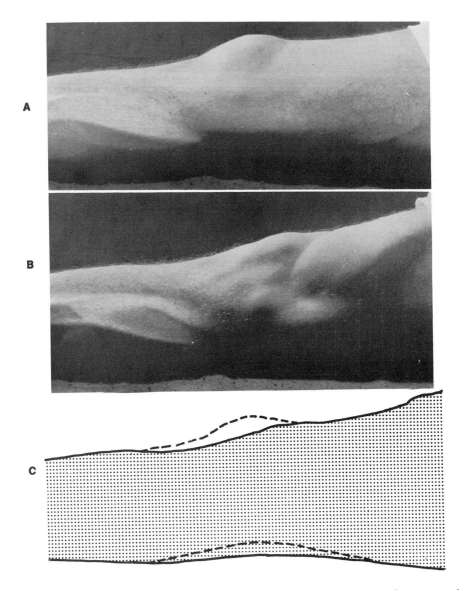

Fig. 3-7. Quadriceps-setting exercise. **A,** Relaxed thigh and knee joint. **B,** Quadriceps muscle located on the anterior thigh is tightened and shortened, moving the patella proximally. **C,** Movement of patella proximally and pressing of popliteal space against the mattress. (**A** and **B** from Gould, M. L.: Amer. J. Nurs. **56:**577-582, 1956.)

early in the course of his care. Such exercises are valuable in improving circulation, in maintaining muscle strength, and in preventing tightness of tendons and limitation of joint motion.

While working with the patient, the nurse should observe whether the patient is able to plantarflex and also if he is able to turn his foot inward (inversion) and to pull his foot up (dorsiflexion). These activities are valuable in preventing drop foot deformity and tightness of the heel cord.

Can the patient tighten the quadriceps muscle? This muscle, located on the anterior portion of the thigh, enables one to extend and stabilize the knee, and it is important in maintaining erect posture. The quadriceps setting exercise is taught with the patient in the supine position and with the limb in extension. He is instructed to contract the muscles on the anterior portion of the thigh so that the kneecap is drawn upward toward the thigh. He maintains the muscle contraction for 5 seconds and then allows the muscle to relax for 5 seconds. The physician may request that the patient do this exercise for 5 minutes every hour during the waking day. Straight leg raising is another exercise frequently prescribed to strengthen the quadriceps muscle. In the supine position, with the knee in extension and the foot in a neutral position, the patient lifts the limb off the bed. At first this is difficult, but with practice the limb is raised to

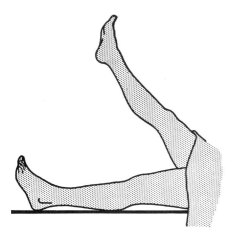

Fig. 3-8. Performing straight leg–raising exercises develops the strength of the quadriceps muscle. (From Gould, M. L.: Amer. J. Nurs. **56:**577-582, 1956.)

approximately a 45 degree angle with the body. This position is held for several seconds, then the limb is lowered slowly (Figs. 3-7 and 3-8).

If tightness of the hamstrings (flexion contracture) is to be prevented, the knee joint should not be supported continuously in a flexed position. The position of extension must be secured at frequent intervals.

Does the patient lie or sit with his limb in a position of external rotation? A sandbag or trochanter roll placed along the lateral aspect of the thigh will encourage him to maintain his limb in a neutral position. Does he like to have the backrest elevated, or does he sit in a chair for long periods? To avoid flexion contractures of the hips, he needs to lie flat (on a firm mattress) with the hips in full extension. Can he abduct and externally rotate his arms to tie his gown strings and comb his hair, or have his pectoral muscles become too tight?

Is full extension of the cervical spine attained at intervals throughout the day and night, or is the patient lying with marked flexion of the neck? Frequently, patients like the flexed position because it enables them to see the ward. However, the nurse should remember that maintaining this position for long periods of time promotes poor posture and impairs normal respiratory expansion.

There is no better place than the ward for the rehabilitation patient to practice activities of daily living. Whether the task is learning to dress, brushing his teeth, getting from the bed to a chair, or performing exercises in preparation for walking on crutches, the nurse who keeps informed of the plan of treatment and the progress that the patient is making can render valuable assistance to the patient and the other members on the rehabilitation team by carryover of the program to the ward.

It is essential that those on the rehabilitation team have knowledge of local, state, federal, and private resources that may be utilized in rehabilitation. During recent years, many facilities have been made available. As the number of personnel trained in rehabilitation increases, assistance to the disabled person will increase in many places. The worker who keeps informed of available resources can offer the patient valuable assistance in meeting his complex needs.

Text continued on p. 140.

EVALUATION OF DAILY LIVING ACTIVITIES
OCCUPATIONAL THERAPY

Name_____Birth date_____Age_____Sex____

Address/Hospital No._____

Diagnosis_____Date onset_____

Vocation_____Handedness_____

KEY
(Scores indicate skill accomplished within a reasonable time)
0—Cannot be accomplished
1—Can be accomplished with human aid
2—Can be accomplished with adaptation of environment (low bed, special toilet
   seat, handrails, ramps, etc.)
3—Can be accomplished with use of mechanical aids (splints, braces, prostheses,
   crutches, wheelchair, etc.)
4—Can be accomplished without aids, adaptation, or assistance
*—Not practical (time, too much supervision required)
N.A.—Not applicable to this patient

Date and √ form on initial test.
Any changes in status from initial test should be dated.

HOME SITUATION
Note suggestions for adaptation next to each line or check when so indicated. In special
instances, diagram of layout will be advisable.

Location: City_____Rural_____

Travel: Own car____Hand controls____Taxi____Bus____

Apartment: Floor____Rooms____Elevator____Self-service____None____Walk up_____

Private house: Floors____Rooms____Stairs____Elevator____Self-service____None_____

Entrance: Door____Step____Railing:____right____left____none____Ramp____

Bathroom: Door____OK for wheelchair____Tub____Shower over tub____Stall shower___

Note type of floors: Bedroom____Living room____Kitchen____Bath____

Information unavailable (explain)

Assistive devices

I. BED ACTIVITIES

	0	1	2	3	4
1. Moving in bed: Roll to right____to left____					
2. Turn onto abdomen____					
3. Come to sitting position____					
4. Sit erect in bed (LSP)____					
5. Sit on edge of bed (SSP)____					
6. Adjust blanket, sheets, etc.____					
7.____					

II. WHEELCHAIR SKILLS

	0	1	2	3	4
1. Bed to wheelchair; wheelchair to bed____					
Method____					
2. Propel chair____					
Number of feet____					
3. Lock/unlock brakes____					
4. Raise/lower footrests____					
5. Open, close, and pass through door____					
Type of door____					
6. Pick up objects off floor____					
7. Transfer to/from straight chair____					
At table____					
Standing free____					
8. Transfer to/from easy chair/couch____					
9. Transfer to/from toilet____					
Method____					
10. Transfer to/from car____					
11. Get from wheelchair to floor, from floor to wheelchair____					
12.____					

III. PERSONAL HYGIENE

	0	1	2	3	4
1. Comb/brush hair____					
2. Set hair____					
3. Brush teeth or clean dentures____					
4. Apply toothpaste to brush____					
5. Shave/put on cosmetics____					
6. Care for fingernails/toenails____					
7. Use handkerchief____					
8. Give self bed bath____					
Unable to reach____					
9. Dry thoroughly with towel____					
10. Use of shower____					
11. Get into/out of bath____					
12. Toilet____					
Method____					
Flush toilet____					
Use of toilet paper____					
Adjust clothing____					
Use urinal/bedpan____					
13. Manage catheter:					
Independent care____					
Clamp off/unclamp____					
Empty SP bag____					
14. Feminine hygiene____					
15.____					

	0	1	2	3	4

IV. DRESSING

1. Put on/remove bra_____
   How? What method_____
2. Put on/remove shorts, panties_____
   Method_____ standing, on bed, seated
3. Put on/remove slipover garments_____
   Method_____ standing, on bed, seated
4. Put on/remove button shirt_____
   Method_____ standing, on bed, seated
5. Put on/remove slacks or pants_____
   Method_____ standing, on bed, seated
6. Put on/remove socks or hose_____
   Method_____ standing, on bed, seated
7. Put on/remove shoes_____
   Method_____ standing, on bed, seated
8. Lace/unlace shoes_____
9. Tie/untie laces_____
10. Hook/unhook garters/suspenders_____
    Front_____
    Back_____
11. Fasten/unfasten buckle_____
12. Button/unbutton_____
    Little_____
    Big_____
    Circle location—front, side, back
13. Fasten/unfasten snap_____
14. Fasten/unfasten zipper_____
    Circle location—front, side
15. Fasten/unfasten hooks and eyes_____
16. Tie/untie necktie_____
17. Fasten/unfasten safety pin_____
    Small_____
    Large_____
18._____

V. APPARATUS

1. Put on/remove braces _____
2. Lock/unlock braces _____
3. Put on/remove splints, feeders, slings _____
4. Put on/remove corset _____
   Type of lacing _____
5. _____

VI. EATING

1. Eat with fingers/sandwich_____
2. Eat liquids with spoon_____
3. Eat with fork/cut with fork_____
4. Cut with knife_____
5. Butter bread_____
6. Drink from glass, cup, paper cup_____
7. Pour liquid from milk carton/pour liquid from
   bedside pitcher_____
8. Open carton of milk_____
9._____
10._____

VII. AMBULATION	0	1	2	3	4
1. Walks _____					
2. Stand and work at table_____					
Regular table_____					
Stand-up table_____					
3. Walks with package_____					
4. Get up from floor when falls_____					
With crutches_____					
Without crutches_____					
5._____					

VIII. UTILITIES	0	1	2	3	4
1. Write:					
Legibly_____					
Name and address_____					
Copy paragraph_____					
2. Turn pages of book/magazine_____					
3. Cut with scissors_____					
4. Open a package of cigarettes_____					
5. Light a match/lighter_____					
6. Pick up change_____					
7. Make correct change_____					
8. Telephone:_____					
Standing_____					
From wheelchair_____					
Hold receiver_____					
Dial_____					
Use coins_____					
9. Wind watch_____					
10. Open/close windows_____					
11. Open/close drawers_____					
12. A.D.L. Board check-out_____					
Height of board_____					

Numbers accomplished

_____ _____
_____ _____
_____ _____

SUMMARY

Therapist's signature _____

FAMILY AND JOB ADJUSTMENTS

Teaching the patient and his family is an important aspect of rehabilitation. The patient is taught that good skin care is essential to prevent pressure areas. He learns that his position must be changed and that wrinkles and crumbs may cause breaks in the skin. He inspects his skin for redness or blisters that may come from shoes or braces. He knows that poor position may result in deformity and that lack of exercise may lead to stiff joints. He recognizes the necessity for adequate intake of fluid for the prevention of kidney stones, and he learns how to care for his bladder catheter properly. He practices applying his brace, dressing himself, and taking care of his personal needs. To be successful, rehabilitation must be a learning process for the patient and his family. The disabled person must learn to accomplish many of the activities of daily living by new methods.

The nurse on the rehabilitation team has an excellent opportunity to know and understand the patient and his family. She recognizes that the family members as well as the patient experience emotional strain and need to make adjustments. How do they react to the situation? Through this period of adjustment a trained clinical psychologist can help the family and patient in resolving emotional problems and apprehensions. However, the rehabilitation worker recognizes that the patient and his family must be realistic about his disabilities. False hopes must not be fostered. It must be realized that certain impairments may persist but that remaining abilities and capacities can be defined, guided, and developed. The regime of treatment should give the patient the opportunity and motivation to do as much for himself as possible. This includes the privilege of making his own decisions and taking responsibility for his own acts. Day-by-day improvement may seem very small. Discouragement and an attitude of futility must be combated from the beginning.

To the extent possible, ordinary activities required for independent daily living must be painstakingly relearned by the patient. These will include sitting, bending, turning, getting out of bed, walking, climbing stairs, putting on clothes and braces, and managing all personal care. The program to develop these skills may be complex. Experience and a high degree of skill are required to teach them effectively. Nurses should know what system of rehabilitation is being employed so that they may constantly encourage and instruct the patient in his struggle for physical independence.

As has been indicated, there are other factors in the total rehabilitation of patients, particularly those concerning family, social, and job adjustments, which are also very imporant. The advancements made since World War II have been heartening. In many types of jobs, it has been discovered that a handicapped person can contribute as much as a physically normal person. Sheltered workshops and shops attached to hospital wards have been set up in some communities and are used by local industries for piecework, such as construction of radio and airplane parts. Weaving, watch repairing, typing, printing, metal and leather crafts, painting, and wood carving may provide work for patients with severe orthopedic handicaps and have, in many instances, given them a means of earning a livelihood. Factories in many communities have sent small machinery to hospital workshops to be assembled by handicapped patients. Watch and radio repairing are within the grasp of all but the most severely affected patients.

Family acceptance of the severely handicapped person, with an understanding of his need to live his own life as much as is possible, is one of the most important factors in the total rehabilitation program. All of the splendid work accomplished in the hospitals and workshops can be nullified in the home if oversolicitousness, rejection, or pity is evident to the patient. Nurses will need the help of social workers and social agencies to work out problems of family adjustment.

The problem of caring for an occasional disabled patient is indeed a perplexing one for nurses. If they are cognizant of the dangers and armed with knowledge of means to overcome them, they will play an important part in his early physical rehabilitation. Their initial efforts may help keep the patient alive. If they are imbued with a determination to help the handicapped patient become as independent as possible, they should be able to secure assistance from others to aid the patient at various stages of his progress.

OCCUPATIONAL THERAPY IN ORTHOPEDICS

By definition "occupational therapy is the art and science of directing man's responses to selected activity to promote and maintain health, to prevent disability, to evaluate behavior and to treat or train patients with physical psychosocial dysfunction."* The primary goal of an occupational therapist for an orthopedic patient is restoration of physical function. For each patient this may include restoring joint motion, regaining muscle strength, or improving coordination. The general aims with all patients are the development of work tolerance, socioeconomic adjustment, and prevocational testing (Figs. 3-9 to 3-17).

Certainly, psychologic manifestations must not be overlooked in the orthopedic patient. The tendency of a patient to withdraw from society or to dwell on pain and problems suggests he has not made a healthy adjustment. The occu-

---

*Official definition adopted by the Delegate Assembly of the American Occupational Therapy Association. Am. J. Occup. Ther. **24:**324, 1970.

pational therapist substitutes an activity for inactivity, thus helping to prevent such regression and promoting a better adjustment.

The media used in accomplishing these objectives are varied. Frequently a wrong impression is created when a patient busy with a craft is observed. The craft is noticed; the activity is not. The *occupational* of occupational therapy is not the project the patient is working on, nor is it his vocation or avocation outside the hospital; rather, it is the *occupation* or activity of mind and body. Use of arts and crafts is a valuable method employed by the occupational therapist, but it is only one of many. Adapted recreational activities and self-help training in bathing, dressing, and feeding skills are other important methods. Writing, use of the telephone, manipulation of doors, latches, and dials, and similar activities of daily living are taught to the handicapped patient (Fig. 3-18). The media are selected with the specific patient in mind. The referring physician's aim and the patient's impairment, interests, background, age, sex, and many other factors must be carefully considered.

Occupational therapy plays a coordinating role in the total rehabilitation of a patient. It bridges the gap from hospitalization to life outside the hospital by enabling the patient to improve his

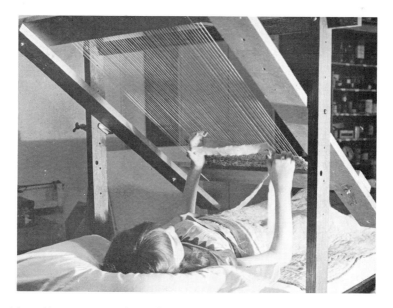

Fig. 3-9. Adjustable rug-weaving frame for use by the bed patient. This type of activity not only appeals to the patient but also provides valuable exercise for fingers, wrists, elbows, and shoulders afflicted with arthritis.

ability to care for himself and to carry out activities utilizing the movements or actions learned in physical therapy. Occupational therapy helps to prevent the disability that often results from disuse; it encourages the development of latent abilities; it trains the patient in prevocational skills, and it develops work tolerance.

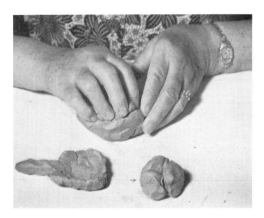

Fig. 3-10. Using modeling clay for finger mobilization. Sponge rubber may also be used to strengthen finger muscles.

DIVERSIONAL THERAPY

The importance of diversional treatment in occupational therapy should be appreciated. The nurse should be aware of the hazards of prolonged, enforced idleness. The handicapped person hospitalized for long periods often has too little to do and too much time to think and worry. This is often associated with depression and excessive complaints and demands. Under such circumstances diversional activity may be invaluable to keep the individual occupied and partially fulfill his need to feel productive. Diversional therapy should not be considered only a frill or luxury. It may be much more therapeutic for the patient than many of the daily nursing routines, such as the bath, which occupy so much of the attention of the nurse. In rehabilitation, activities performed by the patient himself are usually more important than things done to or for him.

EDUCATION FOR THE CHILD WITH A HANDICAP

In considering the future of a handicapped youngster, the nurse should understand that education for the disabled child (Fig. 3-19) is

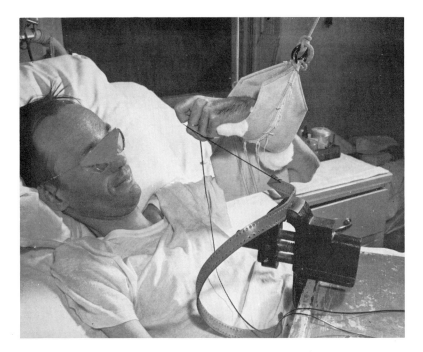

Fig. 3-11. Arrangement of belt-making equipment for the bed patient. This activity provides muscle-strengthening exercises and joint motion for the fingers and arm.

imperative—perhaps more even than for his normal brother. Many means of self-sufficiency and self-support available to the normal person are barred to the handicapped. A handicapped person must be better prepared to fulfill even limited types of occupation. The student should understand that the newest concept of vocational guidance and placement emphasizes the versatility rather than the limitations of crippled individuals. Perhaps the student may one day imbue earnest members of some civic group with an urge to help the handicapped, to take upon themselves responsibility for the higher education of some homebound child. Services are generally available for the homebound child through two-way radio class communication as well as home teacher service provided by the public school system.

PHYSICAL THERAPY

Physical therapy may be defined as the science that deals with the management of disease by means of physical agents such as light, heat, cold, water, electricity, mechanical agents, and therapeutic exercise.

From ancient times the principles of physical therapy have been employed but not always on a scientific basis. The practices of lying in the sun, rubbing a bruised muscle, and bathing a wound in a woodland stream have led through the years to the development of present methods of treatment. These have an important function and are well recognized in most hospitals today.

Thermal therapy

Heat. Heat is a commonly employed form of treatment. It is often used before massage and exercise and seems to enhance the other treatment measures. Physiologic effects of the various types of heat that may be used are similar. External application of heat results in increased temperature of the tissues, vasodilatation, and increased blood flow. Local metabolic activity is increased. Heat tends to relieve pain and muscular tension.

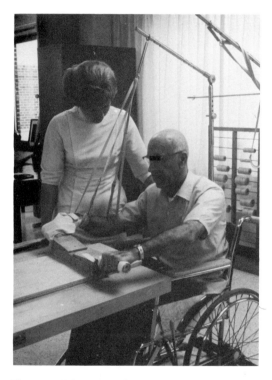

Fig. 3-12. Bilateral sanding used as reciprocal exercise for the arms. The overhead suspension sling supports the weaker arm.

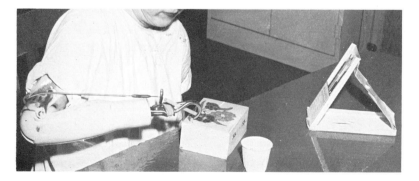

Fig. 3-13. Patient with upper extremity amputation learning to perform fine movements with prosthetic appliance.

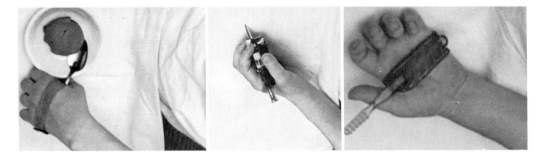

Fig. 3-14. The leather holder with a pocket for holding a spoon, pencil, or other utensil is helpful for the person who has lost the use of the small muscles of the hand but still has some shoulder and elbow motion.

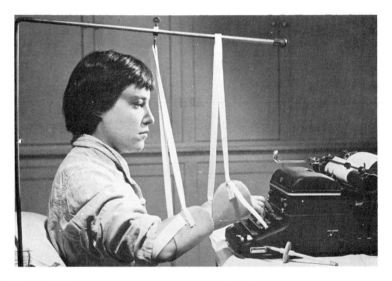

Fig. 3-15. The disabled person who possesses the use of her fingers but has weakness or paralysis of the arm and shoulder muscles may find this supension sling helpful in performing activities of daily living.

SUPERFICIAL HEAT. Any object hotter than its surroundings will give off infrared rays. The infrared lamp is a simple way to apply local heat. There are various kinds and sizes of infrared lamps. The energy output that reaches the patient depends on the wattage of the lamp, the distance from the lamp to the patient, the angle at which the rays strike the patient, and the total area irradiated. Infrared radiation includes the light radiation from 7,700 to 120,000 Å. The amount used in physical therapy usually ranges from 1,200 to 1,500 mμ. This includes no bacteriocidal rays. The main effect consists of heating the local area. Smaller infrared lamps are

usually placed 14 to 18 inches from the skin, larger ones, 24 to 30 inches. The patient should feel comfortably warm but not hot.

Infrared radiation is used in the treatment of arthritis, bursitis, fibrositis, muscle strain, and muscle spasm. It is a convenient way to apply heat at home.

Infrared treatment should not be given following large doses of deep irradiation because serious burns sometimes result.

Hot packs. Many types of hot packs are used in hospitals and at home. One of the most convenient is a very heavy Turkish towel—or two Turkish towels sewed together—heated in boiling water and then quickly wrung out so that as little steam as possible escapes. The pack is then wrapped into a 40-inch square of wool blanket. The patient's skin is not touched by the hot towels but only by the dry wool with the steam coming through it. There is no danger of burning the patient if he is carefully dried between the applications of packs. While one set of packs is on the patient, another set should be boiling. The first set is left on for 3 to 4 minutes, and then the second is applied. Three or four changes are usually needed. These packs are easily applied to almost any area of the body, either by laying the pack on the area or by wrapping it. They have been found very beneficial in treating muscle spasm, strains, sprains, arthritis, and bursitis. Many hospitals prefer hot packs for heat over any other available method (Fig. 3-20).

In addition to the conventional method of applying moist hot packs, commercially prepared compresses or packs with automatic heating units are available. These retain heat for 20 to 30 minutes and eliminate the task of wringing hot water from packs. Such packs are removed from the unit, wrapped in several layers

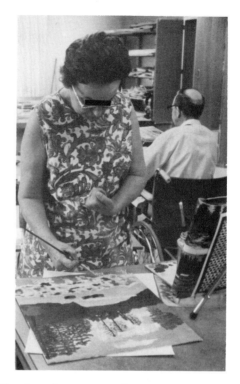

Fig. 3-16. Painting provides practice in fine finger coordination for this patient with posttraumatic cerebral dysfunction.

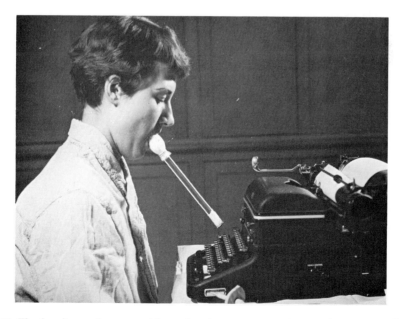

Fig. 3-17. The handicapped person with paralyzed upper extremities may learn to use the typewriter by utilizing a mouth stick. The stick is made of plastic material and has plastic-covered padding, which facilitates holding it in the mouth and provides protection for the teeth.

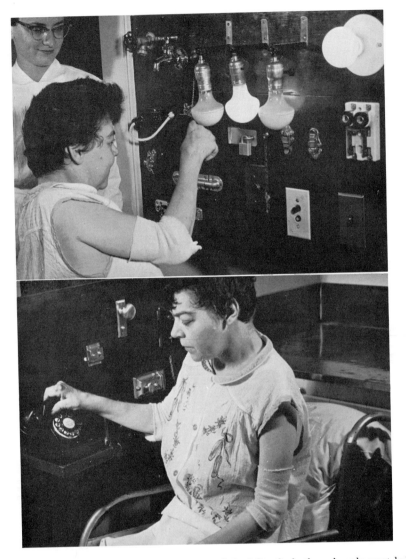

Fig. 3-18. The person with shoulder, elbow, or hand disability finds these boards most helpful in practicing and mastering activities essential to everyday living. The boards may be raised or lowered and contain such articles as light switches, water faucets, doorknobs, locks, and telephone.

of terry cloth, and applied to the desired area. These packs can be obtained in several sizes and are well suited for use in the home as well as the hospital, when there is need for repeated application of moist heat.

Paraffin. Melted paraffin to which mineral oil has been added is very satisfactory as a method of applying heat. The melted paraffin is kept at a temperature between 124° and 132° F. If the paraffin is completely melted and has a little scum on the surface, the temperature is correct. Paraffin is an especially satisfactory method of heating the hand or arm afflicted with arthritis. The extremity is dipped into the paraffin six to ten times until a thick coat (⅛ inch) is obtained. This, carefully wrapped in a bath towel or bath blanket, will hold the heat 20 to 30 minutes. The paraffin can also be painted on the involved area. If alternate layers of paraffin and gauze are used, the resulting pack may hold heat for more than an hour.

Paraffin is used chiefly for arthritis, bursitis, fibrositis, or contractures of the hand. Following the paraffin treatment the treated area is well

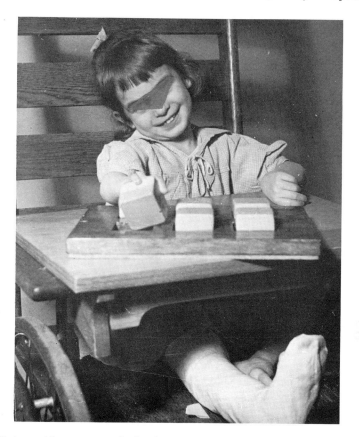

Fig. 3-19. Patient with spastic cerebral palsy using educational toys for eye-hand coordination exercise.

prepared for massage and exercise. Paraffin-dip treatment can easily be carried out at home by heating the paraffin in a double boiler and using the scum test as a temperature guide. A candy thermometer should be used to check the temperature (Fig. 3-21).

DEEP HEAT. Subcutaneous fat is a poor conductor of heat. Superficial heating is inadequate for heating deeper tissues. To obtain deeper tissue heating, certain forms of physical energy are used. They are able to penetrate skin and subcutaneous tissue without damage and are changed into heat in the deeper tissues. Types in common use at present are shortwave and microwave diathermy and ultrasound.

Shortwave diathermy. High frequency current is used for deep heating. The resistance of the tissues to the currents forced through them generates heat. An induction cable is employed to create an electromagnetic field. The cable can be either wrapped around the part to be treated or coiled to make a flat applicator. Shortwave diathermy is limited to wavelengths of 3 to 30 meters with frequencies of 10 to 100 megacycles. As the high frequency current enters the body it tends to spread so a fairly large area is heated. A padding of toweling ½ inch to 2 inches thick is used between the skin and electrodes to absorb perspiration and prevent burning. Physiologically, the effects of shortwave diathermy are identical with the effects of other types of heat. The only difference is that the hyperemia produced by shortwave lasts longer and deeper layers of tissues are penetrated.

Diathermy is used for treatment of chronic sinusitis, mild inflammation of bone, joint, and muscle, chronic osteomyelitis, and various forms of arthritis and bursitis. High-frequency currents are also used surgically. Fulguration and electrodesiccation are used to destroy warts and

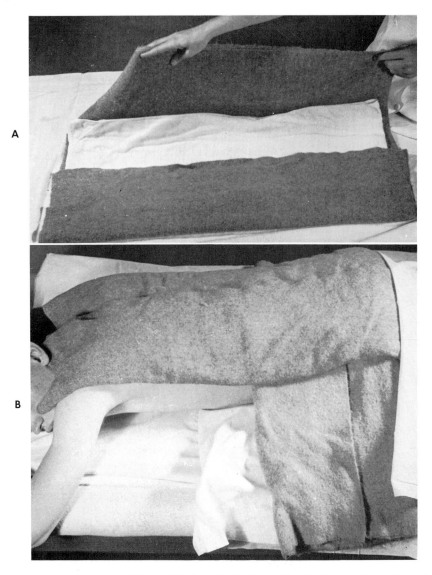

Fig. 3-20. A, A steaming hot towel being folded inside the dry woolen blanket. **B,** Hot packs applied to the back for pain in the lower portion of the back.

small skin blemishes. Electrocoagulation is used to remove larger tumors and to stop bleeding (Fig. 3-22).

Microwave diathermy. Radiated electromagnetic waves are utilized. Machines provide a wave length of 12.2 cm. at a frequency of 2,450 megacycles per second. The director of the machine provides focusing, several inches from the skin surface. The heating effect is greater in tissues with high water content.

Ultrasound. The energy for ultrasound thera-

py consists of mechanical vibrations with frequency from 0.7 to 1 megacycle. These waves do not travel through air, so direct contact with the skin is necessary. A coupling jelly is used between the applicator and the skin. Ultrasound may provide heating of tissue at a depth up to 5 cm. (Fig. 3-23).

Cold. Therapeutic cold has been of more limited value than heat. Local applications of cold causes vasoconstriction, decreased blood flow, decrease in local tissue metabolic activity,

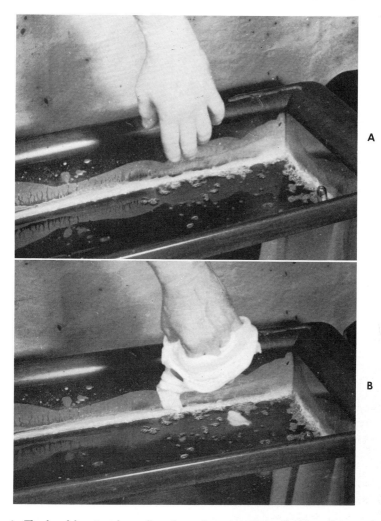

A

B

Fig. 3-21. A, The hand has just been dipped ten times into the melted paraffin. **B,** The paraffin glove is being removed. This may be put back into the paraffin bath and remelted.

and decrease in local temperature. The response varies depending on the nature and temperature of the coolant applied, duration of the application, and the area treated.

Brief application of cold produces transient vasoconstriction followed by vasodilatation, increased blood flow, and local effects that resemble those following heat. Cold is sometimes used to replace heat treatments in patients who tolerate heat poorly.

Ice bags, cold bath, or compresses are often used to minimize the initial reaction of tissues to injury, for example, sprain. Refrigeration of tissues can induce local anesthesia. Intense cold (for example, liquid nitrogen) produces tissue destruction and is sometimes used to treat certain skin lesions.

Hydrotherapy

Hydrotherapy consists of the use of therapeutic pools, the Hubbard tank, whirlpools, contrast baths, sprays and douches, and hot packs.

Therapeutic pools. To be most useful, a therapeutic pool should be 12 to 15 feet wide and 20 to 24 feet long. It should have walking bars and

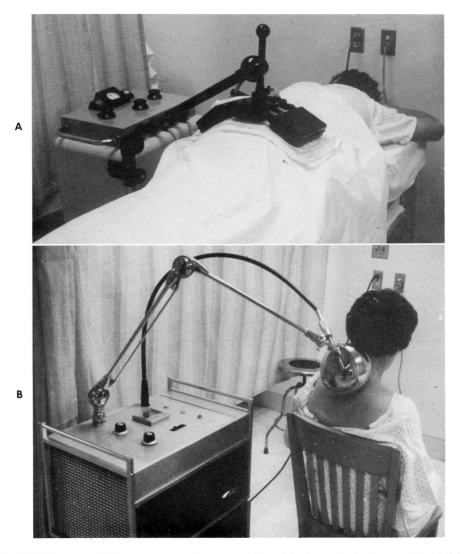

Fig. 3-22. Short wave diathermy treatment being administered for **A,** low back strain and **B,** painful neck muscle spasm.

proper depth to permit walking practice for the patients. The temperature of the water depends on the amount of activity the patient will perform, the age and diagnosis of the patient, and the length of time the patient will be in the water. If the program is one essentially for exercise, the water should be between 80° and 95° F. If a heating effect is desired, the temperature can be as high as 102° F.

Therapeutic pools have proved very valuable in treating patients convalescing from poliomyelitis and children with cerebral palsy. The buoyancy of the water makes it possible for a child to use a weakened muscle through a greater range of motion. Patients can use walking bars in the pool earlier than outside because of the buoyancy of the water. The heat of the water raises the pain threshold so that the patient can tolerate stretching exercises more easily. Both the buoyancy and the heat encourage relaxation of the cerebral palsy patient, and he can perform his exercises with more ease. In addition to the physical and physiologic benefits from a therapeutic pool, the psychologic lift to the patient is very valuable (Fig. 3-24).

Hubbard tank. The shape of the Hubbard

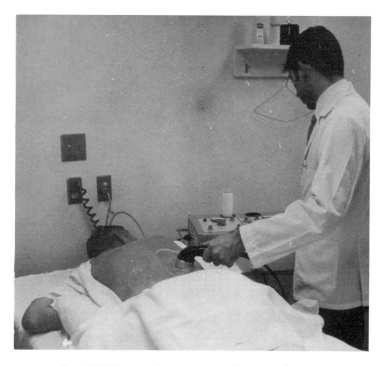

Fig. 3-23. Ultrasound treatment to relieve muscle pain.

tank is such that it permits exercise movements of the arms and legs that are not possible in an ordinary tub (Fig. 3-25). The water temperature is usually kept at about 99° to 100° F. for exercise and 102° F. for heating. Although a Hubbard tank is not as satisfactory as a therapeutic pool for exercise, it is frequently employed. Since it is not necessary for the therapist to be in the pool to treat the patient, as in a therapeutic pool, the Hubbard tank may be more practical as far as the personnel are concerned. Sometimes a whirlpool agitator is placed in the tank.

Whirlpools. The temperature of the water in the whirlpool is maintained between 100° and 110° F, usually 105° F. The air pressure coming into the water gives a swirling, gentle massaging action to the water. Whirlpools are especially valuable in treating patients with fractures or after tendon or ligament surgery. The whirlpool treatment makes it much easier to clean dry scaly skin from affected areas, increases circulation to the part, and tends to relieve pain and stiffness. Whirlpools are also used in the treatment of burns and amputations that are not completely healed. In these cases a mild anti-septic solution is often added to the water. Children can be put into the whirlpool tank for general heating of the entire body prior to stretching and exercises. Whirlpool treatment for patients with arthritis has proved very helpful in relieving pain and stiffness (Fig. 3-26).

Contrast baths. In contrast baths the patient's feet or hands are moved alternately from hot to cold tubs of water. The temperature in the hot tubs ranges from 100° to 105° F. and in the cold tubs from 65° to 70° F. Immersion should begin and end in hot water—4 minutes in hot water and 1 minute in cold water. Seven to nine immersions are usually given. The treatment is generally used for arthritis and peripheral vascular disease and preceding massage and exercise for sprains and contusions.

Ultraviolet radiation

Ultraviolet radiation is in the range of the light spectrum from 1,800 to 3,900 Å. It can be produced by several artificial sources, including the hot quartz mercury lamp, the cold quartz lamp, or the carbon arc. The dosage is governed by the minimal erythema dose (M.E.D.), which

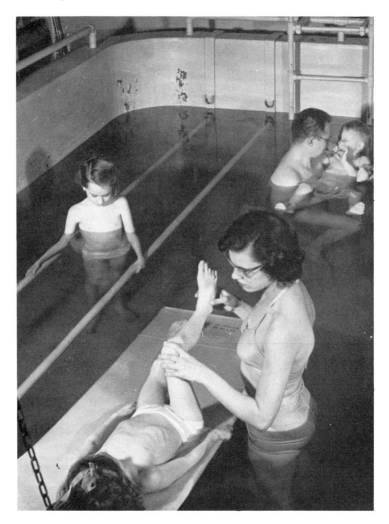

Fig. 3-24. By the use of this canvas table, routine stretching exercises as well as underwater exercises and walking practice can be given in the pool.

is defined as the shortest exposure at a certain distance that will produce a preceptible reddening of the skin that occurs within 6 to 8 hours after treatment and that will disappear within 24 hours. Care must be taken to cover the eyes of the patient with moistened pledgets of gauze or cotton, and the operator must wear goggles. Conjunctivitis could result from neglect of these precautions (Fig. 3-27).

The aforementioned erythema with resulting increase in local circulation and the well-known bacteriocidal effect of ultraviolet radiation govern its indications. It is extensively used in the treatment of decubitus ulcers, infected superficial wounds, and many skin diseases. It has been shown to produce antirachitic effects by increasing vitamin D production in the skin.

Electrical stimulation

Each electrical stimulation machine will give a variety of currents or combinations. The main currents used are galvanic and faradic. Galvanic and direct current stimulates the muscle and therefore causes a response even when nerves have been damaged. Faradic or alternating current stimulates the nerve and stimulates the muscle only when it has a normal nerve supply. These currents and their various combinations and derivatives can be used as testing devices to determine whether or not the nerve to the

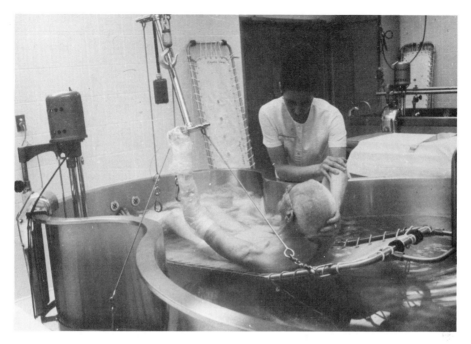

Fig. 3-25. The therapist is giving exercises to the patient in the Hubbard tank.

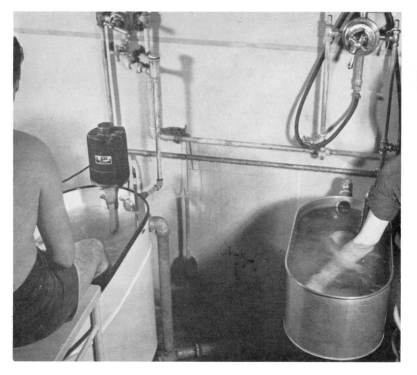

Fig. 3-26. Leg and arm whirlpools.

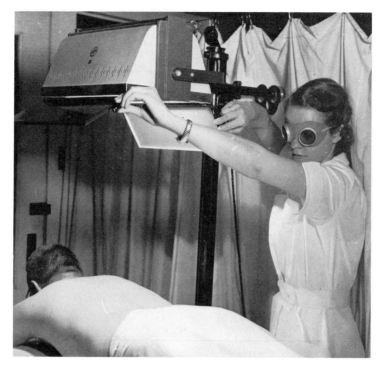

Fig. 3-27. Ultraviolet lamp being opened for an exposure to the back.

muscle is normal. If it is damaged, the extent of the damage and the rate of nerve regeneration can be determined. Electrical stimulation may cause muscle contractions something like voluntary activity, producing approximately the same metabolic effects. This has proved valuable as a form of exercise to avoid muscle atrophy in denervated muscles.

Massage

Massage is the term applied to the systematic and scientific manipulation of body tissues for remedial and restorative purposes. For effective application of massage it is essential that one have (1) adequate knowledge of muscle, joint, and nerve anatomy of the affected part; (2) a knowledge of the desired effects; and (3) a skillfull technique and understanding of the various strokes.

Physiologic effects of massage on the skin include a sedative effect on the peripheral sensory nerves, reflex stimulation of motor nerves, a temporary hyperemia, and a cleansing of the epidermis. The main effect on the muscles is the hastening of the removal of metabolites from the muscle, which helps relieve fatigue and spasm. Massage will not increase muscle strength. Only active exercise can do that. Depending on the intensity of the stimuli, massage can produce either a sedative or a stimulating effect on the nervous system. It has been shown that massage definitely increases the pain threshold; this is apparently related to the counterirritant phenomenon. Since the lymph circulatory system is entirely dependent upon external pressures (normally, muscle contraction and joint movement), massage has proved valuable in moving lymph fluid in patients with edematous conditions. Massage has a minimal effect on venous or arterial flow; the pumping action of the heart is a much more adequate means of circulating the blood. Massage produces no significant change in red or white blood cell count or in the hemoglobin. Massage cannot rub away excess fatty tissue. Massage is highly effective in stretching excessive fibrous tissue in subcutaneous areas.

The massage technique is generally based on the following four strokes:

1. *Effleurage* consists of stroking the surface

of the skin. The amount of pressure is varied to make it a light or heavy stroking.

2. *Petrissage* is the kneading of the soft tissues.

3. *Friction* is applied by rotary movements of the skin over underlying tissue. The thumb or fingers are kept in firm contact with the skin, and the movement is between the skin and superficial tissue and the underlying structures.

4. *Tapotement* consists of a percussion-type movement against bodily tissues. This type of massage has very little place in the treatment of pathologic conditions because it is too heavy.

To get the best results from a massage, the patient should be in a comfortable relaxed position. The part to be massaged must be supported and completely uncovered, and the rest of the patient's body carefully draped. The operator should be in a comfortable working position. Once the massage is started, the therapist's hands maintain contact with the part being massaged until the massage is completed. The stroking pattern generally follows the muscle groups. The rhythm should be slow and steady, the pressure gentle but firm. The heaviest pressure is on the upward stroke (toward the heart, centripetal in direction), and the return stroke is very light. Massage should never be painful. Pain is the prime contraindication for massage. Cold cream is generally preferred as a lubricant, although cocoa butter is often used for burned or scarred areas, and talcum powder is used over hairy surfaces. Any baby oil, olive oil, or mineral oil may be used.

Massage is used in the treatment of patients with arthritis, fibrositis, edema, and traumatic conditions such as sprains and strains, fractures, burns, amputations, and muscle spasm. Massage should not be given to anyone having any acute inflammatory process, skin eruption, malignancy, or fever.

THERAPEUTIC EXERCISE

One of the principal aims of therapeutic exercise is to maintain or restore the functional activities of the individual at the highest level possible. This can be accomplished through various types of exercises. Exercises are classified as follows: passive, active assistive, active, and resistive.

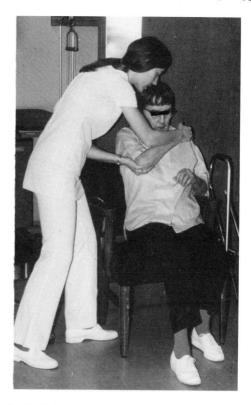

Fig. 3-28. Passive exercise for paralyzed arm is administered with some stretching for proprioceptive stimulation to help elicit reflex muscle contraction.

Passive exercise. Passive exercise is the movement of joints and associated tissues (bones, muscles, tendons, and other soft tissues) of various parts of the body by the application of external force, supplied either manually by the therapist or by some kind of mechanical device. This kind of exercise is employed when the patient is unable to perform active exercises. The chief purposes of passive exercise are (1) to promote circulation in the parts being exercised; (2) to maintain or increase range of motion of the joints; and (3) to counteract the development of adhesions and contractures (Fig. 3-28).

Active assistive exercise. Active assistive exercise is an exercise in which the patient is assisted in the performance of active movement. The assistance may be either manual (provided by the therapist) or mechanical (supplied by pulleys, weights, elastic bands, or slings). Such assistance is usually given to counterbalance the force of gravity acting on the extremity and

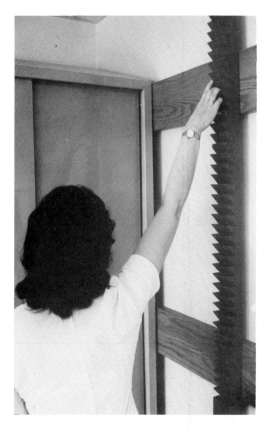

Fig. 3-29. Active shoulder exercises with a finger ladder.

thus assist the weakened muscles in performing the exercise. The assistance should be minimal so that the muscle is performing at its maximum strength.

Active exercise. Active exercise is executed by the patient himself, using his own muscles without additional resistance. Nurses reinforce active exercises when they have the patient bathe himself, take care of his toilet needs, dress himself, and so forth (Figs. 3-29 to 3-31).

Resistive exercise. Resistive exercise is active exercise performed by the patient against an external resistive force (Figs. 3-32 and 3-33). Resistive exercises are either manual resistive exercise or progressive resistive exercise. In early stages of muscle strengthening, manual resistive exercises are the most useful because they allow the therapist to apply and regulate the resistance given throughout the active movement, direct the movement properly, and eliminate any muscle substitution. Progressive resistive exercises employ maximal contraction of muscles. These exercises enable the patient to increase muscle strength and muscle bulk (hypertrophy), increase efficiency of muscle contraction, and improve muscle coordination through facilitation. Progressive resistive exercises may be done with the use of iron weights,

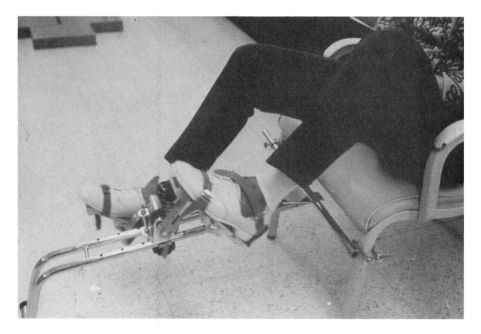

Fig. 3-30. Active reciprocal motion exercise for the legs using a restorator attached to a chair.

sandbags, elastic bands, or vigorous underwater activity. These exercises should be performed in progression after the therapist has determined the maximum load. The pattern of progression is ten repetitions with 50% maximum load, ten repetitions with 75% maximum load, and then ten repetitions with 100% of maximum load. As strength improves, the resistance used is increased in increments.

To obtain the best results from these exercises, the patient should perform them twice daily for as long as is necessary. In many cases the exercises must be continued at home after discharge from the hospital. The therapist will

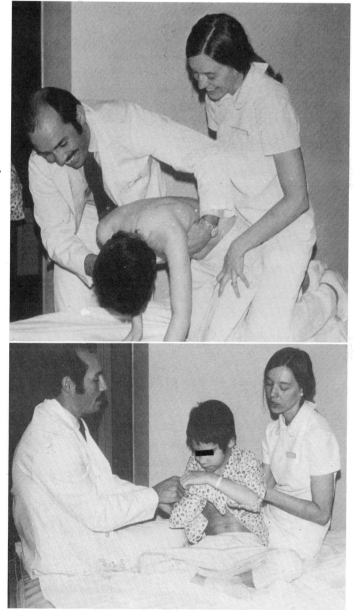

Fig. 3-31. Youngster with brain damage performing active exercise learning to balance in **A,** crawl and **B,** sitting position.

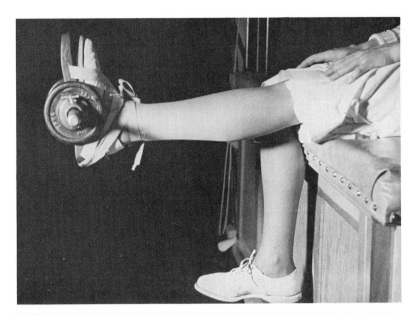

Fig. 3-32. Resistance exercise for the quadriceps muscle. Starting position for this exercise is sitting with the legs over the edge of the table with a rolled towel placed under the knee for proper support. The leg being exercised is then raised to the position shown, held there for a few seconds, and slowly lowered.

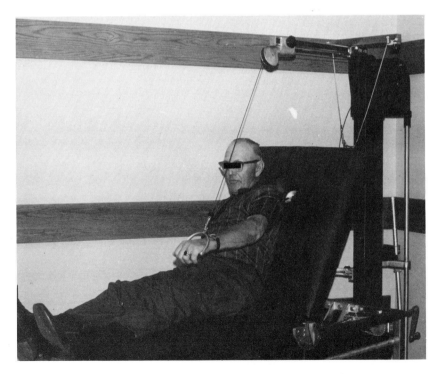

Fig. 3-33. Resistive exercise for shoulder extension. An exercise table is utilized. Resistance can be increased by adding more weights at the head of the table.

instruct the patient or the family concerning both the proper technique to use and the length of time to continue the exercises.

The scope of therapeutic exercise is broad. It includes the following:

1. Coordination exercises for patients with multiple sclerosis, cerebral palsy, or cerebellar ataxia
2. Muscle-strengthening exercises for those with various orthopedic and neurologic disorders
3. Exercises designed to prevent deformity, such as range of motion activity for patient with arthritis
4. Exercises to correct deformity, such as heel cord contracture
5. Activities to maintain mobility of joint and muscle, such as stretching for patients with Guillain-Barré syndrome
6. Exercises given for esthetic effect, as in the treatment of patients with postural defects
7. Exercises used to provide relief from pain, as in patients with pain in the lower portion of the back
8. Exercises given to teach patients to relax
9. Respiratory exercises that will increase vital capacity

In England much work has been done with breathing exercises for patients with asthma. Some patients have been able to increase their breathing during attacks and in many cases to prevent attacks. Exercises given for peripheral vascular disease may improve the efficiency of the circulatory system.

Let us briefly follow a patient in his attempt to ambulate after 4 months in traction because of a hip fracture. During the past several weeks the therapist has had the patient perform a series of arm-strengthening exercises and isometric exercises of the involved extremity in preparation for ambulation. The first step may be use of the tilt table where the patient is acclimated to the vertical position. He may be given crutches to take some of the weight off his feet while on the tilt table. When the patient tolerates the tilt table in a vertical position for 30 minutes, he is advanced to parallel bars, where he learns the proper gait and balance. The bars are more stable than crutches, and thus the patient develops confidence in his walking ability. When he can walk several lengths of the parallel bars, he is fitted properly with crutches. Once he learns the proper gait and develops some skill and endurance in handling crutches outside the parallel bars, he is taught how to get into and out of a chair, to go up and down stairs, to walk backward and sideways, and to open and close doors. A person on crutches can learn to be very independent and capable of taking care of himself in almost any circumstance. This pattern of teaching a patient to be ambulatory is in evidence at many stages every day in a physical therapy department.

CARE OF THE PATIENT WITH SPINAL CORD INJURY

Spinal cord injuries are becoming more common with high-speed automobile accidents and trauma from falls, athletic injuries, and gunshot wounds. With improved techniques of care in the acute phase after the injury, such as better control of shock, tracheostomies to assist breathing and clearing the airway, and treatment of multiple injuries, these patients are surviving to require long-term rehabilitation and ultimately to go home to a new way of life. It is vital that rehabilitative measures be started from the earliest days in the hospital to prevent complicating problems that might severely limit the patient's ultimate functional capacity. The following discussion describes measures that make a great difference in the level of function and quality of daily life the person with a spinal cord injury can achieve. They are primarily preventive and require a great deal of conscientious thought.

A patient with a fractured spine and with spinal cord involvement presents what may be truly called a major nursing problem. Fractures of the spine may, of course, exist without cord injury, but patients do not then constitute so great a nursing problem as those with associated cord injury. Attention will therefore be concentrated primarily on the more severe type of injury where cord involvement is present. Nurses caring for patients who have paraplegia or quadriplegia from spinal cord injury must constantly remember that urinary sepsis and pressure sores are common causes of death in this condition.

MANAGEMENT OF THE BLADDER

Injury to the spinal cord is almost invariably accompanied by disturbances in the bowel and bladder function. Nerves located at or below the spinal cord injury no longer function. Messages to and from the brain are lost. Consequently, the cerebrum does not receive sensations indicating need to empty the bladder. Thus, the person with a spinal cord injury is not able to exercise conscious control of voiding. After injury, a state of spinal shock exists, and during this time the bladder is atonic and incapable of emptying itself. As the patient recovers from spinal shock after weeks or months, reflex activity below the level of injury may develop. As this reflex activity returns, some bladder emptying capacity may be regained. The final result may be a neurogenic bladder that may be spastic or continue to be flaccid. The spastic bladder is very irritable and unable to retain significant urine volume; the flaccid bladder retains large volumes of urine and occasionally partially empties by "overflow."

Protection of the urinary tract from infection and prevention of overstretching of the bladder should begin immediately after admission of these patients. Almost all patients will require catheterization. Usually an indwelling Foley catheter is used. In some centers a straight catheter has been utilized every 4 to 6 hours. However, if the bladder is not catheterized on time,

overdistention may produce permanent damage to the muscle of the bladder wall. Reflux from the bladder into the ureters or residual urine left in the bladder increases the dangers of urinary infection and the formation of urinary calculi. During the period of catheter drainage, measures to prevent urinary infection and the development of urinary calculi are very important.

Aseptic technique is important during catheterization procedures and when caring for the bladder. The newer Silastic catheters result in less encrustation and stone formation. In some cases, a three-channel catheter may be utilized so that a closed system of continuous bladder irrigation can be set up. The bladder may also be irrigated intermittently. Sterile solutions of .25% ascetic acid or other acid mixtures, of dilute aqueous benzalkonium chloride (Zephiran) or of dilute anti-infective agents may be used for bladder irrigation.

A high fluid intake (3,000 to 5,000 ml.) is prescribed to help prevent precipitation of the salts that tend to form urinary calculi. Keeping the urine dilute also helps prevent infection. Maintenance of an acid urine is also desirable since it provides a less favorable medium for growth of bacteria and tends to prevent precipitation of calcium.

Frequent changing of the patient's position is helpful in preventing stasis of urine in the kidney pelvis. Also, it is known that weight-bearing stress decreases the amount of calcium lost from the skeletal system. Thus, the early use of the tilt table is valuable. In addition to the nursing procedures, antibacterial agents are frequently used to prevent or control infection.

After the first few days, some physicians will ask that intermittent drainage be instituted, in contrast to straight drainage. The filling and emptying of the bladder helps preserve the elasticity of the bladder musculature and maintain a usable bladder capacity. However, there is some dispute regarding this point, because some physicians feel that reflux into the ureters may occur while the catheter is clamped for 2 to 3 hours.

A cystometrogram may be performed to determine the amount of bladder muscle function present. If a bladder-training program is prescribed, the indwelling catheter is removed and emptying of the bladder is attempted at regular intervals. The nurse must remember that after removal of the catheter it is necessary to learn whether the patient is emptying his bladder sufficiently. Catheterization for residual urine at intervals may be ordered by the attending physician. If the residual is too great, damage to the kidneys may be caused by vesicoureteral reflux. High residual urine also increases the possibility of infection.

The training process to establish an automatic bladder is slow and requires much patience and continuous effort by the patient, doctor, and nursing personnel. Provision must be made for emptying the bladder at designated times, before the quantity of urine in the bladder induces spontaneous voiding. By trial and error and control of fluid intake, the patient learns how long he can go between voidings and remain dry. He learns to recognize symptoms such as abdominal discomfort, chills, or restlessness as indicative of need to empty his bladder. Micturition may be induced by such measures as manual pressure on the bladder (Credé method), by straining, or by other trigger mechanisms the patient may find effective. For some males a condom catheter may be used if the bladder empties well but the pattern of voiding remains unpredictable.

If the establishment of an automatic bladder is not successful, it will be necessary to resort to the use of continuous catheter drainage. The female will frequently tolerate an indwelling urethral catheter for months or years. Males have much more difficulty because of the high incidence of urethritis. If a urethral catheter is not tolerated, an alternate route of drainage must be provided such as suprapubic cystostomy or an ileal loop or pouch. With the catheter or with any of these other procedures, there remains an increased incidence of infection so that the steps mentioned previously regarding control of infection apply here as well. The appearance of chills, fever, or bloody urine or inability to irrigate the catheter is an indication for the patient to seek medical advice promtly. How frequently a catheter is changed depends upon the kinds of urinary problems the patient is having and the attending physician's orders. The catheter in the suprapubic cystostomy

is cared for in a manner similar to that of the urethral indwelling type. Strict asepsis, twice daily irrigations with a bacteriostatic agent such as 0.25% acetic acid, and cleaning around the orifice followed by a light dressing are required. Ileal loops require an appliance to be glued to the skin around the orifice and held in place by a strap around the trunk. These usually need to be changed every 3 to 6 days, depending on the patient's activity. As with the catheters, they may be connected to a leg bag or to bedside drainage. Either of these diversional drainage devices works well in the prone position as long as the tube is not bent acutely.

BOWEL TRAINING

Like bladder training, bowel training is an essential aspect of the care of the paraplegic or quadriplegic patient. One thing that will help the patient who is on a prescribed bowel-training program is establishing a definite time of day for use of the bedpan, commode, or toilet. The time chosen should take into consideration the patient's work day, his eventual return to gainful employment, and his usual bowel habit. Provision for privacy encourages relaxation, and abdominal massage or pressure downward toward the sigmoid and rectum may be helpful in stimulating peristalsis and defecation. Exercise, as with the normal individual, is beneficial.

The diet should include a normal amount of bulky foods; however, it must be remembered that an excessive amount of high-residue food can cause loose stools and disturb a regulated bowel pattern. A fecal moistening agent is frequently prescribed for the patient with a spinal cord injury.

In establishing a pattern it is frequently found necessary to use suppositories at a regular interval. This can be once daily or at 2- or 3-day intervals. Depending on the amount of sensation or reflex established, the use of bisacodyl (Dulcolax) or glycerin suppository may be required to maintain the habit. With a gloved finger, the suppository should be inserted high in the rectum above the internal sphincter against the bowel wall. As the suppository melts, the rectal mucosa is irritated and peristalsis is stimulated. Twenty minutes to 2 hours may elapse after the suppository is inserted before bowel evacuation occurs.

It is usually important for the patient to establish a routine of exercise and then a relaxed, unhurried period on the bedpan or toilet to develop the habit pattern. It is frequently found that sitting on the toilet or a bedside commode is more conducive to a good bowel movement than is use of a bedpan or disposable diapers. Teaching the patient the technique of inserting the suppository is important in the learning process. Since sensation is generally lacking, visual check of the stool volume and consistency by the nurse and the patient is necessary. Eventually, the bowel evacuation habit may not require the suppository for initiation but may be stimulated by a gloved finger in the rectum, abdominal pressure, or a series of exercises. A bowel movement every second day is usually sufficient. However, impactions are not uncommon among these patients, and at times it may be necessary to gently remove fecal material with a gloved finger. Diarrhea or continuous soiling frequently indicates an impaction. Normal saline enemas may be necessary, but with bowel training the need for enemas is minimized. These should be given with extreme care because the intestine of the paraplegic patient distends easily if too much liquid is given or if it is given too rapidly. On the other hand, some patients may not be able to retain the fluid and it acts more as an irrigation. Since results from the enema frequently continue for several hours after the procedure, protective padding should be provided for the patient. A successful habit without use of enemas is the desired goal.

BODY ALIGNMENT

Special attention to good body alignment, change of position, and range of joint motion is necessary. If skull traction has been applied, the amount of extension of the cervical region must be carefully controlled according to the attending physician's wishes. In the supine position, the lower extremities are maintained in neutral position. External rotation is prevented by the use of trochanter rolls or sandbags. A padded footboard is used to support the feet at right angles, and the heels must be protected to keep decubiti from developing. With the quadriplegic, attention must be paid to the arms; bony prominences, especially the elbows, are protected. The wrist is slightly dorsiflexed. The metacarpo-

phalangeal joints are positioned in flexion, and the thumb should be kept in a position of opposition, with the web space maintained. In the prone position, the ankles are supported on a pillow. This produces some flexion of the knees and keeps the feet in a functional position.

While involved with maintaining correct body alignment, the nurse must not forget that changing the patient's position at scheduled frequent intervals (insofar as this is possible) not only is necessary for comfort but also helps to prevent hypostatic pneumonia and the development of decubiti. (See Chapter 1.)

The prone position should be used to help relieve pressure on the sides and back. It is also advantageous in improving the oropharyngeal airway, improving drainage and ventilation of posterior lung segments, and improving drainage from the renal pelvis. If a pillow is not placed beneath the abdomen, the abdomen moves freely and breathing is easy.

PREVENTING JOINT CONTRACTURES

For the patient with spinal cord injury, maintaining normal range of joint motion is an important aspect of his care. The individual with paralyzed limbs is dependent on someone else to move his extremities (Fig. 3-34). Passive exercises to prevent joint contractures are ordered and supervised by the attending physician. In some larger hospitals, the physical therapist is assigned this responsibility. However, the nurse not only must be cognizant of the need but also must know how to move the paralyzed extremities through a normal range of motion. This can easily be done during the morning bath or as part of other nursing care procedures. (See Chapter 1.)

MUSCLE SPASMS

In patients with spinal cord injury, muscle spasms may produce difficult problems. These may develop as the motor neuron reflex arc returns. Traction, frames, splinting, and even proper bed positioning seems to stimulate reflexes that result in powerful muscle spasms. Apparatus applied to forcibly maintain a desired position frequently causes pressure sores. Pressure sores are also frequently the result of pressure or abrasion of skin against the bedclothes occurring with spasms. As the patient

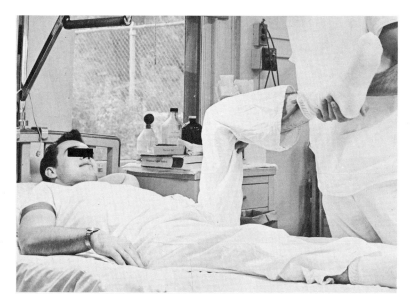

Fig. 3-34. Passive exercise of paralyzed limbs is an important aspect of the care needed by the patient with spinal cord injury.

improves, the tendency toward flexion and adduction deformities often becomes a perplexing problem. Even turning the patient in bed may trigger abnormal motor impulses that are almost impossible to control. Side rails or other protective measures must be used to prevent the patient's falling from the bed. Because mass reflexes are so difficult to combat and are so distressing to the patient, surgery is sometimes performed to eliminate them. Intraspinal resection of the nerve roots (rhizotomy) may be performed. This produces a flaccid paralysis that eliminates the mass flexion and adduction spasms. Other procedures to relieve the spasms, which the neurosurgeon may elect to do, are subtotal spinal chordectomy, subarachnoid alcohol block, or peripheral neurectomy. When relief from the muscle spasms has been obtained, it is possible to institute bladder training and to care for pressure sores more adequately because the bed can be kept dry and the patient can be made comfortable, and deformity can be prevented. Activities of daily living may then be learned, and the previously helpless individual can have a more active and useful life.

EXERCISE PROGRAM

It is imperative that a planned active exercise program be carried out for all nonparalyzed muscles and passive exercises be prescribed for

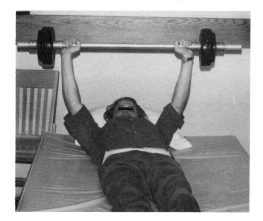

Fig. 3-35. Weight lifting used as a resistive exercise to strengthen upper extremity muscles. This will help the paraplegic patient master transfer and ambulation techniques.

the paralyzed extremities. The patient with cord damage needs more than to maintain normal strength in nonparalyzed muscles. He needs to increase the strength in these muscles so they may help substitute for the function of paralyzed muscles. Strong muscles will make it possible for him to change his position in bed, maneuver himself from bed to chair or chair to toilet, and perhaps manipulate crutches and perform other activities of daily living. All of these things are extremely important for the individual adjusting to a new way of life.

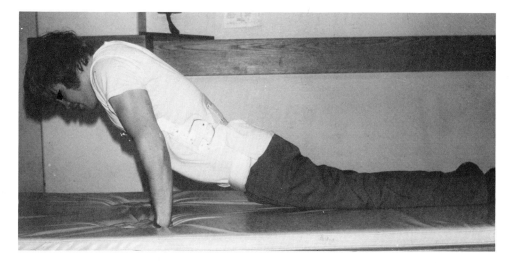

Fig. 3-36. Push-ups are another type of resistive exercise for arm strengthening in the paraplegic.

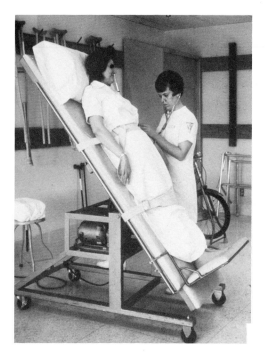

Fig. 3-37. Early use of the tilt table is helpful to the paraplegic patient and aids in overcoming postural hypotension. Weight bearing on the long bones helps to slow the development of osteoporosis.

An exercise program is aimed primarily at strengthening the muscles of the upper extremities, the shoulders, the back, and abdominal muscles, depending upon the level of cord injury. One of the earliest exercises is getting the patient to reach and to turn himself. Another early exercise prescribed may be weight lifting (Fig. 3-35). This helps to strengthen the finger flexors, the wrist extensors, and the elbow extensors. These muscles along with the shoulder depressors are important for transfers and crutch walking. Prone push-ups may also be recommended (Fig. 3-36). The bed patient may be taught to do push-ups in the supine position by raising himself to his elbows and then to a sitting position with palms of his hands on the bed. In this position, the patient may use his hands to elevate his body off the bed. Use of the trapeze strengthens the elbow flexor (biceps) primarily, and is less valuable. Learning to balance oneself in the sitting position should be practiced.

Early use of the tilt table, mentioned earlier, offers many benefits. The patient may not be able to assume a fully erect position initially. Lightheadedness or faintness may result from postural hypotension. To help prevent pooling of blood in the abdomen and legs, an abdominal binder or elastic hose may be utilized. Early weight bearing on the tilt table as described previously not only helps prevent osteoporosis but also serves as a morale booster for the paralyzed individual (Fig. 3-37).

Wheelchair exercises may include push-ups. The patient places his hands on the arms of the chair and raises his buttocks off the seat of the chair. This exercise is desirable for strengthening arm muscles and should be performed at frequent intervals also to relieve and change the pressure on the buttocks area.

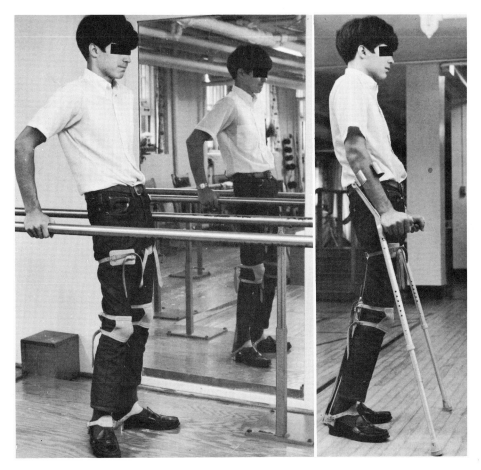

Fig. 3-38. The patient with paralysis of the lower extremities first learns to balance in the standing position and to walk with the aid of parallel bars, then with crutches.

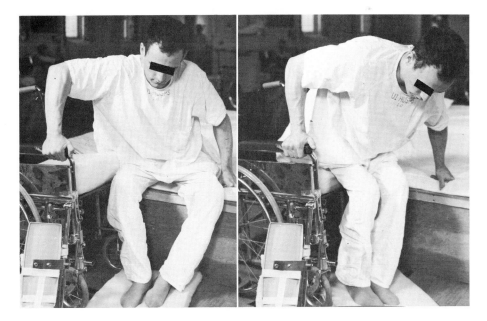

Fig. 3-39. A patient with paralysis of the lower extremities transfers from the mat (bed) to the wheelchair. The chair is placed parallel to the mat, wheels are locked, and the armrest nearest the patient is removed. By placing one hand on the chair armrest and the other on the mat, as illustrated, he is able to lift and support his body weight as he moves to the chair seat.

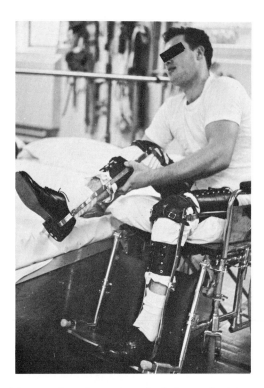

Fig. 3-40. Transferring from the bed to a wheelchair. With the wheels locked and the armrest nearest the bed removed, the patient uses his arm and shoulder muscles to slide across to the chair seat. Then with his hands he moves his legs off the bed and places his feet on the wheelchair footrests.

This can be very helpful in preventing pressure sores. Wheelchair games such as throwing darts or bowling are helpful in strengthening muscles of the upper extremity and to provide active recreation.

When the patient has been fitted with braces, parallel bar exercises may be instituted to develop skills in balancing, weight bearing, and walking (Fig. 3-38). After learning to ambulate in the parallel bars, he advances to the use of crutches. He must learn to balance and also to manipulate the crutches. Becoming fully ambulatory with crutches involves more than learning the crutch gait patterns. To become independent, the individual must also learn to rise from a bed or chair to standing, to open and close doors, to go up and down curbs, ramps, and steps, to sit down, to get off and on a toilet seat, to get in and out of a car, and many other activities he will find necessary for an active life.

BRACES

Many patients with cord injury are fitted with braces. The type of brace prescribed will depend upon the level of the spinal cord lesion and the resulting muscular involvement. Individuals with lesions below the first lumbar vertebra are usually fitted with long leg braces. Patients with a lesion between the tenth thoracic and first lumbar vertebrae will need the long

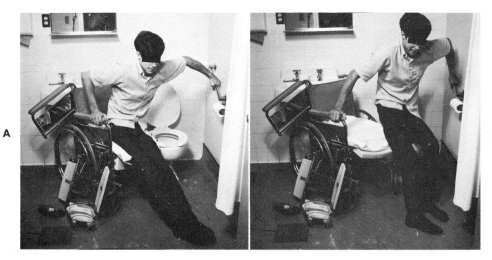

A   B

Fig. 3-41. Transferring from the wheelchair to a toilet seat. **A,** The chair is positioned as illustrated, with wheels locked and the armrest nearest the stool removed. **B,** By using the chair armrest and the wall handle bar, the patient is able to support his body weight and to transfer from the chair to the toilet seat.

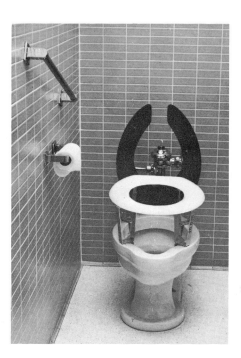

Fig. 3-42. An elevated toilet seat may be very helpful to the disabled individual, particularly the elderly patient or the patient with a hip problem. Note the handle bar.

leg braces with a pelvic band or with a lumbosacral corset. If the spinal cord lesion is at the tenth thoracic vertebra level or above, the patient may need, in addition, a body brace that is attached to the leg braces. The making and fitting of braces requires considerable time and skill. Consequently, braces are expensive. Helping the paraplegic learn how to care for his braces is a necessary part of his training.

The wearing of braces by the patient with sensory loss is not without hazards. The skin must be checked carefully for reddened areas each time the brace is removed. If the alignment of the brace is not correct or if metal rubs the skin, pressure points will occur. Since the paraplegic does not have pain sensation, he must always be cognizant of his problem. As he learns the skills involved in putting on and removing braces (Fig. 3-45) he must be trained to check, each time he removes the braces, the skin for visible signs of pressure. Furthermore, care must be taken that the shoes worn by the patient fit properly and do not cause blisters.

PREVENTION AND TREATMENT OF BED SORES AND TROPHIC ULCERS

One of the chief factors contributing to the development of a pressure sore is impaired circulation. Nerve damage with paralysis and loss

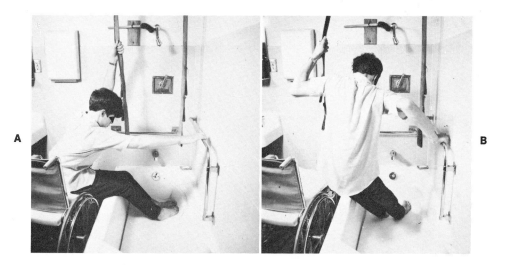

A **B**

Fig. 3-43. Transferring from the wheelchair to the tub. The chair is placed parallel to the tub and the armrest nearest the tub is removed. **A,** The patient uses his hands to turn his body and to place his legs over the side of the tub. **B,** Then, by grasping the overhead strap and wall handle bar, he is able to support his weight and lower himself into the tub.

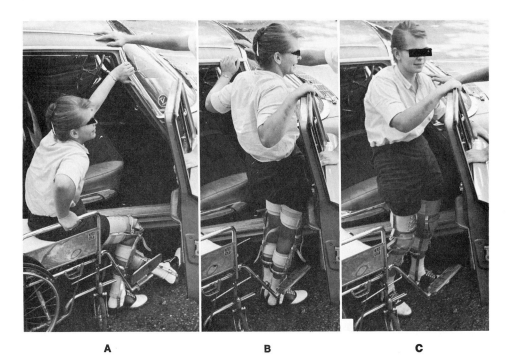

A	**B**	**C**

Fig. 3-44. Transferring from a wheelchair to a car seat. With the car door open, the chair is placed in the position illustrated. **A,** The patient removes her braced legs from the chair supports and slides forward in the chair. The left leg brace is locked in extension. **B,** By use of the arms as illustrated, the standing position is assumed. **C,** The individual pivots and is in position to lower herself onto the car seat with or without unlocking brace. She will then use her arms to turn her body and to place her lower extremities in the car. (Courtesy Physical Therapy Department, University Hospitals, The University of Iowa, Iowa City.)

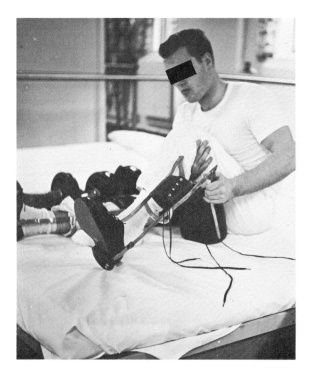

Fig. 3-45. When the patient is able to maintain his balance in a sitting position, he learns to put on his leg braces. As illustrated, he flexes the knee and lifts his leg with one hand and with the other hand maneuvers the brace and places his foot in the shoe. (Courtesy Physical Therapy Department, University Hospitals, The University of Iowa, Iowa City.)

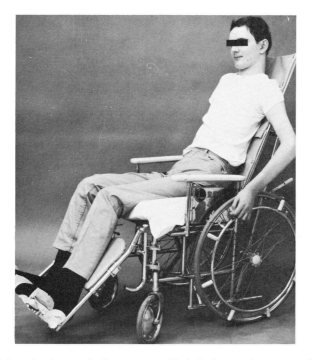

Fig. 3-46. Wheelchair for the quadriplegic patient. High back provides support for the head and shoulders. Wheels are constructed so that chair can be propelled by the patient who has minimal hand function.

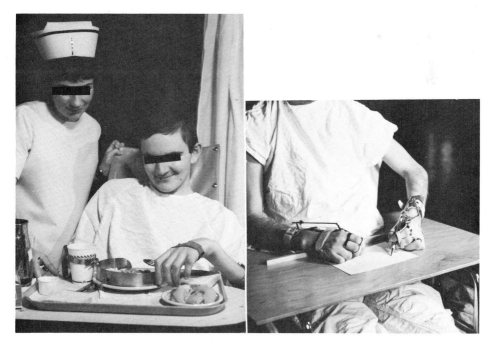

Fig. 3-47. Use of special equipment that may enable the individual with loss of hand function to feed himself and to grasp a pencil or similar object.

of muscular activity results in a diminished blood supply to the part. Since the patient is unable to move at frequent intervals, circulation is further hampered by pressure from the body weight, especially over bony prominences. As a result, nutrition to the part may not be adequate, and breakdown of the skin and underlying tissues will occur unless preventive nursing measures are instituted. Abnormal sweating in many patients with spinal cord injuries may result in maceration and more skin problems. Frequent change of the patient's position plus gentle massage of the skin on which he has been sitting or lying helps stimulate local circulation. The use of flotation pads, Plastazote devices, water beds, sponge rubber pads, acrylic fiber pads (arti-ficial lamb's wool) and alternating pressure air mattresses may be of assistance in distributing weight. Since most patients will not have expensive devices at home, it is preferable to teach proper skin care without dependence on such major devices as alternating pressure pads.

If body pressure is continued on a reddened area, it can result in a pressure sore in a relatively short time. Eliminating pressure on the affected area until all signs of redness or inflammation have disappeared is the best and most effective treatment. This may restrict the patient's activities for a few days. The individual who lacks normal sensation must learn to check visually, by use of a hand mirror, all vulnerable spots.

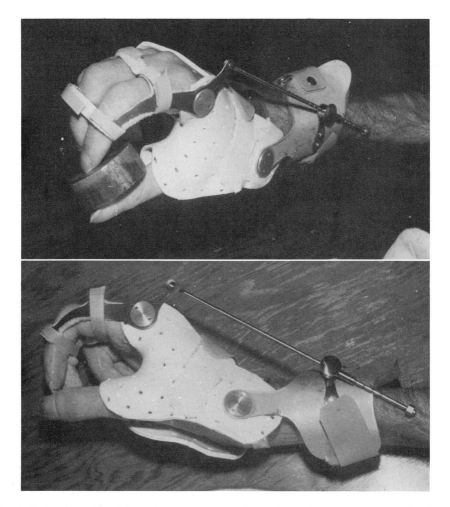

Fig. 3-48. A wrist-activated dynamic splint may permit certain quadriplegics to use the hand more functionally with stronger pinch and finger extension.

SELF-HELP AND CARE

As soon as possible, the patient with a spinal cord injury should begin to help with his own care. This will vary greatly among patients, depending upon the level of the lesion, the individual's attitudes and emotional stability, and the nurse working with the patient. The person who is discovering what it means to be disabled from spinal cord injury nearly always has periods of depression. He frequently has little interest in doing very much for himself at this stage. He may be morose, critical, and demanding. Early activity and signs of progress will help the patient begin to regain some self-esteem and help prevent prolonged feelings of discouragement and dependency. A program of graduated activities needs to be planned with the patient and his family. The activities should challenge the patient, but at each level should be within his capabilities so that he does not feel constantly frustrated. New interests and skill should be fostered and developed. The most desirable goal for the patient is complete independence and self-sufficiency. If feasible, this should be planned. However, for many of these patients, this is not a realistic goal; some dependency may be necessary. In any case, realistic goals should be established, and activities planned to accomplish them (Figs. 3-46 to 3-48).

In the rehabilitation unit, group interchange can be fostered. It has been found that the ward situation, where patients can observe and talk about their own and other patients' disabilities, is often helpful. Competition with and encouragement from others can be invaluable. Patients sharing the rehabilitation unit may learn a great deal from each other, from routines for transfer, exercising, and gait training to managing money, and sexual, and family problems. Recreational activities may be helpful by occupying the patient's attention for periods free of thoughts about his disability (Fig. 3-49).

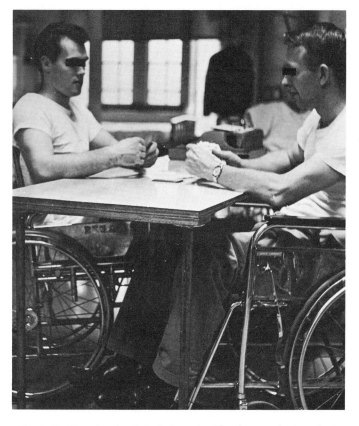

Fig. 3-49. Diversional activity is important for the paraplegic patient.

CARE OF THE PATIENT WITH A CEREBROVASCULAR ACCIDENT

Hemiplegia is a term that means, literally, "paralysis of one side of the body." The brain is particularly vulnerable to changes in circulation. Interruption in the blood supply to the brain, even for as short a time as a few minutes, results in necrosis of the cells of the brain and loss of function in the body area innervated by these cells. This is referred to as a "stroke." The area of the brain damaged varies from patient to patient. The loss of blood supply results, in most cases, from either a thrombus, an embolism, or a hemorrhage within the brain.

Arteriosclerotic changes in the vessel walls are frequently present in the patient who has suffered a stroke as a result of a thrombus. The etiology of the arteriosclerotic conditions is at present unknown. Today cerebrovascular accidents rank third as a cause of death in this country, being exceeded only by heart disease and cancer. Because of the increasing longevity of our population it is expected that the number of people suffering strokes will increase. The outcome for these patients will depend upon the kind of nursing care they receive from the onset of a cerebrovascular accident. Of course, the extent of the brain damage is paramount with respect to the ultimate functional outcome.

PATHOLOGY

The brain is composed of cortical gray matter near its surface, wherein lie cell bodies, and white matter containing axons or nerve fibers. Cell bodies initiate the functions of the brain, and nerve fibers then carry the messages from the cells out to the rest of the body. The brain not only sends out messages to muscles for movement, balance, speech, respiration, and blood pressure, but also receives information regarding sight, hearing, taste, touch, pain, and so forth. It must integrate the incoming information, take appropriate action, and carry on the higher thought processes of memory, problem-solving, and personality development. Many functional areas have been identified in the cerebral cortex.

Occlusion in the distribution of the middle cerebral artery is the most common stroke lesion (Fig. 3-50). Small vessels that supply fibers in the internal capsule are often occluded. In the internal capsule, fibers from the cortex are grouped together to descend the brain stem and spinal cord. With interruption of these fibers there may be loss of motor and sensory function to a major part of the body. Hemiplegia or paralysis of one side results. Since most fibers from one side of the brain cross to the other side of the body, a lesion in the right side of the brain results in left hemiplegia and vice-versa. A stroke may not result in total loss of function. There may be mild, transient weakness; more persistent partial paralysis or severe hemiplegia occurs in different cases. Also, one may have loss of vision, especially in one visual field, changes in balance, sensory perceptual impairment, or changes in blood pressure or respiration. The areas of the brain concerned with speech and language are located in the dominant cerebral hemisphere. A right-handed person with right hemiplegia caused by a left cerebral injury will commonly have trouble with speech (aphasia or dysphasia).

REHABILITATION

Following a stroke, the more severely involved patient will need intensive nursing care. Safety precautions must be taken to prevent injury, should attempts be made to get out of bed. Careful checking of the vital signs is essential. Slowing of pulse and respiration and elevation of blood pressure and temperature may indicate rising intracranial pressure affecting vital centers. If swallowing difficulties are present, intravenous therapy may be necessary to help meet the patient's nutritional needs. During the first few days fluids may be limited and should be given slowly to help prevent cerebral edema. Accurate record of intake and output is an essential part of the care. If the ability to swallow is impaired, aspiration is a great risk if oral feedings are attempted. Stringy foods and foods that

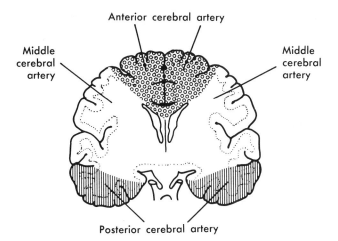

Fig. 3-50. Coronal section of the brain. Most cerebrovascular accidents produce lesions in the area of brain supplied by the middle cerebral artery in one hemisphere.

are difficult to chew should be avoided. Turning the patient to the unaffected side will help him to control liquids and food placed in the mouth. Mouth care should be given at frequent intervals, with particular attention to the paralyzed side. If the patient is accustomed to wearing dentures, he may handle food more easily with the dentures in place. If dysphagia continues to be a problem, a nasogastric tube may be inserted.

If the blink reflex is lost or the patient is unable to close the eyelid, protection for the eye is needed. Irrigation with physiologic saline and instillation of eye drops several times daily are usually prescribed to prevent drying and the development of corneal ulcers. If hemianopsia is present, the patient will have loss of vision in the right (or left) visual field of both eyes. The bedside equipment, eating utensils, and so forth should be placed within the patient's field of vision.

Since many of these patients are unable to move, nursing measures aimed at preventing hypostatic pneumonia should be started at the onset of illness. Frequent change of position and encouraging the patient to breathe deeply and to cough will help prevent stasis of secretions in the lungs. For some patients, suctioning may be necessary to remove secretions from the throat. An oropharyngeal airway may be used, and in some cases a tracheostomy is necessary to maintain an open passageway. The frequent changing of position for the stroke

patient is also necessary to prevent the development of pressure areas. A planned schedule of turning should be included in the nursing care plan.

Rehabilitation efforts should be started early in the course of patient's hospital stay. Efforts to prevent deformities should be initiated and correct positioning should be practiced from the beginning even if the patient is severely ill with shock or coma. If shock is present, the patient must be moved with great care. As the patient's condition improves, more attention can be given to frequent changes of position, proper alignment of body parts, and range of motion exercises to protect the skin and prevent deformities. Because of changes in the level of consciousness, weakness, and reduced or altered sensation, the patient may tend to ignore his affected extremities. A detailed description of the various positions has been presented in Chapter 1. The advantages of the prone position include the following:

1. Reduction in the possibilities of acquiring decubitus ulcers from prolonged lying in the supine position
2. Improvement of the airway as tongue and jaw move forward
3. Better drainage of mucus from posterior lung areas and upper respiratory tract
4. Decreased possibility of aspiration of gastric contents
5. Decrease in problems with pneumonia and atelectasis

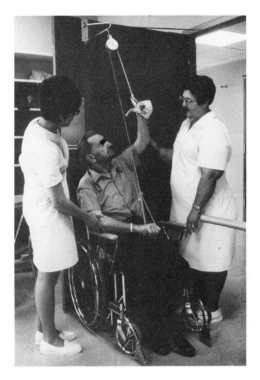

Fig. 3-51. Using a pulley, the hemiplegic patient can give his paralyzed arm range of motion exercises.

It may be difficult for the patient to tolerate the prone position at first. This can be overcome by use of partial front lying position. Positioning may be aided by the use of bedboards, footboards, hand rolls, or posterior leg splints. With each change of position, the patient's skin should be checked for redness or other color changes indicative of too much pressure on a given area. Careful attention must also be given to the axillas, the groin, and the hands for proper skin hygiene. Dependent limbs, such as hands and feet, will become swollen if not elevated and put through range of motion.

As soon as the patient is out of shock, usually within the first 24 to 48 hours, range of motion exercise for all joints is started to prevent deformities. Generally, moving each joint through its complete range of motion two or three times daily will prevent tightness and deformity. This can be done by the nurse while bathing the patient. However, in time, a member of the patient's family may be taught to help with these passive exercises, or in some instances the patient may learn to use his uninvolved arm and leg to move and passively exercise the involved extremities—such as flexing and extending the fingers, dorsiflexing the wrist, and providing flexion and extension of the elbow.

The patient should be encouraged to actively

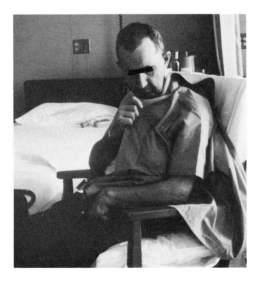

Fig. 3-52. Man with left hemiplegia practicing dressing himself. He should learn to put his paralyzed arm through the sleeve first.

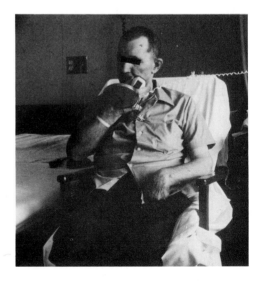

Fig. 3-53. One handed shaving with an electric razor. The mirror is equipped to hang from the patient's neck.

move all unaffected muscles and joints to maintain mobility and strength. The patient's motivation may be increased and his self-pity lessened by these early indications that plans are being made for his recovery (Fig. 3-51).

Another major area in rehabilitation, which the nurse may help carry out on the ward, is training in self-care and the activities of daily living. As soon as the patient's condition permits, he should be encouraged to participate in his

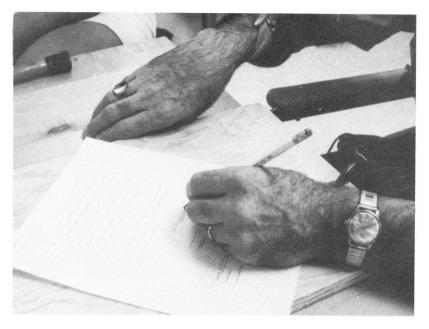

Fig. 3-54. Learning to write with the nondominant hand.

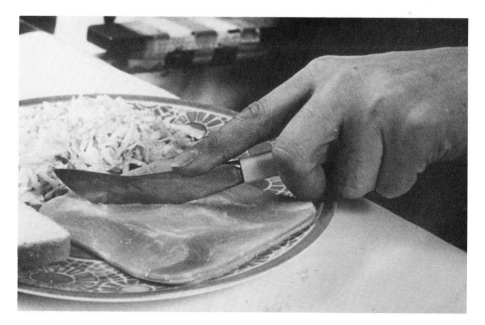

Fig. 3-55. Using a rounded, sharp, "rocking" knife, this patient with right hemiparesis is able to cut meat with one hand.

own daily care. Bathing, combing hair, brushing teeth, shaving, or applying make-up will encourage a sense of well-being and will help improve muscle strength and joint function. The patient will frequently have to be taught to do things with one hand, at least initially. This may be slow and clumsy at first, but the patient should not be hurried or he will become frustrated and discouraged. Nurses should realize that a person who has suffered a stroke may be emotionally labile and may frequently break into tears. When a patient has mastered some of the simpler tasks in self-care, he should be asked to try more difficult and complex activities such as dressing and writing. When the nurse is helping the patient learn to dress himself, it should be remembered that with most clothing the affected arm or leg must be placed in the garment first. In undressing, the garment is removed from the unaffected limb first, and then from the paralyzed side (Figs. 3-52 to 3-55).

It is important that the nurse seek assistance from occupational therapists and physical therapists when such personnel are available. Therapists are especially trained in the techniques for teaching self-care and can also provide ap-

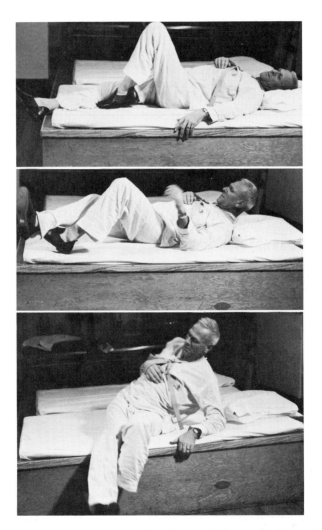

Fig. 3-56. When the patient wishes to transfer from the mat (bed) to a wheelchair, the chair is placed as illustrated near the patient's uninvolved side. The pictures illustrate a patient's use of his normal arm and leg to help him assume the sitting position on the bedside and then to transfer to the chair. For this patient to transfer from the wheelchair to the bed, the position of the chair would be reversed.

propriate exercises based on the results of manual muscle tests of strength, range of motion tests, tests of motor control and coordination. As the patient improves, he may be taught to use his unaffected extremities so that he can sit up in bed and achieve sitting balance with or without support. He may be taught to transfer from bed to chair and vice versa. To transfer, the patient sits up on the side of the bed toward his unaffected side. A chair at bedside should face the foot of the bed at a slight angle. The patient can use his unaffected arm to lock the wheelchair, stand, reach the farther arm rest, pivot on the unaffected leg, and lower himself into the chair using the arm rest to support himself.

When the patient returns to bed from the wheelchair, the chair should face the head of the bed at a slight angle with the unaffected side near the bed. As the patient leans forward to stand and transfer, he is again leading with his normal side (Fig. 3-56).

In most instances, the half side rail and a trapeze are very helpful to the stroke patient when he wishes to shift his position in bed, turn to the side-lying position, raise his body to a sitting position, or assume the standing position. The stroke patient (when lying in bed) is taught to use his normal limb to move his paralyzed one. By placing the toes and forefoot of the strong limb beneath the involved limb at the ankle, he is not only able to shift his position; he may learn also to turn to his side (with help of the side rail) and in some instances to assume the sitting position on the side of the bed.

During the period of learning to do for himself, it is helpful to have tables and working surfaces of convenient height. Placing the patient in a sitting position, when possible, will assist him in managing activities with greater ease.

Achieving bowel and bladder control may be a frustrating experience for the stroke patient. The bladder is frequently flaccid initially after the stroke, and an indwelling catheter may have to be used. Later, the flaccid bladder may become spastic. At this time, a bladder-training program may be initiated, similar to that used for a paraplegic. A bowel-training program also should be initiated. The hemiplegic who re-

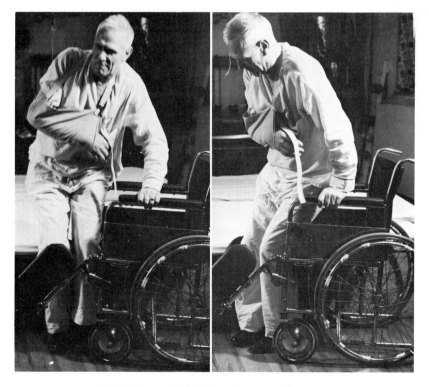

Fig. 3-56, cont'd. For legend see opposite page.

mains incontinent after a month of bowel training is usually a poor candidate for independent living.

Disposable paper diapers are useful for bowel incontinence. The patient must be checked for bowel function daily. Impaction is common but is avoidable when close supervision is given. Laxatives and suppositories are occasionally required. Enemas may be useful on occasion but often are incompletely expelled and cause soilage throughout the day. At least 90% of patients will regain bowel and bladder control with time as sensation improves and confusion decreases with the return of consciousness. Suppositories to establish bowel habits are seldom required for more than a few days. As soon as the patient is well enough, having a bedside commode or bathroom privileges will add to his feeling of well-being.

When there is incontinence of urine, an indwelling catheter is frequently used in the early phase in an effort to keep the patient dry and protect his skin. At first this is usually put to straight bedside drainage; however, intermittent clamping of the tube and drainage at regular intervals is thought to assist in reestablishing bladder function. It should be noted that there are problems with intermittent clamping, and some physicians do not subscribe to this technique. Because of the irritation and increased chances of infection, it is important to remove the catheter as soon as possible. It is important that all care of the catheter and tubing should be done in an aseptic manner to prevent bacteria from entering the system. Clean bedside drainage tubes are just as important as clean catheters.

The patient should learn to use a wheelchair until he learns to walk. Some patients require a wheelchair for extended periods. The patient will usually need some help in learning to propel this chair with one arm. In some instances, it is helpful to remove the leg support on the uninvolved side, so that the patient can use his foot as well as his arm in propelling and guiding the chair. Many times a patient has problems with the weakened foot slipping off the foot support. A chair with a heelrest on the foot support can help this problem (Fig. 3-57).

If the patient has a flaccid arm, a sling support

(Fig. 3-56) should be worn to prevent shoulder subluxation when the patient is in the upright position. If spasticity occurs in the arm, the sling can usually be discarded since the spastic muscle tone will support the shoulder.

The next area of training involves ambulation. It is important for all patients—but especially for the elderly—to begin ambulating as soon as possible. Weakness on one side will be the major problem of stroke patients, but this will frequently be complicated by loss of sensation especially joint-position sense. There may also be cerebellar injury with resultant balance and coordination problems. These will affect the ultimate outcome immensely.

Most hemiplegic patients develop reflex patterns in the affected limbs. In the leg an extensor reflex pattern may allow standing without buckling of the knee. At first the patient learns to sit on the edge of the bed, and then in a chair, and later to stand as he relearns balancing in the upright position. Many patients with nondominant side strokes and left hemiplegia have rather severe impairment of perception. These patients may perceive vertical position of the head and trunk incorrectly and have trouble learning to balance themselves.

When the patient can support his weight standing on the affected leg, gait training should begin in the parallel bars in physical therapy. There he will learn balance and weight shifting. He will then advance to heel-toe walking and a reciprocal gait pattern. In the course of progressing from bed to chair to parallel bars, the patient will both learn transferring techniques and improve muscle strength.

Bracing is commonly necessary in the hemiplegic patient. With a more spastic extensor reflex pattern, the foot will tend to invert at the ankle. The gastrocnemius muscle tends to overpower the foot dorsiflexors, resulting in an equinus or toe-down position. This position makes weight bearing difficult and moving the toe through during a swing phase of gait troublesome. The most commonly used leg brace for hemiplegics is a short leg brace attached to the shoe to prevent the toe-down position. Teaching the patient proper use and care of the brace, as well as means of getting it on and off, can add to the complexity of rehabilitation. Again, it is

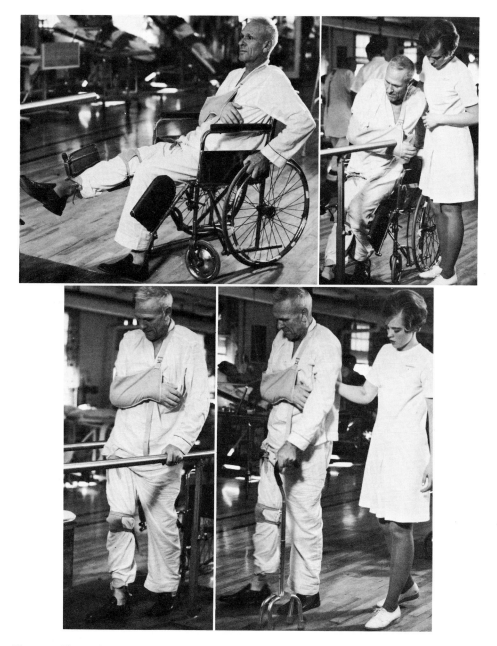

Fig. 3-57. The stroke patient propels the wheelchair with his normal arm and leg. Patient then learns to balance and walk, first with the parallel bars and then with a cane. An up-to-date chart (pp. 136 to 139) of the rehabilitee's accomplishments pertaining to activities of daily living can be most helpful to the nurse. It provides a better understanding of what can be expected from the patient in the realm of self-care, as well as the goals toward which he is working. (Courtesy Occupational Therapy Department, University Hospitals, The University of Iowa, Iowa City.)

important to emphasize an unhurried approach to the patient so that frustration will be kept to a minimum. Long leg braces are seldom required. External supports with a walker, quadriped cane, crutch, or standard cane may also be required. If assistive devices are indicated, early introduction is important for better patient acceptance.

During the first few months, various techniques may be used to stimulate or facilitate the function of muscle groups in the affected areas. Electrical stimulation, brushing, icing, and vibration may improve muscle performance in selected cases as part of the muscle re-education program (Fig. 3-58).

Speech therapy may be helpful for patients with disorders of speech and communication. Some patients are able to speak, but not distinctly, because of poor control of lip, tongue, and throat muscles. Such dysarthria often improves with regular speech therapy and practice. Other patients with lesions of the speech center may have aphasia. Some individuals have expressive aphasia and have problems with speech, writing, or telling time. Others have trouble understanding the spoken or written word or in recognizing familiar objects and have receptive aphasia. Most patients have a mixed type of aphasia with both receptive and expressive deficits. Some individuals have nonfluent aphasia and say very little. Others have fluent aphasia. They talk on in meaningless jargon (Figs. 3-59 and 3-60). It is important to realize that the communication disorder affects only use of language symbols and does not represent a general intellectual deficit. It also should be noted that many older persons have severe hearing impairments that further impair their communication skills (Fig. 3-61).

A speech clinician should be involved to work with the patient. Repetitive drills may be helpful. Memory patterns of words or phrases that the patient has retained will be sought by the therapist in an effort to regain some speech function. Much depends on the effort of the patient. This can be encouraged by the nurse on the ward during bathing, bed making, and other periods of care of the patient. Encourage but do not demand speech. The patient will many times make meaningless or nonsense syllables but they are

attempts. If he lacks functional speech, phrase questions so that a "yes" or "no" answer may be used, for this is at least a start. Allow him to use speech in any way he can (speaking, writing, reading) as much as possible. It is helpful to have him repeat after you words or phrases con-

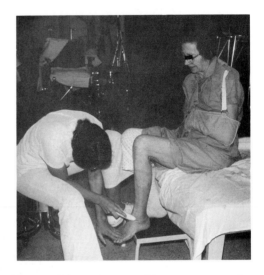

Fig. 3-58. Vibrator being used in an attempt to stimulate some reflex activity and contraction of the ankle dorsiflexors.

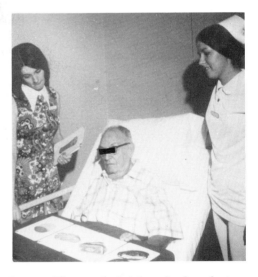

Fig. 3-59. The speech clinician asks the aphasic patient to identify a common object by pointing to the correct picture and then attempting to repeat the word.

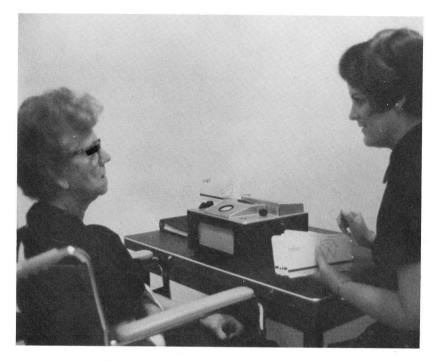

Fig. 3-60. A machine that repeats the name of the object pictured on the card can be used for speech drills in patients with certain types of aphasia.

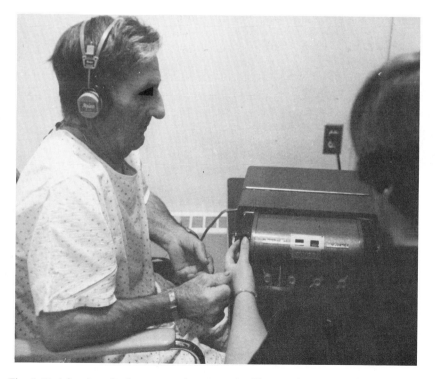

Fig. 3-61. A hearing check may reveal unrecognized hearing loss in an aphasic patient.

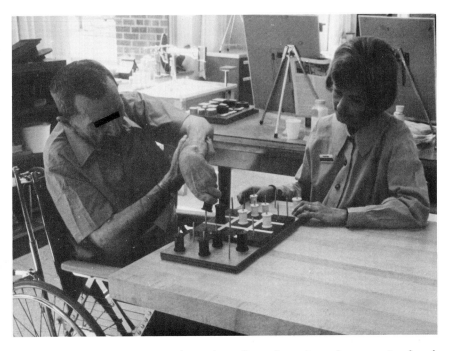

Fig. 3-62. A spool tic-tac-toe game can be used as a form of exercise and as recreation for a hemiparetic patient.

cerning his immediate surroundings and then try to initiate them on his own. Speaking slowly and distinctly will help him understand you. If he becomes fatigued or resists help, it is best to drop the activity for a time. Do not let him struggle overly long when trying to say something, but allow him an unhurried period to work at it before assisting him.

When taking care of the individual problems such as skin, position, bowels, and speech, it is important not to forget the patient as a whole. He needs attention as much as his individual symptoms (Fig. 3-62). Rehabilitation involves thinking about his relationship to his family and society. It is very important to teach the family how to work and live with the patient. They should be encouraged not to be overly helpful to the patient, so that he will become as independent as possible. They should be included in discussions of the long-term planning that involves realistic goals. Every effort should be made to encourage the family and the patient to participate in decisions regarding long-term care of the patient.

Muscle strength, coordination, and balance can be achieved through exercises as well as activities. The patient must also become involved in relearning homemaking activities (Fig. 3-63) using new methods of travel, and exploring possible vocational and avocational avenues. He should be referred to local or state public health, social welfare, and vocational rehabilitation agencies when appropriate. These agencies can often assist in the transition from hospital to home. The public health nurse can be of invaluable assistance in helping the patient and his family make adjustments in the home, which will help the patient maintain his independence and still provide him with needed assistance and understanding. Members of the family may need continued support and reassurance to help them cope with the many problems that arise. It is important to consider age, the severity of the disability, and the patient's interests, as well as social and cultural factors, when planning rehabilitative self-care and vocational goals. It is important to be realistic and not excessively optimistic with the patient.

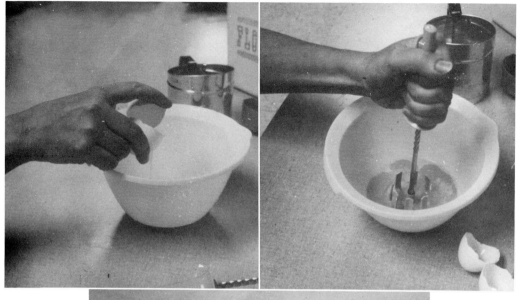

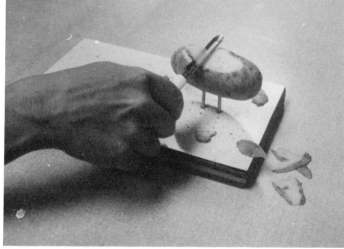

Fig. 3-63. One-handed homemaking activities can be mastered by some hemiparetic patients. **A,** Techniques for breaking an egg, **B,** using a push-pull egg beater, and **C,** spikes to hold the vegetable being peeled can be easily learned.

STUDY QUESTIONS

1. A 21-year-old man has been admitted to the rehabilitation area with a fracture of the tenth thoracic vertebra, resulting in cord injury and paralysis of the lower extremities (paraplegia). Review the following aspects of his care.

   (a) Nursing care will include changing the patient's position at relatively frequent intervals. Describe or demonstrate good body alignment in the prone, supine, and sidelying positions. Explain reasons for frequent turning of the patient.

   (b) Describe the nursing care that will help to prevent the development of pressure sores. Why is the paraplegic patient prone to develop decubiti?

   (c) What urinary problems may be anticipated?

   (d) Passive exercises will be prescribed to help maintain joint motion of the lower extremities. Describe or illustrate range of motion for the ankle, knee, and hip joints.

   (e) Describe the secondary contractures that may be anticipated when the muscles of the lower extremity are paralyzed.

(f) Review some of the physiologic changes that may take place because of the patient's inactivity. Be prepared to substantiate your answers.

(g) Use of the tilt table is frequently prescribed early in the care of the paraplegic. Why is this beneficial?

(h) Active exercises will be prescribed to strengthen the muscles of the upper extremities. Explain.

(i) It will be necessary for this patient to learn to do many things in a new way. Explain some of the activities of daily living that the rehabilitation team will encourage and help him to master.

(j) The patient's morale will greatly influence the success of his rehabilitation. Discuss factors that may influence how the patient feels about what has happened to him and his adjustment to a new way of life.

2. Mr. A. has been admitted to the rehabilitation service with the diagnosis of a cerebrovascular accident. The left side of his body is paralyzed.

(a) Describe or demonstrate various bed positions you would utilize for this patient.

(b) Is the development of pressure sores a problem?

(c) Describe joint contractures that are most likely to develop when a hemiplegic condition is present.

(d) What is meant by a functional position of the hand?

(e) Why has Mr. A. been admitted to the rehabilitation service? What do you think should be gained by a period of treatment and care in this particular unit?

REFERENCES

Allgire, M. J.: Nurses can give and teach rehabilitation, ed. 2, New York, 1968, Springer Publishing Co.

Anderson, N.: Rehabilitative nursing practice, Nurs. Clin. North Am. 6:303-309, 1966.

Barckley, V., and Campbell, E. I.: Helping the handicapped child achieve emotional maturity, Am. J. Nurs. 59:376-379, 1959.

Bedford, J. B.: Beds and tables. In Licht, S., and Kamenetz, H. L., editors: Orthotics etcetera, New Haven, 1966, Elizabeth Licht, Publisher.

Brown, M. E.: Self-help clothing. In Licht, S., and Kamenetz, H. L. editors: Orthotics etcetera, New Haven, 1966, Elizabeth Licht, Publisher.

Campbell, E. B.: Nursing problems associated with prolonged recovery following trauma, Nurs. Clin. North Am. 5:551-562, 1970.

Christopherson, V. A.: Role modifications of the disabled male, Am. J. Nurs. 68:290-293, 1968.

Chronic disease and rehabilitation, Nurs. Clin. North Am., 1, entire issue, Sept., 1966.

Davis, M., Mainwaring, E., Anderson, N., and Ryan, J.: Rehabilitation nursing, a source guide for in-structors, Minneapolis, 1964, American Rehabilitation Foundation.

Deaver, G. G.: Crutches, canes and walkers. In Licht, S., and Kamenetz, H. L., editors: Orthotics etcetera, New Haven, 1966, Elizabeth Licht, Publisher.

Hallburg, J. C.: Teaching patients self care, Nurs. Clin. North Am. 5:223-231, 1970.

Halverson, E. A.: Taking rehabilitation to the patient, Can. Nurse 67:49-51, 1971.

Holmes, J. E.: The physical therapist and team care, Nurs. Outlook 20:182-184, 1972.

Hopkins, H. L.: Self-help aids. In Licht, Sidney, and Kamenetz, H. L., editors: Orthotics etcetera, New Haven, 1966, Elizabeth Licht, Publisher.

Komentz, H. L.: Selecting a wheelchair. Am. J. Nurs. 72:100-101, 1972.

Krusen, F. H., Kottke, F., and Ellwood, P.: Handbook of physical medicine and rehabilitation, Philadelphia, 1965, W. B. Saunders Co.

Lawton, E. B.: Activities of daily living for physical rehabilitation, New York, 1963, McGraw-Hill Book Co.

Licht, S., and Kamenetz, H., editors: Rehabilitation and medicine, New Haven, 1968, Elizabeth Licht, Publisher.

Lowman, E. W., and Rusk, H. A.: Self-help devices. In Rehabilitation Monograph No. 21, New York, 1962, Institute of Physical Medicine and Rehabilitation.

Lowman, E., and Rusk, H.: Self-help devices: communication and vocations: writing aids to compensate for forearm, elbow and shoulder involvement, Postgrad. Med. 35:327-329, 1964.

Lowman, E., and Rusk, H.: Self-help devices: communications and vocations: writing aids for non-functioning upper extremities, Postgrad. Med. 35:423-425, 1964.

Lowman, E., and Rusk, H.: Self-help devices: communications and vocations: positioning typewriter for the physically handicapped, Postgrad. Med. 35:659-661, 1964.

Martin, N., King, R., and Suchinski, J.: The nurse therapist in a rehabilitation setting, Am. J. Nurs. 70:1694-1697, 1970.

Peszczynski, M.: Housing for the disabled. In Licht, S.: and Kamenetz, H. L., editors: Orthotics etcetera, New Haven, 1966, Elizabeth Licht, Publisher.

Plaisted, L. M.: The clinical specialist in rehabilitation nursing, Am. J. Nurs. 69:562-564, 1969.

Rosillo, R. H., Fogel, M. L., and Freedman, K.: Affect levels and improvement in physical rehabilitation. J. Chronic Dis. 24:651-660, 1971.

Rothberg, J. S.: The challenges for rehabilitative nursing, Nurs. Outlook, 17:37-39, Nov., 1969.

Rusk, H. A.: Rehabilitative medicine. In A textbook on physical medicine and rehabilitation, ed. 3, St. Louis, 1971, The C. V. Mosby Co.

Schroeder, C.: Accepting the handicapped pupil, Nurs. Outlook 11:372-373, 1963.

Schwartz, D.: Problems of self-care and travel among

elderly ambulatory patients, Am. J. Nurs. **66:**2678-2681, 1966.

Smolock, M. A.: The nurse's role in rehabilitation of the handicapped child, Nurs. Clin. North Am. **5:**411-420, 1970.

Sorensen, K., and Amis, D.: Understanding the world of the chronically ill, Am. J. Nurs. **67:**811-817, 1967.

Sorenson, L., Ulrich, P., Coles, C., and Grendahl, B.: Ambulation: a manual for nurses, Minneapolis, 1966, American Rehabilitation Foundation.

Stryker, R. P.: Rehabilitative aspects of acute and chronic nursing care, Philadelphia, 1972, W. B. Saunders Co.

Talbot, B.: Automobile modifications for the disabled. In Licht, S., and Kamenetz, H. L., editors: Orthotics etcetera, New Haven, 1966, Elizabeth Licht, Publisher.

Valadez, A. M., Anderson, E.: Rehabilitation workshops—change in attitudes of nurses, Nurs. Res. **21:**132-137, 1972.

Welch, S. R.: Tilt-table therapy in rehabilitation of the trauma patient with brain damage and spinal injury, Nurs. Clin. North Am. **5:**621-630, 1970.

Spinal cord injury

Abramson, A.: Modern concepts of management of the patient with spinal cord injury, Arch. Phys. Med. **48:**113-121, 1967.

Adams, L., and Bluefarb, S.: How we treat decubitus ulcers, Postgrad. Med. **44:**269-271, Sept., 1968.

Barrett, D., and Klibanski, A.: Collagenase debridement, Am. J. Nurs. **73:**849-851, 1973.

Bertrand, G.: Management of spinal injuries with associated cord damage, Postgrad. Med. **37:**249-262, 1965.

Boyarsky, S., editor: The neurogenic bladder, Baltimore, 1967, The Williams & Wilkins Co.

Brownlowe, M. A., Cohen, F., and Happich, W. F.: New washable woolskins, Am. J. Nurs. **70:**2368-2370, 1970.

Culp, P.: Nursing care of the patient with spinal cord injury, Nurs. Clin. North Am. **2:**447-457, 1967.

Decker, R.: What to tell a twenty-year-old quad, Phys. Ther. **51:**1299, 1971.

Delehanty, L., and Stravino, V.: Achieving bladder control, Am. J. Nurs. **70:**312-316, 1970.

Ford, J. R. and Cooke, T. D. V.: Rehabilitation of the quadriplegic, Can. Nurse **67:**37-38, 1971.

Freeman, L. W. and Perkins, L. C.: Care of the paraplegic patient, Bedside Nurse **3:**11-18, 1970.

Frost, A.: Handbook for paraplegics and quadriplegics, Chicago, 1966, Wallace Press, National Paraplegia Foundation.

Gallagher, L.: What do you tell a twenty-year-old quad, Phys. Ther. **51:**914-915, 1971.

Grabenstetter, J.: Synthetic fat helps prevent pressure sores, Am. J. Nurs. **68:**1521-1522, 1968.

Harwin, J., and Hargest, T. S.: The air-fluidized bed: a new concept in the treatment of decubitus ulcers, Nurs. Clinics North Am. **5:**181-187, 1970.

Henderson, G. M.: Teaching-learning for rehabilitation of the spinal cord-disabled individual. Nurs. Clin. North Am. **6:**655-668, 1971.

Holliday, Jane: Bowel programs of patients with spinal cord injury: a clinical study, Nurs. Res. **16:**4-15, Winter, 1967.

Kahn, E., and Rossier, A.: Acute injuries of the cervical spine, Postgrad. Med. **39:**37-44, 1966.

Kemp, B. J. and Vash, D. L.: Productivity after injury in a sample of spinal cord injured persons: a pilot study, J. Chronic. Dis. **24:**259-275, 1971.

Knapp, M.: Spinal cord injury, Part I, Postgrad. Med. **42:**A95-A99, 1967.

Knapp, M.: Spinal cord injury. Part II, Postgrad. Med. **42:**A111-A116, 1967.

Kosiak, M.: An effective method of preventing decubital ulcers, Arch. Phys. Med. **47:**724-729, 1966.

Kosiak, M.: Etiology of decubitus ulcers, Arch. of Phys. Med. **42:**19-29, 1961.

Langford, T. L.: Nursing problems: bacteriuria and the indwelling catheter, Am. J. Nurs. **72:**113-115, 1972.

Levine, Myra, moderator: Quadriplegic adolescent, Nursing '72 **2:**28-32, June, 1972.

Martin, A.: Nursing care in cervical cord injury, Am. J. Nurs. **63:**60-66, 1963.

May, C. M.: Wheelchair patient for a day, Am. J. Nurs. **73:**650-651, 1973.

McElhinney E.: Pressure sores—prevention and treatment, Physiotherapy **54:**283-285, 1968.

Moolten, S. E.: Bedsores in the chronically ill patient, Arch. of Phys. Med. Rehab. **53:**430-438, 1972.

Perrine, G.: Needs met and unmet, Am. J. Nurs. **71:**2128-2133, 1971.

Pfaudler, M.: Flotation, displacement, and decubitus ulcers, Am. J. Nurs. **68:**2351-2355, 1968.

Pratt, R.: The nursing management of acute spinal paraplegia, 7 part series, Nurs. Times **67:**499-500, 537-540, 567-569, 604-606, 638-639, 662-663, 699-700, 1971.

Recent developments in research and in medical care relating to paraplegic and quadriplegic patients, Arch. Phys. Med. **47:**entire issue, July, 1966.

Regina, Sister E.: Sensory stimulation techniques, Am. J. Nurs. **66:**281-286, 1966.

Report of a Conference on the Current Status of the Care of the Spinal Cord-Injured Patient, Committee on the Skeletal System, Division of Medical Sciences, National Academy of Sciences, National Research Council, Oct., 1967, Washington, D. C.

Robertson, C. A.: Manual expression of urine, Amer. J. Nurs. **59:**840-841, 1959.

Robertson, C.: Gel pillow helps prevent pressure sores, Can. Nurse, **67:**44-46, 1971.

Rodgers, Helen M.: A water pillow too, Am. J. Nurs. **68:**2359-2360, 1968.

Rosenthal, A. M., and Schurman, A.: Hyperbaric treatment of pressure sores, Arch. Phys. Med. Rehab. **52:**413-415, 1971.

Ruge, D.: Spinal cord injuries, Springfield, Ill., 1969, Charles C Thomas, Publisher.

Santora, D.: Preventing hospital-acquired urinary infection, Am. J. Nurs. **66:**790-794, 1966.

Saxon, J.: Techniques for bowel and bladder training, Am. J. Nurs. **62:**69-71, 1962.

Siller, J.: Psychological situation of the disabled with spinal cord injuries, Rehab. Lit. **30:**290-296, 1969.

Spence, W. R., Burk, R. D., and Rae, J. W., Jr.: Gel support for prevention of decubitus ulcers, Arch. Phys. Med. **48:**283-288, 1967.

Spieker, J. L. and Lethcoe, B. J.: Upper extremity functional bracing: a follow-up study, Am. J. Occup. Ther. **25:**398-401, 1971.

Sudduth, A. L.: Comprehensive care of the traumatic paraplegic, RN **33:**59-61, 1970.

Thornhill, H., and Williams, M.: Experience with the water mattress in a large city hospital, Am. J. Nurs. **68:**2356-2358, 1968.

Torelli, M.: Topical hyperbaric oxygen for decubitus ulcers, Am. J. Nurs. **73:**494-496, 1973.

Trigiano, L. L.: Independence is possible in quadriplegia, Am. J. of Nurs. **70:**2610-2613, 1970.

Tudor, L. L.: Bladder and bowel retraining, Am. J. Nurs. **70:**2391-2393, 1970.

Wilkinson, M.: Rehabilitation of patients with neurological deficit, Nurs. Times **63:**315-317, 1967.

Winter, C., and Barker, M. R.: Nursing care of patients with urologic diseases, ed. 3, St. Louis, 1972, The C. V. Mosby Co.

Winter, C. C., Roehm, M., and Watson, H.: Urinary calculi, Am. J. Nurs. **63:**72-76, 1963.

Wolf, B. A.: Effectiveness of functional retraining for patients with quadriplegia, Phys. Therapy **51:**283-289, 1971.

Stroke (cerebrovascular accident)

Beeson, P. B., and McDermott, W., editors: Cecil-Loeb textbook of medicine, ed. 13, Philadelphia, 1971, W. B. Saunders Co.

Boulay, R., Cohn, S., Kaplan, L., Shapiro, M., and Winokur, S.: Helping the stroke patient to come back walking, Nursing Updated **2:**3-10, 1971.

Brocklehurst, J. C.: Guidelines for rehabilitating stroke patients. 1, Dysphasia and the nurse, Nurs. Mirror **133:**17-19, 1971.

Bruetman, Martin E., Gordon, Edward E.: Rehabilitating the Stroke Patient at General Hospitals, Postgraduate Medicine **49:**211-215, March, 1971.

Buck, M.: Adjustments during recovery from stroke, Am. J. Nurs. **64:**92-95, 1964.

Burt, M. N.: Perceptual deficits in hemiplegia, Am. J. Nurs. **70:**1026-1029, 1970.

Do it yourself again self-help devices for the stroke patient, New York, 1965, American Heart Association.

Ellis, R.: After stroke—sitting problems, Am. J. Nurs. **73:**1898-1899, 1973.

Elwood, E.: Nursing the patient with a cerebrovascular accident, Nurs. Clin. North Am. **5:**47-53, 1970.

Fowler, R. S., and Fordyce, W. E.: Adapting care for the brain-damaged patient, Am. J. Nurs., Part I, **72:**1832-1835, 1972, and Am. J. Nurs., Part II, **72:**2056-2059, Nov., 1972.

Guerrieri, B.: Survey of the knowledge of the nurse in direct-care services concerning proper bed positioning of the patient with hemiplegia, Nurs. Res. **17:**157-159, 1968.

A handbook of rehabilitative nursing techniques in hemiplegia, Minneapolis, 1964, Kenny Rehabilitation.

Hudson, W. J., Hood, M., and Brock, F.: Hospital management of hemiplegia, Can. Nurse **62:**21-23, 1966.

Hurwitz, L. J.: Sensory defects in hemiplegia, Physiotherapy **52:**338-342, 1966.

Hyman, M. D.: The stigma of stroke, its effects on performance during and after rehabilitation. Geriatrics **26:**132-141, 1971.

Jacobansky, A. M.: Stroke: prevention of further deterioration is a key goal in the nursing care of these patients, Am. J. Nurs. **72:**1260-1263, 1972.

Kelly, Sister P.: Mr. Quinto—a difficult rehab patient, Nursing '73 **3:**27-29, April, 1973.

Kessler, H. H.: Rehabilitation manual for hemiplegia, West Orange, N. J., 1961, Kessler Institute for Rehabilitation.

Klocke, J.: The role of nursing management in behavioral changes of hemiplegia, J. Rehab. **35:**24-27, 1969.

Knapp, M.: The hemiplegic patient—rehabilitation, Postgrad. Med. **39:**A143-A149, 1966.

Knapp, M.: The hemiplegic patient—physical problems, Postgrad. Med. **39:**A125-A132, 1966.

Large, H., Tuthill, J., Kennedy, F. B., and Pozen, T.: In the first stroke intensive care unit, Am. J. Nurs. **69:**76-80, 1969.

Miller, B.: Assisting aphasic patients with speech rehabilitation, Am. J. Nurs. **69:**983-985, 1969.

Mitchell, J.: Guidelines for rehabilitating stroke patients. 2, Early management of the aphasic patient, Nurs. Mirror **133:**19-21, 1971.

Nickel, V. L., editor: Orthopedic management of stroke, symposium. Clin. Orthop. **63:**3-161, 1969.

Perry, J.: Orthopedic management of the lower extremity in the hemiplegic patient, Phys. Ther. **46:**345-356, 1966.

Peszczynski, M.: The rehabilitation potential of the late adult hemiplegic, Am. J. Nurs. **63:**111-114, 1963.

Pfaudler, M.: After stroke—motor skill rehabilitation skills for hemiplegic patients, Am. J. Nurs. **73:**1892-1896, 1973.

Piskor, B. K. and Paleos, S.: The group way to banish after-stroke blues, Am. J. Nurs. **68:**1500-1503, 1968.

Rehabilitative nursing techniques. 2. Selected equipment useful in the hospital, home, or nursing home, Minneapolis, 1964, Kenny Rehabilitation.

Rehabilitative nursing techniques. 3. A procedure for passive range of motion and self-assistive exercises, Minneapolis, 1964, Kenny Rehabilitation.

Rothberg, June: Principles of nursing rehabilitation

for patients with cerebrovascular accident (CVA): Nurs. Sci. **1:**368-385, 1963.

Shafer, K., Sawyer, J., McCluskey, A., Beck, E., and Phipps, W.: Medical-surgical nursing, ed. 5, St. Louis, 1971, The C. V. Mosby Co.

Shaw, B. L.: Revolution in stroke care, RN **33:**56-61, 1970.

Smith, G. W.: Care of the patient with a stroke, a handbook for the patient's family and the nurse, New York, 1967, Springer Publishing Co., Inc.

Stanton, J. H.: Rehabilitation nursing related to stroke, Clin. Orthop. **63:**39-53, 1969.

Stern, P. H., McDowell, F., Miller, J. M., and Robinson, M.: Effects of facilitation exercise techniques in stroke rehabilitation, Arch. Phys. Med. **51:**526-531, 1970.

Stohl, Dora J.: Preserving home life for the disabled, Am. J. Nurs. **72:**1645-1650, 1972.

Suggs, K. M.: Coping and adaptive behavior in the stroke syndrome, Nurs. Forum **10:**100-111, 1971.

Ullman, M.: Disorders of body image after stroke, Am. J. Nurs. **64:**89-91, 1964.

Weisbroth, S., Esibill, N., and Zuger, R. R.: Factors in the vocational success of hemiplegic patients, Arch Phys. Med. **52:**441-446, 1971.

Whitehouse, F. A.: Stroke—some psycho-social problems it causes, Amer. J. Nurs. **63:**81-87, 1963.

Whitehouse, F. A.: Stroke: the present challenge, Nurs. Forum **10:**90-99, 1971.

4

Common painful affections in adults

LOW BACK PAIN

In recent years there has been an increasing number of patients complaining of pain in the lower portion of the back; hence, much attention is paid to this disability in an attempt to determine precisely the origin of pain in each case.

With a detailed history, complete examination of the back, and adequate roentgenography, it is usually possible to determine whether the cause is likely to be infection, tumor, arthritis, or something mechanical in nature. Any disease, injury, or affliction known to involve bones or joints throughout the body is capable of choosing the bones and joints of the lower part of the back. By far the majority of backaches are the result of mechanical stresses, and it is this type of backache that will be discussed.

ANATOMY OF THE LOW BACK

The anatomy of the lower part of the back should be reviewed for an understanding of the nature of mechanical causes of backache. The entire spine is composed of vertebral bodies that are separated by disks. These disks are resilient and capable of absorbing shock much the same as shock absorbers on automobiles. This shock-absorbing mechanism is nature's way of protecting the brain from impact shock, such as might occur in a jump from a height or a fall on the ice in a sitting position. When the disks are injured or chronically strained by repeated heavy lifting, they undergo changes

so that they lose their resilience and become narrowed. This is called degeneration and is commonly painful.

The facets are small joints, one on either side of each vertebral segment, that form the fulcrum for motion when the spine is flexed, extended, rotated, or bent sideward. These facets are covered with smooth articular cartilage that allows easy, gliding, symmetric motion when they are normally placed. Frequently the facets are asymmetric or anomalous in their position as a result of congenital malformation. When this is the case, the cartilage wears out prematurely and can be the cause of pain in the lower back. The pain often begins as "catches" in the back and is referred to as the facet syndrome.

Asymmetry of the facets is only one of the many anatomic variations that can occur in the lumbosacral area. The most frequent anomaly is an incomplete fusion of the lamina of the first sacral segment. Another common variation is sacralization of the fifth lumbar segment (Fig. 4-1), which means that the fifth lumbar segment takes on characteristics of the sacral rather than the lumbar spine.

SPONDYLOLISTHESIS

Spondylolisthesis, or the slipping forward of one vertebral segment on another (Fig. 4-2), constitutes the congenital anomaly most likely to produce backache. The presence of spondylolisthesis does not always cause backache, but perhaps 60% of these disorders do eventuate in symptoms.

POSTURAL STRAINS

Postural strains comprise a group of backaches that are mechanical in nature and occur

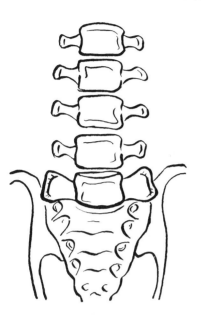

Fig. 4-1. Anomaly of the fifth lumbar vertebra. Note that in this particular case there is sacralization on both sides of the vertebral body. (From Kenney, W. C., and Larson, C. B.: Orthopedics for the general practitioner, St. Louis, 1957, The C. V. Mosby Co.)

in normal spines in the absence of predisposing causes such as anomalies. As the term implies, this type of strain is the resultant effect upon supporting ligaments that resist any poor posture for long periods.

The entire group of mechanical backaches has a similar pattern of treatment. An attempt should be made in all cases to detect the predisposing cause, be it a congenital anomaly or a faulty postural habit. By elimination of the abnormal stresses the symptoms can be controlled.

Eliminating abnormal stresses is accomplished by teaching the patient the correct positional use of the spine—that is, proper standing position, proper lifting habits, proper sitting positions, and the avoidance of twisting motions. Frequently this instruction can be supplemented by his use of a support such as a low back brace or corset (Fig. 4-3) that will act as a reminder rather than a true support for the back. Weak musculature should be built up to proper strength by exercises.

RUPTURED DISK

Perhaps 10% of the backaches that are brought to a physician's attention are caused by a ruptured disk. As the name suggests, a portion of the nucleus pulposus, which is the central part of an intervertebral disk, herniates through the posterior ligament that invests it. This herniated fragment of disk comes to lie within the

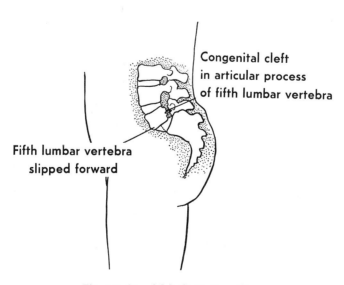

Congenital cleft
in articular process
of fifth lumbar vertebra

Fifth lumbar vertebra
slipped forward

Fig. 4-2. Spondylolisthesis (type II).

spinal canal, and by occupying space it crowds or actually causes pressure on the nerve roots within the spinal canal. Nerve roots when irritated become painful, and the pain is radiated along the entire course of the nerve; hence it is likely that a ruptured disk will cause pain radiating into the leg and foot. This has commonly been called sciatica, but the term is not correct because only one of the many nerve roots that make up the sciatic nerve is affected.

Lifting from a stooped position is the most common cause of rupture of an intervertebral disk. Whenever back pain is associated with radiating leg pain, a ruptured disk should be suspected. Weakness of muscle groups, changes in sensation, and loss of the ankle reflex or the knee jerk are helpful signs to localize the particular nerve root that is irritated. Another way to determine the exact level of the ruptured disk is by the use of contrast media intrathecally. Radiopaque material introduced by spinal puncture technique will be visible in the fluoroscope and reveal a filling defect at the site of the ruptured fragment. This procedure is known as intraspinal myelography (Fig. 4-4).

The treatment for a ruptured disk is likely to be operative, since removal of the protruded fragment of disk (Fig. 4-5) will relieve the radiating pain. Operative treatment is imperative only when there is evidence of increasing nerve root pressure. In milder protrusions nonoperative treatment, namely bed rest, will often relieve the acute symptoms.

In all types of backaches so far discussed, spinal fusion can be done to relieve pain when conservative measures have failed. The pain will be eliminated when there is no longer motion through the affected segments. Fusion is fre-

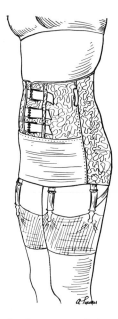

Fig. 4-3. Sacrolumbar support. It is made of brocade, elastic, and straps. It has a pad over the sacrum and is heavily reinforced with corset stays.

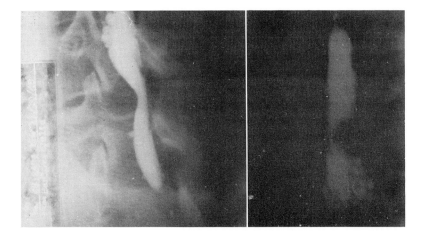

Fig. 4-4. Ruptured nucleus pulposus protruding into a column of radiopaque contrast medium during myelography. (From Kenney, W. C., and Larson, C. B.: Orthopedics for the general practitioner, St. Louis, 1957, The C. V. Mosby Co.)

quently carried out after removal of a ruptured disk in order to stabilize the degenerated level in which the rupture occurred.

NURSING CARE

Early mild back strain is usually treated by recumbency and heat. Adequate recumbency for this condition requires a hard bed and supports under the lumbar spine and knees. The support under the lumbar spine should be a hair pillow or folded sheet. It should be a firm support, so a sheet folded lengthwise is preferable to a feather pillow. If the patient prefers to lie prone, he will usually be most comfortable with a pillow under the lower abdomen and another supporting the feet so that the knees are mildly flexed. Radiant heat may be ordered, or moist hot packs may be used. Prolonged heat, however, will increase congestion, which is extremely undesirable in low back pain. Hot paraffin is sometimes used to supply heat and is put on by brush in repeated applications until a thick coating is obtained. It will maintain heat in the part for as long as 40 minutes. Massage is not usually a part of the physical therapy for patients with back pain, particularly in the acute stage, since muscle spasm is somewhat exaggerated by it. Deep massage in the less severely affected patient is sometimes of considerable comfort, but it must be used with caution. Medications usually consist of aspirin or some other type of salicylate given at 3- to 4-hour periods. Muscle-relaxant drugs are occasionally ordered for relief of muscle spasm.

Back-strapping with adhesive tape frequently provides temporary relief in mild cases. This procedure is performed by the orthopedist, but there are sometimes emergencies in which the orthopedic nurse may be called upon to do this at the request and under the direction of the physician. Adhesive strips 3 to 4 inches in width are used and should be long enough to extend from the anterior iliac spine on one side across the back and beyond the anterior iliac spine of the other side. Considerable traction is exerted on each strip as it is applied, and a lumbar pad of felt to supply pressure over the sacral region may be used under the tape. Three to four strips of adhesive tape are necessary, and these extend from the trochanter level to above the iliac crests. The patient may be standing or may be lying in bed while these are applied. It has been found that the patient, when standing, can provide assistance if he is allowed to stand in a corner and brace himself with his hands against the walls. Strapping gives only temporary relief, but occasionally symptoms may subside and the patient will be able to return to his work. Occasionally, strapping is used in conjunction with recumbency or traction. The main contraindication here is that the use of heat is restricted because of the presence of the tape.

Bed rest is usually ordered for severe pain in the lower portion of the back. The patient is most comfortable in a semi-Fowler position. In this position, with the backrest elevated approximately 20 degrees and the knees flexed slightly (Fig. 4-6), there is less tension of the back muscles

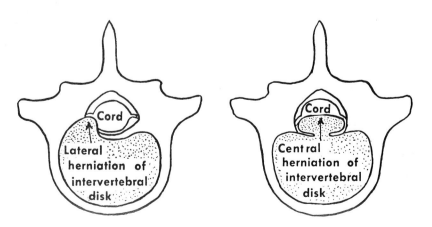

Fig. 4-5. Ruptured nucleus pulposus. Diagram showing mechanism of pressure on cord.

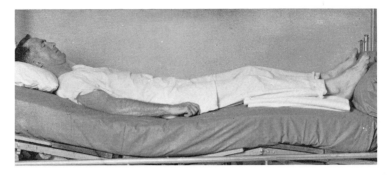

Fig. 4-6. The patient with acute back pain is usually more comfortable with the backrest elevated 20 to 30 degrees and the knees flexed slightly.

and of the hamstrings. At times the attending physician will find it necessary to apply traction to relieve spasm of the thigh and back muscles. Simple Buck's extension can be used intermittently to relieve back pain. In the acute stage of this condition, however, the patient is likely to be uncomfortable in any position, and, for this reason, he is allowed to assume whatever attitude he can find to give him relief. Morphine may be necessary to control pain, which is sometimes so severe that the patient is in continuous agony. Nurses tend to minimize low back pain as one of the minor afflictions until they have cared for a patient with an acute case and watched the intense suffering that he endures.

When the acute pain has subsided, exercises may be ordered for the purpose of improving the patient's body mechanics and thereby building up a resistance against further back strains as the result of postural deviations. Nurses should make an attempt to watch these exercises as they are taught in the physical therapy department. Usually, such exercises are begun by having the patient—first in the lying position and then standing—flatten the lumbar spine by active contraction of the abdominal and gluteal muscles. Diaphragmatic breathing is also emphasized. Sometimes the exercises are done by the patient in bed as often as every hour during the day. He may be taught to contract the gluteal muscles five or ten times, using a steady, slow rhythmic contraction. A second important bed exercise for this condition is one in which the patient lies on his back and raises his head and shoulders a short distance from the bed without using his elbows to brace himself. This also may be done five to ten times an hour until he is doing the exercise a hundred times daily.

Use of the therapeutic corset. Practically all physical therapy after treatment for these patients is designed to create a set of corset muscles sufficiently strong to serve as an internal splint for the low back. Until this can be accomplished, some kind of corset or brace is customarily prescribed. Nurses should understand that a corset for this condition should be prescribed by the physician. Patients who attempt to purchase corsets for low back pain without the advice of an orthopedist frequently spend a great deal of money on garments that are absolutely inefficient and may even exacerbate their condition. Corsets for low back pain have a dual purpose. In the first place they should provide a type of immobilization for the painful back, and secondly they should assist in maintaining the trunk in good posture. Use of the therapeutic corset is often a somewhat perplexing problem to the student who has relatively little chance to obtain experience in its application (Fig. 4-7). Students should be given the opportunity to watch the prescription corsetière doing the final fitting and to observe points of special importance in the construction and application of the garment.

The corset is made to fit the curves of the back so that no loose or gapping spaces occur anywhere. Its length must be sufficient to assist in the control of the buttock muscles, and it should be high enough to approximate the lower portion of the shoulder blades. The front of the corset must be long enough to support the abdomen adequately, and a careful fitting over the

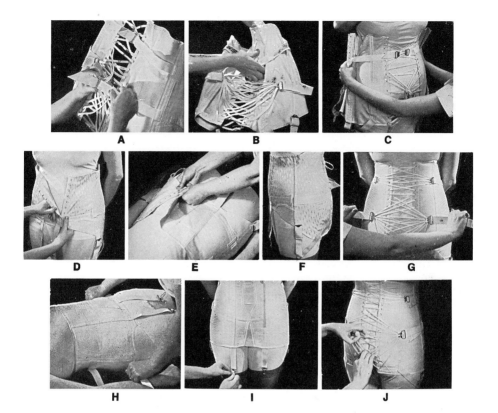

Fig. 4-7. Application of a corset for conditions of the low back. **A,** Release the buckles by turning them backward on the straps, holding the buckle between the first finger and thumb, and slide toward the end of the strap to within 2 inches of the end. **B,** After releasing the buckles it is advisable to bend the corset bones in the top and bottom in the back in order to conform to the curves of the body. **C,** Standing position. Place the support on the body with the center back well down under the gluteus muscles (as shown). The bottom of the front should curve down to the pubic bone; the bones of the support, if any, should not press on the pubic bone. **D,** Hooking the support in the standing position. If the top hook of the support is fastened first, it will hold the support on the body while the fitter hooks the rest of the support from the bottom upward. **E,** Reclining position. Same procedure as in standing position. **F,** Fastening side hose supporters. In both standing and reclining positions, fasten side hose supporters in such a manner that the front portion will draw straight down on the side as shown. **G,** Pulling the adjustment straps in the standing position. Draw, slightly, the top strap or lacer sufficiently to settle the support at the waistline. Then hold the lower straps, one in each hand, and give a steady pull, thus laying a foundation around the pelvis. **H,** Reclining position. The patient must raise her body to enable the fitter to obtain a proper grip on the straps and to give a firm, steady, outward pull. Procedure is the same as for standing position. Caution: always tighten the opposite straps at the same time, one in each hand, and not first one and then the other. **I,** Fasten front hose supporters straight down without tension. **J,** Inspection of fitting. See that there is no slack in any of the lacers; if slack is present, retrace lacers with the fingers. Tuck ends of the adjustment straps backward through the loops designed to receive them. When correctly adjusted, the back opening should not be more than 2 or 3 inches wide; if it is, a garment of larger size should be chosen. Have the patient sit down to make sure that the support is comfortable and that it does not slip from its proper position on the body. (Courtesy S. H. Camp & Co.)

iliac crests is necessary to prevent the garment from sliding up.

Perineal straps are sometimes used to prevent the corset from rolling up, but these are not considered essential if the fit of the garment is adequate. (Sacroiliac belts, however, may frequently have this feature attached.) Pads made of flannelette sewed into place over the sacrolumbar region of the corset are not uncommon, but again these are considered superfluous if the corset is carefully constructed to fit the curves of the back. Back-lacing is considered desirable for proper fitting in therapeutic corsets.

The patient should be observed in a sitting position after the corset is applied to see that it does not slip from its original position. A garment that fits loosely or that rolls up is of no value. The front stays should not press down on the pubic bone because this will cause the patient considerable discomfort. The garters are an important part of any therapeutic corset and should be kept in good condition. The posterior and lateral garters are particularly important for the correct fitting and placement of the corset. Nurses should observe that they are not fastened in such a way that they go off at an angle when attached to the hose. The front garters must be attached to the hose without undue tension, for tension may make it impossible for the patient to stand erect.

Nursing care of the patient with a herniated disk

Conservative treatment. Rupture of an intervertebral disk is a well-recognized cause of pain in the low back. Conservative treatment for this condition may be the same as for any type of low back pain: recumbency, heat, support, and exercise. A semisitting position is sometimes found to be efficacious for the comfort of the patient. The backrest is elevated about 20 degrees, and the legs and thighs are elevated on pillows along their entire length. Forward flexion of the lumbar spine is thereby encouraged. Physicians who prescribe this position do not permit lying in the prone position (hyperextension of the spine) at any time.

Muscle spasms frequently cause the patient great discomfort. The application of heat by means of a hot-water bottle, hot moist packs or, in some instances, a heating pad may give relief.

Pelvic traction or Buck's extension may be applied and muscle relaxant drugs prescribed. In some instances, however, narcotics will be necessary before relief is gained. When this patient is turned, it is important that the shoulders and hips be moved in one plane. Twisting of the spine is avoided by teaching the patient to turn in log fashion. A wide drawsheet that extends from the shoulders to below the hips may be used. A pillow is placed between the patient's thighs. The nurse, reaching across the patient, grasps the rolled drawsheet and gently turns him toward her onto his side. The patient's hips should then be pulled back toward the center of the bed, and the uppermost limb adjusted on the pillow previously placed between the thighs. Another method of turning this kind of patient is described in the discussion of nursing care of the patient with a spinal fusion. The use of a child's bedpan or a bedpan with a tapering back will cause the patient with back pain less discomfort than the ordinary adult bedpan. For placing the patient on the pan, he is rolled onto his side, and the pan and a small pillow or roll to support the lumbar region are placed in position. The patient is then rolled back, onto the pan. Having him use the trapeze should be avoided. A foot support to hold the covers off the feet and to prevent drop foot adds to his comfort and is a necessity if there have been motor or sensory changes in the limbs.

Since conservative treatment usually consists of several weeks of bed rest, the patient with this problem may become quite discouraged and feel that little progress is being made. He may fear being operated upon or question whether he will be able to return to his usual activities without recurrence of the condition.

Prior to ambulation the patient is fitted with a corset or brace that provides support and immobilization of the back. The purpose of the support is to prevent recurrence of the condition. It should be worn when the patient is not in bed. Also, a pair of good walking shoes should be worn when the patient is permitted to begin activity. Another important aspect in preventing recurrence of this condition is instructing the patient in correct body mechanics. Proper methods of lifting and stooping must be practiced and strenuous activity avoided if recurrence is to be prevented. The practice of correct body mechanics also includes use of good sitting posture. The use of a straight-back chair as opposed to the overstuffed chair is recommended for the person with a back problem. Strain on involved nerves may be caused by sitting with the knees crossed or by sitting with the knees in extension—such as when elevating the feet on a footstool or driving a low-seat car. In addition, any sudden twisting movement of the spine should be avoided.

Nursing care after laminectomy. Laminectomy is sometimes necessary for a patient with lesion of an intervertebral disk. This is particularly true if it is a recurrence of previous disk problems. The surgical procedure provides for removal of the portion of the nucleus pulposus that is protruding or ruptured from the intervertebral disk. To do this, a portion of the lamina of one or more vertebrae is removed. The nursing care of a patient after a laminectomy without fusion is a relatively simple problem, quite different from the nursing problem encountered in laminectomy for the person having a fractured spine or a cord tumor. When spinal fusion is not done simultaneously with the laminectomy, the patient is usually permitted to move about in bed at liberty and is encouraged to exercise his feet and legs at frequent intervals. Nurses are instructed to observe the patient's ability to do this after the operation and to record this carefully during the early postoperative period. Blood pressure readings are taken postoperatively at frequent intervals. The patient should be placed on a firm mattress. Maintenance of the supine position may be ordered for the first 24 hours postoperatively. Pressure on the operative area helps prevent formation of a hematoma. The usual precautions in turning patients with conditions of the spine should be observed in the care of each of these patients. The body is turned in one piece, and twisting at the hips is carefully avoided. Face-lying and side-lying positions are often permitted. When the patient lies on his side, a pillow between the legs will prevent strain on back muscles. A pillow to support the upper arm will prevent sagging of the shoulder. Early ambulation is frequently prescribed for the patient who has had a laminectomy. This in itself helps to prevent many postoperative complications, such as retention, distention, phlebitis, and hypostatic pneumonia.

Postoperative care of the patient with spinal fusion

Postoperative care of the patient with spinal fusion will vary somewhat in different clinics, but a general outline will be given here.

Some doctors require their patients with spinal fusion to lie prone for the first few days and be turned only for voiding. This is usually because they fear pressure and necrosis at the operative site. Others prefer that the patient lie flat on his back without being turned for several days. The patient is usually most comfortable if pillows are used to support the legs along their entire length. Some relaxation of the back muscles is obtained by this slight elevation. Furthermore, it is thought by many surgeons to be a means of overcoming a threat of thrombophlebitis in the femoral vessels. When the pillows are arranged, they should not be placed in such a fashion that flexion of the knee is exaggerated. The first pillow should be placed high enough under the thigh to support the limb along the full length of the hamstring muscles. The lower pillows support the knee and lower leg on a slight incline without undue knee flexion.

When a plaster bed is to be used after surgery, allowance should be made for the dressing that the patient will be wearing. This dressing, consisting of gauze sponges and combination pads, is sometimes quite generous and, unless allowance is made, pressure upon the incision is inevitable. The plaster bed must be well prepared for the patient. Wrinkles and ridges should be eliminated. The doctor preparing the bed will have padding inserted at the proper points. The stockinet must be pulled out to cover all the raw edges and taped down securely. Straps are often added to the bed, and its final finishing is done by a brace maker. If this is not done, the nurse is responsible for drying the plaster and for having straps with buckles in readiness. The entire shell may be covered with stockinet sewed on neatly. The area around the buttocks must be protected with a waterproof material. All this should be done before surgery because the patient can seldom spare either section of the shell long enough for repair afterward. The advisability of having the patient lie in the plaster bed for a time before surgery is great. Any points of discomfort incidental to the shell can thus be discovered before the patient is compelled to lie in it permanently.

When a good plaster bed has been made preoperatively, orders will usually be given to turn the patient for morning and evening care. This turning may be done the first evening if the patient's condition permits. A patient in shock, however, will often benefit by being allowed to lie quietly until the next morning. If the patient lies on his back, careful check of the pulse and blood pressure will be necessary to detect hemorrhage, since the dressings are not visible.

There may be a mild and temporary decrease in the tone of the genitourinary and gastrointestinal tracts as a result of the inevitable shock to the sympathetic nervous system. Considerable liberty is allowed the nurse in giving fluids to these patients. Fluids are usually encouraged as soon as nausea is past. Diet is increased as the patient tolerates it.

If the patient is an adult, it is advisable to have sufficient help so that the initial turnings may be accomplished with as little discomfort as possible. He is naturally apprehensive at this time, and everything should be done to give him a sense of security. Later turnings will be accomplished much more easily if this is done. The patient in a well-fitting plaster bed can be turned with relatively little pain to his back. If the graft has been taken from the tibia, slight changes of position in the knee joint will cause muscular pull on the tibia, which causes the patient considerable pain.

After a week or so the pain and muscle spasm in this leg will have subsided, but during the early days it is very acute and is a source of great concern to the patient. At present, however, many surgeons are taking the graft from the crest of the ilium instead of the tibia. Thus, the difficulty in turning and the pain experienced by the patient are somewhat lessened.

The patient is moved all in one plane to the side of the bed. The undersheet is then changed by a nurse on the opposite side of the bed. Pillows are arranged to receive the leg from which the graft has been taken, and a support is made ready for the feet. The plaster shell should be securely fastened at the axillary level and around the hips.

If possible, the arm toward which the patient is to be turned should be placed above the head. For operations on the dorsal spine, however, it is sometimes better to have the arm on which the patient is to be turned stretched downward along the side of the cast. The nurse standing at the side of the bed toward which the patient has been pulled must take responsibility for seeing that this arm is freed immediately after turning is done. Otherwise, the pressure of the heavy plaster bed on the arm may cause considerable bruising. The patient is turned toward the clean side of the bed as a unit, without twisting at the hips or knees. One nurse can accomplish this if the patient is not too large. For a large adult, however, two nurses are advisable. One nurse places her hands on the patient's shoulders and hips, and the other assumes responsibility for the leg operated on, with some assistance from the nurse who stands on the opposite side of the bed.

Once turned, the patient should be made as comfortable as possible. The feet should be supported on a pillow placed under the ankles so that the toes do not dig into the bed. The posterior shell of the cast is removed, the dressings are carefully inspected for signs of hemorrhage or drainage, and the surrounding skin is washed and then rubbed gently with alcohol. The circulation of the back, head, and neck is important for the well-being of patients who have had spinal surgery and should be given frequent attention. Back rubs should include the scalp, neck, and thighs. The patient should be urged to lie prone for as long as he can do so in order to reestablish circulation in the dependent areas of the back and thighs. He may ask to be turned back almost immediately, but a little explanation of the purpose of the position will often help in prolonging the period.

Turning the patient with spinal fusion who is not immobilized. Patients with spinal fusions frequently are not immobilized in plaster. Extreme care and gentleness in turning are essential for these patients to avoid motion of the spine that will be accompanied by excruciating pain. To maintain good alignment, some doctors request that these patients be kept flat and that they lie either on the abdomen (Fig. 4-8) or on the back. In other instances patients are permitted to move and turn as they wish.

When a patient is being turned from his back to his abdomen after spinal fushion, without benefit of cast or brace, the nurse will apply the same technique used with the patient in a plaster cast. First, the patient is moved to one side of the bed. If the bed is made with a wide draw-sheet, the sheet can be used as a slide for the patient. This helps to avoid twisting movements of the spine. Clean linen is placed on the opposite half of the bed. Two nurses stand at the side of the bed toward which the patient is to be turned. The patient's arms are kept close to his side, and he is instructed to make his body rigid. The first nurse places her hands on the patient's far shoulder and arm, and the second nurse grasps the patient's hip and thigh. Slowly and gently, they turn the patient onto his abdomen toward themselves. Following this, it is necessary to move the patient back to the center of the bed. This again can be accomplished with the drawsheet. When the patient lies in the prone position, the dorsum of his feet need to be supported by a pillow. His arms may be placed in any comfortable position.

If the patient is turned on his side, the nurse will remember what constitutes a good side-lying position. The pillow between the legs to prevent adduction of the uppermost limb will avoid added strain on sore back muscles.

During the early days after surgery careless-ness in turning seldom takes place. The patient is so apprehensive that it is necessary to guard one's every movement lest unnecessary pain be caused. After 10 days or 2 weeks, how-

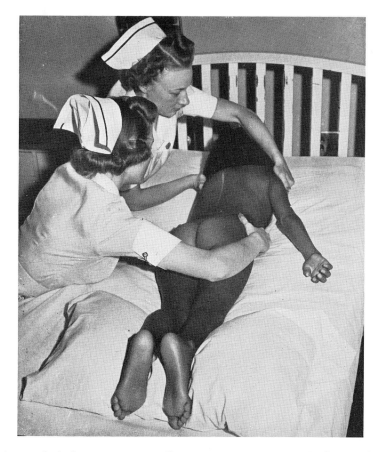

Fig. 4-8. One method of turning a patient (from prone to supine position) after spinal operation, when no supportive apparatus is used. Patient is rolled toward the nurses and, to avoid twisting movements of the spine, the shoulders and pelvis are turned simultaneously. The same method of supporting the shoulders and pelvis may be employed when the patient is turned from the supine to the prone position.

ever, when the patient's general condition is on the upgrade and the acute pain in the leg and back is much diminished, haste and carelessness sometimes do occur, for nurses on busy wards tend to try to turn such patients with insufficient help. Healing in spinal grafts takes place slowly, as does all bone healing, and gentle handling must continue for many weeks. The so-called critical time after spinal operations is considered to be 4 to 5 weeks. Particular care in handling the patient during this time should be observed. Spinal pseudarthrosis can occur because of careless postoperative handling of the patient with spinal fusion. The patient will learn to help the nurse in turning. Fewer persons can then accomplish the same effect for which many persons were needed during the first postoperative days. However, twisting or piecemeal turning, arching, or sagging of the buttocks and shoulders during the procedure should never be tolerated.

Edema of the face sometimes occurs in patients after spinal fusion, particularly if maintenance of shock position is necessary. This can be remedied by lowering the bed as early as seems compatible with the patient's general condition. A temporary impairment of bowel function is often encountered. Enemas are usually ordered between the fourth and sixth days, but they may not be efficacious unless they are preceded by very mild laxatives. Rectal impaction must not be allowed to occur before a cathartic is given. Occasionally, oil enemas will be more successful than large-volume enemas. The establishment of regular habits of elimination will soon help to overcome the need for enemas or laxatives and should be part of the patient's routine. The back and legs of the patient must be supported while he is on the bedpan so that all sections of the body are in the same plane. These patients will have less discomfort if a bedpan with a tapering back is used in place of the regular bedpan. Attention to such details will sometimes pay surprising dividends in helping the patient to resume normal habits of elimination.

Patients who must lie prone are in danger from pressure at areas over the iliac crests. This is particularly true of the thin patient in a bivalved cast. Reddened or bluish areas around the bony crests should receive immediate atten-tion because skin breakdown there is extremely rapid. The areas must be massaged frequently; crescent-shaped pieces of white felt may be lightly taped around the crests and often serve to overcome the hazard of lying prone. Circular doughnuts or pieces of felt with circles cut out of the center are not advisable, for they frequently serve to cut off circulation to the part still further.

The patient's progress and his resumption of normal activities—such as sitting, standing, and walking—will depend upon the diagnosis that made the spinal fusion necessary. Fusions in patients with disabilities of the low back usually progress more rapidly than those in patients who have had tuberculosis or similar infections of the vertebrae. It is urgent that patients who are to remain in bed for a prolonged period have constant intelligent care to parts of the musculoskeletal system that are not primarily affected but important to them when they become ambulatory. The physician may prescribe deep-breathing exercises, exercises for maintaining muscle tone in the feet, quadriceps setting, and, later, flexion and extension of the knees. The feet should be provided for by a support to keep the covers from pressing on the toes and to maintain the normal physiologic position of the feet in standing. Knee hyperextension should be eliminated by a small rolled towel placed under the head of the tibia just below the popliteal space. Outward rotation of the hip, if not controlled by a cast or plaster bed, should be prevented by sandbags or a trochanter roll. Unless contraindicated, the patient should be provided with occupations that will ensure normal varied use of the arms and shoulders.

The patient will usually be provided with a brace before he is allowed out of bed. It is essential that the nurse know how to apply the brace correctly and that she recognize its importance to the patient's ultimate recovery. The physician will usually order the patient to wear the brace at all times, in bed or out, until permission to omit it for short periods is given.

Applying back braces. Nurses should remember that low back braces (Fig. 4-9) and spring back braces may ride up considerably, particularly on heavy women. Perineal straps to prevent this are sometimes used but are never

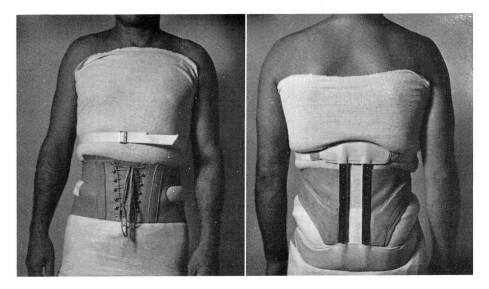

Fig. 4-9. Anterior and posterior views of a low back brace.

very comfortable for the wearer. If the brace has a well-fitting pelvic band, this will often overcome the tendency of the brace to ride up. A safe rule to remember is that in every back brace the pelvic band should fit low enough to hold the upper part of the buttocks adequately. When the brace is applied, the abdominal leather apron must be laced very snugly at the lower portion, diminishing in snugness as the lacing ascends. It is important in applying back braces to observe that the spinal uprights are far enough apart not to press on the vertebral prominences, but also close enough together to fit well between the scapulae.

Another important point to remember is that it is essential that a back brace allow the patient to sit with the hips at right angles, with no impingement of the metal or the leather on the groin. The patient must be able to sit without having the brace pushed up by the chair.

Spinal braces, such as the Taylor back brace, are not infrequently used for postoperative immobilization after fusions of the low back (sacro-iliac fusion, sacrolumbar fusion, or combinations of the two). These supports are often applied in the operating room, and the patient wears them continuously for a period of several months. For back care he is carefully turned in the brace. The metal and leather part of the apparatus is then lifted off the back, but the canvas apron that supports the abdomen is left under the patient as he lies prone, making it easy to reapply the brace once the back is cared for. A thin cotton vest of some knitted material is usually worn beneath the brace.

BURSITIS

LOCATION

Throughout the body there are a number of places where bony prominences are exposed to irritation, either from outward pressure or from the friction effect of tendons, ligaments, and even the skin over these bony prominences. Such prominences are protected by small sacs or compartments that are filled with a lubricating synovial fluid produced from the walls of the sac. This allows the gliding of the various structures over bony prominences without friction. A bursa may develop in an area where none normally exists if persistent irritation continues. The ordinary location of these bursae (Fig. 4-10) is as follows:

1. Shoulder
   (a) Subacromial
   (b) Subcoracoid
2. Elbow
   (a) Olecranon
3. Hip
   (a) Gluteal (under attachment of glueteus maximus)
   (b) Trochanteric (greater trochanter and lesser trochanter)
   (c) Ischial (weaver's bottom)
4. Knee
   (a) Prepatellar (housemaid's knee)
   (b) Pretibial (under patella tendon)
   (c) Superficial pretibial (over tibial tubercle)
   (d) Popliteal
   (e) Bicipital
5. Foot
   (a) Achilles (under the attachment of the Achilles tendon)
   (b) Retrocalcaneal (anterior to the Achilles tendon)
   (c) Inferior calcaneal (under the attachment of the plantar fascia to the heel—policeman's heel)
   (d) Bunion (may develop on either the inner or the outer side of the foot when there is bony prominence of the metatarsal head as seen in hallux valgus)

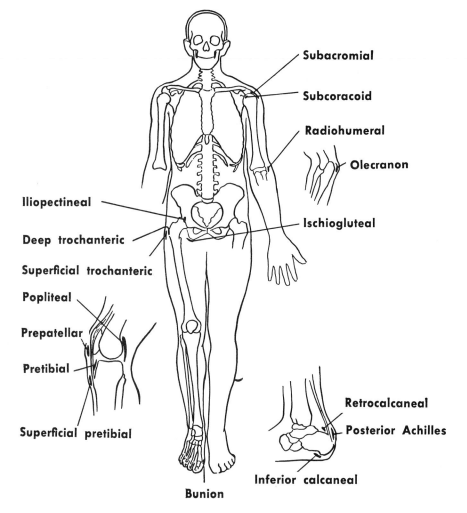

Fig. 4-10. Locations of the most common bursae.

SYMPTOMS

Inflammation of a bursa may develop gradually as the result of a repeated strain or injury or may develop acutely as the result of more severe damage. Pain, swelling, and marked tenderness are present. When active motions involve the function of the bursa, pain is greatly aggravated. Passive motions, however, are usually not so painful as they would be if there were joint involvement.

Acute inflammation of a bursa may develop when bacteria or toxins from remote focal infection settle there.

TREATMENT

The causes of bursitis, such as irritation and infection, should be removed.

In the noninfectious types of bursitis complete rest and the application of heat are important. A sling or a flannel spica applied to the extremities often is effective in giving relief.

Subdeltoid bursitis. Subdeltoid bursitis is one of the commonest forms and may need special treatment. The subdeltoid bursa is situated between the deltoid muscle and the rotator cuff of the shoulder. The inflammation arises in this bursa secondary to degeneration in one of the tendons of the rotator cuff, usually the supraspinatus. Calcium is deposited into the degenerated area, and it is often possible to see a calcific deposit in a roentgenogram of the shoulder that is painful as a result of bursitis. Pain is the outstanding symptom and frequently radiates down the arm. Restriction of motion in the shoulder may be so severe that this condition has been referred to as frozen shoulder.

Treatment of subdeltoid bursitis will depend on whether it is in the acute or the chronic stage. In acute bursitis the treatment is aimed at relief of pain. The simplest way to release the calcium that is under tension and is responsible for the active pain is to insert a needle and wash it out. This can be done with Procaine HCl (Novocain). At times the calcium is inspissated (dried out to form a hard pebble) and may require surgical excision. Many times the acute attack will cure itself by absorption of the calcium; however, this may require a period of a few days, during which time the patient must be well medicated for pain and the shoulder must be immobilized in a sling.

Chronic bursitis does not demand immediate treatment to relieve pain, although pain is present. The main consideration is to stop irritation of the degenerated rotator cuff so that it may heal. Avoidance of extreme motion and lifting, plus use of local heat, may control the symptoms and allow the process to subside. Many physicians prescribe radiation therapy, but the beneficial effect is variable. Pendulum exercises to regain lost motion are perhaps the most important treatment. Local injection of hydrocortisone into tender areas often helps to relieve pain.

DISABILITIES OF THE FEET

ANATOMY OF THE FOOT

The feet, small or large, must take the burden of weight bearing for various sizes and shapes of bodies. They bear the weight of the body when walking or standing and serve as levers in raising and propelling the body forward. The bony structure consists of seven tarsal bones, five metatarsal bones, and fourteen phalanges. At birth much of this structure is soft tissue (cartilage), and for this reason the foot of the newborn infant (when deformity exists) lends itself to corrective measures much better than the foot of an older child. There are two main arches, the longitudinal and the transverse (metatarsal). These arches are present at birth. The baby's foot, however, may appear quite flat because of a fat pad that fills the longitudinal arch space. The medial aspect of the longitudinal arch extends from the os calcis to the head of the first metatarsal. The lateral aspect extends from the os calcis to the head of the fourth and fifth metatarsals. This arch is supported by two groups of muscles: (1) those of the inner and (2) those on the outer side of the ankle. The inner group of muscles consists of the tibialis anticus, normally attached below the internal cuneiform, the posterior tibial muscle, normally attached to the scaphoid, and the flexors of the toes, whose tendons act by leverage under the astragalus (sustentaculum tali) to support the arch. All these muscles work in coordination and are assisted to some extent by the intrinsic muscles of the foot. The outer side of the foot is supported by the peroneal muscles—longus, brevis, and tertius. These muscles tend to balance the arch-elevating effect of the muscles of the inner side of the foot and at the same time work in unison to support the arches of the foot.

The metatarsal arch extends medially from the base of the fifth metatarsal to the base of the first metatarsal. This arch is supported by the balanced action between the flexors and the extensors of the toes combined with the intrinsic muscles of the foot.

When muscle action fails, from disuse or disease, the strain is transmitted to ligamentous structures, such as the plantar fascia, and to other ligaments around the joints. Strain is often accompanied by inflammatory change. Thus, it can be readily understood that the patient who has been at bed rest needs adequate support for his arches when ambulation is permitted. This patient needs a well-fitted shoe and not paper slippers.

MOVEMENTS OF THE FOOT

When caring for the bed patient, it is essential to know the normal movements of the foot and ankle. If these motions are not contraindicated and are performed passively or actively, joint contractures can be prevented. Plantar flexion (equinus position) and dorsiflexion of the foot take place at the ankle joint. Inversion (supination) and eversion (pronation) movements of the foot are made possible by the subastragalar joint. Adduction and abduction motions take place in the midtarsal joints. Flexion and extension of the toes take place at the metatarsophalangeal and the interphalangeal joints.

SHOES

Characteristics of a well-fitted shoe. Properly fitted shoes are an important factor in the prevention of foot deformities. If pain and foot discomfort are to be prevented, the shoe size and shape should conform to the foot. The foot must not be forced into an ill-fitted shoe. The shoe length, with weight-bearing, should extend approximately ¼ to ½ inch beyond the end of the great toe. A shoe that is too short will cause crowding of the toes, and the great toe will be forced into a hallux valgus position. A straight inner last is desirable. Continuous wearing of pointed shoes will result in a hallux valgus deformity and the formation of a bunion. (Fig. 4-11). A properly fitted shoe must have a sufficiently wide sole at the ball of the foot to permit free movement of foot muscles. The length should be proportioned so that the ball of the foot is accomodated at the widest part of the shoe. This part of the shoe needs to be flexible to permit bending of the toes. The shank should give fairly good support. The heavy person or the person who stands for long hours may need a stronger shoe and a more rigid shank than the person who sits for long periods. The shank of a child's shoe, unless ordered otherwise by his physician, should be flexible. The heel should fit the heel of the foot. Sling-strap slippers give little or no support, do not hold the heel in position, and tend to cause blisters and calluses.

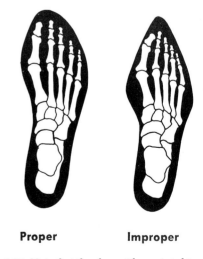

Proper   **Improper**

Fig. 4-11. Note that the shoe with a pointed toe forces the great toe into a hallux valgus position.

The height of the heel depends upon the purpose of the shoe. A shoe that is to be worn when working or walking should have a heel of reasonable height. It is difficult for the person who walks or stands in high heels to attain good posture and to practice good body mechanics. The weight of the body is thrown forward on the ball of the foot. This results in calluses and strain on the metatarsal arch.

Children's shoes. The baby who has not started to walk needs covering for his feet only to keep them warm. These shoes need to have soft soles that permit motion of the feet and use of foot muscles. When he learns to walk, his shoe should have a thin leather sole sufficient to protect his foot but flexible enough to permit normal motion and use of the muscles, particularly at the ball of the foot. The best shoe for a growing infant, especially if there is any abnormality, is of the high-topped variety with a firm sole, narrow heel, and broad toe.

PREDISPOSING CAUSES OF FOOT STRAIN

Foot strain caused by inherently weak muscles can begin with the first steps that a child takes. This weakness may persist and cause foot strain throughout life.

A second common cause of foot strain is ill-fitted shoes. There has been a tendency in the past to conform to style rather than to the shape of the foot, and the result has been high heels, narrow wedging toes, and a narrow sole. Fortunately this is at present being partly overcome, and there is an attempt to make shoes to conform to the shape of the average foot, but such correct shoes are still none too popular. Although ample width is essential in the metatarsal region, a shoe should not be sloppy or ill fitted at the instep and heel. One of the common causes of foot trouble, particularly in women, is the ten-

dency of the manufacturers to make shoes that are sufficiently large in circular dimension, but in which the sole of the shoe is narrower than the ball of the foot (Fig. 4-12). This is likely to cause strain on the metatarsal arch, because pressure is exerted upward along the lateral borders of the foot, and, in spite of the fact that the person has ample room within the confines of the shoe itself, there is no freedom of muscle action. A frequent statement is: "If my shoes were any bigger I couldn't keep them on my feet."

A third cause of foot strain is inadequate muscular and ligamentous support. (The arches of the foot are supported by ligaments, tendons, and muscles.) The child who is growing very rapidly may complain of some foot discomfort. Muscular strength is not keeping up with the growth of the body. Prolonged inactivity will result in weakness and atrophy of the soft tissues supporting the arches of the foot. If weight bearing is permitted in soft bedroom slippers, the patient may develop painful feet. Excessive body weight puts an additional strain on the foot. The muscular and ligamentous support of the arches may become inadequate, and the inevitable result is painful, flattened arches. Excessive exercise in soft rubber-soled shoes, when the individual is not accustomed to such activity, may result in foot strain and pain.

BUNIONS

There are two types of bunions, the acquired and the hereditary. Acquired bunions are definitely caused by wearing shoes that are too pointed and too narrow or too short.

Hereditary bunions are caused at least in part by a congenital abnormality. The space between the first and second metatarsals is increased so that bunion development in almost any type of shoe is unavoidable (Fig. 4-13).

Hallux valgus is an abnormal position of the big toe. Bunion is an overgrowth of bone. The two are commonly associated (Fig. 4-14).

The pain and discomfort from bunions can in most instances be relieved by properly fitted shoes and by support of the metatarsal arch. Arch supports, metatarsal bars, and sufficiently wide shoes are essential. Sometimes the sufferers from these deformities are not willing to accept the type of shoe necessary for relief.

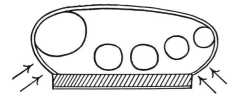

Fig. 4-12. Pressure exerted to cause metatarsal arch strain when shoe is improperly built. Such a shoe may have plenty of room.

Congenital bunion **Acquired bunion**

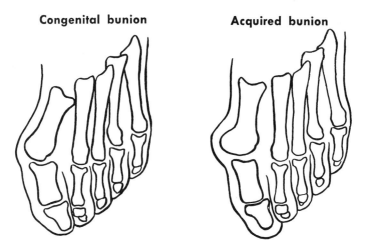

Fig. 4-13. Note difference in angle between first and second metatarsals.

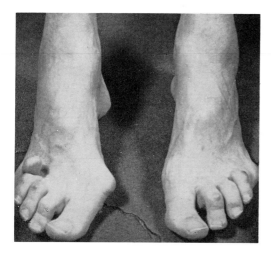

Fig. 4-14. Hallux valgus deformity with bunion, overlapping fifth toe (right), hammer toes, and corns.

Sometimes bunions may be so severe that bony correction is required.

Operative procedures are directed at correction of the abnormal position by various techniques, the commonest of which is removal of the proximal portion of the first phalanx (Keller operation), and the bunion is corrected by removal of bony overgrowth.

In the congenital type, osteotomy at the base of the first metatarsal may be combined with tendon transplantation according to the method of McBride. An osteotomy at the distal end of the metatarsal may also be necessary to restore the alignment.

LONGITUDINAL ARCH STRAIN

The pain in longitudinal arch strain both in children and in adults is usually felt in the arch of the foot and in the muscles of the legs. As a rule the pain that is caused by arch strain is present only after exertion and fatigue. If there is an inflammatory condition accompanying such a strain, it is usually characterized by aggravation of the pain on first arising in the morning or upon sudden activity after short periods of rest. Pain that is present only after activity is usually the result of muscle and ligamentous strain rather than inflammation of the joints and ligaments.

Treatment is designed to relieve the strain on the tibialis anticus and posticus muscles by means of temporary arch supports made of felt and leather and designed to the individual requirement. Felt is used instead of steel because the latter is rigid and tends to decrease the muscle development for correction. Particularly if knock-ankle deformity (Fig. 4-15) is present, a Thomas or orthopedic heel (Fig. 4-16) with an inner elevation may also be added.

A distinction should be made between acute arch strain and permanent or chronic flatfoot. In the latter it is justifiable to use rigid arch supports of stainless steel or Monel metal. In acute arch strain, exercises with temporary lifts and supports may be of distinct value in restoring muscle power after the strain has been relieved. In chronic flatfoot, however, exercises

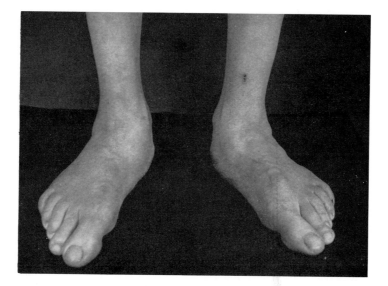

Fig. 4-15. Pronation of the foot. A common postural disturbance. Note flattened or depressed position of the longitudinal arch. If the foot is observed from the back, the Achilles tendon curves toward the midline. Frequently, the patient with pronated feet will complain of backache and of pain in the calves of the legs.

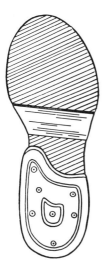

Fig. 4-16. Thomas (or orthopedic) heel often used in combination with a metatarsal bar.

are of little value. It may be necessary at times to use a high-topped shoe to offset the demands on the muscles that also control the ankle.

METATARSAL ARCH STRAIN—METATARSALGIA

The metatarsal arch is supported primarily by muscles, and, when the muscular action fails because of abuse or disuse, strain is placed upon the ligamentous structure and upon the arch. If strain is severe enough, there is a flattening of the arch and weight is taken on the heads of the second, third, and fourth metatarsals. The person with this condition will develop a callus over the ball of the foot, and walking will become quite painful. To relieve this pain, felt or rubber pads covered with leather may be placed just posterior to the heads of the second, third, and fourth metatarsals. The padding gives support to the arch and relieves pressure. The physician may also request that a metatarsal bar (anterior heel) be attached to the shoe. This, again, gives the arch support and relieves pressure on the metatarsal heads.

In strains of either longitudinal or metatarsal arches, a support of felt and leather may be designed from the pedograph or outline of the weight-bearing surface of the foot (Fig. 4-17). It is the object of supports not only to relieve pressure in the area of the foot that does not come in contact during weight bearing but also to distribute the pressure evenly through the area not bearing weight and a small portion of the weight-bearing area.

One of the main requirements in strain of the metatarsal arch is to give sufficient room

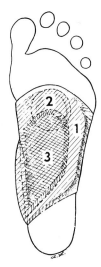

Fig. 4-17. Design for arch support based on the normal weight-bearing surface. The pads are of felt or rubber and covered with leather. Pad **3** fills the normal arch space. Pad **1** distributes pressure evenly over a larger area, and pad **2** increases pressure under the metatarsal arch at any desired point.

for action of the muscles that support the metatarsal arch. Therefore, adequate width of the shoe in the metatarsal region is necessary. Many broad short feet need EE or EEE shoes, which are difficult yet possible to obtain.

EXERCISES

The treatment described is aimed at relieving the symptoms and enabling the person to get about without discomfort. If the condition is to be corrected, however, the strength of the muscles that normally support the arch must be restored. This may be accomplished by active exercises. The following exercises are frequently prescribed to relieve arch strain.

For the metatarsal arch. One exercise prescribed to strengthen the metatarsal arch is the towel exercise. A towel is placed on the floor, and the feet are placed parallel to each other about an inch apart with the heels just over the posterior border. The toes are then contracted alternately one foot with the other so that the towel is gradually accumulated under the arch. Another exercise for the metatarsal arch is the marble exercise. Ten to twelve marbles are placed on the floor, and by action of the flexor tendon they are picked up, moved and released

rhythmically. A pencil may also be used. The toes may also be contracted rhythmically over the edge of a step or a large book upon which the subject is standing (Fig. 4-18).

For the longitudinal arch. In the standing position the feet and toes are inverted so that the weight is borne on the outer border of the feet. This exercise should be repeated thirty times. Another exercise for the longitudinal arch is performed by rising on the balls of the feet, raising the heels, and everting the ankles. This is to be repeated twenty to thirty times.

For contracted heel cords. Two exercises for contracted heel cords are performed as follows: (1) stand on the heel, raising and inverting the forefoot, and (2) stand with the ball of the foot on the edge of a stair and drop the weight downward, stretching the heel cords. These exercises should be done at least twice daily and should be repeated, starting at about twenty times each, and increasing to about fifty.

OTHER DISABILITIES OF THE FEET

There are other causes for disabilities in the foot as a result of disease, trauma, and disturbances in circulation.

Apophysitis. Apophysitis is a disease of the heels of growing children as a result of traumatic and metabolic disturbance. There is an irritation of the posterior epiphysis of the os calcis. Pain and tenderness are characteristic. Treatment consists of removing the counter of the shoe and temporarily raising the heel ½ to ¾ inch. Calcium, phosphorus, and vitamin D should also be administered.

Koehler's disease. Koehler's disease is characterized by pain, tenderness, and slight swelling about the tarsal scaphoid. It is caused by trauma, direct or indirect, and by circulatory disturbances in the bone, causing degenerative changes and compression within the scaphoid. It is relieved by casts or by arch supports and a lift or wedge along the inner side of an elongated heel.

Freiberg's disease. Freiberg's disease is a condensation or infraction in the distal end of the second metatarsal, usually resulting from trauma and aseptic necrosis and characterized by shortening of the metatarsal, tenderness

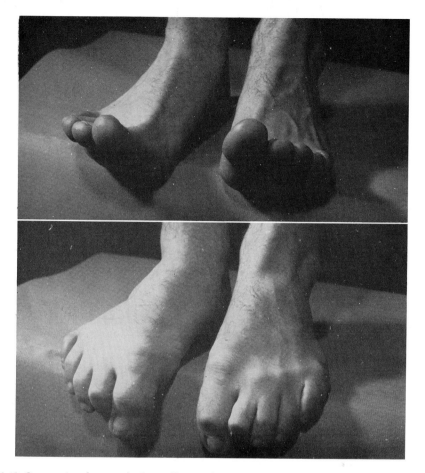

Fig. 4-18. Contracting the toes rhythmically over the edge of a stair step to strengthen foot muscles.

about the metatarsal head, and some strain of the metatarsal arch. It is treated by support of the metatarsal arch.

Clawfoot and hollow foot. Clawfoot (Fig. 4-19) and hollow foot consist of a contracture of the muscles and ligaments of the plantar arch as a result of relative overactivity of the extensors of the toe as compared to the flexor action. This may be influenced or instigated by continued metatarsal arch strain, arthritis, or spastic or infantile paralysis. The condition is frequently accompanied by calluses under the metatarsal heads and by corns on the dorsal surface of the interphalangeal joints of the toes. The treatment may require proper support of the metatarsal arch with arch supports and metatarsal bars, tenotomy of the extensor tendons to the toes, tendon transplantation of the ex-

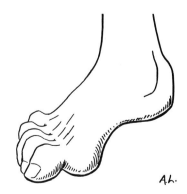

Fig. 4-19. Clawfoot deformity with retraction of the toes and high arch (cavus).

tensor tendons to the metatarsal heads, or, in severe cases, resection of the metatarsal heads or proximal portions of the phalanges.

Hammer toes. Hammer toes (Fig. 4-20) may be either congenital or acquired as a result of contracture of the extensors of the toes. The first interphalangeal joint is usually prominent and flexed. A corn usually develops on top and on the end of the toe. Correction can easily be obtained by resection of a portion of the proximal phalanx so that the toe is shortened and the muscle contracture released.

Knock-ankle and flatfoot deformities. Knock-ankle and flatfoot deformities in children are common and are frequently accompanied by bowlegs or knock-knees and internal rotation of the tibiae so that the child walks with a pigeon-toe and knock-ankle gait. It is difficult to tell whether or not there is a true flatfoot deformity in young children when they are beginning to walk because of the frequent existence of a fat pad under the arch. Arch supports are not often indicated, and the correction can usually be accomplished by lifts and elongated heels. When the internal rotation and pigeon-toe deformity is not severe and the principal deformity is knock-ankle, an elongated heel with an inner lift of ⅛ to ¼ inch will usually correct the deformity within a few months. If a pigeon-toe condition is present, it may be necessary to add to the shoe alterations (⅛ inch or more) for outer elevation of the soles.

When the pigeon-toe deformity is severe with marked internal rotation of the ankle on the knee, it is best to use cable rotators attached to the outside or the inner side of the shoe. They spiral the leg and are fastened to a belt at the waist. (Fig. 4-21). The adjustment of these rotators may exert the necessary tension to maintain correct alignment. In 6 to 18 months the alignment becomes fixed and the deformity disappears.

Bowlegs in children are not uncommon up to the second year and probably compensate for foot deformity, or vice versa. After the bowleg deformity has subsided, a reversion to the knock-knee status may take place and persist to the seventh or eighth year. During this time frequent changes in shoe elevations may be necessary to meet the current requirements of balance.

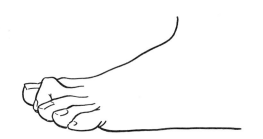

Fig. 4-20. Hammer toe. A corn usually forms on the top and the end of the toe.

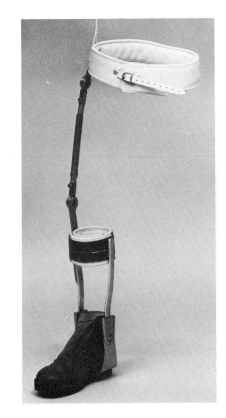

Fig. 4-21. Becker twister. A cable twister between the short leg brace and the pelvic band can be adjusted to aid outtoeing or intoeing, whichever is required. This attachment does not interfere with free motion at the knee and therefore is useful for children.

GOOD HYGIENIC CARE OF THE FEET

Good hygienic care of the feet, daily bathing, and massage will help to relieve tired, aching feet. Contrast baths improve circulation and the tone of foot muscles. The person who spends many hours on his feet may secure relief from aching feet by changing shoes during the working hours. Proper length hose and care in trimming of the nails will help to prevent painful ingrown toenails and dangerous infection. The nails should be trimmed straight across. Irritation and pressure caused by ill-fitted shoes will result in corns and calluses. A corn is an overgrowth of the outer layer of skin and is nature's way of protecting the soft tissue. Pads may be used to relieve the pressure. To secure permanent relief, however, it is necessary that the shoe fit properly and that pressure on the area be relieved. Maintaining clean healthy skin will help greatly in preventing athlete's foot (dermatophytosis). Wearing clean hose and permitting shoes to air and sun is of considerable value. Blisters and abrasions of the skin should have proper care. This is particularly important for the older person who has poor circulation or the person with diabetes whose tissues heal slowly.

STUDY QUESTIONS

1. Conservative treatment of low back pain may include bed rest and intermittent traction. Explain recommended bed position(s) and type(s) of traction used.
2. Frequently a patient with low back pain is fitted with a brace or corset for support and immobilization. Explain why this is helpful and describe correct application of the back brace or corset.
3. The patient with low back pain caused by muscle strain is instructed in correct body mechanics. Why is this an important aspect of his care?
4. A herniated disk may be the cause of back pain. Review anatomy of the spine and explain the meaning of a herneated nucleus pulposus.
5. Explain how care following a laminectomy differs from care following a spinal fusion.
6. After an extended period of bed rest, it is desirable that the patient wear shoes that provide support for the feet. Explain why this is recommended.
7. Exercises may be prescribed in addition to arch supports for the treatment of fallen arches. Explain.
8. Review criteria that may be used in evaluating a properly fitted shoe.

REFERENCES

Adams, J.: Foot problems in adults, Postgrad. Med. **42**:1-6, 1967.

Armstrong, J. R.: Lumbar disc lesions: pathogenesis and treatment of low back pain and sciatica, ed. 3, Baltimore, 1965, The Williams & Wilkins Co.

Brown, H., and Brown, B.: Lumbar intervertebral disk disease, Postgrad. Med. **37**:446-451, 1965.

Bruck, H. O., and Lambert, C. N.: Common foot disabilities, Am. J. Nurs. **59**:1580-1583, 1959.

de Cutierrez-Mahoney, C. G., and Carini, Esta: Neurological and neurosurgical nursing, ed. 4, St. Louis, 1965, The C. V. Mosby Co.

Durbin, F. C.: Affections of the toes, Practitioner **201**: 749-758, 1968.

Fairbank, T. J.: Deformities of the arches of the foot and related conditions, Practitioner **201**:742-748, 1968.

Farni W. H.: Backache relieved through new concepts of posture, Springfield, Ill., Charles C Thomas, 1966.

The foot, Physiotherapy **53**: entire issue, April, 1967.

Gibbens, M.: Diagnosis and treatment of low back pain, Orthop. Surg. **10**:218-221, 1968.

Harrold, A. J.: Laminectomy for disc disorders, Nurs. Times **67**:406-408, 1971.

Hickling, J.: Spinal traction technique, Physiotherapy **58**:58-63, 1972.

Hines, T. F.: Corsets and soft supports. In Licht, S., and Kamenetz, H. L., editors: Orthotics etcetera, New Haven, 1966, Elizabeth Licht, Publisher.

Hood, Lucille B., and Chrisman, D.: Intermittent pelvic traction in the treatment of the ruptured intervertebral disk, Phys. Ther. **48**:21-30, 1968.

Kester, N.: Low back pain: pathomechanics and a regimen of treatment, Arch. Phys. Med. **49**:396-402, 1968.

Knapp, M.: Low back pain. Part I. Diagnosis, Postgrad. Med. **41**:A133-A138, 1967.

Knapp, M.: Low back pain. Part 2. Treatment, Postgrad. Med. **41**:A131-A139, 1967.

Larson, C. B.: Low back pain, Postgrad. Med. **26**:142-149, 1959.

Locke, R.: Foot care for diabetics, Am. J. Nurs. **63**:107-110, 1963.

Lucas, D.: Spinal bracing. In Licht, S., and Kamenetz, H. L., editors: Orthotics etcetera, New Haven, 1966, Elizabeth Licht, Publisher.

Matthews, J. A.: The effects of spinal traction, Physiotherapy **58**:64-66, 1972.

Mercer, W., and Duthie, R.: Orthopedic surgery, ed. 6, Baltimore, 1964, The Williams & Wilkins Co.

Morris, J. M., Lucas, D. B., and Bresler, B.: Role of the trunk in stability of the spine, J. Bone Joint Surg. **43-A**:327-351, 1961.

Musick, Doris T., and MacKenzie, Marguerite: Nursing care of the patient with a laminectomy, Nurs. Clin. North Am. **2**:437-445, 1967.

Pasternak, S.: The patient with a ruptured disk, Am. J. Nurs. **62**:77-80, 1962.

Raney, R. B., and Brashear, H. R.: Shand's handbook of orthopaedic surgery, ed. 8, St. Louis, 1971, The C. V. Mosby Co.

Rothman, R. H., guest editor: Symposium on disease of the intervertebral disc, Orthop. Clin. North Am. **2**:307-592, 1971.

Selke, O. O.: Foot strain, Am. J. Orthop. **2**:48-49, 1960.

Shafer, K., Sawyer, J. R., McClusky, A. M., Beck, E. and Phipps, W. J.: Medical-surgical nursing, ed. 5, St. Louis, 1971, The C. V. Mosby Co.

Simko, M.: Foot welfare, Am. J. Nurs. **67:**1895-1897, 1967.

Stauffer, R. N., Ivins, J. C., Miller, R. H.: The lumbar disk syndrome and its operative treatment, Postgrad. Med. **49:**87-93, 1971.

Wiley, L., editor: Rupture of the cervical disk, Nursing '73 **3:**33-39, April, 1973.

Wiltse, L. L.: The etiology of spondylolisthesis, J. Bone Joint Surg. **44-A:**539-560, 1962.

Yates, D. A. H.: Indications and contra-indications for spinal traction, Physiotherapy **58:**55-57, 1972.

Zamosky, I., and Licht, S.: Shoes and their modifications. In Licht, S., and Kamenetz, H. L., editors: Orthotics etcetera, New Haven, 1966, Elizabeth Licht, Publisher.

5

Trauma to bones, joints, and ligaments

CARE OF THE ACUTELY INJURED PATIENT

Accidental injuries are today one of the most important environmental health problems that face the nation. Injury is the leading cause of death in the first half of man's life span and ranks fourth among causes of death at all ages. One of each eight beds in general hospitals throughout the United States is occupied by the victim of an accident. The needed attention therefore becomes a very important problem to nursing, both in care of the trauma to the musculoskeletal system and in care of the patient with multiple injuries.

Triage. Hospitals have provided accident rooms for the first-line care in surgical emergencies. A surgical emergency is a sudden unexpected medical crisis that requires rapid action, and today most of these are sustained through violence. The location of the emergency rooms must be readily and quickly accessible to all modes of transportation in order that the injured person can receive this immediate attention. Furthermore these emergency rooms, to fulfill their purpose, must provide all the tools that are necessary to save life. Most importantly, the personnel must be on standby alert and ready for triage as a patient enters the emergency room. Triage means sorting, or putting first things first, as the needs of the patient are surveyed when he is transferred from the ambulance.

Treatment priority. In any patient with mul-

tiple injuries, treatment priorities must be rapidly assigned. These crucial decisions are based on the following pattern.

1. Restoration of the cardiorespiratory physiology is of first priority.

2. Then comes the treatment for injuries of hollow viscera such as intestine and bladder.

3. Laceration of the soft parts, head injuries, and closed fractures can await treatment until after the preceding have been managed.

4. Injuries of the bone are next in importance.

For example, in a patient with a combination of skull fracture, femoral fracture, and rupture of hollow viscus, shock is immediately treated. External bleeding is controlled by pressure or ligature, and the fractured extremity is simply splinted. As soon as the vital signs are stable, the patient may be transferred quickly to the operating room for laparotomy to repair the visceral injury and prevent further peritonitis. Coma, unlike shock, does not interdict needed operation.

A team captain must be in charge of the patient who has been acutely injured. Because of the serious problems, this leader is usually a general surgeon or the general practitioner with the widest experience. At the same time he uses all available specialists immediately as the needs indicate. The captain must have the authority to assign diagnostic and therapeutic priorities. This is the essence of triage.

NURSING RESPONSIBILITIES

Obviously of first importance is to note the patient's breathing, which can be determined at a glance. Lack of aeration, evidenced by blueness, means an obstructed airway, especially in the face of gasping efforts of the chest. If an adequate passageway cannot be obtained by proper use of suction and the usual insertion of an airway, more drastic measures may be required. It is important, therefore, to make certain that proper instruments and airways are readily available in the emergency room so that the doctor may proceed with tracheotomy. Syringe and needle may be required for pleural aspiration or to relieve pressure pneumothorax. If the chest is flail, from multiple fractures through the rib cage, mechanical assistance to respiration becomes necessary. As a temporary measure, sometimes a sandbag placed against the flail chest can give some support.

In the presence of obvious external bleeding, the size and location of any wound from which the blood comes is noted and control is instituted by gauze pack pressure held firmly by hand or bandage, and only rarely is a tourniquet indicated.

Once respiration is established, bleeding is controlled, and blood volume replacement has been initiated, further evaluation of the extent of the injury is then more systematic. At this time the patient can be questioned about identification and the circumstance of the injury and the more subtle injuries, such as internal bleeding and bowel ruptures, can be dealt with properly.

SPRAINS, STRAINS, DISLOCATIONS, AND FRACTURES

This discussion will deal with the damage to bones, joints, and ligaments that is produced by external forces such as a blow, twist, pinch, fall, or crush. The skeletal system has a certain resilience for resisting such forces until the force from the outside becomes greater than the strength of the bones, at which point bone will yield and break. The individual bones have differences in strength, depending mostly on their shape and size, to resist these forces. They also vary in shape, size, and strength from one person to another and from one age to another. For example, the bones of children are more flexible and less brittle than those of adults. In the elderly person the strength of the bones diminishes as it does in disease states, such as osteoporosis, so that less external force is required to break them. These external forces will be referred to as trauma. Tissues of the body exposed to external violence or insult can be damaged. The bones, joints, and ligaments of the body are vulnerable to injury, and the effects therefrom can cause serious disablement. Therefore an understanding of the effects of trauma to the body is essential.

The occurrence of accidental injuries is increasing each year on our highways, in industry, in the home, on the farm, and in sports. Constant attention to the prevention of injury has become a national theme. Safety belts in automobiles, safety guards on machinery, nonslip materials in the home, and improved protective gear for football players are examples of the emphasis on prevention. Plans for the care of mass casualties are a part of hospital organization today and indeed are carried out on a national scale through the Federal Office of Civilian Defense.

NURSE'S ROLE IN PREVENTING INJURIES

It would be illogical to outline ways in which nurses may assist in preventing such conditions as tuberculosis, poliomyelitis, and back strain and then to omit emphasizing their part in the prevention of fractures. Their role as health teachers demands that they recognize some of the commonest causes of accidents, particularly those in the home, and know methods by which they may be eliminated.

Accidents in the home are almost as important as motor accidents, in both incidence and severity. Studies have shown that the greatest number of injuries results from falls; indeed, falls are responsible for almost one-half of all injuries in the home.

Because falls play a large part in the etiology of fractures, the home hazards that frequently have been the cause of falls should be recognized by nurses. Many grave accidents take place yearly in the course of going up and down stairs. Waxed stairs and waxed landings are always dangerous. The waxing process of any floor surface should be carefully done, since too much wax or too little polishing tends to make floors slippery. Floor wax on stairs may be particularly treacherous.

Stairs should be provided with handrails. If none are available, the householder should be urged to stretch a cord or rope along the stairs at a suitable level, adequately supported by firm uprights. In homes in which there are young children, gates at the top of stair flights are essential to prevent falls.

Steps should never be cluttered with stray objects, as cellar stairs, for instance, are so likely to be. They should be kept clear for traffic, and all members of the family, young and old alike, should recognize that running down steps is distinctly hazardous. All stairs that lead outside should be covered with coarse salt or sand during icy weather.

Children and adults should be alert for such objects as marbles, clothespins, pencils, and toys left about on stairs, landings, and floors. Every child and adult should recognize the great danger and threat to balance that a round rolling object, like a marble or pencil, presents to the unwary walker. All should be taught to remove them from the floor or sidewalk whenever they are observed.

Small scatter rugs can be very treacherous. They must be well anchored to prevent slipping. This may be done by rug fasteners or by the use of rubber floor mats. Scatter rugs should never be placed at the top or bottom of stairs.

To assist in preventing some of the hundreds of bathroom accidents that take place each year, a rubber mat in the tub is advisable. A railing on the wall near the tub will give more confidence and provide safety for the elderly person taking a tub bath.

Another common cause of home accidents is standing on rocking chairs or on old frail kitchen chairs to reach high shelves or to put up curtains. A small firm ladder should be available for all such household jobs.

If the household includes an elderly person who must get up at night to go to the toilet, it is important that a clear, unobstructed lane be left between his bed and the bathroom. An easily available bedlight will also discourage nocturnal journeys in the dark, which are fraught with so much hazard for the elderly person.

These are only a few of the more obvious pitfalls for the person in the home. The alert and observing nurse will be quick to notice others. Most of these items seem of little importance, but it is from just such a background that many severe fractures originate.

In addition to the prevention of accidents in the home, it also has become very important in recent years for the nurse to aid in the prevention of injuries to hospitalized patients. The commonest causes of injury in hospitals are falling from the bed, rolling off carts, and slipping on waxed floors. Side rails on the bed are mandatory in some hospitals for all patients and should certainly be put to use for those patients who are medicated, feeble, or confused. Transport carts are commonly equipped with straps and side rails for holding the patient to the cart, and these should be utilized. Slippery floors should be avoided when patients are ambulating with crutches or just beginning to ambulate. Highly waxed floors should not be permitted in the hospital area.

SPRAINS AND STRAINS

Sprains and strains are terms used to describe the damage done to ligaments in the body by an injury. Each joint in the body is protected by ligaments, and each may be subject to injury.

The nurse on the orthopedic ward will seldom

have occasion to care for a patient with a sprain. The nurse in the doctor's office, however, or the nurse in an outpatient area may frequently be called upon to assist in the application of support to a sprained ligament and to instruct the patient in the care of the injured area. (Figs. 5-1 to 5-3).

A sprained ankle is the most common joint injury and occurs when the foot is inverted forcibly. Normally, the lateral ligament of the ankle is a dense fibrous structure with a set length. One end is fixed to bone at the tip of the fibula and the other end is fixed to the astragalus. When the foot is inverted, this ligament becomes taut and stops further inversion. If the force acting to invert the foot is greater than the resisting force or strength of the ligament, the ligament must tear. This tear is a sprain. Should the tear be incomplete or, in other words, microscopic in extent, it may be called a strain. If the ligament holds and the giving way occurs at the fixation site to bone with a small fragment of bone attached to the ligament, this would be called an avulsion fracture. Any ligament thus damaged will repair by scar tissue if the torn ends are approximated and held in place for 3 or more weeks, which is the usual healing period.

Treatment consists of providing support and protection of the ligaments until healing can take place. Support is provided by strapping the foot and ankle with adhesive tape or an Elastoplast bandage. To prevent swelling, it is necessary that the extremity be elevated much of the time for the first 2 or 3 days after the injury. Also, the application of an ice bag during this time is helpful in minimizing hematoma.

Shave ankle.

Cover lacerations with sterile dressing before tape is applied.

Paint skin with tincture of benzoin or tincture of rosin.*

Select tape size to fit contour of ankle (1 inch to 2 inches wide).

Hold foot in neutral position in regard to inversion or eversion.

Keep foot as near right angle as pain will allow. ....

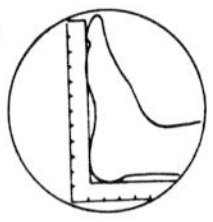

Avoid constrictive circular taping.

Circulation impaired

For subject sensitive to tape:

    use stockinet or wrap with gauze

    before taping.

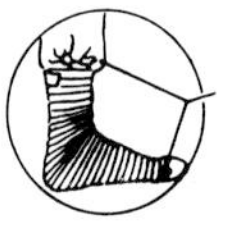

Cover skin with cotton or gauze where tape edges cross; prevents

    blisters and lacerations. ....

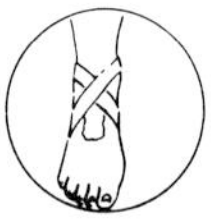

Leave no small areas of exposed

    skin between strips of tape. ......

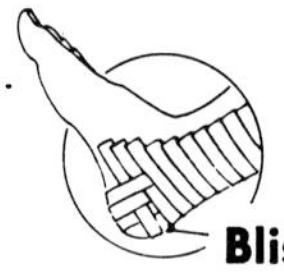

*Tincture of rosin: 1 lb. of rosin

    plus 1 gal. of alcohol (can use

    any alcohol, even rubbing alcohol)

Blister in untaped area

Fig. 5-1. Rules for adhesive taping used for prevention as well as treatment of sprains of the ankle. (From Paul, W. D., and Allsup, D.: Prevention and treatment of ankle sprains, The University of Iowa College of Medicine and Department of Athletics, Iowa City.)

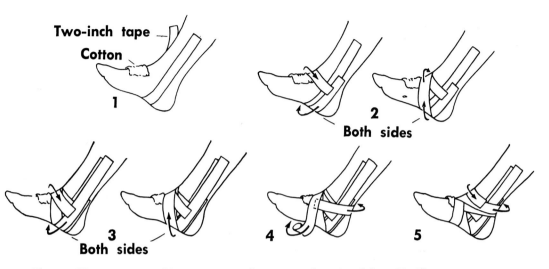

Fig. 5-2. Western wrap used in prevention and treatment of sprains of the ankle. This wrap is easy to apply, prevents inversion and eversion, but allows flexion and extension. It protects ankle mortise. (From Paul, W. D., and Allsup, D.: Prevention and treatment of ankle sprains, The University of Iowa College of Medicine and Department of Athletics, Iowa City.)

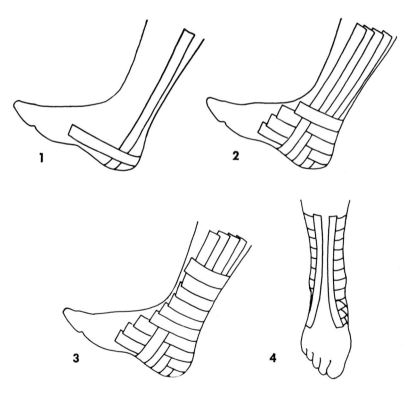

Fig. 5-3. Basket weave used in the treatment of ankle sprains. It is used only in the acute stage to allow swelling but does not protect ankle mortise. (From Paul, W. D., and Allsup, D.: Prevention and treatment of ankle sprains, The University of Iowa College of Medicine and Department of Athletics, Iowa City.)

Although a minimal amount of weight bearing is permitted at first, this is gradually increased as the soreness diminishes. After such an injury the physician will usually request that a roentgenogram be made to rule out the possibility of a fracture.

At the end of a 2-week period, the Elastoplast support is removed, and if the tenderness has disappeared sufficiently, an elastic bandage or support may be applied. This is worn to prevent swelling of the ankle and is gradually discarded as the patient's condition warrants.

Occasionally, the torn ligament ends will curl just enough that the ends cannot be kept together. In such a case there is a chance that healing will be incomplete. An unstable joint or easily recurring sprain of the joint will be the outcome. Recourse to external support or surgical repair of such a ligament is occasionally necessary.

DISLOCATIONS

Traumatic dislocation of any joint occurs when the force of the injury is greater than that which would cause a sprain. A joint is protected by more than a single ligament, and if all the ligaments yield or tear under pressure of the force, the entire joint can separate so that the surface of one bone making up the joint no longer meets or opposes the surface of the other bone making up the joint. This is called a dislocation and is ordinarily described in terms of which way the acting force displaced the distal portion of the joint, for example, posterior dislocation of the hip, which means that the head of the femur comes to lie outside of and behind the acetabulum. In order that any dislocated joint can function properly again, the dislocated portion of that joint must be relocated to its original anatomic relation with its articulating member. Usually, an anesthetic is required to relax the muscles which in their spasm tend to hold the bones in the dislocated position. On rare occasions the dislocation cannot be reduced by simple manipulation because a portion of the torn tissues or some associated soft tissue such as tendon becomes wrapped around the dislocated part in such a fashion as to prevent relocation. In this event a surgical operation (open reduction) is necessary. Once the dis-

location is reduced, whether by open or closed reduction, the damaged joint must be immobilized for 3 or more weeks to allow the torn ligamentous and capsular tissues to heal.

FRACTURES

Mechanical forces in the causation and treatment of fractures

An understanding of the causes of fractures and their management requires some knowledge of forces and how they act. This is a subject that is urgent, as judged by the rapidly increasing rate of accidents, if we consider the question of the type and magnitude of stresses and strains the human body can safely tolerate. Crash injury research groups are collecting data on the speed of the vehicle at the time of crashing, the position of the injured person in the vehicle, the direction the person faced, and the structural part of the vehicle believed to be responsible for the injury. One of the common injuries in survivors is fracture of one or more bones.

The study of stress-strain pehnomena in bones is a problem in biomechanics. During movement, as well as during rest, the bones are subjected to a variety of forces that are primarily the result of muscle action and body weight.

A *force* is simply a push or a pull. There are three kinds of force—*tensile* (pulling apart, like a rubber band); *compressive* (pushing together, like an accordian); and *shearing* (a force acting perpendicular to long axis to produce a twist).

When forces act on a body, there is internal resistance to absorb or transmit that force. The internal resistance, which cannot be seen nor measured, is called *stress. Strain* on the other hand, can be seen and measured as a deformation or change in shape.

If force continues to act on a bone in a longitudinal direction with sufficient magnitude, the bone will bend (strain); if the force continues, the internal resistance (stress) will fail to absorb more force and the bone will break. The force has exceeded the capacity of the bone to absorb it. Practically all materials including bone have an *elastic limit* or point of maximum stress beyond which they will not return to their original shape.

Another important concept is the relation of

force to energy. (Energy is the capacity to do work.) The importance of the idea of work lies in the fact that a body upon which work is done thereby acquires the capacity to do an equal amount of work in returning to its original state. For example, work is done when the main-spring of a watch is wound and the spring acquires energy, which can be measured by the work it does as it unbends. To raise a 10 pound weight 100 feet above the ground, 1,000 foot pounds of work (energy) are required. Once raised, it has gained the power to do that same amount of work in returning to its original posi-tion. At 100 feet above the ground the weight has potential energy. When it falls to the ground, it retains the energy it had but it is now energy of motion. When it reaches the ground, it has lost all its advantage of position but still has power to do work by virtue of its motion, which is called kinetic energy.

Translated into practical terms, this discussion points out that a person riding in an automobile has kinetic energy received from the forward velocity of the automobile. If the automobile comes to a sudden stop, for example, by bump-ing into a stone wall, the person riding continues to move in the same forward direction until another force alters that direction. As the person goes forward and strikes the windshield, the velocity of forward motion becomes zero. If the windshield does not break, the kinetic forces still present in the body are absorbed into each segment of the body until the forward motion of each segment becomes zero. One such segment is the head, which strikes the windshield as though thrown like a baseball. The weight of the head brought to a sudden stop transmits the kinetic energy to the skull. This energy is rapidly absorbed by the internal stress resistance of the bones of the skull. If the amount of stress ex-ceeds the elasticity of the bone, there will be strain failure to return the shape of the skull to normal. The failure will result in a break of the bone in the form of a depressed skull fracture. Any kinetic energy remaining after having been spent to produce the fracture can either depress the fracture further or enlarge the fracture, depending on the amount of energy available. Had the occupant in the automobile been wear-ing a shoulder strap, the continued forward

motion of the body (kinetic energy) would have been transmitted to the shoulder strap, im-parting to the strap a push force. Because the stress resistance of the harness is more elastic than the bone, the strap would absorb all the remaining kinetic energy without exceeding its elastic limit, therefore declerating the body to zero velocity without injury.

Had the occupant been asleep with the knees resting on the forward dash compartment, the forces would act in a different direction on the body. The center of gravity of the body would be in the same longitudinal plane as the thighs; therefore, forward momentum of the body would be directed to the dashboard through the femurs, and the kinetic energy would be absorbed by the internal stress resistance of the thigh bones and one of two events, or both, could occur. The stress in the femur could exceed the limits of strain deformation (the elastic limit of bend), and the bone would break. The break would allow a gradual deceleration of the remaining energy as the bone fragments angulate or shorten the bone. The other possibility would be a failure of the elastic limit of strain at the hip, resulting in a dislocation of the hip.

In these examples, the dissipation of kinetic energy can be compared to a rubber ball thrown at a pile of rocks. As the ball bounces from one rock to another, the distance it bounces becomes less and less as the kinetic energy is dissipated or used up in each bounce. The ball finally comes to rest when all forces acting on the ball are in equilibrium.

Similarly, and injured body will come to rest when the kinetic forces have been dissipated and gravity has neutralized body weight, whether it be by the support of the ground, the floor of the car, or part of each. The center of gravity of each body segment may have altered as a result of the injury. A fracture in the femur, for example, will have added a new center of gravity of the thigh since the fracture has in effect created two thighs out of one. The upper half of the thigh will rest independently on the lower half, thus one could be rotated inward, the other outward. One segment could rest in line with the body and the other at a right angle yet still aligned with the lower leg. What-ever the position, whether with or without deformity, the injured limb very quickly gains equilibrium and remains at rest until shifted by a new force. Any attempt to move the injured limb will create muscle spasm, which becomes a new internal force. The muscle spasm occurs from nerve reflex whose stimulus is initiated by any tension or compression of the injured periosteum. This reflex is also accompanied by acute pain; therefore, both pain and muscle spasm can be controlled by immobilization of the injured part. Obviously first aid immobilization disregards proper reduction of the fracture but does control pain and muscle spasm while the injured person is transported to a hospital.

In the hospital the decision for "setting" the fracture is made. Restoration of the fractured bone to its original length and alignment constitutes a reduction. Because any manipulation causes pain and muscle spasm, the injured patient must have adequate anesthesia, whether general or local. In some fractures, such as in the femur, the powerful muscles continue spasms even in a cast and the reduction of the fracture cannot be maintained. In this instance, a better means of reduction and maintenance of reduction is by traction.

Traction is the act of pulling by external force. The force must have proper direction and proper magnitude to accomplish a reduction of the fracture as well as to maintain the proper length and alignment of the injured bone until it is repaired and healed. The nurse should understand the forces that act on the body when traction is applied. As a reminder, Newton's third law states "with every force there is an equal and opposite reaction force." If the injured person is to remain at equilibrium in bed and the fractured extremity is to be pulled by a force, there must be an equal and opposite force to neutralize the pull. The bed will neutralize the force of gravity. The internal force of muscle spasm will be neutralized by the force of the traction. Obviously none of these forces are acting in the same direction and therefore are not exactly opposed. Any two or more forces acting on a body and not exactly opposed are known as *vectors* of force. If the direction and amount of each force is known, their combined action becomes known as the *resultant* force. The nurse must understand the vectors and the resultant force in order to deal expertly with the patient in traction.

Vectors. A *force* may be defined as that which tends to cause or alter the motion of matter. It can be a push or a pull. Many forces may act on a body to cause motion and any motion that

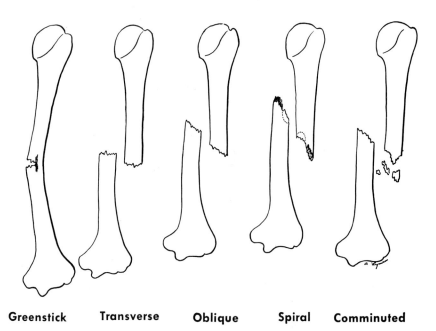

| Greenstick | Transverse | Oblique | Spiral | Comminuted |

Fig. 5-4. Fracture types.

occurs will be the result of the combined action of all the forces. If the forces act in the same direction, their sum will be the strength of a single force acting in one direction. If there are two forces acting in exactly opposite directions, the amount of resulting single force will be the difference between the two whereas the direction of that force would be the same as the larger of the two. If the opposing forces were equal, no motion would occur since the sum of the forces is equal to zero. When the sum of the forces acting on a body equal zero, the body is said to be in equilibrium.

Any two or more forces not exactly opposed or not exactly in the same direction are designated vectors of force—only a part of one force may neutralize a part of another while the direction of the final force will be different from either. Vectors may be added geometrically to determine both the amount and the direction of the *resultant* force acting on the body.

In actual practice the precise amount of force

is seldom if ever computed. With experience and awareness of the objectives of a given traction, both the direction and amount of weight can be estimated. Furthermore there is a daily change in the demands on the traction as muscle spasm subsides and the muscles actually fatigue; this, combined with a patient shifting position in bed, makes correction somewhat trial and

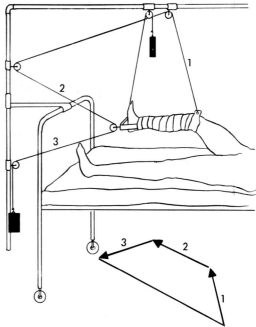

Fig. 5-6. Russell traction. The pull is applied through adhesive strips to the skin over the leg. The limitation for uses of this skin traction is the tolerance of the skin to tension stresses over a period of time. This traction illustrates the vectors of force and the *resultant* direction and amount of pull in the long axis of the femur. The single weight suspended at the foot of the bed provides the total energy while the pulleys determine the directions of pull provided through one weight. The weight at the top of the bed simply prevents drop foot and has no relationship to the original traction. If a 5-pound weight were pulling at the foot of the bed, there would be in effect a 5-pound pull at 3 as well as at 2 and, therefore, a total of 10 pounds pulling on the leg. A single force of 5 pounds would be lifting the knee at *1.* An irregular polygon can be drawn to unit scale with the forces connected by representative lines each parallel to the force it represents. In the diagram 3 corresponds to 3 and so on, leaving the unmarked line as the direction and amount of *resultant* force acting nearly in line with the femoral shaft.

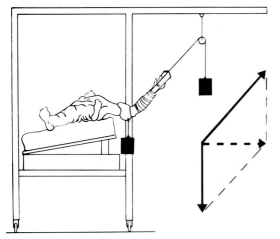

Fig. 5-5. Dunlap traction. The humerus has a fracture just above the elbow. The traction is applied to pull the humerus to its proper length (reduce the overriding of the fragments) and to restore the proper longitudinal alignment of the humeral shaft. One weight pulls the forearm up and out. Another weight pushes the humerus downward by means of a sling. The parallelogram shows one arrow parallel to the line of pull on the forearm, the other arrow parallel to the downward push on the humerus. These are the vectors of force, whereas the heavy interrupted arrow (the diagonal of the parallelogram) indicates the direction and amount of the resultant force.

error until the situation stabilizes after a week or so. During this unstable period the direction and amount of pull on the traction can be adjusted according to need indicated by repeat roentgenogram or other examination findings. Particular care must be exercised to prevent overpull since this will distract the fragments in the case of fracture.

Types of fractures

A fracture is a break in the continuity of a bone. To understand and discuss fractures it is necessary to use terms that describe type, location, and other features pertinent to the problem (Fig. 5-4).

Each bone in the body is highly developed to carry out a specific purpose. It is logical, therefore, that each bone has it own characteristics. In general, the long bones (femur, tibia, humerus, radius, and ulna) are tubular with variations relating to internal stress patterns of

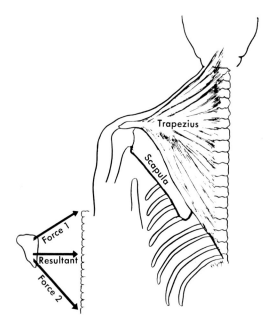

Fig. 5-7. The action of the trapezius muscle on the motion of the scapula provides another example of force vectors as they relate to bodily functions. *Force 1* is the direction of pull when the upper fibers of the trapezius contract, *force 2* is the direction of pull for the lower fibers. The *resultant* force indicates the direction the scapula will move when the upper and lower fibers contract essentially equally.

trabeculas as well as variations in cortical thickness from one end to the other. These variables are explainable on the basis of stress, since nature provides the necessary strength (resistance) when it is needed to bear weight, resist muscle pulls, and so forth. The cortex of the tibia in a football player or weight lifter will be thicker than that in a man of similar size in a sedentary occupation. If such tibias were tested by strain gauges and breaking points determined, it would require more force to break the tibia with the thicker cortex. Nonetheless, every bone has a point at which it can no longer resist applied force without breaking. This is the basis of all fractures. Because bones are adapted to ordinary stresses of day-to-day living, it would take a stress greater than that to produce a fracture. Most fractures are the result of instances in which there is no control of the amount of force involved.

Since injuries are not deliberately sustained, they occur when least suspected and when one is not prepared to resist them. Consequently, the forces that occur come from any direction and in variable amounts. This accounts for the fact that of the thousands of fractures that occur no two are exactly alike. Another factor that adds variability is that of muscle pulls in effect at the time of the fracture. An example of the latter accounts for the gymnast who can dive over a bar to a hard floor and absorb enough of the shock by well-timed muscular relaxation to break the impact. The type of fracture produced in this instance would be by indirect force and could be located at any point from the wrist to the shoulder. The direction of the line of fracture would most likely be long oblique.

Direct force, such as that supplied by a lead pipe falling across the forearm, allows more accuracy in the prediction of a transverse fracture line exactly at the point of impact of the lead pipe.

When a bone is fractured, it means that a single unit becomes two units, and each unit is spoken of as a fragment. The fragment nearest the cephalad end of the body is referred to as the proximal and the other as the distal fragment. These two fragments ordinarily become separated at the site of the fracture in various ways. Imagine a piece of bamboo 2 feet long with a strong rubber band stretched from one end to the other and fastened. On the other side another but weaker stretched rubber band is placed. If the bamboo were cut transversely in its middle, it would bend immediately from the overpull of the stronger elastic. This is the mechanism of a transverse fracture. The angle at the fracture site will furnish the identifying description for this particular fracture, for example, a transverse fracture in the middle third with lateral angulation (if the apex of the angle points away from the midline of the body) of 30 degrss (or whatever angle the distal fragment has moved from the original bone alignment).

To construct another possibility, return to the bamboo and this time cut the bamboo on a 4-inch diagonal instead of transversely. Upon completion of the cut, the two fragments will slide by one another until the original length of the bamboo becomes shortened enough to release the tension in the elastic bands. Because one band was shorter than the other, the stronger side will also angulate similarly but less than it did with the transverse cut. This fracture will be described then as an oblique fracture of the middle third with a 2-inch overriding (or whatever amount the total length has been shortened) and lateral angulation of 10 degrees.

These two example will account for the majority of fractures, but because minor variations are possible, additional descriptive terms are needed. The fracture site may be splintered, in which case there may be multiple fragments. Instead of a transverse or oblique fracture, it would be called a comminuted fracture. Should the fracture line be oblique and follow a spiral course as it involves a tubular bone, it will be referred to as an oblique spiral, followed by the usual description of location, overriding, and angulation.

Occasionally, when a long bone is fractured, the fractured end of one fragment will be driven into the surrounding muscle mass. It will not only override and angulate but will also be displaced sideways a bone's width or more from its fellow fragment. In this instance it will be described as a transverse fracture with overriding, angulation, and 1 inch (or whatever amount) lateral (medial, anterior, or posterior

referring to the distal fragment) displacement. In a vertebral body in which the diameter of the bone nearly equals the length and the most force applied is compression (as one would squeeze an orange between two hands), the bone will yield by collapsing into itself. This is described as an impacted or compression fracture. In disease states in which bone is weakened, such as in osteoporosis, metastatic bone lesions, or osteogenesis imperfecta, a fracture can occur with as little force as that required during a sneeze or a twist in bed. This is termed a pathologic fracture.

General principles of fracture treatment

The objectives of treatment of any fracture are threefold: (1) to regain alignment and length of the bony fragments (reduction), (2) to retain alignment and length (immobilization), and (3) to restore function to the injured part.

The surgeon has at least three commonly used means to accomplish reduction of the fracture: (1) closed manipulation, (2) traction, and (3) open reduction by surgical procedures. Most fractures can be reduced by closed manipulation, which means that the fracture ends can be brought into opposition by manual manipulation. The muscle spasm that tends to shorten the bone by overriding must be overcome. This can be accomplished by traction alone if it is maintained long enough to fatigue the muscles. However, the swelling, stretching, and rubbing of the periosteum at the site of injury is painful. In order to spare pain and also obtain muscle relaxation, an anesthetic is most often employed. It is seldom under these circumstances that reduction cannot be accomplished. If for any reason reduction cannot be performed as soon as the patient has been evaluated, the fractured part should at least be immobilized until reduction can be carried out.

Traction becomes the treatment of choice when the surgeon finds that any reduction he is able to obtain cannot be maintained by a plaster cast. This situation is common in fractures other than those of the transverse variety. Anticipating this difficulty, the surgeon may elect to utilize the traction not only to maintain but also to accomplish the reduction, thereby obviating the need for closed reduction and anesthesia. The traction is provided by a Kirschner wire or other metal pin placed through the bone distal to the fracture, by means of which constant weighted pull can be maintained for weeks if necessary. This is known as skeletal traction. There are many modified methods of use, some of which are incorporated in combination with plaster casts. However it is used, the traction pin need be used only until sufficient callus is evident to maintain alignment. Plaster cast immobilization will be sufficient to complete the healing process.

To reduce a fracture by surgical methods is seldom necessary except in those fractures that are known to be impossible to reduce or maintain with either closed or traction methods. Intra-articular fractures, fracture of the medial epicondyle of the humerus in children, fractures of both bones of the forearm in adults, and fractures of the neck of the femur are examples. Except as indicated, open reductions are practically never indicated in children. Many surgeons elect open reductions at times when other methods would give satisfactory results. These are justified on the basis that hospital time will be reduced, and joints above and below the fracture can be kept mobile, since immobilization is provided mechanically by rods, plates, screws, and other devices rather than by plaster casts that would have to extend to immobilize the joint above and that below the fracture. The advantages must outweigh the possible complications of operative infection and delayed union, which are hazards in any operative attack on the fracture site.

A more recent technique of operative fixation makes use of compression plates. It is thought that healing may be more certain and also hastened if the bone ends at the fracture site are held snugly against one another by actual compression. An apparatus has been in use which does mechanically accomplish this. It is applicable mostly to the long bones in the case of transverse fractures.

Restoration of function is as important as any other part of treatment. Well-planned treatment and avoidance of complications give a head start toward regaining function of a fractured extremity. Prolonged immobilization that allows for atrophy of disuse and stiffening of joints to occur is to be avoided. Although a fracture heals in good position, the function is not restored until the soft tissues are free of contractures and have regained flexibility and strength. This process, if well managed, can be accomplished in weeks. If it is neglected, a patient can be handicapped for months. Well-directed physical therapy is helpful at this stage.

Fracture healing

The sequence of events in tissue repair from the time of injury to complete healing of the fracture is quite well understood. As soon as the bone fractures, bleeding occurs from the damaged bone ends and from periosteal and soft tissue disruption around the fracture site. The bleeding produces a hematoma that is the basis for subsequent events. During the first week after injury the hematoma becomes invaded and replaced by granulation tissue that is organized into fibrous tissue after 3 weeks. The cells called fibroblasts transform into cells capable of producing a matrix or cement substance called osteoid. Into the osteoid are deposited mineral salts that are apparent by roentgenography. This is bone callus (early bone). In children it can be seen in the roentgenogram within 3 weeks of the time of fracture, whereas in adults, especially in the bones with poorer blood supply, the appearance may be delayed until 2 to 3 months after injury. The callus is usually fusiform in shape and forms a continuous bridge across the fracture site. After the callus has made its appearance, it then becomes remodeled into a stress pattern that resembles that of the parent bone. The callus is often more abundant than is seemingly necessary, but in the remodeling stage (which may require a year) the excess amount is absorbed, leaving only an amount sufficient to withstand the stress needs of the bone.

Certain factors are known that can disturb this healing process. Delayed union is the term for the healing process that is slowed to the extent that months are required to complete union. In some instances firm union is never produced (nonunion), and a false joint with fluid present as well as motion (pseudarthrosis) may actually tend to form. Repeated manipulations of the fracture after the first 7 to 10 days can be one cause, and inadequate immobilization is another. Inadequate immobilization can be a matter of degree since it is quite impossible to ensure absolute immobilization by any means. The occurrence of infection will delay and sometimes prevent healing of fractures. Disturbed metabolism, especially of protein as in chronic debility or deficiences of either vitamin C or vitamin D, will delay callus.

Complications

Fracture complications include nonunion, malunion, infection, nerve damage, circulatory disturbance, epiphyseal damage, posttraumatic arthritis, kidney stones, and emboli.

Nonunion. Nonunion may be caused by any one of several factors. Inadequate immobilization can cause delayed union or nonunion of the fracture. Inadequate reduction may be a factor. If less than half of the bone ends are in contact with each other, nonunion usually results. If the bone ends are held too far apart by traction, it is evident that callus formation will not span the space. If the blood supply to the fracture line has been damaged, it is possible that the nutrition to one of the bone fragments may be inadequate and callus formation will not take place. When fracture occurs in certain areas (the lower one-third of the tibia, neck of the femur, and carpal scaphoid bone), healing may be slow or difficult to accomplish because of the disturbed blood supply and poor nutrition of the affected area. Also, if soft tissue becomes lodged between the bony fragments, union is not likely to take place.

To correct nonunion, the surgeon may perform a surgical procedure to freshen the bone ends and drill numerous holes near the fracture site in hopes of improving the circulation. In some instances the extremity may be braced and activity increased in order to improve the blood supply to the part. Bone grafting to the affected area may be necessary. Bone from the tibia or the iliac crest is placed across the fracture site. This is known as an onlay graft. Another method of bone grafting is that of inserting the graft directly into the medullary canal.

Malunion. With the complication of malunion, union of the bony fragments takes place but in a position of deformity. Numerous factors, such as inadequate reduction, an improperly applied cast, or a cast that has softened and permitted movement of bony fragments, may cause this.

Infection. Infection is always a possibility when a compound fracture occurs. Also, with open reduction of a fracture there is some risk that infection can occur and complicate the healing process.

Nerve damage. Nerve damage may be caused by the sharp edges of the bone fragments or by the injury that caused the fracture. Motor power of the muscles of the extremity and the sensitivity of the skin should be checked carefully. Damage to the peroneal nerve may result in drop foot, or injury to the radial nerve may result in wrist drop.

Circulatory disturbance. Circulation in the part distal to the fracture should also be checked carefully. This is particularly important with fractures around the elbow. Volkmann's contracture may result from a disturbance of the circulation in the elbow region. Nail beds of the fingers of the affected extremity should be observed, and the radial pulse should be taken at frequent intervals.

Damage to the epiphysis. If the fracture causes damage to the epiphysis of a child, growth may be arrested in that extremity or in a portion of the extremity. This, of course, results in deformity as the child grows.

Posttraumatic arthritis. When an intra-articular fracture causes damage to a joint surface, a painful posttraumatic arthritis may result. In some instances an arthroplasty or an arthrodesis may be performed to alleviate the pain.

Kidney stones. Kidney stones can occur when total body immobilization is carried out. They result when disuse causes excessive loss of calcium from the bones. Maintaining a high fluid intake is helpful in eliminating the calcium, but maintaining prophylactic muscular activity is better treatment.

Emboli. Occasionally, in compound fractures or in simple fractures in which clotting has taken place in a vein, a portion of the clot may break off and be carried throughout the circulation to various parts of the body. Air emboli also occur. If an embolus makes its way to a vital organ, such as the lung, heart, or brain, there may be disastrous consequences, even death.

The patient usually develops a rapid pulse and evidences of shock that come on abruptly. Death may occur within a few minutes or within a few hours after the onset of symptoms. Treatment other than preventive by adequate immobilization is of no avail. Those patients with emboli in the less vital areas may have the symptoms and signs in a milder degree and yet recover. The emboli are more frequently pulmonary than any other type and may occur as late as 6 to 8 weeks after the injury.

EVALUATION OF THE INJURED PART

The trauma resulting from a single force, such as a blow to the forearm, is a matter for examination of the single injured part. Such a direct blow can be expected to break the bones at the site of impact and produce an angulation like a bent twig. Landing on both feet in a fall from a height produces indirectly transmitted forces that can injure bones and joints at a distance from the point of impact, such as the collapse of a vertebral body in the upper lumbar spine. Crushing injuries from cave-ins increase areas of damage further because they involve both direct and indirect forces. Crushing injuries commonly involve tissues, such as internal organs in addition to bones, and thus internal hemorrhage can occur and produce shock that demands immediate detection and treatment. An associated head injury may render the person unconscious, which complicates the picture of shock. The forces on the chest might have fractured enough ribs to produce paradoxical breathing that interferes with proper ventilation. When poor ventilation, unconsciousness, and shock are present simultaneously, the evaluation and treatment of the injured bones and joints are of secondary concern. Any person with multiple injuries requires immediate evaluation by a physician well versed in all aspects of trauma, and seldom in medicine does the situation call for more astute, careful, complete, yet quick analysis to institute proper treatment in proper sequence to ensure first things first.

First aid and fractures. In first aid, any contaminated open fracture should be dressed and splinted in the exact position in which it was found so that proper precautions can be taken when the patient reaches a hospital or other point where he can receive adequate surgical attention. Some surgeons contend that because a thorough debridement is necessary in any open fracture, the additional amount of contamination occuring when the bones are pulled into line when first seen does not materially increase the chances for infection of the compound wound. This contention is doubtful.

It is preferable that a clean dressing, handkerchief, or sheet be applied at the site of injury and that the limb be splinted in the position of the existing deformity. The use of strong irritating antiseptics such as iodine, Lysol, or carbolic acid is contraindicated. Alcohol, Mercurochrome, Mercresin, or Scott's solution may be used with little chance of local damage or coagulation of the tissues.

If the patient is in shock, all possible attention should be paid to this. Intravenous saline infusions, transfusions, or blood plasma may be necessary.

There are a few simple rules that apply to first aid in fractures.

1. Keep the patient at rest in a horizontal position as long as he is unconscious or until the extent of his injury can be determined.

2. If he must be transported while still unconscious, continue the horizontal position until consciousness is regained sufficiently for the injured person to signify points of pain and tenderness.

3. In a person with a back injury every precaution should be taken to avoid motions of the spine, particularly such as would occur if the person were brought into a sitting position, because this may lead to damage to the spinal cord by fragments of bone protruding into it or pressing upon it.

4. When there is injury to the spine or to the limbs, it is of particular importance that the surgeon know definitely whether or not any paralysis was present immediately after the injury. This cannot be determined in the unconscious patient with a head injury, but it can be determined in other patients. The knowledge of this fact may decide the ultimate recovery or loss of function in a limb or limbs. This is also true in compound fractures. Written records of

what has been found and done should accompany each patient to the hospital or surgeon's office.

5. There is considerable debate at present as to the advisability of using a tourniquet, since the prolonged use may lead to death of the tissues in the extremities beyond its point of application. In open fractures it is preferable to use a piece of sterile or clean bandage or string to tie off the bleeding vessel if it is exposed or to apply local pressure to the vessel by means of a pad of sterile gauze and a sterile bandage. If a tourniquet must be used on a patient with violent bleeding, it should be removed every 20 to 30 minutes and the bleeding should be observed. If coagulation has occurred in the vessel, the tourniquet may be left loosened but there should be constant observation for return of bleeding.

6. Emergency immobilization and transportation depend on the anatomic location of the injury (Figs. 5-8 to 5-13).

(a) In injuries of the spine or head the recumbent position is essential. If a rigid stretcher such as a plank, a door, a ladder, or two poles and a blanket cannot be obtained, it is advisable to roll the patient horizontally onto his face and transport him in the arms of two or three persons to a truck or the back seat of a car. He should never be brought into a position that will flex the spine.

(b) In injuries of the clavicle, ribs, shoulder,

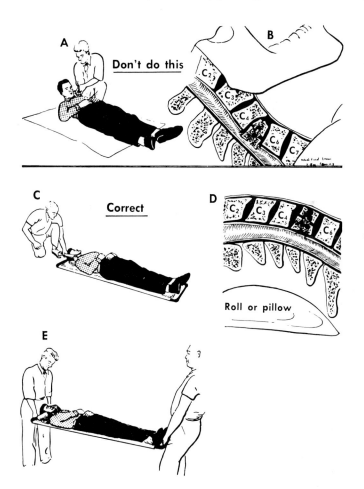

Fig. 5-8. Do's and don't's in the transport of patients with injuries of the cervical vertebrae. (From White, J. C.: Injuries to spinal cord and cauda equina. In Cave, E. F., editor: Fractures and other injuries, Chicago, 1958, Year Book Medical Publishers, Inc. Illustrated by Mrs. Murial McLatchie Miller.)

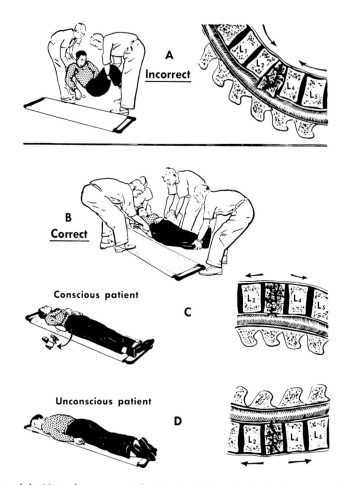

Fig. 5-9. Do's and don't's in the transport of patients with injuries of the lumbar and lower thoracic vertebrae. (From White, J. C.: Injuries to spinal cord and cauda equina. In Cave, E. F., editor: Fractures and other injuries, Chicago, 1958, Year Book Medical Publishers, Inc. Illustrated by Mrs. Murial McLatchie Miller.)

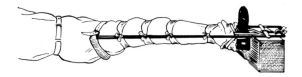

Fig. 5-10. Keller-Blake splint for first aid immobilization of a fractured femur. The ankle is carefully padded, and the leg is supported in the splint by encircling strips of cloth. The shoes and clothing are not removed in order to avoid unnecessary painful movement of the damaged extremity. Traction is maintained by means of a strip of cloth that is secured around the ankle, tied over the end of the splint, and twisted taut by means of a stick. The distal end of the splint is supported to give some elevation. (From Brown, T.: Fractures of the femoral shaft. In Cave, E. F., editor: Fractures and other injuries, Chicago, 1958, Year Book Medical Publishers, Inc. Illustrated by Mrs. Murial McLatchie Miller.)

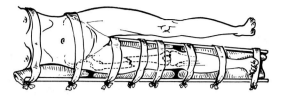

Fig. 5-11. Improvised splint, made of boards or sticks, for fracture of the femoral shaft. The lateral splint extends distally from just below the axilla and is secured to the trunk; the medial splint extends distally from the groin. All splints are padded to avoid pressure over bony prominences. (From Brown, T.: Fractures of the femoral shaft. In Cave, E. F., editor: Fractures and other injuries, Chicago, 1958, Year Book Medical Publishers, Inc. Illustrated by Mrs. Murial McLatchie Miller.)

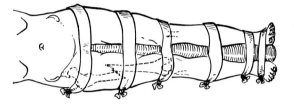

Fig. 5-12. Improvised immobilization for fracture of the femoral shaft when no splints are available. Legs are secured together with padding in between. Feet are also bound together in order to control rotation. (From Brown, T.: Fractures of the femoral shaft. In Cave, E. F., editor: Fractures and other injuries, Chicago, 1958, Year Book Medical Publishers, Inc. Illustrated by Mrs. Murial McLatchie Miller.)

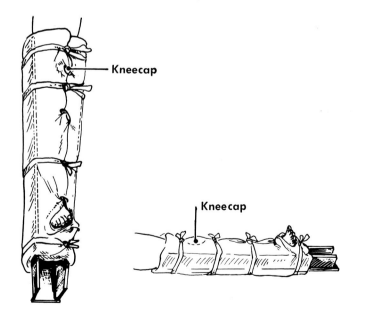

Fig. 5-13. The pillow-and-side splint as applied to the ankle. One strap extends above the knee and one below the foot. (From Aufranc, O.: Ankle injuries. In Cave, E. F., editor: Fractures and other injuries, Chicago, 1958, Year Book Medical Publishers, Inc. Illustrated by Mrs. Murial McLatchie Miller.)

and elbow, splinting can best be done by bandaging the arm to the side of the chest. This may be done with any materials obtainable, such as a torn sheet, a shirt, or other clothing. Two triangular slings work well if obtainable.

In fractures around the elbow and forearm, one or two wooden splints from the axilla to the fingertips may be tied to the arm with handkerchiefs or strips of clothing.

(c) In injuries of the hip, thigh, knee, and leg, immobilization may be obtained by narrow boards placed on either side of the leg and held together by a bandage or strips of clothing. When the hip is injured, the splinting should extend from the heel up to the side of the chest and the bandage should encircle the chest and the leg. All injuries of the bone should, if possible, be immobilized to include the joint above and below the injury. If no splinting material is available, fairly adequate immobilization can be obtained by tying the injured leg to the uninjured one with a series of bandages from the thigh to the foot.

(d) For fractures of the ankle and the lower leg the most satisfactory temporary splint is the pillow bandage. The limb is laid longitudinally on a pillow so that the heel is just above the edge. The lateral edges of the pillow are then brought together over the limb and pinned. When the ankle is reached, the lower ends of the pillow are crossed under the foot, brought upward, and pinned so that a compact splinting effect is obtained. In all splinting of fractures the bony prominences should be protected by cotton batting if obtainable or by any soft material.

(e) The Thomas splint for the leg and the Jones splint for the arm are easily applied and give good immobilization for transportation. They are carried by almost all first aid stations and ambulances, either civil or martial.

7. Shock is the result of a disturbance in the vasomotor system that allows relaxation in the peripheral circulatory system, thereby decreasing the amount of blood returning to the heart. The heart pumps from an empty system and is unable to fulfill the requirements for blood exchange to itself and other parts of the body. Shock may be the result of hemorrhage or a complete temporary disarrangement of the nervous system as a result of the injury. Fear may be an element in its production. It may be fatal. The blood pressure is greatly lowered, and the pulse is rapid and weak. The skin becomes pale, and the injured person may become listless or even unconscious. If hemorrhage is the cause, it should be stopped as promptly as possible and fluid should be administered in replacement. Stimulants such as coffee or tea may be used. Morphine and its derivatives tend to restore the balance between the peripheral and central circulations. Complete rest must be given in a recumbent position. As soon as infusions and blood or plasma transfusions are available, they should be given. Shock is usually caused by pain due to movement at the point of fracture and from hemorrhage rather than from malposition.

Hospital treatment in open fracture. To prepare an open wound for operation, soap and water should be used. A brush or sponge will help the effectiveness of this. Benzine is used to dissolve greasy materials. The skin and wound are then painted with a noncoagulating antiseptic, and draping is applied. The wound is flushed clean with several quarts of saline solution under low pressure. This is done with an elevated bottle and a glass nozzle on the end of rubber tubing. All loose, bruised, or contaminated portions of tissue are then removed with knife or scissors. Bone should be preserved if possible.

The antibiotic drugs have aided greatly in lessening the fight against infection. They are placed directly into the wound after the cleansing and debridement. In addition, a specific antibiotic is given orally or intramuscularly over a period of 3 to 7 days after the injury. They have served to lessen the occurrence of infection tremendously.

This should not be considered a substitute, however, but merely an adjunct to adequate debridement.

Antibiotics do not eliminate the necessity for giving both tetanus antitoxin and gas bacillus antitoxin as prophylactics for all patients with compound fractures. Immobilization after open reduction of open fractures is an essential part in the avoidance of infection and other complications. All patients with open fractures who arrive at the hospital for treatment within 6 hours after injury are considered clean and are treated by debridement, flushing with quantities of sterile saline solution, instillation of an antibiotic, reduction, closure, and the application of a cast.

Open fractures occurring longer than 6 hours before the patient gains admission are considered primarily infected in spite of the most careful debridement and other precautions, including antitoxins. In these patients, drainage is instituted and, if necessary, because of pain and elevation of temperature for a 24- to 48-hour period, the cast should be bivalved or a window made and the wound inspected. Otherwise, the open wound is left undressed within the cast.

The odor of gas bacillus infection is characteristically sweet and pungent, and air bubbles may be seen exuding from the wound. The presence of air in the tissue may also be demonstrated roentgenographically. The pulse is rapid, and the temperature is variable. Removal of the cast may be necessary, since the fracture is now of secondary importance. Multiple incisions into the tissue for adquate air penetration and drainage may be needed. In addition to the administration of gas gangrene antitoxin, the complication may call for hyperbaric oxygen therapy. This therapy consists in administering 100% oxygen in an environment (hyperbaric chamber) that provides for an increased atmospheric pressure.

FRACTURES OR DISLOCATIONS OF THE FACE, JAW, SKULL, CLAVICLE (COLLAR BONE), AND SHOULDER

In the statistics of World War II, fractures of the skull were relatively infrequent, and when they occurred they were problems for the neurosurgeon and required special instruction from him concerning nursing care. Similarly, serious injuries to the face involving the nose and sinuses were problems for the nose and throat specialist, whose ingenuity was often taxed in evolving methods and apparatus capable of restoring and maintaining the position of misplaced fragments.

Fractures involving the jaw usually call for the special attention of a dental surgeon. However, certain principles in the treatment can be mentioned. Loose teeth near the fracture line should not be removed unless absolutely necessary. Sometimes the alignment of the teeth and jaw may be obtained by using wires or rubber bands to hold together the teeth of the upper and the lower jaw. Occasionally the fragments of the jawbone may have to be held together by wires through the bone. Sometimes metal bands may be required to supplement

wiring, and sometimes plates fastened along the teeth, attached to a plaster of paris headgear by means of wires and elastic bands, may be used for adequate correction.

DISLOCATIONS OF THE JAW

Cause. Dislocation of the jaw is usually caused by violent yawning or yelling or by blows against the chin.

Anatomy. The dislocations may be unilateral or bilateral and usually consist of the forward or inward displacement of the condyles of the mandible from their articulating surface on the skull.

Symptoms and signs. Forward protrusion of the chin and inability to close the mouth are symptoms of dislocation of the jaw. If the dislocation is unilateral, the chin is displaced away from the dislocated side. There is usually rather severe pain and muscle spasm, and the lips and tongue become dry.

Treatment. Simple dislocations of the jaw can usually be reduced without anesthesia.

The surgeon swathes his thumbs in gauze and bandage to prevent being bitten. Pressure is exerted against the lower molars with increasing force downward and backward until reduction takes place. Following reduction, the upper and lower jaw should be held together by bandages around the head (Barton four-tailed bandage) for a period of 2 to 3 weeks so that habitual dislocation does not develop.

FRACTURE OF THE CLAVICLE (COLLAR BONE)

Fracture of the clavicle is one of the commonest of fractures. It may occur in any part—inner, middle, or outer. Treatment may be different for each type.

Cause. A fall on the shoulder or outstretched hand, exerting the entire force on the clavicle, and occasionally a direct blow may cause a fracture of the clavicle.

Anatomy. The pectoral muscles and weight of the arm bring the shoulder downward, inward, and forward, with overriding of fragments. The clavicle is the only bony connection between the chest and shoulder girdle.

Problem. The length of the clavicle must be maintained by keeping the shoulder up and held backward during healing (Figs. 5-14 to 5-16).

Healing period. A healing period from 4 to 8 weeks is usually required for fractures of the clavicle. Children under 10 years of age heal rapidly.

Treatment. In children the figure-of-eight dressing will usually suffice for the full treatment until union is shown to be present clinically and roentgenographically. The dressing is changed for cleanliness only. Zinc sterate powder is used to prevent chafing.

In adolescents and adults it is usually preferable to use a Velpeau dressing for 10 days to 2 weeks. This can be followed by a figure-of-eight dressing.

In obstinate cases, adolescent or adult, and especially in girls, when perfect alignment is necessary, side traction should be used for 3 to 4 weeks and followed by a figure-of-eight dressing.

Occasionally, when proper alignment cannot be obtained conservatively, an open reduction

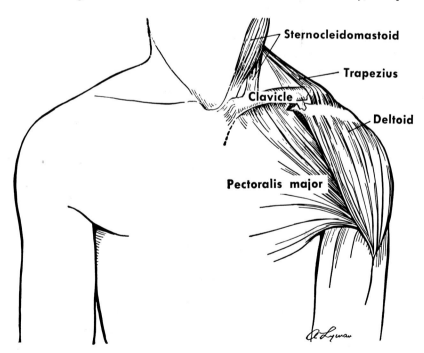

Fig. 5-14. Muscle mechanics of fracture of the clavicle. The sternocleidomastoid pulls upward on the proximal fragment while the weight of the shoulder pulls down and the pectoral muscles pull inward and forward, tending to override the fragments.

may be performed. Wiring with stainless steel or the use of Kirschner wire inserted into the medullary canal can, except for the scar, give perfect results.

FRACTURE-DISLOCATIONS AND DISLOCATIONS OF THE ACROMIOCLAVICULAR JOINT

Fracture-dislocations and dislocations of the acromioclavicular joint are the result of the same type of injury as that causing fracture of the clavicle. Roentgenograms frequently do not show the extent of the injury.

Problem. The shoulder must be kept upward and backward.

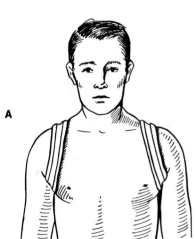

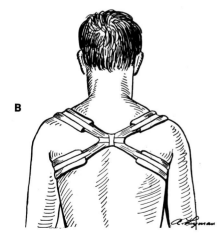

Treatment. A figure-of-eight bandage with adhesive strapping from the chest to the back and a pad over the clavicle is frequently employed in treatment of these fractures. The use of compound tincture of benzoin aids greatly in preventing skin irritation from the use of adhesive tape. Adhesive tape is changed often to prevent skin irritation. Immobilization must be maintained long enough to allow complete healing (6 to 10 weeks).

Patients with severe cases may require operative repair of the acromioclavicular joint as well as the ligament between the clavicle and the coracoid process.

In chronic painful dislocations the resection of the outer inch of the end of the clavicle usually leads to relief of symptoms and restoration of function (Mumford). Recovery occurs in about 3 weeks. Metallic fixation by a nail or Kirschner wire may be used in some instances.

DISLOCATIONS OF THE HEAD OF THE HUMERUS

There are several types of dislocation of the head of the humerus, but the most common is a forward and downward displacement.

Cause. Dislocation of the head of the humerus is usually caused by a fall on the outstretched

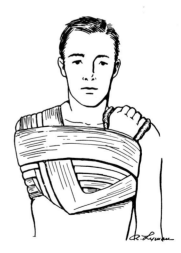

Fig. 5-15. A, Front view of figure-of-eight dressing. **B,** Back view. Felt, bias flannel bandage, and adhesive tape are used. Dressing should be changed every week or 10 days for cleanliness.

Fig. 5-16. The Velpeau bandage is used temporarily to immobilize clavicle, shoulder, humerus, elbow, or forearm. Wherever skin comes in contact with skin, a protective pad should be inserted.

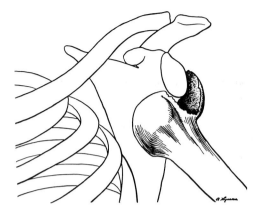

Fig. 5-17. Fracture-dislocation of shoulder. Greater tuberosity is torn off (subglenoid type).

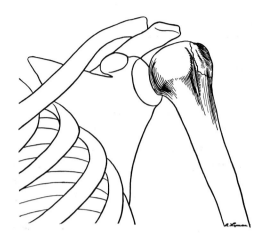

Fig. 5-18. Dislocation of shoulder reduced. Tuberosity has resumed normal position.

arm. Abduction of the shoulder joint is possible to only 90 degrees. At this point the humerus presses against the acromion process. This levers the head of the humerus downward or forward. The capsule of the joint is torn either anteriorly or at its attachment to the glenoid fossa. The head of the humerus enters the space below the glenoid fossa and rests under the coracoid process.

Symptoms and signs. The major symptom is pain. The arm cannot be brought against the side of the body, and there is a depression under the acromion process where the head of the humerus should be. The dislocation may be accompanied by fracture of the tuberosity (Figs. 5-17 and 5-18).

Reduction. Reduction should be performed with the patient under complete anesthesia to prevent further damage to the head of the humerus and to allow free movement so that the capsule will again close over the head allowing it to fall back into its normal position.

Problem. It takes about 3 to 4 weeks for ligamentous structures to heal. Motion that does not put strain on the healing area in the torn capsule, however, does not retard healing but maintains flexibility. Therefore, the problem with simple dislocations of joints is to begin motion within a few days. In dislocation of the shoulder the problem is to keep the elbow constantly forward to the shoulder plane on the affected side. If there is a detached fragment from the head to the humerus, it usually falls back into position during the reduction.

Treatment. Frequently a Velpeau dressing is used for a few days after reduction, and then this may be replaced with a neck-wrist strap. This strap must keep the wrist close to the chin so that only forward flexion and forward roation can be accomplished. As more complete healing takes place, this distance between the neck and wrist can be increased.

When habitual dislocations occur through placing strain on the healing capsule too early or through repeated dislocation, operative repair is needed. This may be done by passing the tendon of the long head of the biceps muscle through the head of the humerus (Nicola), or by suturing the capsule and labium to the anterior inferior lip of the glenoid fossa (Bankart).

FRACTURES OF THE NECK OF THE HUMERUS

Cause. Usually a fall directly against the shoulder with the arm against the chest or incompletely abducted is the cause of fracture of the neck of the humerus.

Anatomy. The pectoral muscles pull the distal (controllable) fragment inward and forward (Fig. 5-19), and the deltoid pulls it upward. They are the strongest muscles of the shoulder girdle group. The three types of fracture of the neck of the humerus are transverse, oblique, and comminuted.

Reduction. In all patients except those without displacement there should be an immediate attempt to restore perfect anatomic replacement under general anesthesia. With the transverse

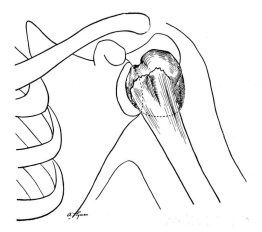

Fig. 5-19. Fracture of the neck of the humerus showing anterior and upward displacement of the distal fragment. The fracture line of the head is angled forward.

type this can usually be accomplished. In the other types, however, reduction may be difficult or impossible by this means.

Problem. The elbow must be kept close to the midline of the body to relieve the pull of the pectoral muscles. Some form of traction that will relax the deltoid and thereby prevent overriding and anterior angulation, the two salient factors necessary to reduction, must be provided.

Treatment. In fractures within or in close proximity to the shoulder joint, early motion is of great importance. Whenever anatomic reposition can be accomplished, motions can be started 10 days or 2 weeks after injury. In some instances, however, reductions are difficult to obtain and maintain, and it may be necessary to use a Velpeau dressing for 3 to 4 weeks or a lateral traction apparatus that maintains forward flexion and traction.

As soon as gluing of the fracture is present after the most nearly perfect position has been attained, active motion is started. This may require 2 to 4 weeks, depending on the appearance of the primary and subsequent roentgenograms and the estimated mechanical difficulties.

Usually a cast extending from the axilla to the wrist with a neck-wrist strap can be applied early (Figs. 5-20 and 5-21). The weight of the cast (which can be augmented by sheet lead at the elbow) will give the necessary traction, and the neck-wrist strap can be adjusted to give the required anterior flexion of the shoulder. In

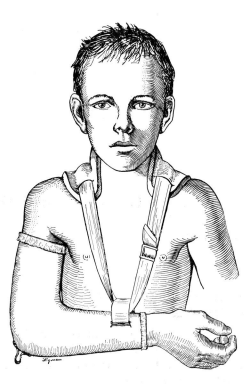

Fig. 5-20. The pendulum method of treatment of fractures in the region of the shoulder or shaft of humerus; this is the so-called hanging cast. Frequently, the cast is not essential, and efficiency depends on the neck-wrist strap combination. Loop at elbow for night traction.

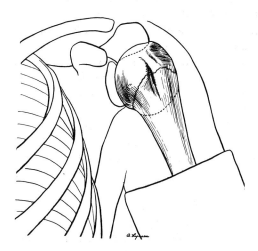

Fig. 5-21. Fracture manipulated under anesthesia and pendulum cast applied. For additional traction along with a neck-wrist band a 3-pound lead weight was incorporated in the cast at the elbow.

this way early motion without strain in the fractured area may be started.

Healing period. The healing period is from 6 to 10 weeks.

STIFF SHOULDER

In all kinds of fractures of the shoulder, arm, elbow, forearm, or wrist, delayed return of func-tion is frequently caused by adhesions about the shoulder joint as a result of disuse. It is best, therefore, with the approval of the surgeon in charge, to begin shoulder motion early in all patients with fractures of the extremity. This should consist of external rotation and forward flexion of the arm two or three times daily.

FRACTURES OF THE ARM, FOREARM, ELBOW, AND WRIST

FRACTURES OF THE SHAFT OF THE HUMERUS

Cause. Direct violence, such as a blow from the side, or indirect violence, such as a fall on the outstretched hand, may cause fracture of the shaft of the humerus.

Anatomy. There is usually overriding, es-pecially when the fracture is above the attach-ment of the deltoid muscle. There is also a tendency toward outward bowing. If the frac-ture is in the middle third of the humerus, special observation is indicated at once because of the proximity of the radial nerve to the bone. (Fig. 5-22). If the radial nerve is injured, it may be in one of three ways, which may be recognized as follows:

1. Severance of the nerve may be indicated by immediate inability to extend (raise) the hand at the wrist. Prognosis is poor for recovery without suture.

2. Contusion is made obvious by paralysis, which may occur gradually, with wrist drop as soon as the swelling and edema have reached a sufficient stage. Prognosis for recovery is good with rest.

3. Paralysis as a result of bony overgrowth in healing is evidenced by the gradual develop-ment of wrist drop 2 to 3 months after injury. Prognosis is good with removal of bony over-growth, freeing the nerve.

Problem. Maintaining traction and restoring the best alignment of the fragments are usually the chief problems in treating this type of frac-ture. There is often a tendency toward outward bowing that can be overcome either by more traction or by a pad between the elbow and the body.

Treatment. This fracture, if transverse, may be treated by immediate reduction with the pa-tient under anesthesia, or in a few instances it may be plated or wired. Usually, a cast from the axilla to the wrist is most satisfactory to the comfort of the patient and adds to the sim-plicity of treatment in all fractures in the shaft of the humerus. A loop of webbing or tape may be incorporated at the elbow so that traction by weights and pulleys can be maintained when the patient is lying down (Griswold) (Fig. 5-20).

Those fractures that occur a few inches above the elbow must have special consideration, since there is a great tendency to angle outward as a result of the combined pull of the biceps and triceps muscles. This causes a loss in the carry-ing angle at the elbow if it is uncorrected. The tendency may be overcome to some extent by applying a cast from the axilla to the fingers with the forearm in a position of extreme and forced pronation (palm down).

Healing period. Fractures of the shaft of the humerus may be slow to heal. In about 10% of the patients either delayed union or nonunion occurs. Ordinarily, however, a fracture of the

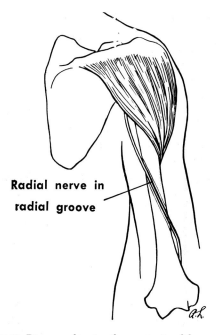

Fig. 5-22. Diagram showing the proximity of the nerve to the bone, with accessibility to injury.

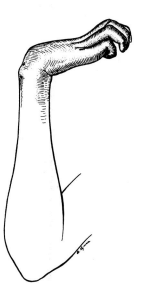

Fig. 5-23. Well-established Volkmann's contracture with clawhand and flexion of wrist and fingers. Note atrophy of forearm.

humerus will heal sufficiently for elbow motion in about 4 to 8 weeks. Complete recovery may occur in 8 to 10 weeks. In delayed union it may take as long as 3 to 6 months. In nonunion a bone graft operation is usually the most satisfactory way to obtain union.

When patients are in casts, usually little nursing care is required except to watch for complications. The nurse should attempt, however, with the consent of the surgeon, to maintain freedom of motion in as many of the neighboring joints as possible by means of massage around the joints and assisted active motions.

FRACTURES NEAR THE ELBOW

Cause. Fracture near the elbow is most common in two forms of injury: (1) in falls with the elbows extended (children) and (2) in direct violence exerted against the elbow (adults). There may be the impact from a passing car when the elbow is out of the window or there may be a fall on the elbow. The type of fall that in an adult would likely cause a dislocation of the elbow as a result of leverage of the olecranon process in the olecranon fossa would cause a supracondylar fracture in a child.

Anatomy. The elbow cannot normally extend beyond 180 degrees. Forcing beyond this point will cause either a dislocation of the elbow joint or a fracture just above the joint. The ulnar nerve runs downward just behind the inner posterior side of the joint, and the medial nerve runs just in front of the joint. Either is likely to be damaged at the time of injury or in reduction. With ulnar injury there may be an immediate or a delayed loss of sensation in the little and ring fingers. With medial injury there may be an immediate or delayed loss of sensation in the index and middle fingers. Any swelling or edema occurring within the firm capsule of the joint or within the aponeurosis (muscle covering) may cause great tension to be exerted from within. This may lead to (1) paralysis of the median, ulnar, and radial nerves, causing disturbance of motion and sensation in the forearm and hand, and (2) extravasation of blood into the fibers of muscle tissue so that they go through a stage of swelling and, later, scar formation (Volkmann's contracture) (Fig. 5-23). There is frequently much swelling after fractures and other injuries near the elbow joint, and symptoms of constriction of vessels and injury to muscles may be apparent within 4 to 48 hours after injury. Patients with injuries around the elbow joint, therefore, should be under hourly observation for at least 48 hours whether the fracture has been reduced or not. During this time notation by the nurse of any excessive swelling or loss of sensation should be made constantly. If such should occur, there should be immediate release of tension by complete freeing of any pressure caused by the cast or by incision of the superficial tissues by operation. The fracture should be disregarded until a circulatory balance is re-established.

Some of the most severe and complicated fractures the surgeon has to deal with occur in the elbow sideswipe injuries. They are usually compounded, and the humerus, the ulna, and the radius may be shattered. Nerves and tendons are frequently damaged. The repair is tedious and consists of thorough debridement, suture of nerves and tendons, and restoration of bone and joint alignment. The latter frequently requires internal fixation with wires, screws, or plates. Some patients, however, may be treated after repair by lateral traction in recumbency.

Treatment. Supracondylar fractures (Fig. 5-24) and dislocations should be reduced with the patient under anesthesia. It is usually ne-

cessary to place the elbow in a position of flexion to maintain reduction. The amount of flexion must be determined by the ability of the circulation to tolerate it. In fractures in young children the flexed position may be necessary for only 2 to 3 weeks. This is true of dislocations in young and old, but older persons may need a longer period for complete bone healing. If swelling is severe in patients treated early, or if reduction has not been accomplished to a satisfactory degree after 7 to 14 days, lateral traction either by adhesive traction or skeletal traction through the olecranon process should be instituted. In the majority of patients it will be successful, provided the surgeon and nurse are vigilant in the application of forces to correct the deformity.

Healing period. Motion should be begun within 3 to 6 weeks, depending on the stability at the time of reduction. Complete healing of the fracture requires approximately 8 weeks, but return of complete motion may require 3 to 6 months.

Fractures of the olecranon process

Cause. Fracture of the olecranon process (Fig. 5-25) is usually caused by a direct blow.

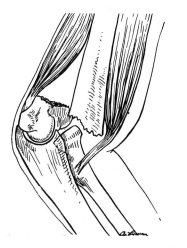

Fig. 5-24. Supracondylar fracture of the humerus. There is posterior displacement of the distal fragments with tension on nerves, tendons, and vessels. The fracture is within the capsule of the elbow joint.

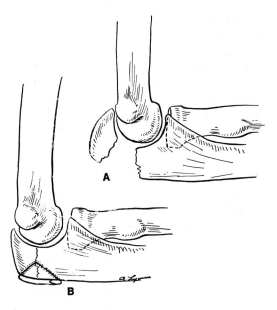

Fig. 5-25. Fracture of the olecranon process, which always requires open reduction if the fragments are separated. **A,** Fracture. **B,** Wire suture, which should be fairly superficial for best results.

Symptoms and signs. Pain, swelling, and inability to extend the elbow forcibly are symptoms of fracture of the olecranon process. Before swelling has occurred, a groove may be felt between the fragments.

Treatment. Open reduction is the treatment of choice in all patients who manifest any perceptible separation of the fragments. Reduction may be obtained by wiring or nailing, or it may be maintained by a removable beaded screw.

FOREARM FRACTURES

Cause. Forearm fractures may be caused by either direct or indirect violence, usually the latter.

Anatomy. Pronation and supination are the essential functional motions in the forearm. To preserve these motions after fracture, the bones must be replaced so that they will be parallel to each other and of equal length. There must be no obstacle or obstruction between them. The width of the interosseous space varies according to the tension or relaxation of the controlling muscles that rotate the forearm from pronation to supination (Fig. 5-26). Therefore, when the fracture occurs near the elbow, in the mid-arm, or near the wrist, the governing factor determining the position in which the controllable distal portion of the fractures is placed in relation to the uncontrollable or fixed proximal fragments depends on the location of muscle attachments and the various tendencies of their pull.

Treatment. In fractures above the pronator radii teres there is outward rotation of the upper fragment of the radius by the biceps tendon. Therefore, the forearm must be placed in outward rotation (supination). In fractures below the pronator radii teres the forearm must be placed in a position of inward rotation (pronation) to match the muscle action above.

The radius, probably because it has a better blood supply, usually heals faster than the ulna, but nonunion in the bones of the forearm is not uncommon and may require bone graft operations to stimulate bone union. Some irreducible fractures may be treated by bone plating or by intramedullary nailing.

Problem. Rotatory motion of the forearm must be restored as soon as sufficient union to tolerate the strain has been demonstrated

roentgenographically. The cast must extend from the fingers to the shoulder. The nearer the fracture is to the wrist, the sooner the cast can be cut to below the elbow. Daily full ranges of motion of the shoulder and, as soon as possible, of the elbow should be carried out to prevent adhesions.

Healing period. The healing period varies considerably with the amount of soft tissue damage at the time of the injury, the age of

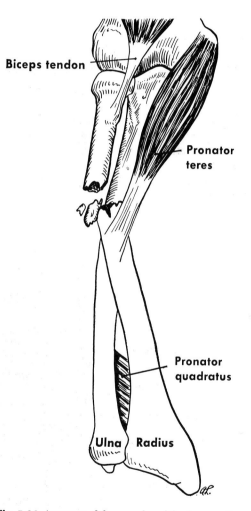

Fig. 5-26. Anatomy of the muscles of the forearm that influence pronation and supination. In fractures above the pronator teres the uncontrollable upper fragment is rotated outward (supinated). In fractures below the pronator teres the upper fragment is rotated inward (pronated). Fractures are placed in the fixed position to meet the upper fragment accordingly. The pronator quadratus always has a tendency to pull both bones together.

the patient, and the individual speed of healing (factors unknown). Solid union cannot be expected (except in children) in less than 8 to 12 weeks. In some patients in whom there is delayed union, immobilization must be maintained for 3 to 4 months. This causes considerable delay in the return of motion and function in the joints and muscles.

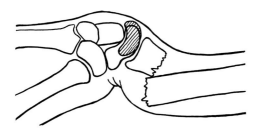

Fig. 5-27. Colles' fracture. Lateral view showing overriding and posterior displacement of controllable fragment.

FRACTURE OF THE WRIST (COLLES' FRACTURE)

Colles' fracture is one of the most common and classic fractures (Figs. 5-27 and 5-28).

Cause. Colles' fracture is caused by a fall or by breaking a fall with the outstretched hand.

Anatomy. The far end of the radius is broken off and displaced backward. The typical silver fork deformity results. Muscles play no particular part except to cause overriding by spasm. With the posterior displacement of the end of the radius, several other complications usually occur, such as (1) shortening of the forearm, which tends to make the ulna impinge on the carpal bones, (2) fracture of the styloid process of the ulna, and (3) posterior facing of the wrist joint, which interferes with action of the flexor tendons.

Problem. Reduction may be maintained by the use of (1) the circular cast; (2) anterior and posterior splints that are molded and held in the correct position by bandage, preferably bias flannel or elastic; (3) commercial splints, which

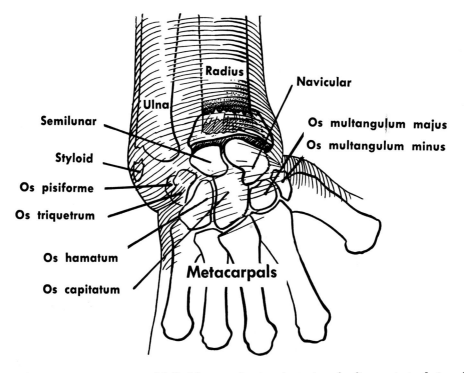

Fig. 5-28. Anteroposterior view of Colles' fracture showing shortening of radius, posterior facing of joint, and fracture of styloid process.

as a rule are not dependable except in a few patients with fractures in which fragments are not much displaced and forcible maintenance of corrective position is not necessary; or (4) skeletal traction that may be essential to good reduction with some patients with comminuted fractures. A Kirschner wire may be passed through the olecranon and another through the metacarpal bones of the hand. These are incorporated in the cast after reduction. This method may also be used when both bones of the forearm are broken.

Anesthesia. One of several types of anesthesia may be used: (1) local injection of Procaine HCl (Novocain), 1% to 2%, into the area of hemorrhage within the fracture site, (2) intravenous injection of Pentothal sodium, and (3) general anesthesia with gas, gas-ether, or ether.

In a few patients who are given treatment immediately, reduction may be performed without anesthesia because of nature's temporary anesthetizing effect.

These methods may be employed in the reduction of all fractures and may be selected according to the condition of the patient. The level of blood pressure, senility, and length of anesthesia time must be taken into consideration.

Treatment. In reduction it is important that the lines of the deformity be the determining factor in the application of the traction force. The flexed elbow offers a satisfactory means of countertraction when a nurse or assistant applies a firm grip there. Traction on the fingers and hand must be exerted first in the line of the deformity. When sufficient traction has been obtained to overcome muscle spasm and to free the impacted serrated bone ends, correction of the deformity will be easy if the distal portion is brought into a position that meets the proximal portion of the fracture. It is essential to proper reduction that these three requirements be fulfilled: (1) restoration of the length of the radius, (2) restoration of forward facing of the joint surface of the radius, and (3) ulnar deviation of the wrist to restore reposition of the styloid process and ensure adequate space in the ulnocarpal region.

Convalescent treatment, combining exercise, heat, massage, and splinting (Fig. 5-29), hastens the return of function.

ROUTINE TREATMENT FOLLOWING FRACTURES

As a general principle, cold applications or ice caps should be used in all injuries—fractures and sprains—within the first 24 or 36 hours to lessen swelling and relieve pain. After this, heat is more soothing.

In most patients with bone and tissue injury, aspirin or some form of salicylate is effective for relief of the aching pain. When muscle spasm is present, however, some of the morphine derivatives may be used fairly freely at first. This is particularly true when the injury is associated with shock.

NURSING CARE

Fractures occurring through the neck or upper third of the humerus that are reduced by traction offer some perplexing problems to the nurse. For traction the bed must have a firm hard mattress, and some method of countertraction must be devised. Usually, elevating

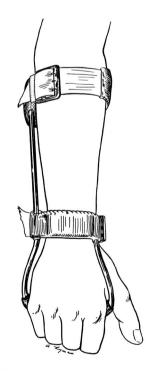

Fig. 5-29. Three-point splint for wrist drop; also used for protection of the wrist after fractures of the carpal bones on lower end of the radius. Allows free use of fingers and thumb.

the bed by shock blocks under the head and foot of the affected side will provide sufficient countertraction, although occasionally some type of restraint jacket secured to the unaffected side may be necessary also. The traction is applied in two parts with the arm flexed. Two adhesive straps that extend to a board and pulley extending from the side of the bed are used for the upper arm. Another set of adhesive straps is applied to the forearm and attached to a spreader that is a considerable distance beyond the ends of the fingers. From this spreader a rope extends to an overhead pulley and then to the weights. Some type of padded handle suspended from this spreader is useful, inasmuch as it enables the patient to flex his fingers and hand over it. Extension on the forearm is used to eliminate its dependent weight as well as to relax muscle spasm in the upper arm (Fig. 5-30).

Although the rest of the patient's body is unencumbered, he is usually not permitted to turn, and for that reason considerable discomfort in the upper back and shoulders may occur. Frequent alcohol rubs for these areas will be of use in eliminating this discomfort. Changing the undersheet must be done with great dexterity to prevent movement of the patient's body and disturbance of the traction. Because pressure points tend to form rather easily around the bony prominences of the wrist, this area should be inspected frequently.

Fractures above the condyles of the humerus—the elbow fracture of common parlance—are very common in active youngsters. Such patients do not often remain long in the hospital. They are frequently brought in for reduction and dismissed in a few hours. It is essential that the parents be warned of the danger of circulatory impairment from subsequent swelling and that they be told how to detect such a complication. They must understand that the fracture itself should not occasion severe discomfort for the child and that continued crying or repeated complaints may indicate that there is an obstruction in circulation. Not long ago a small boy with such a fracture was taken to his home 5 miles out of town after reduction of a supracondylar fracture that had been performed in the hospital outpatient department. The child

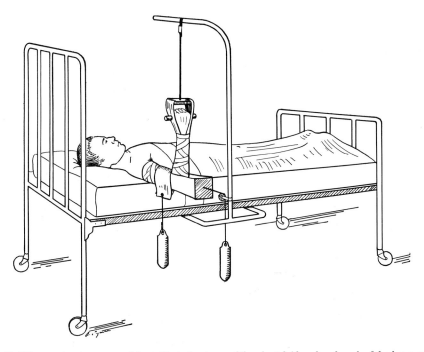

Fig. 5-30. Side-traction apparatus. Adaptable to fractures of the clavicle, head and neck of the humerus, shaft of the humerus, and supracondylar fractures.

complained bitterly for 24 hours before the parents realized this was not the normal sequence of events after a fracture. When he was brought back to the hospital, a fully developed ischemic contracture of the kind described by and named by Volkmann had occurred, and 10 months of constant treatment were necessary to bring back even partial use of the hand.

Coldness, pallor, and cyanosis of fingers may be the first indications that there is circulatory impairment. Swelling and pain often follow rapidly, and some paresthesia may be detected on touching the digits. Since all fractures are accompanied by some degree of swelling, observation should be constant and vigilant in these cases. Too often this may be neglected because the patient seems to need relatively little nursing care and, for the most part, looks after his own wants.

A good test for circulation is the blanching sign that determines patency of blood flow. The nail of the thumb is momentarily compressed, and the return of blood to the nail is observed. If the return is immediate, circulation is thought to be adequate. Sluggishness in the return of the blood to the part is indicative of some degree of impairment and should be reported to the physician. One authority warns in huge letters in his textbook on fractures: "WATCH THE HAND FOR SWELLING AND BLUENESS OF THE NAILS. CAUTION ALL CONCERNED THAT IF THIS OCCURS THE FIXATION APPARATUS SHOULD BE REMOVED AND THE ARM BROUGHT INTO EXTENSION. THE FRACTURE CAN ALWAYS BE REDUCED THE SECOND TIME BUT A VOLKMANN'S CONTRACTURE IS A PERMANENT DISABILITY."*

Surgeons make it a rule to disregard the fracture in any circulatory emergency.

Elevation of the arm by pillows or by suspending the arm in an overhead sling may sometimes reduce the swelling considerably. With the first evidence that circulation is not normal, however, the nurse should be on guard. No excuse can possibly be made for delay in reporting the condition to the surgeon, and this

means at night as well as during the day. When no doctor is available, the nurse may have to split the cast throughout its entire length. The constriction may be caused by tight bandages or padding beneath the cast, and so these also must be cut. The skin must be visible from one end to the other. The cast, once split and spread, can be taped together temporarily, because it usually does not need to be removed to relieve the symptoms. Nurses are warned not to be satisfied with splitting the cast half-way, since this is usually inadequate to release the constriction. Unless they are specifically ordered by the surgeon, windows should not be cut in casts. The swelling and edema that may occur through a window will only exacerbate the existing trouble.

Releasing the constricting cast and bandages may not reduce the symptoms, particularly if they are caused by callus formation that involves the nerve. For this reason frequent inspection of the digits should follow the spreading of the cast.

Occasionally, the surgeon will order a small window cut out over the radial artery before the patient is brought back from the plaster room after reduction of such fractures. This allows the nurse caring for the patient to check

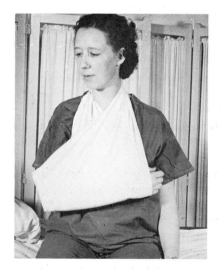

Fig. 5-31. Correct application of arm sling. Note support of wrist. The sling ends are crossed on the posterior aspect of the neck and pinned in two places. The double pinning helps distribute the weight, and there is no pressure from a knot.

*From Magnusson, Paul B.: Fractures, Philadelphia, 1949, J. B. Lippincott Co.

frequently on the circulation in the extremity. It is of great importance that the pulse be carefully taken and recorded at stated intervals, perhaps as often as every 15 minutes. A faint disappearing pulse may indicate pressure on the artery and should be reported. Comparison with the pulse of the unaffected arm will be of assistance in gauging the seriousness of the constriction.

Nurses notifying physicians of circulatory impairment should chart the notation and the time at which the physician was called.

A word should be said in regard to slings that are frequently used after injury to the forearm or wrist (Fig. 5-31). If the sling is applied in the common fashion with the long bias edge encircling the wrist and the ends going over alternate shoulders, do not use a knot to fasten the ends at the back of the neck. Such a knot places considerable strain on the back of the neck, and for relief the patient allows his shoulders to droop forward. Small safety pins used to pin the ends distribute the weight of the sling more evenly. Some surgeons object to a sling being passed around the neck at all. They prefer that it be passed over the opposite shoulder and under the arm, because if the sling is placed around the neck it is possible for the patient to lower his arm by simply lowering his head. A sagging sling that does not support the wrist and allows the forearm to droop beyond a right angle is a very sloppy, inefficient apparatus. The patient who is wearing a sling to support the arm must be given instructions regarding movement of the shoulder joint. This joint should be taken through a normal range of motion several times daily to prevent tightness or limitation in shoulder motion.

FRACTURES IN THE HAND

FRACTURES OF THE CARPAL SCAPHOID

Fracture of the carpal scaphoid, when encountered alone or in combination with dislocations of the wrist, deserves special comment. The disabling possibilities are often underestimated, and treatment if often insufficient or lacking.

Cause. Falling on the outstretched hand is usually the cause of fractures of the carpal scaphoid.

Anatomy. The bones of the wrist are peculiar in that the greater part of their surface is covered with articular cartilage. This means that the supply of circulation is correspondingly limited.

An interruption of the circulation by fracture or loss of continuity means starvation to one or another portion of the injured bone with resulting disintegration or death of bone (aseptic necrosis).

Diagnosis. Diagnosis is based on roentgenographic findings. Four views should be taken. Sometimes, the fracture line does not show up for 2 or 3 weeks. There are pain and tenderness in the "snuffbox."

Treatment. Complete reduction by adequate manipulation is the first requirement. Adequate and prolonged immobilization in a cast or splint is next. If nonunion should occur, drilling holes through the fracture line or a bone graft may lead to healing; or the removal of one or both of the fragments may improve function and relieve pain.

Healing period. A fracture of the carpal scaphoid requires immobilization in a cast or splints for 8 to 10 weeks for union to take place.

FRACTURES OF THE METACARPALS

Cause. Fractures of the metacarpals are caused by (1) direct violence or crushing injuries, and (2) indirect violence, such as striking a blow with the closed fist.

Anatomy. Most of the muscle power in the

hand is on the palmar surface (interossei and lumbricales). These muscles act to bow the metacarpal bones backward in the event of fracture.

Problem. The metacarpals must be immobilized adequately in a position that will overcome the tendency toward posterior bowing.

Reduction. Manipulation under anesthesia is often necessary to restore normal position. To maintain this, several methods are used.

A plaster cast may be employed to apply pressure posteriorly along the shaft and anteriorly on the palmar surface under the head, or the metacarpophalangeal joint.

Skeletal traction is another method used to maintain reduction of the fracture. By passing a small pin through the phalanx or by using the miniature ice-tong apparatus, sufficient traction may be applied through elastic bands and the banjo splint to maintain proper position of the fragments. This is particularly adaptable to the overriding oblique or spiral fracture.

At the critical time of about 3 weeks, roentgenographic examination must be carried out to see that proper reduction has been maintained.

Healing period. The healing period is 4 to 5 weeks.

FRACTURES OF THE PHALANGES

Fractures of the phalanges comprise two types: the transverse and the oblique fractures of the phalanges and the chip fractures of the posterior surface of the distal fragment of the distal phalanx.

Transverse and oblique fractures of the phalanges

Anatomy. The lumbrical muscles tend to cause palmar angulation of the fragments.

Treatment. The problem of reduction as well as treatment is to keep the fingers in flexion until the critical time has passed. This may be done by binding the fingers over a rolled bandage. When bandages are removed, motion should be re-established.

Chip fractures of the posterior surface of the distal fragment of the distal phalanx

Anatomy. The tendon of the long extensor is attached to the posterior surface of the distal fragment of the distal phalanx. Injury causes an inability to extend the distal phalanx and grave loss of an important function. A stiff joint or an amputation is less disabling than this deformity (baseball finger).

Treatment. Complete, exaggerated, and prolonged (4 to 6 weeks) hyperextension of the distal joint of the finger is the treatment of choice. This gives, as a rule, sufficient time for complete reattachment of the tendon and a return of function. Suture by operation is occasionally necessary.

FRACTURES AND DISLOCATIONS OF THE SPINE AND PELVIS

FRACTURES OF THE CERVICAL, THORACIC, AND LUMBAR SPINE

Fractures or dislocation of the spine are divided into the following groups in the order of severity: (1) fractures or dislocations with extensive displacement and immediate paralysis of the nerves below the point of fracture, (2) fractures or dislocations with displacement and delayed paralysis below the point of fracture, (3) fractures with compression of the vertebrae but with no neurologic disturbance, and (4) fractures of the accessory processes (such as spinous or lateral processes) without any evidence of nerve pressure.

Cause. Causes of fractures of the spine are as follows: (1) a fall in the sitting or stooped position, (2) a jackknife type of injury such as occurs when force is exerted against the shoulders and pelvis at the same time, (3) a direct blow against the back or flank, and (4) certain diseases that cause softening or disintegration of the bones of the spine, such as hyperparathyroidism and malignant metastasis. In this last the break may occur spontaneously or with minimal strain.

First aid. There is a great lesson to be learned in the treatment of acute injuries, which is particularly exemplified in fractures of the spine. Usually, such injuries occur in auto accidents, in athletics, as the result of falls in construction work, or under similar circumstances.

The treatment should be started at the scene of the injury. Obviously, the victim of such an accident may have spicules of bone that could cause damage to the tissues of the spinal cord if he is improperly transported.

Anatomy. The spinal cord is encased in a tube or channel of bone. The abnormal position of the vertebra may cause complete shearing severance of the cord at the time of injury, or the cord may be subjected to damage from spicules of bone or the pressure from surrounding hemorrhage and congestion. If severance occurs, paralysis is immediate below the fractured vertebra. If the damage results from pressure alone, the paralysis is delayed in its development.

Problem. If paralysis occurs but is not immediate or complete, laminectomy (decompression of the spinal cord) and the removal of bone fragments are sometimes indicated. In complete immediate paralysis laminectomy has no value. In uncomplicated compression fractures the problem is to restore the normal contour of the spine.

After injury to the spine (Fig. 5-32), there is almost invariably a shock to the sympathetic nervous system. With this shock comes disturbance of intestinal and bladder activity, and the most serious immediate problem of the patient with spine fracture often directly results from these factors.

The presence of pain often requires morphine sedation, which exaggerates internal stasis and sluggishness of bladder muscles to such an extent that enemas and catheterization

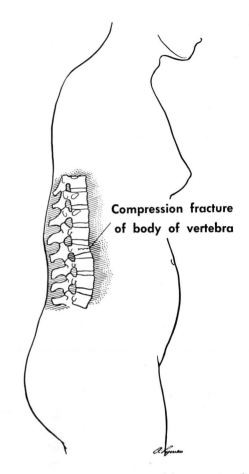

Compression fracture of body of vertebra

Fig. 5-32. Compression fracture of the spine. Angulation or gibbus may occur over the spinous process of the fractured vertebra or the one above.

are frequently necessary for several days. Strong cathartics should not be used because they may cause increased discomfort. The use of a rectal tube and gastric suction is advocated. An indwelling catheter is occasionally necessary for 5 to 7 days.

Treatment. Providing for and maintaining extension of the spine may be accomplished in several ways.

A frame or Gatch bed may be used in the treatment of these patients. Its angle is gradually increased within 4 to 14 days. Maintenance of reduction is checked roentgenographically. After reduction a body cast is applied.

Early reduction under anesthesia is accomplished with the patient suspended by his feet and shoulders, face down. Pressure is exerted

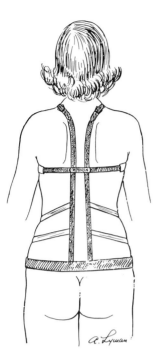

Fig. 5-33. Taylor back brace used for support of the spine in many conditions, such as convalescent fractures and tuberculosis, epiphysitis, arthritis, malignancy, and round-shoulder deformity.

on the spinous processes at the point of fracture until correction has been obtained. Roentgenographic examination may be used to confirm the reduction before the cast is applied. The cast should extend from the hips to the neck to maintain correction. The higher the fracture in the spine, the more difficult it is to maintain the correction. In fractures above the fifth dorsal vertebra, it is necessary to carry the cast on up to the head and chin.

Some spine fractures that have healed with persistent pain need internal fixation by some form of bone fusion or graft or other apparatus to stabilize the spinous processes and laminae in the correct position.

Fractures or dislocations of the cervical spine are best treated by the use of the Crutchfield tongs. These allow weights of 30 to 40 pounds to be used for reduction.

Treatment in the extension cast is usually carried out for 3 to 6 months, according to the severity of the fractures. This is followed by use of an extension brace such as the Taylor back brace (Fig. 5-33) for an additional 4 to 6 months.

Healing period. The healing period of vertebrae is from 6 to 12 months.

NURSING CARE OF THE PATIENT WITH FRACTURE OF THE SPINE WITHOUT CORD INJURY

(For rehabilitative care of patient with spinal cord injury, see Chapter 3.)

Upon arrival in the emergency room, the patient with a back injury and possible cord damage should be kept on the ambulance cot until preliminary evaluation of his injuries can be made by the attending physician. All unnecessary transfers should be avoided. Prior to moving the patient to a bed, the nurse should have specific instructions from the doctor pertaining to the type of bed and equipment needed. In some instances, to facilitate turning and maintenance of desired position, the patient is placed on a lateral or vertical turning frame. If increased extension of the spine is desired, the doctor may request an extension device to be placed on the bed. Also, to secure a firm surface, it is usually necessary to place a fracture board beneath the mattress. Unnecessary moving of the patient can be avoided if these needed articles are in readiness.

When transferring the patient with back injury from the ambulance cot to the X-ray table or the bed, it is advisable to use a "three-man lift." (Fig. 5-34). By keeping the pelvis and shoulders level, flexion and rotation of the spine are avoided. If there is a cervical injury, a fourth person is needed to support the patient's head, preventing flexion or rotation of the cervical vertebrae. Sandbags placed at either side of the head will help maintain the desired position. When removing the patient's clothing, it frequently is necessary to cut garments to avoid motion at the site of injury. All of the above efforts are directed at preventing possible trauma to the spinal cord, which could affect the ultimate outcome.

Upon admission the patient's vital signs are checked and recorded. The rate and type of respirations and the presence of any cyanosis should be noted. If the injury is in the cervical region, respiratory embarrassment caused by involvement of the phrenic nerve may be anticipated. For this reason, equipment for trache-

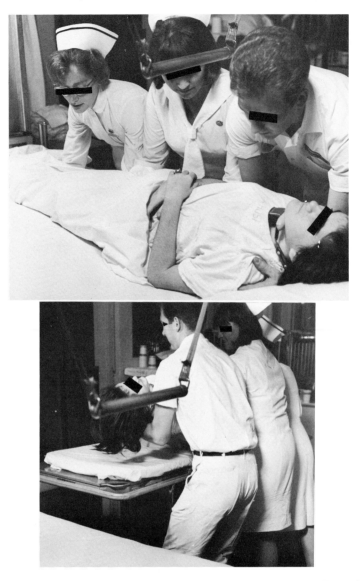

Fig. 5-34. When immobilization of the spine is necessary, the "three-man lift" may be used to transfer a patient from the bed to a cart or vice versa. If immobilization of the cervical spine is necessary, a fourth person should support and control the position of the head. Note that all the "lifters" assume positions at the same side of the bed. The first nurse slips his arms beneath the patient's shoulders and chest region, the second nurse places arms beneath the patient's lumbar and buttocks areas, and the third nurse supports the patient's lower limbs. The cart is usually placed at a right angle to the foot end of the bed. (This may vary depending on the situation.) With the "lifters" working in unison, the shoulders, hips, and lower extremities of the patient's body are moved simultaneously to the edge of the bed. As the second step in the transfer process, and again in unison, the "lifters" raise the patient's body from the bed and move in a circular direction to place him on the cart. (Before starting the procedure, it is advisable to lock the bed and cart wheels.) In some instances as the patient is lifted from the bed, it may be permissible to roll his body toward the "lifters." Carrying a weight close to the body provides for more efficient use of muscles. However, if immobilization of the patient's vertebral column during the moving process is essential, omitting this step may be desirable. Another point to remember is that the use of good body mechanics by the workers is an important aspect in preventing back strain.

ostomy must be available for immediate use, as well as equipment for administering oxygen. Frequently, suction is necessary to maintain a patent airway and to prevent aspiration of secretions. Equipment and facilities for giving intravenous infusions or blood transfusions are necessary items; drugs for combating shock, such as ephedrine or Phenylephrine hydrochloride (Neosynephrine), must be administered as directed by the physician. Pain medications that depress the respirations and those which tend to mask neurologic signs are usually withheld.

Hyperthermia apparent a short time after a cervical cord injury may be of central origin. Intracranial involvement may be detected by checking pupillary reaction of the eyes to light. Signs of confusion or amnesia denoting the patient's level of consciousness should be recorded. The patient with a fracture of the vertebral column must be checked for bladder distention. Usually the doctor asks that a Foley catheter be inserted and secured in place. The amount and appearance of the urine should be noted and a specimen saved. The physician may wish to do a spinal puncture, either to determine if there is bleeding into the subarachnoid space or to determine whether there is a block of the cerebrospinal fluid.

Fracture or dislocation of the cervical spine

Skeletal traction, applied by tongs inserted in the parietal eminences of the skull, is usually used for reduction of fractures and dislocations of the cervical (Fig. 5-35) vertebrae. In some instances it may be necessary to use rather large amounts of weight to reduce the fracture. Progress of reduction is checked roentgenographically; when complete reduction has been obtained, the amount of weight is decreased.

The stab wounds through which the tongs are introduced into the skull are usually dressed with small circular sponges. Very little danger of infection exists, although occasionally this does occur. Inspection of the wound dressings should be made each day, but the dressings are not disturbed without order of the surgeon. Tightening of the tongs is usually done by the surgeon or his assistants.

Although such emergencies are not common,

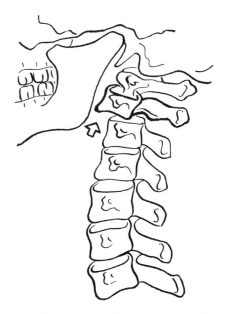

Fig. 5-35. Dislocation of the cervical spine. (From Kenney, W. C., and Larson, C. B.: Orthopedics for the general practitioner, St. Louis, 1957, The C. V. Mosby Co.)

skeletal traction in the skull has sometimes become loose and actual slipping out of the tongs may result. For this reason a set of alternate equipment should be kept on hand, which the nurse may apply until the physician can be reached. A chin halter, a spreader, some rope, and a few sandbags will suffice to maintain the desired position until the tongs can be replaced in the skull.

With the Crutchfield skull traction (Figs. 5-36 and 5-37), careful turning of the patient for back care may be permitted. (Permission and instruction pertaining to turning should be obtained from the attending surgeon.) The patient must be watched for signs of cyanosis during the process and for dyspnea, which might indicate damage to the cord.

Body alignment should be carefully maintained during the turning process, and the patient should be turned as though he were a log and would not bend. Head, shoulders, and pelvis must be turned simultaneously. Flexion of the cervical spine is not permitted. A pillow should be placed in front of the patient's chest to support the shoulder and arm, and another should be placed between the thighs and legs to prevent sagging of the hip. Either of these conditions, sagging of the hip or of the shoulder in the side-lying position, will inevitably alter the position of the spine and should be avoided.

When longitudinal traction is maintained by skeletal tongs, it may be necessary to adjust the position of the cervical spine to accomplish alignment—especially in extension. This may be accomplished by several methods. Two mat-

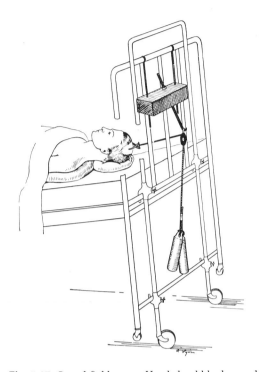

Fig. 5-37. Crutchfield tongs. Head should be low and shoulders high. The upper end of the bed should be elevated. Traction weights of 25 to 35 pounds may be used safely and comfortably.

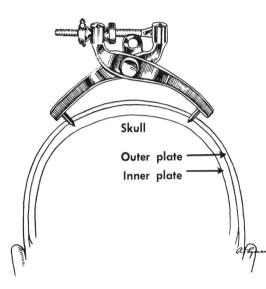

Skull

Outer plate

Inner plate

Fig. 5-36. Crutchfield tongs apparatus.

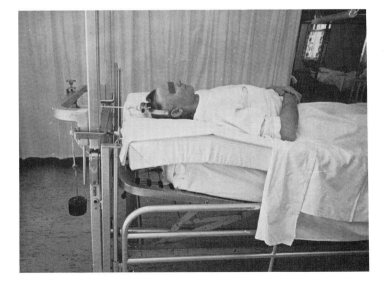

Fig. 5-38. Vinke tongs applied to patient with cervical fracture. Note arrangement of mattresses to provide for extension of the cervical region.

tresses may be placed on the bed; one is in the usual position and another—the upper one, which may be a youth mattress, is positioned so that it reaches only to the patient's shoulders (Fig. 5-38). A thin pillow or pad may be used under the head to help provide the desired position. The same effect can be obtained by placing a sponge rubber mattress on top of the regular mattress as in Fig. 5-38. Extension of the cervical spine may also be obtained by placing firm pillows under the patient's back, from the sacrum to the shoulders. When any of the above methods are being used to maintain the desired position of the cervical spine, turning of the patient is usually not permissible. If *only* longitudinal traction is necessary, the patient may be placed on a bed frame that provides for lateral or vertical turning. (See Chapter 2.)

The cervical fracture patient with head traction will be dependent upon the nurse for many of his needs. If cervical extension is being maintained, soft foods that are easily chewed will be less likely to cause choking than liquids. Liquids should be taken slowly until the patient becomes accustomed to swallowing in this position. As a precautionary measure, since the patient's head cannot be elevated or rotated, it is advisable to have suction equipment available at the bedside. The individual with head traction will not be able to feed himself and, in some instances, may have a poor appetite. Consequently, provision for feeding, plus a relaxed unhurried atmosphere at mealtime, is desirable. Adequate intake of needed nutrients is important.

During the first few days, the patient with compression fracture of the spine or injury to the cord is likely to have a troublesome stasis of the gastrointestinal tract, due to a paralytic ileus. The abdomen may be ballooned to drumlike tenseness by distention of the bowel, and respiratory embarrassment is present because of pressure on the underside of the diaphragm. Relief may be gained by the insertion of a rectal tube, and neostigmine (Prostigmin) may be prescribed to help produce peristalsis. However, it frequently is necessary to use a nasogastric tube and suctioning to provide relief for the patient. During the time that suction is being used, the patient is maintained on intravenous feedings.

Careful observation for change in skin sensation and for loss of motion or muscle strength (handgrip) is an essential aspect of the care needed by the patient with a fracture of the spine without cord damage. Such symptoms can be indicative of pressure on the cord and should be reported to the surgeon. The pressure may be caused by increasing edema or by a change in the position of the bone fragments.

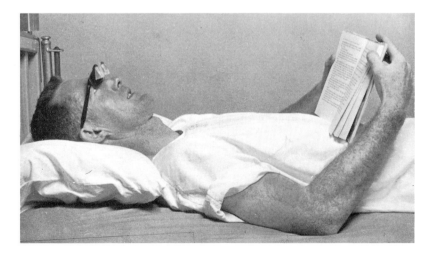

Fig. 5-39. The use of prism glasses makes reading and watching television possible for the patient who cannot have the backrest elevated.

Surgery may be indicated to relieve pressure and to prevent permanent cord damage.

Because of the traction apparatus and the injury, turning may not be permitted, and positioning of the patient is more difficult than with most patients. Thus, frequent encouragement of the patient to breathe deeply is helpful in moving secretions and preventing hypostatic pneumonia. Likewise, skin care and the prevention of pressure sores become a challenge. To prevent skin breakdown, it is usually desirable and necessary to use such aids as sponge rubber pads, acrylic fiber pads (artificial lamb's wool), or perhaps an alternating pressure mattress. Use of these "aids," however, does not lessen either the need for maintaining a wrinkle-free and crumb-free bed or the need for massage to vulnerable spots. Even though turning may be limited, massage to the back can be given at frequent intervals. Pressure placed on the mattress with one hand enables the nurse to slip her other hand beneath the patient's back and give massage to the sacral and scapular areas, likely spots for pressure necrosis.

Placement of the patient on the bedpan presents additional problems. The fracture bedpan, which has a low tapering back, can usually be slipped under the buttocks if pressure is placed on the mattress at each side of the buttocks. Two nurses can do this with less discomfort for the patient than one nurse alone.

Changing the bed linen is easier if two drawsheets are used instead of one full-length sheet. Pillowcases or towels may be placed at either side of the head. When these are soiled, they can be changed without disturbing the head position. During this period of bed rest, active or passive exercise of the arms and legs (as prescribed by the surgeon) is necessary to ensure maintenance of normal joint motion.

Time passes slowly for this patient. Prism glasses may help him to read and to watch television or other activities in the area (Fig. 5-39).

When roentgenograms indicate that sufficient healing has taken place to permit ambulation, the patient is fitted with a neck brace (Fig. 5-40). When traction has been removed and a brace applied, the brace must be worn continuously until permission for its removal is given by the

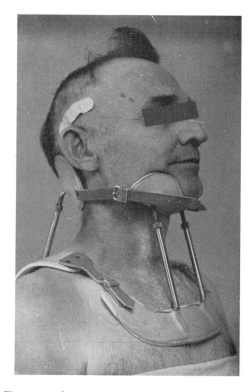

Fig. 5-40. After removal of the Crutchfield tongs the patient is fitted with a brace designed to provide support and immobilization of the cervical vertebrae.

surgeon. Ambulation for this patient must be a slow and gradual process. Assistance with walking is necessary until danger of falling is past.

Fractures of the lumbar and thoracic regions of the spine

In fracture of the spine that is not accompanied by permanent cord injury or spinal fluid block the patient is sometimes placed on a sponge rubber mattress that is superimposed on an ordinary firm felt mattress and bed boards. The feet are kept in the normal physiologic position, the knees are relaxed with a knee roll, and the limbs are cradled so that the weight of the bedclothes is eliminated. The spine is maintained in a position of extension. At other times, extreme extension is ordered. This may be obtained by placing a blanket roll beneath the felt mattress at the desired position, or the patient may be placed in a Gatch bed with his head at the foot of the bed and the knee rest elevated (Fig. 5-41). This will provide for extension of

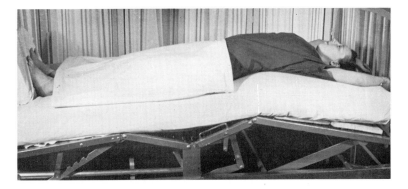

Fig. 5-41. The spine is maintained in a position of extension by use of the three-crank Deckert bed. The amount of extension can be increased or decreased according to need. The same position can be secured with the ordinary Gatch bed by placing the patient's head at the foot and then elevating the knee rest.

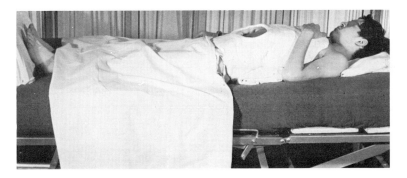

Fig. 5-42. A body cast that has been applied to maintain the spine in an extended position.

the spine and has the advantage of being easily alterable. The elevation of the knee rest is usually about 3 inches at the beginning of the treatment. It may be increased 2 inches daily until a maximum elevation of approximately 10 inches has been reached. Occasionally, reverse peristaltic action accompanied by vomiting may occur during this process. If this happens, further elevation of the Gatch bed should not be attempted.

Patients in extension casts (Fig. 5-42) may be given a regime of exercises designed to strengthen the body musculature, particularly the back extensors, which will be of great importance when the cast is finally removed.

The patient may be kept in a position of extension for approximately 2 months. At this time if roentgenograms show satisfactory results, he may be allowed out of bed in some type of back brace (Fig. 5-43) prescribed by the physician. If

bowel and bladder disturbances were present at the outset, the patient will usually have regained control by this time.

FRACTURES OF THE SACRUM AND COCCYX

Cause. Fractures of the sacrum and coccyx are usually caused by direct violence and are very painful. Falling on ice in a sitting position is a common cause.

Symptoms. Pain that is aggravated by sitting down or arising and tenderness over the sacrum or sacrococcygeal joint are symptoms of fracture of the sacrum and coccyx.

Treatment. After the patient has spent a period of rest in bed with the affected area supported on a rubber ring and much time lying prone, low adhesive strapping or a low girdle may be used to relieve muscle pull. Sitting on hard surfaces should be avoided. Repeated massage of

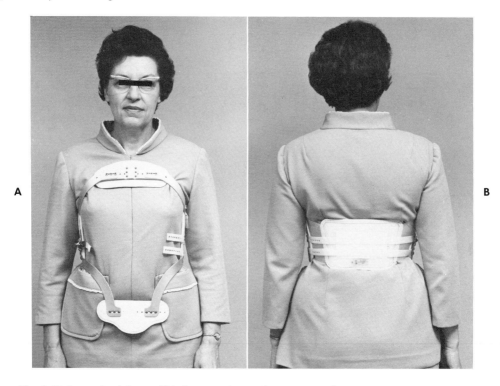

Fig. 5-43. Jewett back brace. This brace is designed to maintain the spine in extension; it is particularly adapted for the ambulatory treatment of compression fractures of the vertebral bodies. It applies the three point pressure principle—pressure backward on sternum and pubis, pressure forward on midback.

the piriformis muscles (rectally) often gives relief. Occasionally, as a last resort, the coccyx may be removed.

FRACTURES OF THE PELVIS

Cause. Fractures of the pelvis usually result from crushing between two forces with considerable violence.

Anatomy. The pelvis is a ring composed of the sacrum posteriorly, the ilia on either side, and the symphysis pubis in front. The weakest spots in this ring are the rami of the pubis. Most of the pelvic fractures occur in the rami (Fig. 5-44), but they may occur in the ilia with displacement of the pelvis.

Complications. At the time of injury there may be damage to the pelvic organs as a result of the direct force or spicules of bone. The urethra is most frequently damaged; the bladder is next. There may be damage to the rectum. If the bladder is full at the time of injury, damage is more likely.

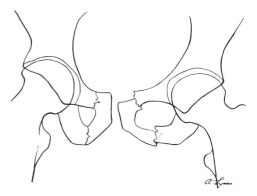

Fig. 5-44. Fracture of both rami of both sides of the pubis. Note the asymmetry of the pelvis. Abduction of both thighs is necessary for correction.

There are two main reasons for restoration of the symmetric ring of the pelvis: (1) to avoid future abnormal strain on the sacroiliac joints and (2) to restore the normal birth canal in women.

Treatment. Overriding of the fragments may

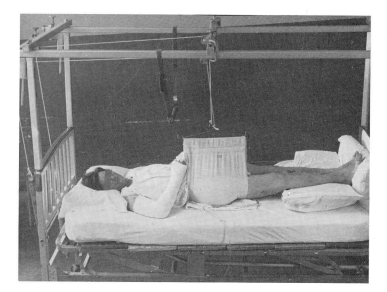

Fig. 5-45. Pelvic sling used in the treatment of fractures of the pelvis.

be overcome by the use of Buck's extension or skeletal traction on the leg of the fractured side. Traction automatically causes abduction and pull at the same time, although side traction may also be necessary.

When sufficient correction has been obtained through traction, a hip spica of plaster of paris is applied with the hip in abduction. It is usually necessary to apply it only down to the knee.

Healing period. Healing usually takes place in 6 to 8 weeks. Weight bearing on the affected side should be avoided during that time. Crutches may be used. Patients with this injury are likely to have persistent trouble in the sacroiliac joint. It is wise to use some form of pelvic girdle for protection during the early months of weight bearing to prevent permanent damage to the sacroiliac joint.

Nursing care. Under the classification of pelvic fractures are fractures of the ilium, pubic bone, sacroiliac, and acetabulum. They are of varying degrees of severity, but in all the nurse should be aware of the danger of internal injuries, particularly to the bladder, urethra, or rectum. A urine specimen by catheterization is usually ordered immediately. A soft rubber catheter should be used—never one made of metal. A rectal examination is also carried out by the physician to rule out injury to the lower bowel.

The most common fracture of the pelvis is that occurring in the pubic bone, and it is often caused by a compression between two solid objects or a fall in which the patient lands on the hip.

After reduction of a fracture of this nature the patient may be placed in a canvas sling attached to an overhead frame (Fig. 5-45). Buck's extension is usually applied to the leg of the injured side. Compression of the pelvis is obtained by fastening the ends of the canvas sling together over the front of the patient. If compression is not desired, the canvas sling may have wooden spreaders at either side and be supported by separate ropes and pulleys on the overhead frame. The hammock should be about 5 feet long and 2 feet wide. It should extend from the upper border of the lumbar vertebrae to midthigh. Just enough weight to keep the pelvis off the mattress is used, and for nursing care the hammock may be pushed or folded back over the buttocks. This type of hammock-sling accomplishes lateral compression on the sides of the pelvis, forcing the separated pubis together at the symphysis. It is usually continued for about 6 weeks.

To care for the toilet needs of a patient who is wearing a pelvic sling presents problems. With the female patient, the doctor may prescribe that a Foley catheter be inserted and used at least during the first portion of the time that traction is necessary. If a catheter is not inserted, the use of a female urinal is helpful. For bowel movements, the use of a small flat pan or a child's fracture pan will cause the least discomfort to the patient, and the least disturbance of the traction apparatus. In some instances, the doctor may permit partial release of the traction to provide for adequate bathing of the buttocks and perineal areas.

When there is no separation of the fragments, the patient may be placed on a firm mattress, with Buck's extension applied to the legs. Unless orders are specifically given to turn the patient, back care is given by elevating the patient either with the aid of an overhead trapeze or with the assistance of another nurse.

Scultetus or abdominal binders are sometimes used instead of hammocks, particularly if there has been no involvement of the acetabulum. The binder should extend from the iliac crest to 2 or 3 inches below the pubis. If the binder is made of canvas, it is wise to insert a lining of flannel cloth or other soft material between the skin and the binder. Instructions given for application of the binder in different types of pelvic fractures are usually as follows:

1. For fracture of the iliac bone, the binder is applied without snugness.

2. For fracture of the ischium or pubic bones, it is applied snugly.

3. If there is separation of the symphysis pubis, the binder is applied as tightly as possible.

FRACTURES AND DISLOCATIONS OF THE HIP

FRACTURES NEAR THE HIP

Cause. Fractures in the upper end of the femur may be near the head. These are called intracapsular. If fractures occur farther out in the neck of the femur, they are called extracapsular; those occurring still farther out, in the region of the trochanters, are called trochanteric or intertrochanteric (Fig. 5-46). To the laity, all of these are broken hips; but to the orthopedic surgeon, they are very different in regard to treatment and prognosis.

Anatomy. The hip is a ball-and-socket joint. To allow free ranges of motion the capsule that surrounds the joint is quite flexible and extends a considerable distance out along the neck. This means that the blood vessels that supply nutrition must enter outside the point of attachment of the capsule. Unfortunately, the ligament between the head and the acetabulum (ligamentum teres) carries little or no circulation to the head. Most of the circulation enters the neck of the femur through nutrient foramina and reaches the head inside the bone. Fractures of the neck cause a tearing of these vessels, and the head within the capsule may be left

with little or no circulation. This anatomic fact is the chief cause of the percentage of nonunions that occur in spite of perfect reduction (20% to 25%). This is also the cause of the necrosis and disintegration that may occur in the head of the femur. When the fragments have been separated by the injury, the strong gluteus medius muscle pulls the distal portion upward. The iliopsoas tends to rotate outward, as does the gluteus maximus. Immediately after the accident, therefore, the leg is usually found in the position of helpless eversion. There are both some shortening of the extremity and considerable pain and muscle spasm on any attempt to move the patient.

Reduction. Reduction is accomplished by applying traction, preferably the Russell traction, maintaining the alignment of the knee in a neutral plane and the hip in flexion. About 10 pounds of weight are used (20 pounds' pull). Reduction usually takes place automatically in 3 to 5 days. During this time the patient is likely to have a great deal of abdominal distress and possibly some difficulty in voiding, as do patients with spinal injuries. Sedatives that

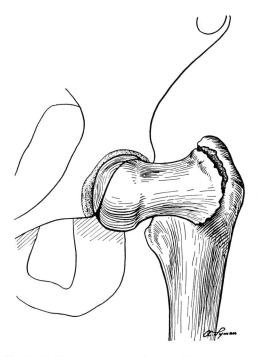

Fig. 5-46. Fracture at base of neck of femur (intertrochanteric type). Note decrease in angle of neck and eversion. The lesser trochanter shows up prominently, denoting outward rotation.

tend to make elimination more sluggish should be avoided if possible. By the injury, the patient has in most cases been forced abruptly from an active to a completely inactive existence, adding to the digestive difficulties. Foods that tend to form gas should be avoided.

Treatment. After reduction by traction or by the manipulative method of Leadbetter, the type of treatment must be determined by the proximity of the fracture to the head, the estimated amount of damage to the circulation to the head, and the general condition of the patient.

When there is a fair amount of neck connected with the head fragment, nailing the femur with a three-flanged Smith-Petersen nail or other device offers many advantages. Complete union may be possible in 5 to 8 months.

After the nailing the patient may be allowed in a wheelchair for well-tolerated intervals on the first or second day. In a few weeks he may be allowed on crutches without weight bearing. Weight bearing should not be allowed for 3 to 5

months and then only if roentgenographic examination shows sufficient union.

When the fracture is very near the head or when circulatory damage appears to be severe, it is advisable, if the patient's condition is satisfactory, to treat the fracture by bone graft. The graft may be taken from the upper part of the same femur, or from either tibia. It is passed through a drill hole of appropriate size, through the trochanter and the neck, and well into the head. In addition to acting as a circulatory stimulus, it also acts as a means of fixation. A Smith-Petersen nail may be used for better stabilization; when this is used, a cast is seldom needed. Union sufficient for weight bearing does not usually occur sooner than 4 to 6 months.

Intertrochanteric fractures almost invariably heal. With the strong pull of the muscles, however, they tend to heal with a loss of the normal angulation between the shaft and the neck of the femur. This leads to deformity. Shortening, external rotation, and adduction often result.

Problem. To prevent deformity, the fracture must be held by an apparatus that will overcome these tendencies until solid union is present. Intertrochanteric fractures have been a problem from the standpoint of hospitalization and also of the health of the patient, because a safe amount of union may not occur before 10 to 12 weeks, and complete union requires 4 to 8 months. The treatment of choice has been a long period of immobilization in Russell traction or other immobilizing apparatus.

Several types of apparatus for internal fixation have been devised. Most notable of these are the Neufeld angled nail (Fig. 5-47), the apparatus of Austin Moore, and the multiple-pin technique of Roger Anderson and others. When the Neufeld nail or the Smith-Petersen nail with the McLaughlin attachment is inserted into the neck of the femur after reduction, the handle is fastened to the shaft of the femur by means of thread-cutting screws. The patients may be allowed to be in a wheelchair in 2 to 3 days and to go through the same routine of convalescence as those patients with nailing of fractures of the neck of the femur.

Early ambulation. The early ambulation of postoperative patients as described by Leithauser cannot be entirely adapted to orthopedic patients.

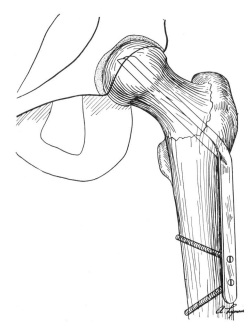

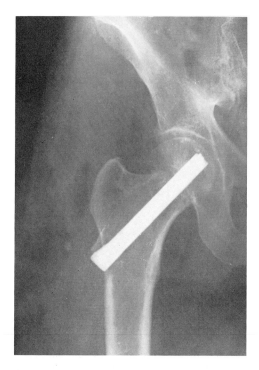

Fig. 5-47. Open reduction of intertrochanteric fracture with Neufeld nail inserted into neck and head and down shaft of femur with divergent screws. This nail is a one-piece stainless steel nail with V-shaped flanges into the neck and head.

Fig. 5-48. Smith-Petersen flanged nail used for internal fixation of fractures of the neck of the femur.

Fracture treatment requires a complete immobilization of the part. The general condition of the patient must, of course, be taken into consideration. The mobilization of patients as related to their general health must be considered first. The things most feared are (1) atelectasis, (2) embolism, and (3) thrombosis. Most of these can be avoided by early ambulation. This does not necessarily mean getting the patient out of bed immediately after operation, but it does mean putting the patient in the most erect position possible after recovery from anesthesia and frequent turning after operation.

Internal fixation in fractures of the neck of the femur and intertrochanteric fractures of the hip has made it possible to mobilize patients at a very early period. The patient who is classified as a poor surgical risk may be up in a chair as early as the following day, occasionally the same day. Postoperative deaths have been cut by more than half, and the danger of operation upon the aged person has been minimized.

Nursing care. Since fracture of the upper end or neck of the femur, the hip fracture as it is

commonly called, presents more nursing problems than any other type of femoral fracture, emphasis will be placed on the nursing care required for this condition. The methods of reduction and of maintaining reduction are still complex. The patient may be placed in one of several types of suspension traction, or he may be treated surgically by internal fixation.

Internal fixation apparatus (the Smith-Petersen flanged nail shown in Fig. 5-48, the Neufeld nail, the Jewett nail, or the Austin Moore pins, to mention only a few) has become the accepted method of treating hip fractures. Nursing problems after such procedures are greatly simplified. The operation itself is not considered a serious threat unless the patient is in very poor physical condition. The complications of old age, however, such as kidney dysfunction, cardiac impairment, and hypostatic pneumonia, make any operation somewhat hazardous and should not be forgotten in any method of treatment.

PREOPERATIVE NURSING CARE. The patient with this type of fracture will complain of pain in the hip region, and any movement of the involved limb causes increased pain and spasm of the thigh muscles. Thus, during the admission procedure, unnecessary transfers should be avoided; when movement of the patient is necessary, manual traction applied to the involved limb lessens the pain by immobilizing the bone fragments. In addition to the patient's complaint of pain, the nurse may note that the involved limb is slightly shorter than the other limb and that it is held in a position of external rotation. Many of these elderly patients have other chronic health problems. The hip fracture is complicated by or perhaps complicates an existing cardiac condition, a diabetic problem, or other health deficit that frequently accompanies the aging process. In some instances, reduction and internal fixation of the fracture is delayed 24 to 48 hours to permit a complete medical evaluation and treatment of any existing health problems. If surgery is delayed, the application of skin traction (Buck's extension or Russell traction) will lessen muscle spasm and the patient is more comfortable with the immobilization produced by the traction. When the muscle spasms have been relieved, an attempt should be made to gently roll the limb to a neutral position. A trochanter roll or sandbag is then used to maintain the correct alignment of the limb.

Pressure sores are a constant threat when the elderly person is confined to bed. The heel of the involved limb is a particularly vulnerable spot; if protection is not provided, a blister or reddened area indicating a beginning pressure sore will develop within a few hours. The use of an alternating pressure pad beneath the patient is helpful in changing pressure points, and the placement of foam rubber pads or squares of synthetic sheep's wool beneath the sacrum and heels has proved very helpful in securing a more even distribution of the body weight and in preventing pressure sores.

Provision for activity and change of position will result in increased patient comfort, as well as the prevention of pressure areas and hypostatic pneumonia. If the bed is equipped with a trapeze, the patient can be taught and encouraged to frequently shift his position. By flexing the hip and knee of his uninvolved limb, and pushing with his foot as he pulls with his hands, the patient finds that he can assist with his care and have a small degree of independence. The activity provides for active exercise of the uninvolved extremities, and encourages self-care. These are aspects of his care that the nurse will want to foster throughout his hospitalization. Bed positions can also be altered by raising and lowering the headrest, and in some instances (when Buck's extension has been applied) the doctor may ask that the patient be turned to his well leg side. Maintaining a correct "line of pull" can be accomplished by moving the traction pulley (in the same direction the patient is turned) and by supporting the involved limb as the patient is rolled onto his well leg side. As the patient is turned, the involved limb is maintined in the same relationship to the patient's body and is supported in a neutral position with pillows.

Encouraging and teaching the elderly patient to cough and to deep-breathe should be included in his preoperative care. This will help prevent hypostatic pneumonia by removing secretions and mucus from the lungs and bronchial tubes.

Accurate intake and output records will help the nurse to know if the patient is drinking sufficient fluids. Assisting and encouraging the patient to take fluids is frequently necessary to prevent dehydration. Also it is not uncommon for the patient with a fracture of the hip to have bladder distention with overflow incontinence. Early detection of these problems is necessary to prevent additional complications. The use of a fracture bedpan which can be slipped under the buttocks with little or no elevation of the hip region, will cause less discomfort than the regular bedpan. When the patient is placed on the pan at frequent intervals, incontinence may be prevented. Needless to say, any nursing care that will prevent the need for insertion of a catheter is desirable. The catheter is a source of worry to the older person and may contribute to urinary tract complications.

POSTOPERATIVE NURSING CARE. Care of the patient following internal fixation may vary considerably. The amount of activity permitted is determined and ordered by the attending physician. If the hip is considered unstable, Buck's extension or some type of suspension traction in combination with a half-ring Thomas splint may be applied for a brief period. The traction pro-

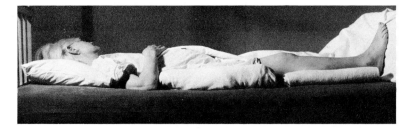

Fig. 5-49. Good supine position for postoperative patient with internal fixation of a hip fracture. Footboard provides support for the feet, and heel pressure is relieved by a small pad beneath the calf of the leg. Neutral position of limb is maintained with a trochanter roll, and full extension of hip joint is encouraged by lowering the headrest. It must also be remembered that continuous pressure over the head of the fibula, on the lateral aspect of the leg, may cause paralysis of the peroneal nerve, resulting in an inability to dorsiflex the foot. This pressure may be caused by permitting the leg to remain in a position of external rotation or by pressure from sandbags, casts, or traction.

vides for temporary immobilization, helps overcome muscle spasm, and increases the patient's comfort. If the hip is considered stable, the patient is usually given much latitude with regard to movement in bed (Fig. 5-49), and as early as the first postoperative evening he may be turned to the side-lying position for back care. The patient with an internal fixation of a hip fracture may be turned to either side. If turning is done toward the extremity operated upon, the bed acts somewhat as a splint, and the patient will be fairly comfortable. However, many times the patient will prefer to be rolled on the uninvolved limb, with the limb that has been operated on kept uppermost. Good body alignment can be maintained with the use of pillows. Two nurses working together can turn the patient to the side-lying position, causing him a minimum of discomfort. He is moved in the bed toward the side operated on; one pillow is placed between the thighs and a second between the legs and feet. The side rail is raised, and the nurses go to opposite sides of the bed. The first nurse places her hands on the patient's far shoulder and hip (using care to avoid the operative site), and the second nurse slips one hand beneath the knee of the leg that has been operated on and the other hand beneath the patient's ankle. As the patient's body is rolled toward his "well leg" side, the operated limb is rolled on the pillows that have been placed between his legs. Careful handling and control of the involved limb are necessary to prevent

pain and discomfort. If the patient desires further support when he turns, he may steady himself by placing his upper hand on the nurse's shoulder. Adjustment of the patient's hips, and the pillows between his legs will provide for a comfortable position and good body alignment. To prevent strain on the fracture site in the side-lying position, it is necessary to maintain the hip and knee in the same plane. Frequently, additional support in the groin area will increase the patient's comfort. (Fig. 5-50).

Many physicians instruct the patient to begin knee movement the day after fixation of the hip. The patient is turned to the side of the fractured extremity so that his knee may be flexed while the hip is kept in the extended position. There may be muscle spasm in the muscles of the thigh, particularly in the quadriceps, when this is first attempted. Nurses should seek complete instructions from the surgeon regarding this treatment and the rate of progress expected.

HELPING THE PATIENT TO BE AMBULATORY. Postoperatively, if there are no contraindications and the patient has not been placed in traction, the surgeon usually requests that elderly patients be up in a chair the morning after surgery, with no weight bearing on the affected extremity. If the patient is able to stand on his uninvolved leg, and pivot to sit in a chair, this method should be used in preference to lifting him out of the bed. Standing provides exercise for the muscles and joints of the uninvolved

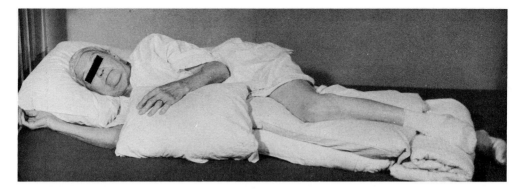

Fig. 5-50. Good side-lying position for the postoperative patient with an internal fixation of a hip fracture. Entire length of the uppermost limb is supported with pillows. Hip and knee are maintained in the same plane, and pressure on the lower limb is avoided.

limb, and secondly the older patient's morale is given a "boost" when he learns that he is able to stand at the bedside and to sit in a chair. However, the nurse should remember that the patient's endurance has been somewhat lessened by the surgical procedure and that several short periods of time spent in a sitting position are better than one long period, which may completely exhaust the patient. Assisting the patient to a chair after hip surgery should be an unhurried activity. Adequate explanation of the procedure will help allay some of the fears and doubts the elderly patient may have about his ability to get out of bed. In addition, he should understand that his weight should not be placed on the involved limb. If available, the patient's hose and shoes should be worn, and a chair with armrests is desirable.

When the order has been given for the patient to be up in a chair, he should first roll onto the side of the sound leg. When this has been accomplished, the knee and hip of the normal leg should be flexed to a right angle, approximating the position of the body in sitting. If the patient is able to partially flex the hip and knee of the affected side, this should be done, but it must be remembered that this leg will require the most gentle handling at all times and that the joints should never be forced beyond the point of pain. Some physicians prescribe the application of an elastic bandage or elastic hose to the injured extremity before the patient is allowed to sit. This support prevents the trouble-

some edema and mottling that occur when the extremity becomes dependent.

To bring the patient to the sitting position, place one arm under the patient's shoulder and the other arm under the knees, gently swiveling the patient to the sitting position. If the fractured leg is extremely sensitive, another nurse may be needed to support it.

Check your own body mechanics carefully for this procedure, being sure to assume the foot-forward position with knees and hips flexed and back straight. Considerable strain and torsion may be placed on the back if resistance from the patient is encountered, and you should be prepared for this before beginning the procedure.

Pivot or swivel the patient to the sitting position, slowly at first in order to prevent faintness. When the sitting position has been obtained, continue to support the patient's back until he is steady. Permit the patient to sit on the side of the bed for several minutes, and at this time instruct him to lift the chest, to practice breathing exercises, and to contract the gluteal and abdominal muscles. The most universal tendency of the elderly patient is to sit on the side of the bed with shoulders sagging, chin on chest, and head and shoulders drooped. Unless efforts are made to overcome this at the outset, this type of posture may become permanent. If there are no signs of dizziness or weakness, assist the patient to the standing position.

Place your hands under the axillae and allow the patient to place his hands firmly on your shoulders. In this way he is assured of adequate support for his first standing experience. Place the chair parallel to the bed, and guide the patient gently toward it turning him in such a fashion that his back is toward the chair seat. As he lowers himself, flex your knees and hips and permit the patient to retain his hold on

your shoulders until he is safely seated in the chair (Fig. 5-51).

When constant attendance with the elderly person is not possible, it is frequently advisable to apply a restraint or "safety belt," which will prevent the patient from falling from the chair or attempting to walk by himself. While in the sit-

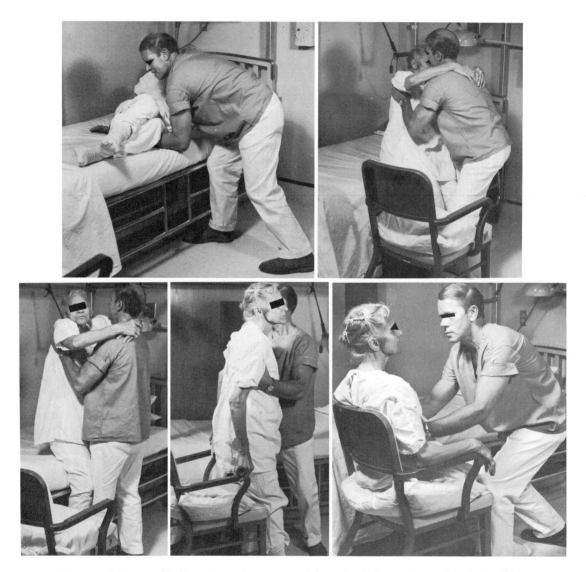

Fig. 5-51. When an elderly patient is being assisted from the bed to a chair, a low bed will be helpful to the patient but may pose a hazard for any nurse who uses poor body mechanics. As the nurse assists the patient to a sitting position on the side of the bed, strain to his own back muscles is minimized if he assumes the foot-forward position and flexes his hips and knees. The nurse shown is in a position to give an unstable patient considerable support and assistance in assuming the standing position, without strain to his back. The patient pivots and may place her hands on the armrests preparatory to sitting in the chair.

ting position, the patient should be encouraged to comb his hair and care for his teeth; if being up in a chair can be arranged at the mealtime, eating becomes a much more pleasurable event. Remember also, that the elderly patient needs more than physical care. Nursing care which shows understanding and respect for the individual as a person, and which supports the older person's self-esteem will help stimulate a desire for independence and recovery. This is very necessary when caring for the older person.

Later the patient can be taught to come to a standing position from the chair without too much difficulty, and his confidence in his ability will be greatly increased once he has accomplished this. The chair must be steady, propped against the bed or wall. The patient is instructed to bend forward from the hips, to place the unaffected leg backward until an acute angle of the knee is formed, and to have the knee on the affected side flexed as much as possible with the foot flat on the floor. The patient places his hands on the armrests of the chair with the elbows slightly flexed to assist in elevating himself. Weight is taken entirely by the normal foot as the patient comes to the erect position.

Complications. Problems that are common in the elderly patient need special attention.

CONTRACTURES. Prevention is accomplished by supporting the body in good alignment and by encouraging activities that enable the patient to exercise his extremities. The deformities to be guarded against are flexion and adduction of the hips, flexion of the knees, and an equinus position of the feet. Full extension of the hip and knee joints should be encouraged by lowering the backrest and by discouraging the use of pillows beneath the knees. Sandbags or a trochanter roll, can be effective means of preventing external rotation of the leg. Proper positioning of the patient in relation to a footboard and encouraging him to dorsiflex his foot several times daily will prevent the development of a drop-foot deformity.

PNEUMONIA. A high percentage of the patients with fractured hips are elderly. The problems involved in this type of nursing are geriatric as well as surgical in nature. Many complications of advanced age may be present, including car-diovascular disease, renal dysfunction, diabetes, and obesity. Hypostatic pneumonia is always a threat if these patients are put to bed even for short periods. We are told that one-half of the deaths that occur after fracture of the femur in elderly patients are brought about by pneumonia. For this reason, prophylactic antibotic therapy is sometimes instituted after fractures and continued for a week or longer. The patient does not feel the development of lung complications. The cough may be painful and the patient may resist it, but the accumulation of mucus in the bronchi may still be present in the form of increasingly solid masses. The longer the process goes on, the more difficult it is to get rid of the plugs by coughing. Often, coughing causes pain at the operative site, and the patient resists the coughing mechanism. The erect position of the body stimulates the elimination of these bronchial plugs. Hence, it is especially important in postoperative patients to avoid this serious complication by early institution of the erect position of the body. If standing is permissible, it is preferred; but this is not always possible, especially if the patient is in traction. In such patients, frequent change of bed position is desirable. Elevation of the head of the bed, protection from drafts, and solicitude in keeping the patient well covered during bathing and turning are essential nursing measures. This patient should be encouraged to breathe deeply and to cough up mucus. Frequent observation must be made to detect evidences of beginning cyanosis and dyspnea.

THROMBOPHLEBITIS. Another common cause of death after fracture of the femur in elderly patients is thrombophlebitis with embolus. As a prophylactic measure against this, an anticoagulant medication may be prescribed.

DECUBITUS ULCERS. Skin care for the older patient is of the utmost importance. A daily bath and the use of strong soaps may increase the dryness of his skin and tend to cause discomfort. A complete bath every other day or twice a week is usually sufficient. Frequent cleansing of the hands, however, and of the perineum and buttocks region is essential in the care of the elderly person. The use of baby oils or lotions will aid in preventing dryness and irritation of the skin. Frequent massage of the buttocks region improves circulation and will help to prevent the development of decubitus ulcers.

Maintaining a clean dry bed is essential if pressure areas are to be prevented. If the patient is very old, if evidences of chronic malnutrition are present, or if there is circulatory impairment as a result of arteriosclerosis, the fight to prevent pressure areas must be particularly vigilant. It must be begun the moment the patient enters the hospital. Patients of this type are not usually placed in an apparatus that would make turning them too difficult, and the responsibility for seeing that decubitus ulcers do not develop is completely in the hands of the nurse. Where circulatory impairment is present, it is an extremely difficult problem. Nothing, of course, will be as beneficial as frequent changes of position. This means that the patient must be turned every 2 hours or even more often. An air mattress may be useful in preventing excessive pressure at any one point of the body. Airfoam sponge rubber under threatened areas has proved very helpful in preventing pressure sores on the sacrum and heels, and unclipped sheepskin is also excellent for this purpose. The sheepskin should be washed frequently with a mild soap and water, rinsed, and dried carefully to keep it soft and pliable.

GASTROINTESTINAL DISTURBANCES. Obstinate constipation is almost invariably present in these patients. The management of this feature can be extremely troublesome if strong cathartics have been used too frequently during the early course of immobilization. Distention is not infrequent, and rectal tubes may sometimes be necessary to overcome this. Careful attention to the patient's diet for roughage, vitamins, and elimination of foods that cause distress will help to overcome constipation. Fecal moistening agents are usually prescribed. Enemas or suppositories may be necessary occasionally, and a laxative may be ordered as needed. Attention to regularity is, of course, essential.

NUTRITIONAL PROBLEMS. A large number of these patients will have eating problems. They may have no teeth and may be unable to see or hear well. Often, they have definite food likes and dislikes, and it is difficult for them to understand hospital routines and methods. The thoughtful nurse can help to make mealtime a pleasant occasion for these older patients.

Because the rate of repair in fractures has been shown to be greatly influenced by the deficiency diseases and malnutrition that are so often present in elderly patients, considerable thought must be given to the diet to include the necessary food elements. Sufficient vitamin and protein intake is particularly important. To build tissue resistance and hasten repair, protein supplements may be given. Protein hydrolysates and amino acid mixtures are procurable for this purpose when the patient is unable to eat sufficient foods containing these substances. Vitamins B and C are also considered important in fracture healing. If these patients are unable to take sufficient diet orally, supplementary feedings containing the essential proteins and vitamins may be given in a formula through a polyethylene tube. The polyethylene tube is a small plastic tube that is inserted through the nostril into the stomach. This tube is taped to the nose and is left in place.

It must be remembered, also, that anything that affects the patient's general condition will be likely to affect the healing of his fracture. Age, of course, plays a large part in the rate at which a fracture will heal. A fracture of the femur in a very young baby will heal firmly in 4 weeks, whereas in a person 50 years of age or older the time required may be 3 or 4 months or longer. As has been stated, deficiency diseases, chachexia, and senile osteoporosis will definitely retard the rate of bone union. Blood chemistry determinations are ordered by the physician when the progress of healing is slow. Serum calcium of 10 to 12 mg. per 100 ml. of blood and phosphorus concentration of 3.5 to 4 mg. are considered normal. Milk and a calcium medication or a parathyroid solution and synthetic vitamin D are sometimes ordered. Vitamin D is usually considered not to be effective unless a sufficient intake of phosphorus-containing foods is given.

UROLOGIC COMPLICATIONS. Elderly patients are particularly prone to develop urologic complications during a period of immobilization. This is sometimes caused by an unwillingness to take sufficient fluids and by an already existing renal impairment. Scantiness of output, discomfort on voiding, concentrated urine, suppression, incontinency, or edema should be reported to the physician. Intake and output should be estimated daily in elderly patients with fracture of the femur until it has been ascertained that kidney function is normal.

All patients, whether young or old, are in danger of developing renal stones if they are extensively immobilized or are inactive for a considerable period of time. This is true whether the immobilizing apparatus is a cast or traction or merely continuous bed rest. Intelligent nursing care can play an important part in diminishing this danger. A large fluid output is essential to overcome renal stasis and to ensure a steady flow of urine. The nurse will need to encourage the patient to take an adequate diet and increased amounts of fluids. This is not always an easy task, since the appetite is often very sluggish. Furthermore, the patient must be moved frequently and with sufficient variation in bed or chair posture that no part of the urinary tract is left undrained for too long a time.

The regime described is usually continued for as long as 3 months after the patient is ambulatory, and roentgenograms every 3 to 4 months thereafter may be ordered. Any symptoms of pain or distress referable to the urinary tract should be reported. Renal stones may occur as early as a month after recumbency.

MENTAL ASPECTS IN THE NURSING CARE OF THE PATIENT WITH A FRACTURED HIP. Frequently the older patient with a fractured hip becomes disoriented. The pain and shock suffered coupled with a strange environment are sufficient to cause mental confusion. This confusion may not be apparent in the daytime, but at night the patient will attempt to get out of bed and his speech will be incoherent. The nurse must realize that this may be expected, and side rails or other protection should be provided for the patient.

Elderly patients with fracture of the hip rarely escape serious mental depression. The prospect of inactivity is in itself a heavy burden to bear, and when it is accompanied by financial worry, it is extremely difficult to prevent attitudes of depression and melancholy. Furthermore, these patients frequently have a pessimistic outlook regarding their own recovery. The nurse caring for them needs to develop considerable understanding and sympathy for their problems. She will be confronted by sessions of tears and hopelessness, not once but

periodically during the time the patient is inactive. Good mental hygiene demands that the patient be given something to do, and constructive occupational therapy is almost indispensable in caring for these patients. Although the trained occupational therapist is highly desirable for assisting with the daily program of the fracture patient, the bedside nurse can help by urging him to do as much as he can for himself, even though he is confined to a chair. It is not always easy to secure cooperation, because considerable apathy and indifference may exist. If the nurse makes it clear to the patient that the desire to have him do things for himself stems from interest in his progress, he will be much more likely to cooperate and less likely to feel neglected when he is urged to care for his own wants as far as it is possible for him to do so. Many physicians order a series of gentle bed exercises to be carried out under the nurse's direction several times during the day to prevent loss of muscle tone and to prepare the patient for successful ambulation at as early a date as possible.

PROBLEMS IN THE PREPARATION FOR WEIGHT BEARING. The amount of time the patient will be kept without weight bearing varies according to the progress of union. It may be from 12 to 16 weeks or longer. As has been stated, bed exercises are frequently prescribed. These may be muscle-setting exercises for the abdominal, gluteal, and guadriceps muscles; dosiflexion and inversion exercises for the feet; and rhythmic breathing exercises. Exercises to strengthen the arms and shoulder muscles are usually added before the patient is ready to walk in order to prepare these muscles for crutch walking. Since the period of inactivity is long, considerable encouragement may be necessary to motivate the patient to continue the exercises over the period when he is nonambulatory. Explanation of the importance of these exercises may need to be repeated at frequent intervals.

Even though exercises are faithfully carried out, there is still a tremendous hill for the patient to climb. Unexpected weaknesses and stiffness of many parts of the body that were not involved in the fracture may be present. These will alarm and depress the patient if he is not forewarned of them. For instance, it is not uncommon to have the patient complain that his knee feels worse than the hip that was fractured. This may be a source of great concern to him, and nurses should take the opportunity to teach the patient something about the mechanics of the quadriceps muscle and its action on the knee and hip in walking.

The nurse who can help the patient understand that his weaknesses and the stiffness in his joints are the natural outcome of his fracture and inactivity and not a permanent sequela to it, will aid greatly in bolstering his failing courage. Nothing should be done that will make him more apprehensive. Any rough or hurried movement while carrying out the prescribed exercise for increasing motion in hip or knee or any enthusiastic increase in the range of motion beyond which the patient has previously gone will also be conducive to much loss of courage. Furthermore, acute muscle spasm around the hip will make it impossible to do anything further in the way of mobilization at that time. Support should be placed under the lumbar spine, the knee, and at the foot, and the limb should not be allowed to lie in outward rotation.

Instruction in crutch walking for the elderly patient may be delayed until partial weight bearing can be permitted. Then the three-point gait is taught. This delay in crutch walking is necessary because the danger of falling and of bearing weight on the affected extremity is too great.

When ambulation and weight bearing are permitted, the use of a walker (Fig. 5-52) may be preferred to crutches. The elderly patient feels more secure with the walker and is less likely to fall.

NEED FOR HOME CARE AFTER FRACTURE OF THE HIP. After a fracture of the hip there is one question that always seems to arise and that causes the patient much worry: "Where am I to go when I leave the hospital?" With the increasing number of elderly persons in our population, the need for adequate convalescent care has become a major problem. The patient with a fractured hip can no longer take care of his needs and be independent. His elderly mate is physically unable to assume this added responsibility. It will be 10 or 12 weeks before he is able to begin weight bearing, barring any com-

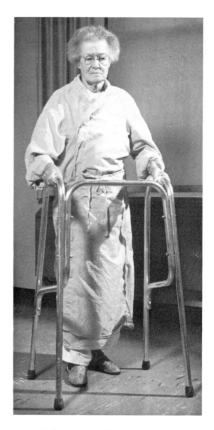

Fig. 5-52. A lightweight adjustable aluminum walker may be used by the elderly patient when ambulation is permitted.

plications. We know that good care is essential during this convalescent period if the elderly person is to maintain his strength and the desire to walk again. Will some member of his family be able to care for him, or will plans for care in a nursing home or an extended care facility be arranged? Whatever plans are made for his convalescent care, the assistance that the public health nurse gives the family and patient at this time may mean the difference between failure and success—a patient who later is able to walk, care for his own needs, and live an independent life.

NONUNION AND ASEPTIC NECROSIS. It is necessary that provision be made for adequate follow-up care for the patient with a fractured hip. Early detection of loss of position, nonunion, or aseptic necrosis makes it possible to institute corrective measures (Fig. 5-53). When nonunion persists after adequate reduction, the sur-

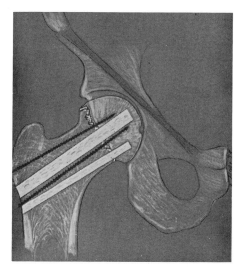

Fig. 5-53. Bone graft with threaded Steinmann pin fixation may be used in the absence of union after nailing procedure. (From Ziffren, S. E.: Management of the aged surgical patient, Chicago, 1960, Year Book Medical Publishers, Inc.)

geon may wish to insert a tibial bone graft in the freshened nail tract; or, when aseptic necrosis has taken place, he may wish to replace the head of the femur with a Vitallium prosthesis. The ball part of the prosthesis (Fig. 5-54) fits into the acetabulum. Some studies of this last surgical procedure have been encouraging. Others report that in some instances there is bone resorption, resulting in loosening of the prosthesis and loss of functional results.

Nursing care following insertion of hip prosthesis. To help prevent dislocation after the insertion of a hip prosthesis, it is usually ordered that the involved limb be maintained in a neutral position with slight abduction. If the hip is unstable, the patient may be placed in suspension traction or in a hip spica cast to maintain the desired position. However, at other times the patient is returned to his bed after surgery with no supportive apparatus. This patient needs to understand the correct position for his limb, and such aids as the trochanter

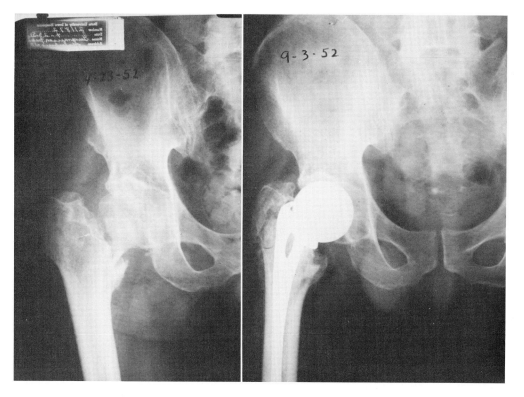

Fig. 5-54. Hip prosthesis. When aseptic necrosis of the head of the femur occurs after a fracture of the neck of femur, prosthesis may be inserted, thus making weight bearing possible.

roll and sandbags may be used to help maintain the desired position. If turning him to the side-lying position is premitted, slight abduction of the involved limb is maintained by placing pillows between the thighs and lower legs. The patient is then turned to the uninvolved side in the same manner as the patient with a hip nailing. If turning is not permitted, back care may be given in the same manner as for the patient with suspension traction. By using the trapeze and the uninvolved limb, the patient is able (with assistance) to lift his hips off the bed for care and linen changes. (See Chapter 2.)

During the first few postoperative days, frequent positioning is necessary and good nursing care is of the utmost importance if the complications so common to the elderly patient are to be prevented. Also during this period the patient is instructed and encouraged to do upper extremity exercises, preparatory for crutch walking. Abdominal, quadriceps-setting, and gluteal muscle–setting exercises may be included. Approximately 14 days after surgery, the cast or traction is removed, and ambulation is started. This should be a relatively slow process, allowing time for the patient to adjust to the sitting and standing positions. When dizziness and weakness are overcome, crutch walking (three-point gait) with "touch" weight bearing is usually permitted. (A walker may be substituted for the crutches.) As the individual progresses with crutch walking, he is encouraged to resume normal activity. The elderly patient may find it necessary to use the crutches or a cane for an extended period of time. Follow-up care should include periodic examination by the orthopedic surgeon.

TRAUMATIC DISLOCATIONS OF THE HIP

There are several types of hip dislocations, but the most common ones are posterior dislocation with or without fracture of the acetabulum and anterior or obturator dislocation.

Cause. Posterior dislocation with or without fracture of the acetabulum is caused by force against the knee with the hip flexed and adducted (dashboard dislocations). There may be damage to the sciatic nerve.

Anterior or obturator dislocations are caused by forced abduction of the thigh with the hip in flexion. The head of the femur is displaced forward and enters the depression of the obturator foramen. There may be damage to the obturator nerve with weakness or paralysis of the adductor muscles.

Symptoms and signs. It is characteristic of the posterior upward dislocation that the patient cannot abduct, extend, or externally rotate the limb. This is in contrast to fractures near the hip joint. There is a mass (the head of the femur) palpable on the ilium.

With the obturator dislocation, the mass is felt in the groin, and the patient is unable to abduct or internally rotate the limb before reduction. Both conditions are very painful during the period of dislocation because of muscle spasm.

Reduction and problem. In posterior dislocation, general anesthesia is necessary. Reduction can be accomplished by placing the patient on his back and exerting manual traction with the hip in full flexion (surgeon's shoulder under patient's knee). Relaxation is essential. If this method fails, the method of Lorenz for congenital dislocations may be successful, that is, extreme flexion and abduction to bring the head into the catyloid notch, then further abduction combined with a decrease in flexion to force the head upward into the acetabulum.

In obturator dislocation exertion of forceful traction in the line of deformity and then adduction as the head engages in the acetabulum accomplish reduction. All reductions of dislocations of the hip are usually accompanied by relaxation of the muscles, freedom of movement, and great relief of pain. A thud can usually be heard and felt as the head enters the acetabulum. The clinical signs should not be relied upon to indicate adequate reduction. Evidence should be established by roentgenograms taken in two directions.

Treatment. Hip dislocations are comparatively easily treated after reduction. It is comforting to the patient with ligamentous injuries to have Buck's extension (with about 5 to 10 pounds of weight) for 2 or 3 weeks—long enough for ligamentous healing. During this time daily exercises of all joints should be carried out as soon as the patient is able to tolerate them.

In fractures of the acetabulum the same treatment is used, but traction should be prolonged for 2 to 3 additional weeks. A wheelchair, crutches, and gradual weight bearing with crutches (then cane) follow, over a period of 6 to 10 weeks.

Attention has been drawn to the possibility of permanent damage to the head of the femur as the result of ligamentous tearing and distur-bance in the blood supply to the head. Aseptic necrosis may occur if the damage is great. Such necrosis may manifest itself after several years by degenerative change in the joint. There may be degeneration of the cartilage and partial or complete ankylosis. Patients with dislocations uncomplicated by fracture, however, usually re-cover in 6 to 8 weeks without further trouble.

FRACTURES OF THE FEMUR

FRACTURE OF THE FEMUR BELOW THE TROCHANTERS

Anatomy. Fracture of the femur below the trochanters is one of the most difficult frac-tures to treat successfully. The fracture occurs above the stabilizing attachment of the ad-ductor muscles so that the upper fragment is controlled entirely by the intrinsic muscles of the hip (Fig. 5-55). The proximal fragment is brought into acute flexion by the action of the iliopsoas. It is brought into abduction by the gluteus medius and into external rotation by both the iliopsoas and the gluteus maximus. Con-sequently, it tends to project forward at a right angle to the body and to abduct and rotate outward.

Problem. The problem is to bring the con-trollable distal fragment into a position which will meet the position of the uncontrollable proximal fragment in flexion at about 80 degrees and abduction and external rotation.

Reduction. Reduction can often be accom-plished with skeletal traction and suspension of the limb in a half-ring Thomas splint with a Pearson attachment. Lateral traction of 5 to 10 pounds may be necessary to bring the distal fragment outward to engage the proximal frag-ment. Alignment may be obtained and demon-strated in anteroposterior and lateral views roent-genographically. If not, additional changes in the apparatus may be made.

If alignment does not take place this way, however, some means of internal fixation may be used, such as properly arranged and fixed steel pins, Vitallium or stainless steel plates, or pos-sibly intramedullary pins.

Healing period. Healing is slow. Solid union does not usually occur in less than 10 to 12 weeks. We are, again, frequently confronted with a hospitalization problem. Internal fixation does not always obviate the necessity of im-mobilization but may make the treatment of the fracture a more flexible one in regard to hos-pitalization and the necessity for bed treatment.

FRACTURE OF THE SHAFT OF THE FEMUR (MIDDLE THIRD)

Cause. Direct or indirect violence is the cause of fracture of the middle third of the shaft of the femur.

Anatomy. The action of the gluteus medius has some tendency to pull the upper fragment outward, and the strong pull of the adductor muscle group tends to cause outward bowing at the point of fracture. In this fracture there is a general tendency to develop inward rotation of the lower fragment and outward bowing. This, if allowed to develop, constitutes an awkward de-formity and is quite disabling.

Use of traction in treatment of fracture of the femur. Some form of traction is required that will maintain pull. Russell or suspension traction usually fulfills the requirements. Ab-duction and external rotation of the distal frag-ment must be maintained. Roentgenograms should be taken frequently to check the position.

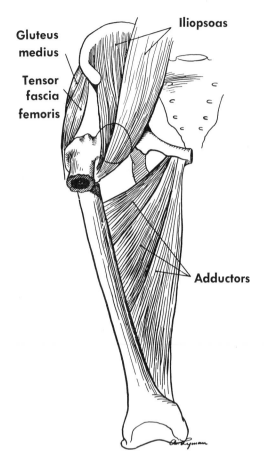

Fig. 5-55. Muscle action in subtrochanteric fractures of the femur.

If there is anterior or posterior angulation or if there is inward or outward bowing, the apparatus must be adjusted with proper slings and weights to counteract and correct the tendency toward deformity. Here again the critical period is important before the callus has developed so firmly that it cannot be molded into correct alignment. Necessary correction must be made before this state occurs. Skin traction obtained by moleskin adhesive or skeletal traction obtained by use of a Kirschner wire or Steinmann pin may be used to secure the desired position of the fragments and to provide for immobilization. Skeletal traction and suspension applied by means of the Thomas, Hodgen, or Keller-Blake splint are frequently used. Skeletal traction is preferred to skin traction because a considerable amount of weight must be applied to overcome spasm of the thigh muscles. When reduction of the frac-

ture has been secured, the amount of weight is reduced to prevent separation of the bone fragments. Traction must be continued until sufficient healing has taken place to permit crutch walking or until sufficient callus has formed to permit the application of a hip spica cast. Care of the patient in traction has been discussed previously. It should be remembered, however, that an overhead trapeze will make it possible for the patient to lift himself for back care and to be placed on the bedpan with less difficulty.

Also, because there is evidence that a high incidence of kidney stones occurs after long periods in traction, nurses should do everything in their power to eliminate this danger. Patients in traction should have a high fluid intake and as much postural variation as is possible without disturbing the apparatus. Frequent urinalyses for patients in traction are usually considered advisable.

The child under 6 years of age with fracture of the femur is usually placed in Bryant traction for approximately 6 weeks. After this a hip spica cast is applied and is worn until roentgenograms show that there is solid union at the fracture site. Care of the patient in Bryant traction has been described previously.

Treatment by means of the cast-brace. The ambulatory treatment of lower extremity fractures is not a new concept. Dr. H. H. Smith reported great success with this form of treatment in seven patients with femoral shaft fractures in 1855.

However, the concept of weight bearing during fracture healing was not revitalized until the post-World War II era. Dr. Dehne popularized the concept of early weight bearing of tibial fractures in long-leg walking casts. The rate of nonunion of tibial fractures decreased markedly, and the time required for solid bony union to occur was significantly shortened.

The idea of early weight bearing of femoral shaft fractures could not be successfully revived until the mid 1960s. The success of the treatment was the result of the new techniques and principles developed in the care of amputees.

The appliance designed for the early weight bearing of femoral shaft fractures is the cast-

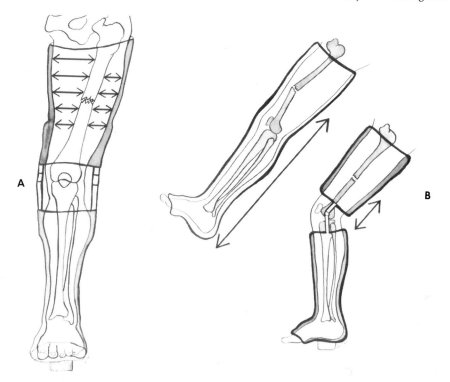

Fig. 5-56. A illustrates the three components of the cast-brace; **B** illustrates comparative lengths of the lever arm distal to the fracture site, with a long leg cast and with the cast-brace.

brace. This is made up of three components: (1) the thigh cuff with its quadrilateral opening superiorly, which controls the rotation of the proximal fracture fragment and creates an increase of the thigh soft tissue hydrostatic pressure to dynamically immobilize the fracture fragments; (2) the short leg walking cast that provides support for the thigh cuff and controls leg edema; (3) the polycentric hinges at the knee level joining the thigh cuff and short leg cast, which serves two functions: first, they allow active motion of the knee, and secondly they decrease the length of the lever arm distal to the fracture whose forces could prevent healing (Fig. 5-56).

The weight bearing of tibial fractures in long leg walking casts is started once the initial soft tissue swelling has subsided. This is also true for the femoral fractures. The patient is treated in balanced skeletal traction for the first 2 to 3 weeks to allow soft tissue healing and resolution of swelling. The cast-brace is then applied with-

out anesthesia. The patient is instructed on quadricep exercises and weight bearing with crutches. The cast-brace immobilization of the fracture to produce solid bony union usually requires from 6 to 8 weeks. By the end of that time the patient can usually walk without crutches and has at least 90 degrees of active knee flexion in the appliance. Consequently, after the removal of the cast-brace, the extremity is readily rehabilitated to a functional level.

Surgical treatment in fracture of the femur. Other satisfactory methods of treatment are those requiring operation. The ones most commonly employed are the following: (1) reduction and insertion of an intramedullary nail (Fig. 5-57), (2) reduction with internotching of the fragments so that they cannot slip off, (3) plating with slotted stainless steel or Vitallium plates and screws, and (4) distraction.

TREATMENT BY INSERTION OF INTRAMEDULLARY NAIL. Fracture of the shaft of the femur

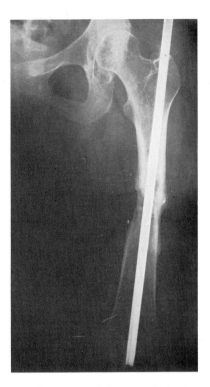

Fig. 5-57. Treatment of fracture of the femur by means of the intramedullary nail. Following reduction of the fracture, the nail is driven down through the shaft of the femur across the fracture site. This type of internal fixation permits increased activity and earlier ambulation.

may be treated by the insertion of an intramedullary nail. After open reduction the metal pin is inserted distally through the greater trochanter and across the fracture site.

Postoperatively, support for the limb is usually provided by means of suspension traction. The traction helps to prevent rotation of the limb until the patient is able to actively control the position of his leg. If traction is not applied postoperatively, sandbags placed along the lateral aspect of the limb will help to prevent external rotation. During the time that the patient is in suspension traction, quadriceps-setting and gluteal muscle–setting exercises are performed. These exercises help maintain muscle strength, prevent distraction, compress fragments, and stimulate callus formation. When the postoperative pain has lessened and the patient has developed sufficient muscle power to control the position of his limb, partial weight-bearing (three-point gait) crutch walking is usually

permitted, but crutches should be used until roentgenograms show bony union at the fracture site.

INTERNOTCHING OF FRAGMENTS. In reduction with the internotching of the fragments, stainless steel wire may be used to prevent slipping. Open reduction may be followed by the application of a hip spica cast extending from the chest to the toes of the affected side with the leg in abduction and external rotation.

PLATING. In plating with slotted stainless steel or Vitallium plates and screws, it must be remembered that muscular and mechanical stresses are great and that it may be necessary to have plates on two sides of the bone, preferably at right angles to each other. The screws should penetrate both cortical surfaces of the bone.

DISTRACTION. Distraction is accomplished by inserting pins above and below the fracture in such a manner that reduction is accomplished by a ratchet and maintained by incorporating the pins in plaster of paris or steel bars (Haynes or Stader) so that overriding or angulation may not take place during healing. Some pressure contact must always be present to prevent nonunion.

Healing period. In children femoral shaft fractures heal quickly. There is frequently solid union in 3 to 4 weeks. In adults solid healing sufficient to avoid deformities from constant muscle pull may not take place in less than 10 to 16 weeks. The likelihood of deformity must be judged clinically according to the age of the patient, the type of the fracture, and the speed with which the individual produces callus, not only visible in the roentgenogram but also recognized clinically by its tendency to shrink and solidify.

It should be remembered that whatever the method used, the speed of healing is not changed, and whatever apparatus chosen by circumstances for the individual case must be kept functioning until complete healing has occurred.

FRACTURE OF THE LOWER END OF THE FEMUR (SUPRACONDYLAR)

Cause. Direct or indirect violence causes fracture of the lower end of the femur.

Anatomy. Fracture of the lower end of the

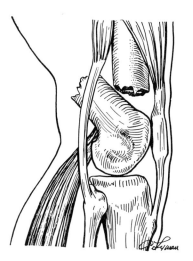

Fig. 5-58. Supracondylar fracture of the femur (transverse). Note the pull exerted by the gastrocnemius.

femur (Fig. 5-58) is distinctive because there is always a tendency toward deformity. It may be serious and permanent if the mechanical principles are not recognized. The gastrocnemius group of muscles is attached above the knee joint and between the condyles of the femur in the popliteal space. The only other muscles that influence the position of the lower fragment in this fracture are the thigh muscles, which cause overriding. Therefore, flexion occurs. This varies according to the distance of the fracture above the joint. Flexion may approach 90 degrees.

Problem. Traction on the leg must be applied with flexion of the knee joint (to release gastrocnemius pull).

Reduction. Usually reduction is accomplished by means of adhesive or skeletal traction with the knee in a flexed position.

If the fracture is of the transverse type, reduction may be accomplished immediately with the patient under anesthesia and maintained by a plaster cast with the knee in flexion. This is true also in young persons in whom there is an epiphyseal separation of the lower femoral epiphysis rather than a fracture.

Healing period. These fractures heal rather rapidly. Complete immobilization is usually necessary for only 4 to 6 weeks. Physical therapy is often valuable in restoring free motion in the joint. Full development of union and function usually takes place in 6 to 10 weeks.

FRACTURES INTO THE KNEE JOINT (FEMORAL CONDYLES)

Cause. Direct force either against the inner or the outer side of the knee joint usually causes fractures into the knee joint.

Anatomy. Such fractures may involve either condyle of the femur or may be of the plateau type involving either of the articular surfaces of the tibia. They are characterized by a tendency to produce a knock-knee (genu valgum) or bowleg (genu varum) deformity of the leg. Muscle pull plays very little part in the treatment, but the lateral and internal ligaments of the joint play a considerable part.

Problem. The contour of the joint must be restored as nearly perfect as possible, and the tendency toward deformity must be slightly overcorrected. Wherever there is damage within a joint as a result of fracture, the prognosis should be guarded, because the healing process in itself may be the source of irregularities that can lead to future irritation and disturbance of joint function.

Reduction. In some instances reduction may be accomplished spontaneously by manipulation with or without anesthesia and the position maintained by a plaster of paris cast. If the fracture is badly comminuted, the cast may need to be extended from the waist to the toes. Usually, however, it need not extend above the thigh.

Knee joint fractures heal better in traction with adhesive tape from the knee down. Often lateral traction is used to correct any tendency toward lateral deformity in the knee. This treatment has the advantage of allowing active motion of the joint during healing of the fracture, but of course it adds to the number of hospital days.

Open reduction is used in patients with severe fractures. This usually consists of the removal of small fragments that prevent apposition of the main fragments. Fixation by the use of nails or threaded wires may be necessary to hold the fragments together during healing.

Healing period. These fractures usually heal rapidly, but strength and stability are lacking for 3 or 4 months. Early motion is important in the knee joint, but protection from the development of knock-knee or bowleg deformity using a long leg brace may be necessary during the healing period of 3 to 4 months.

FRACTURES AND DISLOCATIONS ABOUT THE KNEE, ANKLE, AND FOOT

FRACTURE OF THE PATELLA

Causes. Direct violence is usually the cause of fracture of the patella. Muscular action is another cause.

Types. The three types of patellar fracture are (1) transverse, (2) comminuted (stellate), and (3) linear.

Anatomy. The action of the quadriceps may separate the fragments as much as several inches when the injury occurs. It is important to recognize the significance of this in considering the damage to the capsular ligaments of the knee joint. The repair of lateral tears should be an important part of the treatment.

Treatment. Only linear fractures or stellate fractures without separation of the fragments should be treated conservatively (Fig. 5-59). Conservative treatment can be accomplished by immobilization in a cast in extension for 3 to 6 weeks.

When there is separation of the fragments with tearing of the capsule, open reduction is always indicated. It is preferable in open reduction around joints to delay the operation 3 to 6 days to allow the traumatic reaction to subside and to permit tissue resistance to develop. This lessens the chance for infection. Open fractures may need to be treated immediately.

As a rule it is best to remove small fragments of the patella and leave only one main fragment to which the patella or quadriceps tendon is sutured. There is no longer a fracture to heal, but only the ligamentous attachments. Therefore immobilization time is greatly reduced. When severe comminution with separation occurs, the entire patella is removed, with restoration of good function.

ACUTE AND HABITUAL DISLOCATIONS OF THE PATELLA

Causes. Acute dislocation of the patella is usually caused by direct force against its inner side when the knee is flexed.

Habitual dislocation may start from the same mechanism, but there may be other factors, such as (1) too shallow a groove in the femoral condyles, (2) ball-like shape of the patella, and (3) knock-knee. Here the pull transmitted from the quadriceps tendon to the attachment of the patella tendon on the tibia is not in a straight line, and therefore it places abnormal tension on the ligamentous structure of the inner side of the knee.

Symptoms and signs. The patella can be seen displaced to the outer side of the knee. There is severe pain and muscle spasm, and the knee cannot be actively extended.

Treatment. Reduction occurs automatically when the knee is extended, but sometimes an anesthetic is necessary to accomplish reduction.

When reduced, primary dislocations are immobilized in a well-molded plaster cast from the ankle to the groin. This cast should be worn about 4 weeks. After this an elastic support with

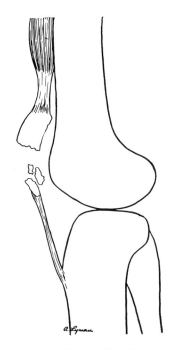

Fig. 5-59. Fracture of the patella with comminution of the lower fragment. This was removed.

stays should be worn for 2 or 3 weeks longer.

In the habitual type some form of operative fixation is necessary. The commonest methods are (1) transference of the patella tendon and its bony attachment inward on the tibia to create a direct-line pull, (2) osteotomy and wedging to deepen the femoral groove if it is shallow, and (3) tendon or fascia lata fixation of the patella to the inner condyle of the tibia.

FRACTURE AND DISLOCATION OF THE TIBIA BELOW THE KNEE (BUMPER FRACTURE)

Cause. Usually direct violence is the cause of fracture and dislocation of the tibia below the knee. They are frequently caused by a person stepping between two cars that are in motion toward each other and are commonly known as bumper fractures. Sometimes they are compound. The section immediately below the knee is usually involved.

Anatomy. The tibia is composed of two plates or surfaces that articulate with the two condyles of the femur. The knee joint has four important ligaments and two semilunar cartilages. The lateral ligaments protect the knee joint from any instability when it is completely straight. When it is extended, both lateral ligaments are tight and prevent any lateral motion of the knee joint.

The internal cruciate ligaments are those in the center of the knee joint and are designed to prevent the leg from displacing itself either forward or backward on the femur. To become acquainted with the direction of these ligaments, remember the direction of the anterior cruciate ligament by placing your right hand, with fingers spread, directly over the right patella when the knee is in flexion. The index finger will give the direction of the anterior cruciate ligament that goes from behind forward and is attached to the anterior tibial spine. The posterior ligament goes in the opposite direction; that is, from the inner condyle of the femur backward to the posterior spine of the tibia. These four ligaments are responsible for the stability of the knee joint in all directions.

The test for injury or tearing of the anterior cruciate ligament is to force the knee completely straight into extension. The anterior ligament becomes tight and hyperextension is not possible when the ligament is intact. If the ligament is torn, however, the joint may be carried to a position beyond 180 degrees.

If the posterior ligament is damaged or torn or if there is a detachment of the ligament with a small amount of bone from the posterior spine of the tibia, the knee joint, when it is placed in a position of 90-degree flexion, may be displaced forward on the femoral condyles to the extent of ½ to ¾ inch. Rotary motions are also increased.

The tendency for deformity is toward the collapsed or fractured side of the tibial condyles (Fig. 5-60). Should it be the outer condyles, there is a tendency toward the development of a knock-knee deformity. Should it be the inner condyle, there is a tendency toward the development of a bowleg deformity. Both of these are preventable.

Problem. The deformed leg must be maintained in proper alignment to the normal leg, and normal joint motion must be re-established at the earliest possible time. Restoration of the most perfect contour of the joint surface is another important problem to be dealt with.

Treatment. In most instances when there are

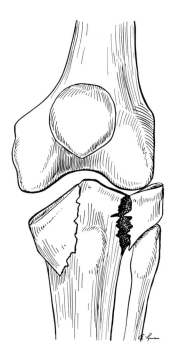

Fig. 5-60. Fracture of the condyles of the tibia into the knee joint. Open reduction done.

fractures of the upper end of the tibia involving the knee joint, conservative treatment is best.

Conservative treatment consists first in the use of moleskin adhesive traction from the knee down, with 5 to 8 pounds of weight. If there is a tendency toward knock-knee deformity, a sling may be arranged so that lateral traction may be applied at the inner side of the joint, using 5 to 8 pounds of weight over the outer side of the bed. The side traction is flexible, as is the traction in the vertical line. Therefore, during the process of healing and repair, the patient is able to carry on motions that will greatly facilitate the speed of recovery of joint motion. As was said before, in all fractures involving any joint, the patient or his relatives should be advised of the possible difficulties in re-establishing joint motion.

In spite of the fact that the knee joint is the heaviest weight-bearing joint in the body, the results of fractures into the knee joint are often more favorable than might be expected from the severity of the fracture affecting it.

It is sometimes necessary, because of the interposition of small fragments between the main fragments of the condylar fractures of the tibia, to perform an operation in which the area is approached, the fragments are removed, and the condyles are brought together in the best possible alignment of the joint surface. Occasionally, it may be necessary to employ a threaded bolt that penetrates both condyles and buckles them together by means of nuts properly arranged and properly designed to exert their pressure. The semilunar cartilages that are frequently mentioned in the literature as a source of trouble in these fractures seem rarely to be the cause of any serious trouble. The scar developed during healing usually anchors them sufficiently to assure future stability.

In some types hospitalization time may be shortened by the application of a cast in an overcorrected position. For example, if the inner condyle is fractured and there is a tendency toward the development of bowleg deformity, the cast can be applied in a position of knockknee.

If the opposite is the case, then the cast must also be applied from high in the groin to the toes in a slightly exaggerated position of bowleg. In either case the cast should be bivalved at an early period with daily motion of the knee joint. Throughout the course of treatment positive active motion and a slight range of assisted passive motion should be practiced.

Healing period. In cancellous bone, such as that found in and near the joint, there is a stage of rapid primary healing, but the stability of the callus so formed is insufficient to withstand much strain in less than 3 or 4 months. This allows the early establishment of motion in the joint, but there is not strength enough for early stress, strain, or weight bearing without danger of the development of deformity.

Condylar fractures of the tibia may heal within 3 or 4 weeks sufficiently for guarded motion with a split cast. Weight bearing on crutches should not be undertaken until the roentgenogram shows a fair amount of union.

It is desirable at times, particularly when early weight bearing is necessary, to use a brace that extends from the ischium to the heel of the shoe with a strap on the inner or outer side of the knee joint (depending on the tendency toward deformity) to prevent abnormal strain.

From the industrial standpoint, it usually takes from 4 to 6 months for patients with this type of fracture to recover sufficiently to return to their normal occupations. The amount of permanent disability is variable. Many patients with severe fractures may return to their normal occupations without any permanent disability. In some, however, whether mildly or severely affected, there may be partial permanent disability and the development of traumatic arthritis.

If the ligaments of the knee joint are sufficiently damaged to create permanent instability of the joint and interfere with the normal function, it may be necessary to operate, using ligamentous structures, such as tendons or tensor fascia lata (from the outer side of the thigh), to stabilize the joint. The procedure requires hospitalization of a patient for 3 to 6 weeks.

FRACTURE OF THE SHAFT OF THE TIBIA

Cause. The cause of fracture of the shaft of the tibia (Fig. 5-61) may be either direct or indirect violence. When there is direct violence, the fracture may be open. A twisting injury may

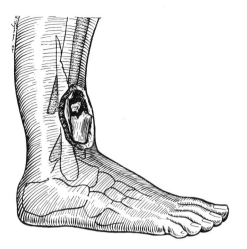

Fig. 5-61. Open fracture of the tibia and fibula at junction of middle and lower thirds.

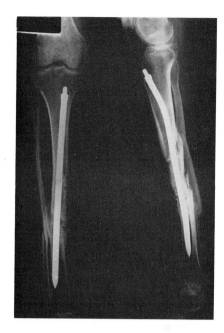

Fig. 5-62. Roentgenograms showing internal fixation of fracture of the tibia by insertion of an intramedullary nail (Lottes' nail). Fracture of the distal third of the tibia is frequently complicated by delayed union or nonunion.

cause a spiral fracture. Fracture of the tibia is one of the most common in automobile accidents, and the percentage of open fractures is greater than in almost any other region of the body. Fractures that occur in automobiles, industry, and war are most often caused by direct violence. The tibia may be broken by the direct impact of the penetrating force or may be broken in such a way that the points of the fracture penetrate the skin.

Anatomy. The tibia is the main weight-bearing bone of the leg. It is well covered with muscle tissue in the upper and middle parts, except over the shin, but sparsely covered with subcutaneous tissue and skin in the lower third. For this reason circulation is poor and healing is slow. Nonunion is relatively frequent in the middle and lower portions. The relation of the planes of the knee joint and those of the ankle are important in reduction. The injured leg should be compared with the uninjured leg before reduction is attempted so that the proper position in regard to rotation may be obtained.

Problem. The problem depends largely on the nature of the fracture—whether transverse, oblique, or comminuted. The problem is to reduce the fracture and maintain reduction by the simplest possible means. Any deviation in alignment must be avoided.

Treatment. With the patient under anesthesia, simple transverse and many oblique fractures may be manipulated into position and treated in

a long leg cast. Roentgenograms should be taken at frequent intervals during the first few weeks to see that slipping does not occur. If severe swelling should occur shortly after reduction, the cast should be split its full length and spread sufficiently to relieve circulatory embarrassment. It can be brought together again after swelling subsides.

If fractures of the tibia are difficult to hold in position, they may be treated by intramedullary nailing (Fig. 5-62), by plating, or by skeletal traction. In the oblique type two or more screws may maintain reduction by transfixing the fracture site. In either case a cast is used for immobilization during the healing period. The fixation apparatus is incorporated.

When nonunion occurs, bone grafting will usually stimulate union. The onlay full-thickness graft held in place by metal screws seems to be the most popular method.

POTT'S FRACTURE

Cause. A blow against the outer side of the ankle when the foot is in contact with the ground

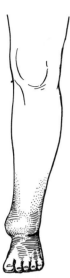

Fig. 5-63. Pott's fracture showing posterior and outward displacement of ankle joint. Ordinary joint contours disappear.

or twisting the ankle when slipping or falling may cause Pott's fracture (Fig. 5-63).

Anatomy. The ankle joint forms a mortice with the internal and external malleoli acting as stabilizing forces to prevent lateral motion. The astragalus acts as a gliding hinge against the lower articular surface of the tibia, allowing only plantar movement and dorsiflexion. All lateral movements occur in joints below the ankle joint. The classic Pott's fracture, frequently called trimalleolar, consists of a fracture of the internal malleolus and of the lower end of the fibula, combined with a backward and outward displacement of the astragalus. Frequently, the posterior lip of the tibia (posterior malleolus) is also broken.

Problem. Proper alignment and contact of the various fragments must be restored by manipulation with the patient under anesthesia. The ease or difficulty with which this reduction may be performed depends on two main factors. (1) If the inner malleolus is fractured near the tip rather than at the base of the malleolus, the proximal portion can serve as a barrier against overcorrecting the fracture inwardly. (2) If the fracture of the posterior malleolus involves as much as one-third or one-half of the posterior surface of the tibial part of the joint, the difficulty in maintaining the forward reduction of the

dislocation is very great and some form of open fixation is usually necessary.

Reduction. In addition to an accurate interpretation of the roentgenograms of Pott's fracture, a comparison between the fractured and unfractured sides should be made. In some persons the ankle joint and the knee joint work in the same plane, whereas in others the ankle joint may be outwardly or inwardly rotated. If reduction is attempted without taking this into consideration, the internal and external malleoli may not come in close contact at the points of fracture.

Treatment. Under fluoroscopic control the fragments are manipulated into a position that gives the closest contact. This usually consists of forced inversion, dorsiflexion, and lateral pressure through the ankle to restore accurate contact of the internal malleolus with the astragalus and of the external malleolus with the tibia. A circular plaster of paris cast is applied to maintain this position and must extend from the toes well up on the thigh with the knee moderately flexed in order to maintain the corrective amount of rotation. When the fracture line of the internal malleolus is at the same level of the joint surface or above it, fixation of the internal malleolus by nailing may be necessary.

Healing period. Healing usually requires from 8 to 12 weeks. As a rule, the portion of the cast above the knee may be removed at the end of 8 weeks, and frequently the lower portion may be bivalved for daily motion at the same time.

When the fracture is the favorable type, weight bearing with the use of a walking iron or similar device incorporated into the cast may be begun as early as 4 to 6 weeks. There may be some permanent disability as a result of traumatic arthritis in the ankle joint.

NURSING CARE IN FRACTURES OF THE BONES OF THE LOWER LEG

Nursing care of a simple fracture of either or both bones of the lower leg after reduction has been obtained and a cast applied presents no very troublesome features to the nurse. If there is considerable swelling, the patient may be admitted to the hospital for a short period before reduction is attempted. Ice bags are frequently used to reduce edema. These bags should not be

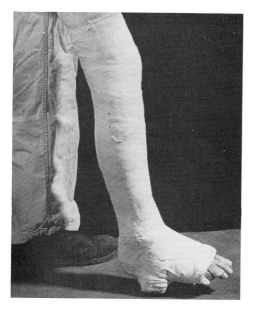

Fig. 5-64. Long leg walking cast.

too heavily filled with ice, and air should be eliminated before the bags are closed. The pressure of several very tightly filled ice bags on a swollen and painful ankle has been known to cause great discomfort to the patient as well as considerable interference with circulation. Attention to the underlying skin to eliminate the danger of ice burns is important. Ice bags should not be applied without some material between the patient's skin and the rubber, even in an emergency. Heat is usually substituted for the ice after 24 to 36 hours.

Walking casts (Fig. 5-64) are sometimes applied to patients with simple fractures of the leg in order to allow the patient to continue his normal occupation. The manner of applying these casts varies somewhat in different clinics. Reinforcements on the sole either with additional layers of plaster or with some type of flexible wood may be used. Stirrups or walking irons of metal may be incorporated into the plaster on the plantar surface of the cast. The patient should wear some type of protective sock to keep the cast and foot clean, and a coat or two of shellac when the cast is thoroughly dried is advisable.

COMPLICATIONS OF OPEN FRACTURES

Tetanus and gas bacillus infection are two complications of open fractures with whose symptoms every nurse should be familiar. Gas gangrene will first be noted at the site of infection as local edema, discoloration, and puffiness. Increase of the pulse rate is a constant systemic manifestation. The complete clinical picture is one of severe localized pain, increase in the size of the limb, rise in temperature, continued acceleration of the pulse rate, and a general picture of severe illness. The coppery color of the skin, which caused Velpeau to name the disease bronze erysipelas, is a characteristic of a very advanced state. Crepitation, which is caused by gas bubbles beneath the skin, is usually present. After some trauma has broken the patient's skin, any of these symptoms is extremely grave and demands immediate surgical attention.

General symptoms of tetanus may be absent. The earliest symptoms observed may be muscular twitchings and spasms that are tonic in nature. Frequently, there is difficulty in opening the mouth. This symptom may occur early in the course before any other symptoms have been noted.

Both diseases are caused by anaerobic bacteria, and surgical debridement of the wound is usually performed immediately. When gas bacillus infection is suspected, the wound is opened wide and all muscle planes in the affected part are exposed. Formerly, deep radiation was employed, followed by irrigation through rubber tubes placed so that they came in contact with every section of the muscles involved. Hydrogen peroxide, Dakin's solution, and other antiseptics were used for continuous irrigation. Amputation was frequently required. Antigas gangrene (polyvalent) serum was administered intramuscularly as often as every 6 to 10 hours in doses of 10,000 units. Local use of penicillin and the sulfonamides has largely replaced the radiation treatments and irrigations formerly employed. Serum is still used in large doses, although faith in it as being of specific value is questionable.

Wounds infected by tetanus are also opened wide, and very large doses of tetanus antitoxin may be given intramuscularly, intravenously, or into the spinal canal. In both diseases supportive treatment is extremely important and intake is kept up by fluids given parenterally. In tetanus the convulsive states are managed with sedative drugs.

FRACTURE OF THE ASTRAGALUS

Cause. Usually indirect violence, such as landing on the foot in a fall, is the cause of fracture of the astragalus.

Anatomy. The astragalus articulates with several bones, and a large portion of its surface is covered by articular cartilage. The area in which the blood supply may reach it is therefore small. In many instances fractures will damage the blood supply to such an extent that healing is delayed. Disintegration of the bone through aseptic necrosis is not infrequent, or there may be nonunion.

Treatment. Perfect reduction of the fracture is essential. To maintain reduction, nailing or bone graft may be required. Occasionally, removal of the astragalus is indicated.

Immobilization in a plaster of paris cast is advocated. The ankle should be placed in a right-angle position so that, if ankylosis should occur, the best function will ensure.

Healing period. Healing is slow, and weight bearing cannot be allowed until union is demonstrated roentgenographically. However, the cast may be bivalved in 6 to 8 weeks, and some motion, heat, and massage may be started for the restoration of joint function. When the cast is discarded, the arch should be supported for weight bearing. Total healing may not occur sooner than 10 to 14 weeks.

FRACTURE OF THE OS CALCIS (CALCANEUS)

Cause. Direct violence, usually from falls in which the victim lands on his heels, is the cause of fracture of the os calcis. Frequently, these injuries are bilateral and may be associated with compression fractures of the spine. They are common in explosions on shipboard.

Anatomy. The os calcis (or calcaneus) is composed almost entirely of spongy bone. When the outer surface is broken, the inherent strength of the bone is lost.

Displacements that occur from the injury are usually in three directions. Lateral compression shoves the fragments out under the external malleolus and tends to cause a flatfoot deformity. Upward displacement of the posterior portion tends to exaggerate the flatfoot tendency. This is increased by the pull of the Achilles tendon. Outward rotation also occurs.

In the usual anteroposterior and lateral roentgenograms of the foot and ankle, the true degree of displacement is not shown. This has led to disastrous undertreatment of these fractures. Because of their disabling effect they are usually much more formidable than they appear. Therefore, roentgenograms should be taken from behind the leg at a 45-degree angle so that a true picture of the lateral displacement and outward rotation of the fragments will be shown. For this view the foot is in complete contact with the X-ray plate.

Treatment. There are several methods of treatment, but the essential factor of all is that the bone be restored to as near its normal shape as possible. This requires lateral impaction of the fragments and downward displacement of the heel. The latter can be accomplished through lengthening of the Achilles tendon and downward replacement through leverage in skeletal traction. The arch must be restored and all corrections must be maintained by the proper application of a plaster of paris cast.

Healing period. Weight bearing cannot be allowed in less than 6 to 8 weeks and then only with the arch well supported to prevent weight being exerted on the os calcis. The degree of permanent disability is usually determined by (1) the extent of involvement of the subastragsloid joint, (2) the amount of residual lateral displacement under the external malleolus and against the peroneal tendons, and (3) the residual flattening of the longitudinal arch.

The rule in many clinics is that, if the pain persists beyond the 6-month period, the accumulation of bone under the external malleolus should be removed and the subastragaloid joint, and possibly others, should be ankylosed by operation.

FRACTURES OF THE METATARSAL BONES AND TOES

Cause. Usually, fractures of the metatarsal bones and toes are caused by direct violence.

Anatomy. The metatarsal heads comprise the anterior arch and one of the main weight-bearing surfaces of the foot. The muscles and tissues here are sparse. Restoration of length and alignment, therefore, particularly in the anteroposterior plane, are the main problems of reduction and treatment because a prominence of bone on either the plantar or dorsal surface of the foot could lead to irritation from weight bearing or shoes. The treatment following the necessary amount of reduction is usually the application of a plaster of paris cast from the calf to the end of the toes. Skeletal traction may be necessary occasionally.

Healing period. These bones usually heal in about 4 weeks. After the removal of the cast, protection must be maintained for several weeks by the use of an arch support within the shoe and a metatarsal bar on the outside.

PHYSICAL THERAPY IN THE TREATMENT OF FRACTURES

Physical therapy after any type of fracture is recognized to be of great importance regardless of what type of reduction has been used. Although nurses will not be required to carry out these treatments as a rule, it is important that they have a good concept of the treatment and its purpose.

The main purposes of physical therapy after fractures are (1) to encourage absorption of traumatic hemorrhage and exudate, (2) to relax muscle spasm and thereby eliminate discomfort and possible deformity, (3) to promote normal circulation in the part and thus to hasten the healing process, and (4) to restore muscle tone and flexibility so that normal functioning is possible.

Heat in some form is almost always part of the treatment. It may be given by means of an electric light bulb suspended from a cradle, by hot packs, by a therapeutic lamp, or by means of a whirlpool bath. It is exceedingly important that nurses recognize the fact that heat has a greater value if administered at low intensity over a long period than if it is given at high intensity for a shorter period of time.

When massage is given, it is usually of the light stroking variety, with slow steady strokes given in the same direction—in the long axis of the muscle and in the direction of venous flow.

Muscle stimulation to encourage muscle contraction is usually part of the physical therapy program. This may be done through electric stimulation or through the patient's own voluntary effort. (Voluntary effort is usually considered preferable.) Although this voluntary effort is possible even though the patient is encased in a plaster cast, many orthopedists provide some type of fixation that allows guarded use of contiguous joints while controlling the fracture site. Traction, hinged splints, or bivalved casts are particularly useful for this purpose.

Active or active assistive exercises with gentle stretching are frequently prescribed for the patient in traction or splints. It is exceedingly important during the first few weeks after fracture. Development of muscle power is recognized as essential if normal function is to be regained. The method of DeLorme, known as the heavy resistance, low repetition method, has worked well in the hands of experienced physical therapists. This method differs from older methods that concentrated largely on low resistance exercises repeated a great number of times. Although this method served to develop endurance, it did not always develop muscle power sufficient for the demands of normal function.

Some type of apparatus to assist the patient in active exercise of the hip may be attached to the bed. This may consist of an overhead frame, skin or ankle traction, and a series of ropes or pulleys that permit the patient to exercise his leg in adduction, abduction, flexion, and extension. The patient is taught to do this by himself, although supervision of his activities is repeated at frequent intervals.

STUDY QUESTIONS

Mrs. S., a 77-year-old lady, has been admitted to the hospital following a fall in her home. She complains of pain in the hip region, and roentgenograms reveal a fracture of the neck of the femur.
1. Describe typical position of the limb after fracture of the neck of the femur.
2. Moving this patient from the ambulance cot will cause increased pain at the fracture site. Describe the method of transferring the patient that will cause the least discomfort.
3. Traction may be applied to the involved limb. What type(s) of traction will most likely be applied? Explain. Describe desirable position of the limb following application of the traction.
4. Surgical treatment of this type of fracture usually consists of a closed reduction with internal fixation. Explain.
5. Review preoperative and postoperative nursing care of the elderly patient with a fracture of the hip pertaining to:
   (a) Prevention of pressure sores
   (b) Prevention of hypostatic pneumonia
   (c) Bowel and bladder problems

(d) Bed positions and activity

(e) Prevention of joint contractures

6. Explain or demonstrate method(s) of helping the postoperative patient from the bed to a chair.

7. What is meant by "aseptic necrosis"? If aseptic necrosis occurs, what surgical procedures may be performed to provide the patient with a functional hip?

8. Review the problems associated with providing continuous care for the patient after her discharge from the hospital. This may include provisions for care in a nursing home, an extended-care unit, her own home, or other available facilities. What financial assistance is available to the elderly individual pertaining to health needs?

REFERENCES

The aged in our society, Nurs. Outlook, vol. 12, entire issue, Nov., 1964.

Alba, I. M., and Papeika, J.: The nurse's role in preventing circulatory complications in the patient with a fractured hip, Nurs. Clin. North Am. L:57-61, 1966.

Amburgey, P. I.: Environmental aids for the aged patient, Am. J. Nurs. 66:2017-2018, 1966.

Anderson, H. C.: Newton's geriatric nursing, ed. 5, St. Louis, 1971, The C. V. Mosby Co.

Boyd, H.: Nonunion of the shafts of long bones, Postgrad. Med. 36:315-320, 1964.

Bradley, D.: Fractures of the ankle joint, Nurs. Times 68:1115-1119, 1972.

Bradley, D.: Fractures of the patella, Nurs. Times 67:1531-1534, 1971.

Bradley, D.: Fractures of the pelvis, Nurs. Times 68:376-379, 1972.

Bradley, D.: Fractures of the upper end of the femur—clinical features, Nurs. Times 66:1523-1525, 1970.

Bradley, D.: Fractures of the upper end of the femur—treatment, Nurs. Times 66:1552-1555, 1970.

Bray, A. P., and Thomas J.: Severe fat embolism syndrome following multiple fractures, Nurs. Times 65:109-110, 1969.

Cave, E. F., editor: Fractures and other injuries, Chicago, 1958, Year Book Medical Publishers, Inc.

Cave, E. F.: The healing of fractures and nonunion of bone, Surg. Clin. North Am. 43:337-349, 1963.

Committee on Trauma of American College of Surgeons: An outline of the treatment of fractures, ed. 8, Philadelphia, 1965, W. B. Saunders Co.

Crenshaw, A. H., editor: Campbell's operative orthopaedics, vol. 1, ed. 5, St. Louis, 1971, The C. V. Mosby Co.

Davenport, R.: Tube feeding for long-term patients, Am. J. Nurs. 64:121-123, 1964.

Davis, R. W.: Psychologic aspects of geriatric nursing, Am. J. Nurs. 68:802-804, 1968.

Dehne, E.: Immediate weight bearing as treatment of tibial shaft fractures, J. Bone Joint Surg. 47A:1085, July, 1965.

Devas, M. B.: Stress fractures in athletes, Nurs. Times 67:227-232, 1971.

Francis, Sister M.: Nursing the patient with internal hip fixation, Am. J. Nurs. 64:111-112, 1964.

Gartland, J.: Fundamentals of orthopaedics, Philadelphia, 1965, W. B. Saunders Co.

Hawkins, L. G.: Hip prostheses, J. Iowa Med. Soc. 56:465-471, 1966.

Hirschberg, G. G., Bard, G., and Robertson, K. B.: Rehabilitation: a manual for the care of the disabled and elderly, Philadelphia, 1964 J. B. Lippincott Co.

Hulicka, I.: Fostering self-respect in aged patients, Am. J. Nurs. 64:84-89, 1964.

The impact of medicare on nursing services, Nurs. Outlook, 14, entire issue, June, 1966.

Knapp, Miland: Keeping the elderly active, Postgrad. Med. 44:203-206, 1968.

Lam, S. J.: Fractures: general principles 1, Nurs. Times 62:410-412, 1966.

Lam, S. J.: Fractures: general principles 2, Nurs. Times 62:446-447, 1966.

Lindhl, K., and Rickerson, G.: Spinal cord–injury: you can make a difference, Nursing '74 4:41-45, Feb., 1974.

Mayo, R. A., and Hughes, J. M.: Intramedullary nailing of long bone fractures; nursing care after intramedulary nailing, Am. J. Nurs. 59:236-240, 1959.

Mendelson, J.: Sprains and strains, Am. J. Nurs. 61:45-50, 1961.

Michele, A.: Principles of fracture care, Am. J. Orthop. 9:34-37, 1967.

Mooney, V., Vernon, N., Harvey, P., and Snelson, R.: Cast-brace treatment for fractures of the distal part of the femur, J. Bone Joint Surg. 52-A:1563-1578, 1970.

Neufeld, A.: Surgical treatment of hip injuries, Am. J. Nurs. 65:80-83, 1965.

Patrick, M.: Care of the confused elderly patient, Am. J. Nurs. 67:2536-2539, 1967.

Patton, F., Behlore, D., and Pechth, P.: Treatment of hip fractures in the geriatic patient, J. Am. Phys. Ther. Ass. 42:314-318, 1962.

Peszezynski, M.: Why old people fall, Am. J. Nurs. 65:86-88, May, 1965.

Ring, P. A.: Fractures of the pelvis, Nurs. Times 61:732-734, 1965.

Roberts, J. M.: New developments in orthopedic surgery—fractures, Nurs. Clin. North Am. 2:386-387, 1967.

Robinson, M., and Van Volkenburgh, S.: Intermaxillary fixation: immediate postoperative care, Am. J. Nurs. 63:71-72, 1963.

Sandick, H.: Priorities must be established in emergency care of the injured, Am. J. Nurs. 62:93-96, 1962.

Sarmiento, A.: Functional bracing of tibial and femoral shaft fractures, Clin. Ortho. 82:2-13, 1972.

Scully, H. F., and Stevens, M.: Anesthetic management for geriatric patients, Am. J. Nurs. 65:110-112, 1965.

Simpson, H. A. S.: Fractured femur and patella complicated by cerebral fat embolism, Nurs. Times **68:** 431-434, 1972.

Slater, R. R.: Triage nurse in the emergency department, Am. J. Nurs. **70:**127-129, 1970.

Stafford, N. H.: Bowel hygiene of aged patients, Am. J. Nurs. **63:**102-102, 1963.

Storlie, F. J.: When they need me, Am. J. Nurs. **65:** 100-101, 1965.

Surgery of the lower extremity, Surg. Clin. North Am. **45:**5-117, 1965.

Trippel, O., Jurayj, M., Staley, C., and van Elk, J.: Surgical use of the hyperbaric oxygen chamber, Surg. Clin. North Am. **46:**209-221, 1966.

Turek, S. L.: Orthopaedics—principles and their application, ed. 2, Philadelphia, 1967, J. B. Lippincott Co.

Wagner, M. M.: Assessment of patients with multiple injuries, Am. J. Nurs. **72:**1822-1827, 1972.

Ziffren, S. E.: Management of the aged surgical patient, Chicago, 1960, Year Book Medical Publishers, Inc.

6

Arthritis

Rheumatism is a general term that includes disorders in which pain and stiffness of the muscles or skeleton are prominent features. It ranks second only to mental and nervous diseases as a cause of time lost from work.

Arthritis is a form of rheumatism in which the joints are the structures primarily affected. It has been estimated that four and one-half million people in this country have arthritis and that 190,000 of these are totally disabled. Over one-half of the disabled persons are less than 45 years of age. With the associated social, economic, and emotional burdens on the families of arthritic patients the importance of the nursing care of the patient with arthritis becomes obvious.

Arthritis is a chronic disease causing varying degrees of disability, frequently quite severe. Unfortunately there is no cure for most of the forms of arthritis. The desired goal in the care of the patient with arthritis must be to help him function efficiently as a human being and as a member of society. It follows, then, that the treatment program must consider the patient's physical health, emotional health, and any social problems that may be present, especially as they relate to family members and economic situation. If the treatment program does not include all these, it is inadequate and will fail to achieve the goal that common sense tells us is the only logical objective. Indeed this should be the kind of attention and desired goal in the care of any patient, no matter what his ailment may be.

The described objective in the care of the patient with arthritis cannot be adequately achieved by any one person. The combined efforts of a number of specially trained persons—the patient's personal physician, consultant physicians, nurses, physical therapist, occupational therapist, social worker, and vocational counselor—will be needed at various times. The overall program is directed by the physician who has the responsibility for the patient's long-term care and who must know all the facets of the patient's problems.

The physician who has the primary responsibility for the patient's care must not only attend to his medical needs but also must assist the patient in other areas. The role of the nurse, as will be shown, is very important in the total program of treatment. The physical therapist has close contact with the patient and similarly contributes a great deal. Many patients have disabilities that make it difficult or impossible for them to perform everyday tasks that we take for granted in our lives, such as putting on shoes or socks. The occupational therapist can help the patient by showing him ways of adapting to his disabilities, by demonstrating techniques for simplifying everyday tasks, and by providing devices to aid the patient in performing these activities. The social worker can help in working out family problems, in providing contact with special service agencies, and frequently giving moral support to the patient who has emotional problems contributing to his disability. The vocational counselor contributes a real service when he helps the patient find a new occupation when the patient can no longer continue at his previous work because of his disability.

There are numerous types of arthritis. The following three are relatively common. Other, less common types usually resemble clinically one of these three, and the principles of nursing care can be applied accordingly.

RHEUMATOID ARTHRITIS

Rheumatoid arthritis is a chronic systemic disease of unknown cause. It is to be emphasized that this is a generalized or systemic disease and not strictly a joint affliction, although the joint involvement is the major clinical feature. Varying degrees of deformity and destruction of joints commonly occur, causing different kinds and amounts of disability. The joint damage may be so severe in some instances as to result in complete invalidism. Rheumatoid arthritis occurs more commonly in women than in men, in a ratio of two or three to one. It may occur at any age, from infancy to advanced old age, but most often appears between 20 and 50 years of age.

The prominent symptoms of rheumatoid arthritis are stiffness, especially upon arising in the morning, and joint pain and swelling, involving multiple joints. The joint swelling is caused by inflammation of the synovium, the tissue lining the joint capsule, and by accumulation of fluid within the joints. There is a definite tendency for involvement of the same joints on both sides of the body, and the arthritis usually affects more joints as time goes on. Although any joint in the body may be involved, there is a predilection for the small joints of the hands and feet. The wrists, elbows, ankles, and knees are commonly involved also.

As a result of the chronic joint inflammation, important anatomic changes may occur, with consequent limitation of joint function. Involvement of the joint capsule and supporting ligaments may cause weakness, stretching, or rupture of these structures, resulting in instability. When the instability is severe, partial dislocation of the joint, referred to as subluxation, may occur. In other instances there is scarring of these supporting tissues, causing limitation of motion. This is termed contracture of the joint capsule or ligament. When scarring occurs within a joint, limitation of motion also occurs and is called ankylosis. It may be so severe as to result in a completely motionless joint. Actual destruction of cartilage and bone within the joint is often found in rheumatoid arthritis.

When severe, it may result in greatly impaired joint function. Muscle weakness is common and may contribute to the patient's disability.

The course of rheumatoid arthritis usually is one of periods of increased disease activity alternating with intervals of decreased disease activity. There may be great variation in the intensity and duration of the periods of increased disease activity from time to time. It is very difficult, therefore, to predict the course of the disease in an individual patient. A small percentage of patients with rheumatoid arthritis will have a mild course with little disability. Most patients will have varying degrees of disability that increase with the duration of the disease. These patients remain largely independent of others for self-care and are usually able to pursue occupations not requiring vigorous physical

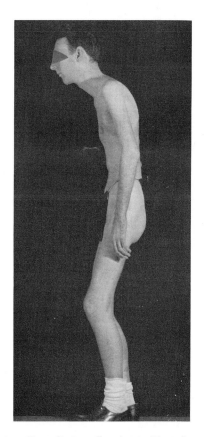

Fig. 6-1. Marie-Strümpell arthritis. Typical posture in ankylosing arthritis of the spine. Hip and shoulder joints may also be involved. (From Smith-Petersen, M. N., Larson, C. B., and Aufranc, O. E.: J. Bone Joint Surg. **27:**562-571, 1945.)

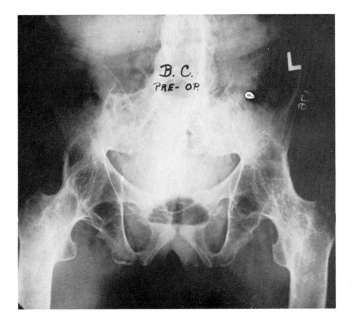

Fig. 6-2. Marie-Strümpell arthritis. Both hip joints, both sacroiliac joints, and the zygapophyseal joints have been destroyed and have undergone bony ankylosis. Note the calcification of the vertebral ligaments. No motion in this portion of the back and in the hips is possible. (From Kenney, W. C., and Larson, C. B.: Orthopedics for the general practitioner, St. Louis, 1957, The C. V. Mosby Co.)

activity. Severe incapacitation will occur in relatively few patients.

Ankylosing spondylitis, also known as rheumatoid spondylitis and Marie-Strümpell arthritis, is a chronic form of arthritis affecting primarily the sacroiliac joints and spine. Frequently it leads to severe ankylosis or limitation of motion of the back (Figs. 6-1 and 6-2). It affects men approximately four times more frequently than women and usually occurs between 16 and 40 years of age. Pain and stiffness of the back are the common symptoms of this disorder. Involvement of the extremity joints occurs in some patients and is usually less severe than in typical rheumatoid arthritis. The course of ankylosing spondylitis is variable, just as in rheumatoid arthritis. It is usually a progressive disease involving more of the spine with the passage of time.

Treatment and nursing care, general considerations

Because rheumatoid arthritis is a chronic systemic disease, consideration must be given to the care of each patient's general health as well as to the treatment of the joint problems. Adequate rest, relief of pain, prevention of deformity, proper nutrition, treatment of other diseases when present, and assisting the patient to understand his disease and develop a proper attitude toward it are the important general features of treatment. There is no cure for rheumatoid arthritis, and it must be clearly understood that all treatment is directed at maintaining good general health and helping the patient to function at his best possible level.

Years of experience have shown that a successful basic treatment program for rheumatoid arthritis must include adequate rest, relief of pain, and a regular exercise program. The patient with rheumatoid arthritis requires 8 to 12 hours' sleep each night and, when the disease is more active, frequent rest periods during the day. In the event of an acute flare-up of the arthritis, several days of bed rest are helpful in reducing joint inflammation and systemic symptoms. However, remaining in bed for prolonged periods of time is undesirable because it leads to increased muscle weakness and limitation of joint motion.

No drug has been found to be more desirable than aspirin for relief of pain, and this is the basic ingredient of the drug therapy portion of the treatment program. Aspirin often controls pain satisfactorily when given in adequate dosages—eight to sixteen or more 0.3 gm. tablets daily. Many patients will not require any other medication. In other patients additional drugs are needed, but the aspirin is continued as the basic drug.

Physical therapy is a basic part of the treatment program for most patients with rheumatoid arthritis. It should consist primarily of therapeutic exercises having one or both of the following objectives: (1) improvement or maintenance of muscle strength, (2) improvement or maintenance of range of motion of joints. Efforts directed at the first objective, especially, should be the major concern of the physical therapist. Therapists often apply heat to painful joints for temporary relief of pain and stiffness. Since the duration of beneficial effect of such treatment is quite brief and since rheumatoid arthritis is a protracted disease, this method of pain relief has limited practicality in the long-term management of these patients. More appropriate pain relief can usually be obtained by adjustment of the drug regimen. When combined with other intensive physical therapy techniques, for example, just before a patient begins a therapeutic exercise period, heat therapy may offer justifiable benefit to the patient.

Other factors must be considered in the basic treatment program for a patient with rheumatoid arthritis. Adequate nutrition is accomplished by a balanced diet having sufficient caloric intake to maintain normal weight. Overweight, even of moderate degree, is deleterious and should be corrected by diet. The adverse effect of obesity must be clearly explained to the patient, and the importance of weight reduction, when needed, should be strongly emphasized. Special diets, supplements, or vitamins have no value in the treatment of rheumatoid arthritis. Treatment of other diseases that are present should be done to improve the patient's general health.

Because rheumatoid arthritis is a chronic disease and the patient often has pain and is limited in the performance of daily activities,

it is common for him to become discouraged and to develop a poor outlook for the future. Moral support for the person with this disorder is a very important aspect of treatment and can mean the difference between success and failure of the overall program. It is important that the patient develop the proper attitude toward his disease. Obviously, a give-up or hopeless reaction on his part is undesirable and, when severe, may be a major factor in causing disability. On the other hand, failure to acknowledge the limitations placed on him by the disease can cause the patient much difficulty, too. The person who adopts a realistic attitude toward his disease, lives within the limitations imposed by it, and follows advice for treatment definitely does better than the one who does not. Physicians, nurses, and others concerned with a patient's care have a great deal of responsibility in this regard because it is from them that he derives many of his ideas and attitudes concerning his illness. Those who care for the arthritic patient must have a realistic but hopeful approach to the patient and his disease. Frequent contact with the patient provides the nurse with ample opportunity to benefit him in this area. Attitudes of pity or unconcern will certainly have an undesirable effect.

Prevention of deformity is of the utmost importance; when deformity is severe, it may be the major cause of disability in an arthritic patient. Many components of the treatment program contribute to this aspect of therapy, such as rest of an inflamed joint, medication to relieve pain, and physical therapy treatments to maintain joint motion and muscle strength. Braces or splints to support the joints may be indicated. Some are used only when the patient is resting or sleeping and others only when the patient is up and about. Specially designed or modified shoes may be very helpful in relieving foot pain caused by deformity.

An often neglected but very significant area for the prevention of deformity is the arthritic patient's bed, in which he spends one-third to one-half of his time. The mattress must be firm with a bed board between it and the spring. The pillow should be thin so as to cause minimal flexion of the neck (Fig. 6-3). Pillows should never be placed beneath the knees because this

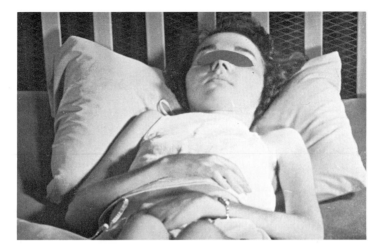

Fig. 6-3. Position frequently assumed by arthritic patients: shoulders adducted, elbows and wrists flexed.

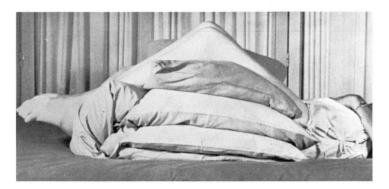

Fig. 6-4. Permanent flexion contractures of the knees and hips caused by the continuous use of pillows to support the knees in a flexed position—common deformities in arthritis.

will very likely lead to the development of flexion contractures of the hips and knees (Fig. 6-4), which is a serious deformity. A pillow placed between the knees to separate the legs slightly, however, is definitely helpful in preventing adduction deformity of the hips. The bed should be relatively high because often the arthritic patient has weak leg and hip muscles. The use of a footboard on the bed to prevent contracture of the heel cord (drop-foot deformity) and to keep the bed covers off the feet is important. Maintaining proper body alignment when resting is helpful in preventing deformity. The arthritic patient should lie with the joints extended as far as is comfortable a good portion of the time. A sandbag or a trochanter roll placed along the lateral aspect of the lower extremity helps to maintain a neutral position of the hip joint. This prevents external rotation of the limb, an undesirable position for the patient with acute hip involvement.

Daily nursing care. Many aspects of daily nursing care that the nurse learns to do routinely require modification or individual attention for the arthritic patient. Simple things that are ordinarily done without thinking, such as going to the bathroom, turning in bed, or even moving an extremity, may be ordeals for an arthritic patient because of pain or disability. He frequently requires a great deal of time. To hurry him or become impatient will only cause him unnecessary pain or dissatisfaction with the nurse. This will retard or prevent the nurse's development of satisfactory rapport with the patient. In the morning especially, or after a period of rest, the arthritic patient moves slowly because of the stiffness so characteristic of the disease. Pain is also frequently increased at these times. It is worthwhile for the nurse to listen to the patient, for often he has learned special ways of taking care of his needs that make it easier for him. Because there is an almost infinite variety in the types and degrees of disability in arthritic patients, care must be individualized, according to each patient's needs. It is important to determine what the patient can and cannot do by himself. He should be expected to do those things of which he is capable, but he will require assistance in others. There is a distinct tendency for some patients to grow increasingly dependent on others, even for those things that they can do for themselves. This, of course, is to be discouraged, and the patient should be led to do more and more for himself as his therapy progresses.

Standard nursing care activities such as bathing, shaving, brushing teeth, and making up beds are necessary parts of the patient's care and are not to be ignored. Because of disability, assistance may be required but should be given only if needed. The patient should be encouraged to establish a daily routine for performing self-care. Because arthritic patients may spend considerable time in bed, special attention to skin care is important. Cleanliness, with skin lotion when necessary, is most helpful. Careful attention must be given to pressure points located over bony prominences, such as the elbows, spinous processes of the vertebrae, sacrum, trochanters, ankles, and heels to prevent decubitus ulcers. Soft foam-rubber pads will offer some protection for these areas, but the most important preventive measure is frequent change of position. Observation of the patient performing his daily activities will give clues for making his efforts easier or less uncomfortable. A trapeze can be placed over the patient's bed to aid him in turning and in getting in and out of bed. The patient with troublesome weakness or pain in the legs will benefit from

the use of a chair with a relatively high seat. It is much easier for him to get in and out of such a chair than from a low one. Armrests give additional assistance in getting in and out of a chair. If troublesome hand deformities are present, eating utensils with modified handles may be beneficial. Likewise, a chair in the shower to enable the patient to sit down while bathing, a bath sponge on a long handle, a long-handled shoehorn, or a rod with a hook at one end to help in putting on socks may be very helpful to the patient.

Many routine daily activities present potential injury hazards for the arthritic patient because of his weakness or instability. The bathtub and shower should be provided with handrails and non-slip floor mats. Wheelchairs, when the brakes are not applied, can be treacherous; all patients should be firmly warned of this. The rubber tips of crutches and canes are essential for safe use of these walking aids. Without them, or when they become worn, the danger of a serious fall is always present. Therefore, they should be checked frequently. Stairways must have handrails. Some of these precautions may seem unnecessary or obvious, but for the arthritic patient they are very important.

Special forms of treatment

Drugs. No matter what medications are used in the treatment of rheumatoid arthritis, it must be remembered that none are curative. They are useful only to aid in the relief of pain and stiffness, and probably none have an effect on the disease itself. Therefore, these medications are never a substitute for the basic treatment program; they are additions to it and are of less importance than the basic program itself. Because pain in active arthritis is caused by inflammation, it follows that most of the drugs are used to suppress inflammation. Medications that have this effect include aspirin, phenylbutazone, indomethacin, the antimalarial drugs chloroquine and hydroxychloroquine, gold, and the various cortisone-like drugs that are frequently called corticosteroids or steroids.

Aspirin is the basic drug in treatment of rheumatoid arthritis. It is definitely helpful in the large majority of patients, quite safe for long-term use, and well tolerated by most patients.

Plain aspirin is the desirable form for most patients and the least expensive. Most patients require relatively large doses, 0.6 to 1.5 gm. four times daily on a regular schedule. In many patients, the maximum tolerated dose is necessary, just short of that dose which causes symptoms of aspirin excess. Greater effectiveness is achieved by the patient's taking aspirin regularly, four doses daily, than when it is used sporadically. A convenient schedule for most patients, and one that minimizes abdominal distress, is a dose with each meal and at bedtime, the latter with a snack or milk. The difference in effectiveness between small and large doses of aspirin is often significant and warrants careful adjustment to determine the maximum dose tolerated by the patient in order to gain the greatest benefit.

The common symptoms of salicylism (aspirin toxicity) are tinnitus (noises in the ears), decreased hearing acuity, vertigo, headache, lassitude, drowsiness, dimness of vision, nausea, vomiting, hyperventilation, and depressed mental function. Of these, tinnitus and hearing loss are the most common and are usually the first to appear. Chronic aspirin therapy causes gastritis in a significant number of patients and gastric ulcer in a lesser but still important number. Both of these problems most commonly occur with epigastric pain. Not all patients taking aspirin who have such pain necessarily have gastritis or ulcer, however. Minor epigastric distress may be eliminated by the use of buffered aspirin. Those patients known to have previous gastritis or gastric ulcer and those who cannot tolerate buffered aspirin should be given enteric-coated aspirin.

For many patients with rheumatoid arthritis, aspirin is not adequate for control of pain and stiffness resulting from joint inflammation. In these cases, additional drugs are necessary. It is strongly emphasized that aspirin be continued in the maximum tolerated dose and that other drugs be added. Of the several drugs listed previously, one or more may be used in combination with aspirin. All are compatible, one with any other. The particular drug chosen will depend on several factors: previous attempts at therapy, severity of disease, cost to the patient, and others.

Phenylbutazone is an anti-inflammatory drug of relatively low potency and may be helpful in some patients. A 1-week trial of therapy is adequate for assessment of efficacy. If no benefit has occurred, it should be discontinued. If helpful it may be continued. The initial dose is 100 mg. four times daily for 1 week, followed by the smallest effective amount. Adverse effects include salt and water retention, which occurs in all patients. This may lead to edema formation, worsening of hypertension, or congestive heart failure in patients with serious heart disease. Abdominal distress similar to that described for aspirin is common. Less frequently, dermatitis or stomatitis occurs. The serious forms of toxicity, although uncommon, involve the bone marrow, causing agranulocytosis or aplastic anemia; the latter is especially serious because approximately 50% of cases end fatally. Long-term therapy with this drug is not recommended if at all avoidable. If done, monthly blood counts must be obtained. Even then, severe toxicity may occur unpredictably.

Indomethacin is an anti-inflammatory drug helpful in some patients with rheumatoid arthritis. The usual initial dose is 25 mg. twice daily, increasing by 25 mg. every 4 days to 25 mg. four times daily. Maintenance doses are 75 to 150 mg. daily. A 3-week trial of therapy at 100 mg. daily is adequate to determine effectiveness in most patients. If beneficial, it may be given for a prolonged period of time relatively safely. Serious adverse reactions are rare although gastritis and gastric ulcer, similar to distress from aspirin may occur. Less serious but distressing side effects frequently requiring that the drug be stopped include headache, dizziness, vague but unpleasant mental symptoms, abdominal distress, and diarrhea.

Two antimalarial drugs, *chloroquine* and *hydroxychloroquine*, have been found to be beneficial in treatment of some patients with rheumatoid arthritis. Their efficacy is approximately equal. Hydroxychloroquine is thought by most to be less toxic. The usual dose of this drug is 400 mg. daily for 6 weeks; then 200 mg. daily, given at bedtime to minimize nausea. A 3-month trial period is required to determine whether it is effective. If so, treatment may be continued. Nausea, flatulence, blurring of vision, and diplopia may occur initially. Usually these require only temporary reduction of the dose and are transient. Deposition of the drug on the cornea causes a gritty sensation in the eye. This clears if the drug is stopped for several weeks. Treatment may then be resumed at a lower dose. Dermatitis and leukopenia occasionally occur, requiring that the drug be stopped. The most serious and least frequent adverse effect is retinal toxicity. It is insidious, unnoticed by the patient until serious visual loss has occurred, and is irreversible. This toxic effect requires that, prior to starting treatment and every 6 months while the drug is given, the patient's eyes and visual function be examined by an ophthalmologist. Only with this precaution is the use of the drug safe.

Gold compounds have been used for approximately 35 years in the treatment of rheumatoid arthritis. Like most of the drugs mentioned, gold is not beneficial in all cases. An adequate trial requires treatment for 20 to 25 weeks. The dosage schedule is an initial dose of gold sodium thiomalate or gold thioglucose of 10 mg. intramuscularly, followed by weekly injections of 40 to 50 mg. until a total of 1,000 mg. has been given. If beneficial, 40 to 50 mg. is then given every 3 to 4 weeks for maintenance therapy. The common adverse effects of gold therapy are dermatitis, stomatitis, and proteinuria. Less frequently, leukopenia, thrombocytopenia, or anemia occur. Precautions to detect adverse reactions promptly should be taken. In most instances, stopping gold therapy is the only treatment needed, but serious reactions require vigorous treatment.

Corticosteroids have been used in the treatment of rheumatoid arthritis for nearly 25 years. They are potent drugs with respect to their capacity to control joint pain and stiffness and also in their capacity to cause adverse effects. The large majority of patients with active arthritis have a favorable response to these drugs with prompt reduction of pain and stiffness.

A large variety of preparations is available, but none has been shown to be more effective or to cause fewer adverse effects than prednisone. It also is less expensive than most of the other forms. The recommended initial dose is 2 mg. three or four times daily. After 1 month,

if there has been good control of pain, reduction of the daily dose by 1 mg. at 3-week intervals is begun, reducing to the smallest dose which gives good control of pain. In patients with more severe arthritis larger doses may be necessary, occasionally up to 20 mg. daily. Rarely, if ever, is a larger dose required.

The numerous adverse effects of corticosteroid therapy are related to the dose and duration of treatment. The most frequent effect is obesity with redistribution of body fat to the trunk and face, resulting in cushingoid faces. With some preparations, salt and water retention lead to edema, hypertension, heart failure in some patients with heart disease, or electrolyte disturbances. Increased susceptibility to infection is a common problem. Glaucoma and cataracts may occur, as may serious emotional disturbances, diabetes mellitus, and osteoporosis. Peptic ulcer disease has long been held to be caused by corticosteroid therapy, but there is little sound evidence to support this impression. Interference with healing of an ulcer, however, is likely, as is delayed healing of any wound. With the small doses often effective in treatment of rheumatoid arthritis, 8 mg. daily or fewer of prednisone, the risk of many of these complications is minimal.

Corticosteroids are also often effective when injected into an inflamed joint. This form of treatment has none of the risks associated with systemic therapy, but the beneficial effect is confined to the treated joint, and the effect is temporary, averaging 2 to 3 weeks. A recently available preparation, triamcinolone hexacetonide, gives significantly longer duration of beneficial effort. The doses of the various preparations vary greatly, and the information supplied by the manufacturer should be followed.

Braces, splints, and traction. As a result of the weakening and stretching of the joint capsule or supporting ligaments, or because of severe destruction of cartilage and bone within the joint, troublesome instability of the joint may be present. This may cause severe pain or result in a joint that is too unstable to function properly. The use of a movable brace to give added support to the joint can be quite helpful at times. They are most often used for support of knees and ankles.

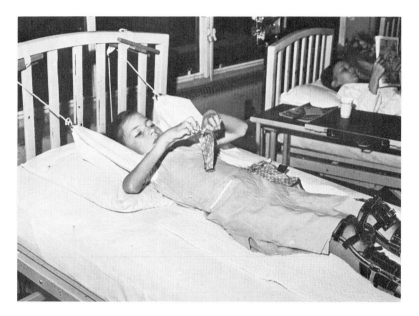

Fig. 6-5. Method of maintaining abduction of arms without interfering with activity of hands.

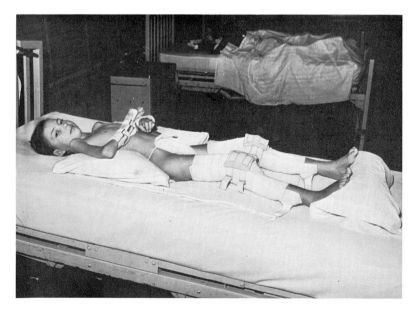

Fig. 6-6. Rest position with pillow under dorsal spine. Adducted position of arms is undesirable for long periods and should be alternated with positions of abduction and external rotation. Note night splints applied with Ace bandages to prevent flexion contractures of the knees. Bars attached at the ankle area prevent rotation of the limbs.

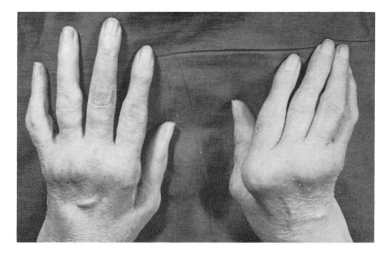

Fig. 6-7. Arthritic hands. Note the enlarged metacarpophalangeal joints and the spindle-shaped fingers that are seen with swelling of the proximal interphalangeal joints. The ulnar deviation of the fingers on the right hand is a common deformity.

During treatment for relief of joint contractures, the use of a rigid support that places a mild, steady stretching force on the contracture is of definite benefit. Such a support is referred to as a splint. Splints are most frequently used on the knees but can be used for contractures of other joints (Figs. 6-5 and 6-6). Splints are also of benefit when used to support an acutely inflamed and painful joint. In this instance the support gives relief of pain and aids in the prevention of a contracture. Recent development of effective rigid splints for support of unstable wrists and knuckle joints of the hands offers promise for effective relief of this difficult problem (Figs. 6-7 and 6-8). Such splints can be worn when working.

Proper application of braces and splints to the extremities is important for their proper function and for the prevention of pain and pressure sores. In this respect the nurse has an important responsibility to the patient using these devices. Early recognition of these problems will prevent unnecessary discomfort or a troublesome complication for the patient. The nurse should become thoroughly familiar with proper use of braces and splints.

Occasionally, when severe contractures are present, traction is used in an attempt to relieve them. This may be applied either to the skin or to the skeleton. A patient in traction

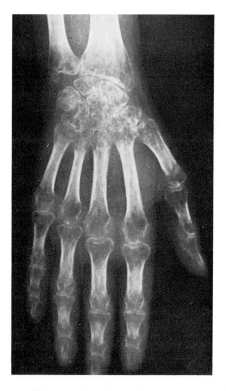

Fig. 6-8. Rheumatoid arthritis showing bone atrophy and narrowing of the joint space. (From Kenney, W. C., and Larson, C. B.: Orthopedics for the general practitioner, St. Louis, 1957, The C. V. Mosby Co.)

requires meticulous nursing care in order to prevent complications. One of the most common is pressure sores resulting from contact with either the bed or the traction apparatus. Because of pain, stiffness, and his resulting reluctance to move, the arthritic patient is quite vulnerable to decubitus ulcers. Therefore, his care requires strict attention to details on the part of the nurse. Important are such simple things as frequent changes in the patient's position in bed, providing at all times clean bed linens that are kept smoothly in place, minor adjustments in the position of the traction apparatus, and protective sponge rubber padding over pressure points when necessary.

Surgery. Surgical treatment of rheumatoid arthritis is indicated in many patients. Operations are performed for removal of swollen synovial tissue in joints around tendons, repair of severely weakened or ruptured ligaments and tendons, and release of severe contractures. Joints that have severe destructive changes may require the insertion of a prosthesis (an artificial joint or joint portion), a repair procedure (arthroplasty) or, at times, bony fusion. The principles and details of nursing care pertaining to both arthritic and orthopedic surgical patients must be applied simultaneously in these patients—sometimes a challenging task.

DEGENERATIVE ARTHRITIS (OSTEOARTHRITIS, DEGENERATIVE JOINT DISEASE)

Degenerative arthritis, as the name implies, is the result of joint deterioration, specifically of the joint cartilage and underlying bone. This process results in varying degrees of joint destruction, but usually not of great severity. The weight-bearing joints of the lower extremities are most often affected and as a rule only one or a few joints are involved. The cause of degenerative arthritis is not known, although there is clearly an association with the aging process of joint cartilage. It is not a systemic disease but is confined to the joint. The onset of this disease is usually during middle or old age.

The major complaint of patients with degenerative arthritis is joint pain upon weight bearing or motion, which is relieved by rest. Frequently there is also stiffness of the involved joint that is relieved by a few minutes or less of activity. The joint may appear to be normal on examination. Frequently, however, there is grating during motion, and there may be bony enlargement. Accumulation of fluid is not uncommon, but the amount is usually not large.

When degenerative arthritis with significant pain has been present for a relatively long period of time, mild to moderate contracture of the joint capsule often occurs along with muscle weakness. This results in limitation of joint motion. Although relatively uncommon, severe joint destruction when it does occur may result in marked limitation of motion and more severe pain.

One of the most common sites of occurrence of degenerative arthritis is in the distal finger joints, those nearest the fingertips. The bony enlargement of these joints has been given the name of Heberden's nodes (Fig. 6-9). The cause for involvement of these small nonweight-bearing joints is unknown. Women are affected approximately twenty times oftener than men, and there is a definite hereditary factor in this form of arthritis. Frequently there are no symp-

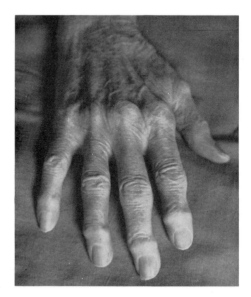

Fig. 6-9. Heberden's nodes. In degenerative arthritis the distal interphalangeal joints may become painful and deformed. (In rheumatoid arthritis the metacarpophalangeal joints and the proximal interphalangeal joints are involved.)

toms. It is not uncommon, however, for these patients to have mild aching pain. Hand function is seldom significantly affected.

The course of degenerative arthritis usually progresses very slowly. The severity of symptoms parallels fairly closely the amount of use of the involved joint. Most patients have mild to moderate restriction of activity, largely because of pain; relatively few patients have severe limitation of physical activity. Rarely will a patient be severely incapacitated because of degenerative arthritis.

Traumatic arthritis is degenerative arthritis occurring in a joint that has been previously injured. The injury may have been in the nature of infection, repeated dislocation, fracture, or another type of arthritis. There is an interval of time, months or even years after the injury, before the degenerative arthritis appears. It may be mild or severe, depending upon the severity of the previous injury and other factors.

Treatment and nursing care. Because degenerative arthritis involves only a few joints, patients with this form of arthritis are usually more easily cared for than those with rheumatoid arthritis. Occasionally patients with severe involvement—for example, of both knees or both hips—will have considerable disability. The presence of other diseases affecting their general health may cause, in conjunction with their arthritis, disability more severe than would result from the arthritis alone. In patients with heart disease that limits physical endurance, the presence of moderately severe degenerative arthritis in a hip or knee may cause walking to be much more laborious with the result that endurance is further reduced. Very often patients with this form of arthritis are elderly and may require modification of care and treatment routines.

The basic principles of treatment are the same for degenerative arthritis as for rheumatoid arthritis, including rest, relief of pain, and physical therapy. Because degenerative arthritis is not a systemic disease, these patients require no more bed rest or sleep than if they did not have arthritis. Rest of the involved joints, however, is very desirable because it provides for relief of pain. Usually this can be accomplished by resting in a chair. Some patients, however,

must lie down for relief of pain, especially when the hips are involved. Frequent interruption of activity with short rest periods is much more effective than occasional long periods of rest.

The need for medication to relieve pain is usually not great. Two or three aspirin tablets three or four times daily usually is sufficient. At times, when aspirin alone is not adequate, the addition of phenylbutazone or indomethacin for a 5- to 10-day period is often helpful. The other drugs used in the treatment of rheumatoid arthritis have no value in this disease. Specifically, steroids, the cortisone-like drugs, should never be given orally. Injection of a steroid into a joint with troublesome pain, however, is frequently helpful in relieving symptoms. The same doses are used as in rheumatoid arthritis.

A large proportion of patients with degenerative arthritis are cared for in the home. Mild degrees of the condition are very common among the population beyond middle age. These persons will usually be hospitalized only when reconstructive surgery is necessary, although they may enter the hospital briefly for corset or brace fittings or for periods of physical therapy.

The health supervision the nurse can give in the home may be an important detail. Health supervision will include attention to details for improvement of the patient's posture and general habits of working, sitting, and standing. Constant sitting, for a patient with degenerative arthritis of hip or spine, is a bad practice. It often leads to flexion contractures of hips, adduction of hips, and a tendency toward dorsal kyphosis. Within the limits of the patient's tolerance, activity is to be encouraged. A person with this kind of arthritis is not one who should be encouraged to assume a life of idleness or a sedentary occupation when other activity is possible.

If shoe corrections have been prescribed, nurses should check frequently to see that these do not become worn down and useless. Shoe corrections provide support and comfort to pronated feet, which are common in this condition, and they may have a great deal to do with improvement in posture. If a brace or corset has been ordered, frequent inspection of the apparatus and supervision of its application are important. If postural exercises have been prescribed, the nurse should have a full understanding of these in order to assist and encourage the patient in their performance.

Another point of importance in which the nurse may play an important role is that of giving reassurance. Worry is not an uncommon feature encountered in patients having this condition. They should be brought to understand that degenerative arthritis does not tend to cause rigid joints and that it does not go from one joint to the other as does rheumatoid arthritis. When the patient understands this, a great burden is sometimes lifted from his mind, particularly if he has a secret fear of becoming a helpless cripple, having perhaps seen a friend or relative crippled with rheumatism.

Physical therapy plays an important role in the treatment of this form of arthritis. The objectives are the same as in rheumatoid arthritis. This aspect of the treatment program is a major factor in preventing increasing disability by maintaining muscle strength.

Local treatment may consist of heat, best given in the form of hot packs applied to the affected joints and adjacent painful muscles. Therapeutic exercise to strengthen muscles and improve joint motion should be done in most cases following the application of heat.

The use of a cane or crutches is often helpful in relieving pain by decreasing the amount of weight borne by the joint. Contractures causing limitations of joint motion are not uncommon. Frequently contractures can be greatly improved with exercises and, at times, night splints. Occasionally surgery will be required. Marked joint destruction associated with severe pain or limited motion, or both, may require surgical treatment. This is usually in the form of an arthroplasty, a repair of the joint.

GOUTY ARTHRITIS

Gout is a disease resulting from the abnormal metabolism of uric acid. In gout there is an increase in the amount of uric acid in the body, which is reflected in an increase in its concentration in the blood. The clinical picture of gout is characterized by this elevation of blood uric acid concentration along with recurrent attacks of acute, severely painful arthritis. In some patients with gout, deposits of uric acid known as tophi occur in various places in the body (Figs. 6-10 and 6-11). Approximately 95% of the patients with gout are men. There is no doubt of an hereditary factor in this disease. In approximately one-half of the cases a history of gout in family members can be obtained. The age of onset, determined by the first attack of acute gouty arthritis, is usually between 20 and 60 years of age.

The typical acute attack of gout begins rather

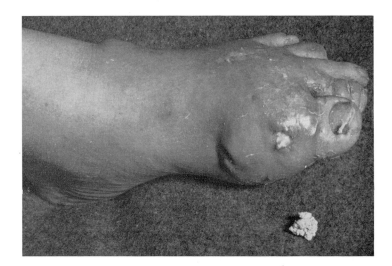

Fig. 6-10. Gouty arthritis with involvement of the first metatarsophalangeal joint, urate crystals, and a draining sinus from a large tophus.

abruptly. There is severe constant pain and the joint becomes swollen and red. The usual attack lasts for 3 to 10 days when untreated.

For unknown reasons the large joint of the great toe is involved much more commonly than any other joint. Other joints in the foot, the ankle, and the knee are also commonly affected. Any joint in the body, however, may be involved.

The course of gout is quite variable, ranging from one or a few attacks during a lifetime to a progressively severe disease with marked crippling, when untreated, in some patients. Most patients, however, fall between these two extremes. With proper treatment attacks of acute gout are infrequent and crippling deformities do not occur.

Treatment and nursing care. Few patients with gout require hospitalization for orthopedic treatment. Medications are available that are very effective in controlling the disease. Colchicine is the traditional drug of choice for treatment of the acute attack. It is given in the dose of one tablet (either 0.5 or 0.65 mg.) every hour until the attack improves; until nausea, vomiting, or diarrhea occurs; or until a total dose of twelve tablets has been taken. Relief of the attack is almost always striking. Phenylbutazone is equally effective for relief of the acute attack, or it may be combined with colchicine in a stubborn attack. It is given in a dose of 600 to 800 mg. on the first day, followed by reducing doses for 3 to 5 days. Indomethacin may be used in a similar fashion, beginning with 400 to 600 mg. on the first day.

Colchicine is also important for prevention of recurrent attacks, and the dose is usually two or three tablets daily. Probenecid (Benemid) is an equally important drug used in the treatment of gout. Its function is to increase excretion of uric acid by the kidney, reducing the total amount of this substance in the body. It has no effect on the acute attack of gout. For it to be effective, probenecid must be taken regularly, every day.

Allopurinol is another drug that is effective in reducing the concentration of uric acid in the body. Its mechanism of action is that of decreasing the production of uric acid in the body, a mechanism quite different from that of probenecid. Allopurinol, too, must be taken regularly in three or four daily doses for maximum effectiveness.

Severe dietary restriction, once a standard

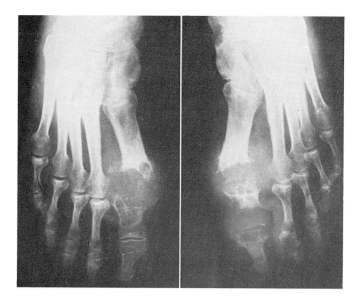

Fig. 6-11. Gout. Note the predilection for involvement of the first metatarsophalangeal joint. (From Kenney, W. C., and Larson, C. B.: Orthopedics for the general practitioner, St. Louis, 1957, The C. V. Mosby Co.)

part of the treatment program, is no longer advocated because it does not contribute greatly to reducing the amount of uric acid in the body. Avoidance of foods high in purine content—such as liver, kidney, sweetbreads, sardines, anchovies, and meat gravies—is a reasonable measure.

When properly treated, gout rarely causes deforming arthritis. The untreated or inadequately treated patient, however, may develop a variety of deformities and contractures of joints. In addition, there may be severe destruction of multiple joints in the late stages of chronic gouty arthritis. These problems require the same principles of treatment and nursing care as those in other forms of arthritis.

STUDY QUESTIONS

1. What is the basic objective in the care and treatment of a patient with arthritis? What are the roles of the various people who may be involved in the patient's care?
2. What are the principles that guide the nurse in her care of a patient with arthritis?
3. What is the fundamental difference between rheumatoid arthritis and degenerative arthritis?
4. What are the basic ingredients of a treatment program for a patient with arthritis?
5. To what details of care and arrangement of the patient's bed must the nurse give attention? What is the objective?
6. What are the two ways in which rest is beneficial to a patient with rheumatoid arthritis? How does this differ in a patient with degenerative arthritis?
7. Contractures are to a large degree preventable. What important contributions can be made by the nurse in this regard?
8. The patient with arthritis who lives within the limitations imposed by his disease does better than those who do not. How may the nurse help the patient to adopt this attitude?

REFERENCES

Abruzzo, J. L.: Rheumatoid arthritis: reflections on etiology and pathogenesis, Arch. Phys. Med. Rehabil. **52:**30-39, 1971.

Ansell, B. M., and Bywaters, E. G. L.: Rheumatoid arthritis (Still's disease), Pediatr. Clin. North Am. **10:**921-939, 1963.

Ball, B., moderator: Helping patients adjust to rheumatoid arthritis, Nursing '72 **2:**11-17, 1972.

Barckley, V., Bettinger, A., Guenther, L., and Ross, R.: Arthritis and a narrow perspective do not mix, Nurs. Outlook **6:**638-639, 1958.

Besson, P. B., and McDermott, W., editors: Cecil-Loeb textbook of medicine, ed. 13, vols. 1 and 2, Philadelphia, 1971, W. B. Saunders Co.

Bergersen, B. S.: Pharmacology in nursing, ed. 12, St. Louis, 1973, The C. V. Mosby Co.

Brassell, M. P., Schaal, F. M., Rossky, E. G., and Spergel, P.: Helping patients adjust to rheumatoid arthritis, Nursing '72 **2:**11-17, 1972.

Brewer, E. J.: Rheumatoid arthritis in childhood, Am. J. Nurs. **65:**66-71, 1965.

Bryan, R. S., guest editor: Symposium on rheumatoid arthritis, Orthop. Clin. North Am. **2:**600-771, 1971.

Campbell, E. B., Hogsed, C. M., and Bogdonoff, M.: Lupus erythematosus, Am. J. Nurs. **62:**74-77, 1962.

Dixon A.: Progress in clinical rheumatology, Boston, 1969, The Williams & Wilkins Company.

Flatt, A. E.: The care of the rheumatoid hand, St. Louis, ed. 2, 1968, The C. V. Mosby Co.

Giest, H.: The psychological aspects of rheumatoid arthritis, Springfield, Ill., 1966, Charles C Thomas, Publisher.

Grahame, R.: Rheumatoid disease 1, Clinical aspects, Nurs. Times **67:**664-667, 1971.

Grahame, R.: Rheumatoid disease 2, Caring for patients, Nurs. Times **67:**701-704, 1971.

Harris, R.: Plaster splints for rheumatoid arthritis. In Licht, S., and Kamenetz, H. L., editors: Orthotics etcetera, New Haven, 1966, Elizabeth Licht, Publisher.

Henry, J. B., and Pinals, R. S.: Evaluation of tests for rheumatoid factor, Postgrad. Med. 48:49-52, **1970.**

Hermann, I., and Smith, R.,: Gout and gouty arthritis, Am. J. Nurs. **64:**111-113, 1964.

Hollander, J. L., editor: Arthritis and allied conditions, ed. 7, Philadelphia, 1966, Lea & Febiger.

Holt, P. J. L.: Surgery in rheumatoid arthritis 1, Nurs. Times **65:**1393-1395, 1969.

Holt, P. J. L.: Surgery in rheumatoid arthritis 2, Nurs. Times **65:**1417-1418, 1969.

Jaschik, E., and Olsen, C.: Nursing care of the arthritic patient at home, Am. J. Nurs. **55:**429-432, 1955.

Knapp, M.: Ankylosing spondylitis, Postgrad. Med. **43:**231-233, 1968.

Knapp, M.: Rheumatoid arthritis, Postgrad. Med. **42:**A99-A104, 1967.

Lamont-Havers, R. W.: Abthritis quackery, Am. J. Nurs. **63:**92-95, 1963.

Larson, C. B., Flatt, A. and Cooper, R. R.: Surgery for the arthritic patient, J. Am. Phys. Ther. Ass. **44:**604-619, 1964.

Lockie, L. M.: How to recognize and treat gout, Postgrad. Med. **43:**98-101, 1968.

Lockie, L. M.: Current evaluation of drugs for treating arthritis, Postgrad. Med. **49:**100-104, 1971.

Loxley, A. K.: The emotional toll of crippling deformity, Am. J. Nurs. **72:**1839-1840, 1972.

Management of arthritis, Postgrad. Med. **51:** entire issue, May, 1972.

Marmor, L.: Hand surgery in rheumatoid arthritis, Arthritis Rheum. **5:**419-427, 1962.

Marmor, L.: Surgery of rheumatoid arthritis, Philadelphia, 1967, Lea & Febiger.

Mayer, J.: Nutrition and gout, Postgrad. Med. **45:**277-278, 1969.

Newton, M.: Surgery in arthritis of the lower extremity, Surg. Clin. North Am. **45:**201-215, 1965.

Nickel, V., Kristy, J., and McDaniel, L.: Physical therapy for rheumatoid arthritis, Phys. Ther. **45:**198-204, 1965.

Primer on the rheumatic diseases, prepared by a committee of the American Rheumatism Association, J.A.M.A. **190:**127-140, 425-444, 509-530, 741-751, 1964.

Rheumatic diseases, Postgrad. Med. **45:** special issue, Jan., 1969.

Rheumatoid arthritis, Med. Clin. North Am. **52:** entire issue, May, 1968.

Rheumatoid arthritis; Parts 1 and 2, Physiotherapy **56:** Sept. and Oct., 1970.

Robinson, W. D.: Rheumatoid arthritis. In Beeson, P.D., and McDermott, W., editors: Cecil-Loeb textbook of medicine, ed. 13, Philadelphia, 1971, W. B. Saunders Co.

Rodman, M. I. Drugs for rheumatic disorders, RN **31:**55-66, 1968.

Seegmiller, J. E. Goals in gout, Postgrad. Med. **45:**99-103, 1969.

Shafer, K., Sawyer, J. R., McCluskey, A. M., Beck, E., and Phipps, W. J.: Medical-surgical nursing, ed. 5, St. Louis, 1971, The C. V. Mosby Co.

Simmons, E. H., and Brown, M. E.: Surgery for kyphosis in ankylosing spondylitis, Canad. Nurse **68:**24-29, 1972.

Smyth, C.: New drugs for arthritis, Postgrad. Med. **44:**77-85, 1968.

Suppes, F. T., Moskowitz, R. W., Lockie, L. M., and Hollander, J. L.: Arthritis, Postgrad. Med. **47:**160-167, 1970.

U. S. Department of Health, Education, and Welfare in collaboration with the Arthritis and Rheumatism Foundation: Strike back at arthritis, Washington, D. C., 1960, Public Health Service Publication no. 747.

Walike, B., Mammor, L. and Upshaw, M. J.: Rheumatoid arthritis, Am. J. Nurs. **67:**1420-1433, 1967.

Williams. R.: Osteoarthritis and rheumatic disease, Postgrad. Med. **42:**334-338, 1967.

7

Bone tumors

Three types of tumors occur in bone: (1) benign (nonmalignant), (2) malignant, and (3) metastatic from other tissues or organs. The benign type grows slowly and does not tend to destroy surrounding tissues or spread to other parts of the body through the bloodstream or lymphatic system. This includes osteocartilaginous exostosis, enchondroma, chondroblastoma, hemangioma, osteoid osteoma, and giant cell tumor (Figs. 7-1 to 7-3).

A malignant tumor (sarcoma) is usually rapid in growth and may be of considerable size before it is recognized by the patient. It often spreads to other parts of the body through the bloodstream before it is brought to the attention of a surgeon.

Tumors metastatic from cancer of other tissues, such as the breast, prostate, lung, kidney, or thyroid, are quite common because bone marrow has a rich blood supply and cancer cells are easily spread through the bloodstream.

BENIGN TUMORS

Generally, the cause is not known for all types of benign tumors. Some of the benign tumors are thought to be aberrations of the growth and development of tissues. The osteocartilaginous exostosis is considered to be caused by displacement of cartilage cells at the epiphyseal plate. As bone growth takes place, the displaced cells cause enlargement near the ends of long bones that may be bumped easily because of their prominence. Some patients may have exostoses of many bones. At times malignant change takes place in one of these tumors. All of the other benign tumors have little or no visible external manifestations because they are confined within bone.

The symptoms in these patients are generally mild pain in the affected bone or prominence, as in the patient with an exostosis. The diagnosis is made with the aid of roentgenograms and surgical biopsy.

Treatment is simple removal, excision, or curettage. Therefore, the nursing care involves routine postoperative management of a patient in a plaster dressing or soft bandages.

MALIGNANT TUMORS

Most bone sarcomas are classified according to the type of tissue formed by the malignant cells; examples are osteosarcoma (Fig. 7-4), fibrosarcoma, chondrosarcoma, hemangiosarcoma, and round cell sarcomas (Ewing's sarcoma, reticulum cell sarcoma, and multiple myeloma, Fig. 7-5). As is true for benign tumors, the cause is generally not known. Certain preexisting conditions, such as Paget's disease of bone, may cause bone sarcoma to develop. At times irradiation therapy given for nonmalignant lesions may induce malignant tumors after a latent period of several years or more.

Diagnosis and treatment. A history of intermittent pain that is particularly troublesome at night, tiredness, a limp, and swelling of a part of an extremity without previous trauma or obvious infection may lead one to suspect a tumor (Fig. 7-6). Such a combination of symptoms requires immediate medical attention. Sometimes the parent will belittle the symptoms as being the result of some recent fall or trauma. The patient frequently looks deceptively well when admitted to the hospital for the first time. The night pain may increase in severity. Roentgenograms are a helpful adjunct to proper diagnosis. In certain of the bone sarcomas,

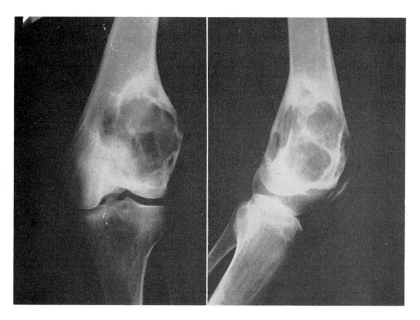

Fig. 7-1. Giant cell tumor (osteoclastoma). It is usually benign but difficult to differentiate from certain malignant osteogenic sarcomas even after biopsy. Characteristically, these tumors expand the shaft, show little bone reaction, involve the epiphyses of the long bones, and seldom break into a joint cavity. (From Kenney, W. C., and Larson, C. B.: Orthopedics for the general practitioner, St. Louis, 1957, The C. V. Mosby Co.)

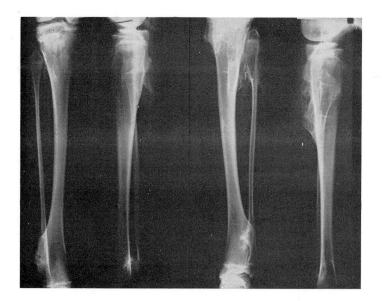

Fig. 7-2. Multiple cartilaginous exostoses. These exostoses are capped by cartilage that tends to mature when normal epiphyses close. The tumors are familial and benign but can produce symptoms if mechanically injured. Rarely (after incomplete surgical removal or with repeated trauma) they may become malignant. (From Kenney, W. C., and Larson, C. B.: Orthopedics for the general practitioner, St. Louis, 1957, The C. V. Mosby Co.)

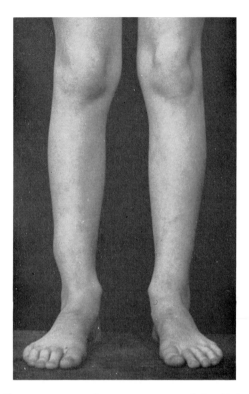

Fig. 7-3. Osteocartilaginous exostosis of the fibula. Note enlargement of lower end of the right leg. This tumor is painless unless bumped.

laboratory work is of value. For instance, osteosarcomas tend to produce a high alkaline phosphatase in the blood serum. Because the treatment and prognosis of bone sarcoma vary with the type of tumor, a surgical biopsy is the surest way to establish an accurate diagnosis. A roentgenogram of the chest will help to determine whether or not obvious metastases are present in the lungs. Metastases, however, may not be visible at the time of the initial examination but may be manifested after treatment has been instituted.

The treatment of malignant bone tumors is surgical removal either by wide local resection (when it is both technically feasible and consistent with conservation of function) or by amputation. In the upper extremity it is more frequently possible to perform a local resection without amputation or disarticulation. In the lower extremity when tumors are present near the knee joint, function is usually better after amputation and the use of an artificial limb. At the midshaft of the femur and the upper end of the femur, resection and replacement either with a metallic prosthesis or an intramedullary rod with supplementary bone transplants may provide function without sacrificing the extremity. When metastasis can be demonstrated,

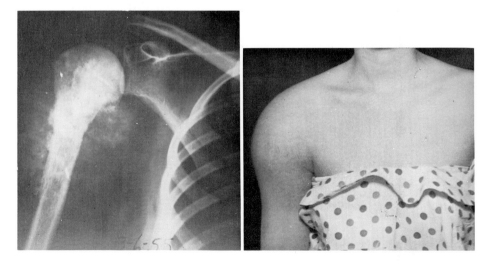

Fig. 7-4. Osteogenic sarcoma of the humerus. This is a primary malignant tumor of bone. It occurs in late childhood or in young adults and is usually located in a long bone near the end of the diaphysis. Early symptoms are severe pain and swelling. This type of bone lesion metastasizes early and the prognosis is poor. Treatment consists of amputation or extensive local resection, and in some instances roentgen therapy is advised.

as in the chest, surgical removal of the original tumor obviously will not cure the patient, but it may be necessary, to control pain and to prevent the local tumor from becoming an ulcerated, fungating, foul-smelling mass.

X-ray irradiation or radioactive cobalt irradiation will be used in patients in whom the tumor is radiosensitive. Some tumors, such as Ewing's sarcoma (Fig. 7-7), can be controlled for many months by this treatment. Reticulum cell sarcoma may be cured by this method. Irradiation is often helpful to relieve pain in tumors even though it may not be curative. In the far advanced stages of malignant bone disease and in tumors from other parts of the body that have metastasized to bone, drugs have been and are being tried in an effort to find one that might control the growth of the tumor cells.

METASTATIC TUMORS

Tumor that is metastatic to bone from cancer of other tissues is the most common tumor found in bone. It usually occurs in patients over 40 years of age when cancers of the breast, prostate, intestinal organs, lungs, and other tissues are most common. The cancer deposit is most frequently found in those bones rich in red marrow such as the spine, pelvis, and ribs (Fig. 7-8). As a rule this site of deposit is the cause of pain, but occasionally the first indication of bone involvement comes when a fracture occurs as a result of some trivial accident. Compression fractures of the spine are common when cancer cells have weakened the structure of the bones of the vertebrae, or there may be pathologic fractures of the hip, shoulder, or pelvis. Proper diagnosis of the type of cancer is essential to proper treatment. Therefore, one needs information afforded by the roentgenogram and, if it is possible to obtain tissue from the metastasis, the histologic diagnosis. In certain locations needle biopsy may be necessary rather than an open surgical biopsy. Metastases from breast or prostate may be controlled for variable periods

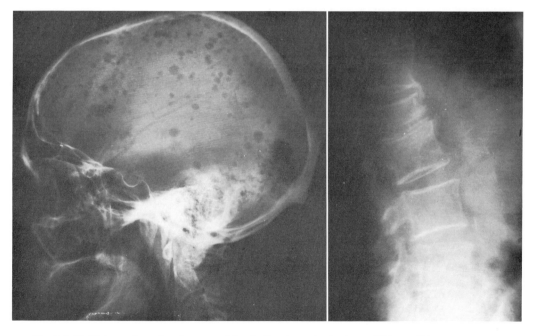

Fig. 7-5. Multiple myeloma involvement of the skull and vertebral column. This condition occurs in an older age group (40 to 60 years) and most commonly involves the axial skeleton (skull, vertebrae, sternum, and ribs). Roentgenograms of involved bone reveal punched-out areas. Multiple myeloma begins in the medullary cavity, is malignant, and can progress rapidly. Pain from pathologic fracture may be the first symptom, or pain in the back region may cause the individual to seek medical care. Bence Jones protein when found in the urine is diagnostic of multiple myeloma. Irradiation of involved areas is often helpful and drug therapy may have a palliative effect. The prognosis, however, is not favorable.

of time by the use of hormones, but in most instances X-ray irradiation and analgesic drugs are necessary for control of pain.

Nursing care. Nursing care of patients with malignant bone tumors does not differ greatly from the care given to a patient with malignancy of any part of the body. Very few of the

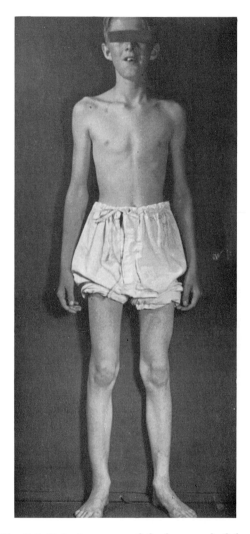

Fig. 7-6. Ewing's sarcoma of the lower end of the right fibula. This type of tumor usually occurs during the early "teen" years, is of medullary origin, and develops in the shaft portion of the long bones. Many times the patient has a history of trauma to the area. Symptoms usually consist of pain and tenderness, fever may be present, and laboratory studies reveal a leukocytosis. Response to irradiation is usually favorable for a period of time; then metastasis occurs. The prognosis for life with this type of tumor is poor.

features will be unfamiliar to the orthopedic nurse experienced in the care of bone infections. The postoperative care of patients who have had amputations or disarticulations will correspond to that of patients with amputations for any cause. If a local resection has been performed, the patient undoubtedly will be in a plaster dressing and the care is the same as that for one in a plaster cast. The real problem develops in patients who have had local recurrence or metastases from the original bone tumor.

The prognosis for these patients is poor. One watches week by week the local and general progress of malignant disease. The patient's own outlook at first is hopeful. Whether or not amputation takes place, he usually displays early desire and determination to get well. Since he presumably knows little about the moribund nature of the disease, one wonders sometimes at the gradual change that comes about in the morale. Consciously or unconsciously, these patients seem to know the outcome. It has been said that the attitude of parents, visiting friends, and even nurses toward the patient tells him the whole story quite clearly. This is probably not entirely true. But there is enough truth in it so that the nurse needs to help his relatives understand the necessity for self-control in the presence of the patient. This is a stern lesson but an important one, and it is just as important for the nurse to learn it as for parents and the other relatives.

False hope must not be given the cancer patient and his family. Providing for comfort measures and helping the patient realize that pain can be controlled may relieve some of his fear and concern about the future. Assistance in planning for home care may lessen anxieties and provide for a happier situation. The nurse who is able to help the patient cope with problems day by day as they arise is offering the cancer patient a reassuring and helpful relationship.

Splinting of the extremity may be done to prevent pain or injury to the affected part. The chance of pathologic fracture occurring at or near the site of the tumor is to be kept in mind, for very little trauma or manipulation is necessary to bring about such fractures. This should be remembered during the bed-making process or when the patient is being turned, and especially if he is allowed out of bed. In the latter case he should be carefully protected against bumps or falls. Fracture may occur from a relatively trivial mishap, and complaints of pain in the area may be considered due to the lesion unless the nurse is vigilant in observation.

Symptoms that the nurse should recognize as particularly indicative of progress of the disease are signs of chest involvement, since the chest is the most common site of metastasis.

Coughing, pain in the chest, and expectoration of blood are serious and should be reported immediately.

Radiation therapy. Although not curative, radiation therapy is helpful in the treatment of some types of bone malignancy. Cancer cells are destroyed and relief of pain may be apparent early in the course of treatment. When radiation therapy is prescribed, instructions should be sought from the radiologist regarding the

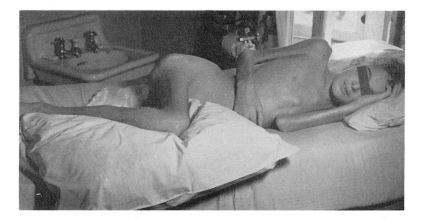

Fig. 7-7. Ewing's sarcoma, terminal stage.

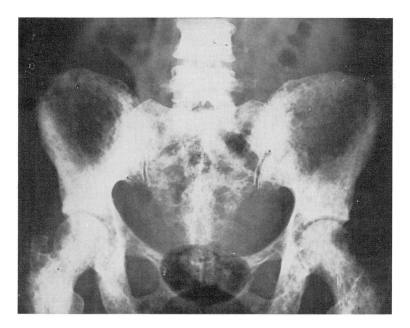

Fig. 7-8. Carcinoma of the breast, metastastic to bone. Solitary metastases usually are to the vertebrae or femur. The more common type of lesion is osteolytic, but occasional cases show bone formation and resemble metastatic carcinoma of the prostate. (From Kenney, W. C., and Larson, C. B.: Orthopedics for the general practitioner, St. Louis, 1957, The C. V. Mosby Co.)

patient's care. Marks on the skin made with an indelible pen indicate the area to be treated, and these should not be washed off. It is important that the skin area involved be protected from trauma such as friction caused by harsh linens or tight garments. The use of soap or lotion on the area is omitted. Adhesive tape applied to hold a dressing in place is very traumatizing to the sensitive skin and should be avoided. Sunbathing is not permitted, since the patient's skin at this time is particularly sensitive to light. The application of either heat or cold is, also, contraindicated. In some instances the patient receiving radiation therapy can be made more comfortable and his skin protected by placing him on a square of sheepskin. This is particularly true if he is emaciated and unable to be out of bed. If breaks in the skin do occur, the physician should be informed of the problem, and any ointment prescribed should be applied to a surgical dressing, which is placed on the involved area. Rubbing of the skin is avoided. As treatment progresses, changes in the skin become apparent. Helping the patient understand that the redness (erythema), the scaling (desquamation), and the crusting are expected may help to lessen his concern about the treatments he is receiving. Maintaining adequate nutrition for the patient with a malignancy can be a very real nursing problem. It is important that his food intake include vitamins, proteins, and other blood-building foods to counteract the advancing anemia. The patient's appetite is frequently poor, and there is the added fact that radiation treatment may cause nausea and vomiting. An anorexia diet may help, and sometimes frequent small meals are tolerated better than the usual three. Drugs that help to combat nausea may relieve some of the discomfort and thus help the patient maintain an adequate intake of food and fluid. Complete blood counts at fairly frequent intervals are ordered for the patient receiving radiation therapy. A white blood count may be taken daily. Subsidiary personnel are usually assigned to transport the patient to and from the radiation therapy department. These individuals need to understand both that a patient who is receiving radiation therapy to a bone lesion may have severe pain with movement and that pathologic fractures may occur. Gentleness and proper support are necessary when the patient is being transferred from cart to bed and vice versa.

Antineoplastic drugs. A few of the antineoplastic drugs have been used in treating certain malignant bone lesions. These drugs have not been curative but, in some instances, have had a palliative effect. The antimetabolites are chemical compounds that interfere with the utilization of essential metabolites, thus interrupting cell growth. One example of this type of drug is 5-fluorouracil (5-FU). The alkylating agents slow the growth of cells by reacting with molecules within the malignant cell. These drugs are toxic to healthy cells as well as to cancerous cells. Mechlorethamine (nitrogen mustard) is an example of this kind of drug. Route of administration varies with the agent. Some may be given by mouth, other by infusion, and some by arterial perfusion. Careful observation of the patient receiving antineoplastic drugs is necessary to detect early signs of toxic reaction or any physical discomfort the patient may be experiencing.

STUDY QUESTIONS

1. Differentiate between malignant and benign bone tumors. List several benign tumors.
2. Review symptoms, diagnostic procedures, and treatment as they relate to Ewing's sarcoma, osteosarcoma, multiple myeloma, and metastatic bone lesions.
3. Discuss nursing care of the patient receiving radiation therapy to a metastatic lesion of the spine.
4. Review complications that the patient with a metastatic bone lesion may encounter.
5. List several primary cancerous lesions that frequently metastasize to bone.

REFERENCES

Barckley, V.: The crisis in cancer. Am. J. Nurs. **67:**278-280, 1967.

Barckley, V.: What can I say to the cancer patient? Nurs. Outlook **6:**316-318, 1958.

Bergersen, B. S.: Pharmacology in nursing, ed. 12, St. Louis, 1973, The C. V. Mosby Co.

Blair, S.: Tumors of bones and muscles of the lower extremities, Surg. Clin. North Am. **45:**247-259, 1965.

Bouchard, R., and Owens, N. F.: Nursing care of the cancer patient, ed. 2, St. Louis, 1972, The C. V. Mosby Co.

Bright, F., and France, Sister M. L.: The nurse and the terminally ill child, Nurs. Outlook **15:**39-42, 1967.

Brindley, H., Murray, R., and Pisar, D.: Management of metastatic lesions of bone. Part I. Orthopedic and radiotherapeutic aspects, Postgrad. Med. **39:**535-539, 1966.

1968 Cancer facts and figures, New York, 1969, American Cancer Society, Inc.

Edwards, P.: Regional cancer chemotherapy, Canad. Nurse **63:**41-43, 1967.

Ellison, R.: Treating cancer with antimetabolites, Am. J. Nurs. **62:**79-82, 1962.

Ferguson, A.: Orthopaedic surgery in infancy and childhood, ed. 3, Baltimore, 1968, The Williams & Wilkins Co.

Fox, J. E.: Reflections on cancer nursing, Am. J. Nurs. **66:**1317-1319, 1966.

Fox, S. A., and Bernhardt, L. C.: Target: cancer. Chemotherapy via intra-arterial infusion, Am. J. Nurs. **66:**1966-1968, 1966.

Henderson, I. W. D.: Current status of cancer chemotherapy, Canad. Nurse **63:**37-40, 1967.

Hoffman, E.: Don't give up on me! Am. J. Nurs. **71:**60-62, 1971.

Jacobs, P.: Tumours of bone, Nursing Times **68:**1572-1375, 1972.

Karnofsky, D. A.: Cancer quackery: its causes, recognition and prevention, Am. J. Nurs. **59:**496-500, 1959.

Leach, R. E., and Torgerson, W. R.: The management of metastatic disease in the skeletal system, Surg. Clin. North Am. **47:**757-767, 1967.

Levine, L.: Intra-arterial chemotherapy, Am. J. Nurs. **64:**108-110, 1964.

Lichtenstein, L.: Bone tumors, ed. 4, St. Louis 1972, The C. V. Mosby Co.

Livingston, B. M.: How clinical progress is made in cancer chemotherapy research, Am. J. Nurs. **67:**2547-2554, 1967.

Livingston, B. M., and Krakoff, I. H.: L-asparaginase, a new type of anticancer drug, Am. J. Nurs. **70:**1910-1915, 1970.

Mangen, Sister F. X.: Psychological aspects of nursing the advanced cancer patient, Nurs. Clin. North Amer. **2:**649-658, 1967.

McKinnie C.: Multiple myeloma, Am. J. Nurs. **63:**99-102, 1963.

McLeod, M.: Osteogenic carcinoma, Canad. Nurse **60:**49-52, 1964.

Meinhart, N. T.: The cancer patient: living in the here and now, Nurs. Outlook **16:**64-69, 1968.

Mercer, W., and Duthie, R. B.: Orthopedic surgery, ed. 6, Baltimore, 1964, The Williams & Wilkins Co.

Nowak, P.: Nursing care in isolation perfusion, Am. J. Nurs. **64:**85-88, 1964.

Raney, R. B., and Brashear, H. R.: Shand's handbook of orthopaedic surgery, ed. 8, St. Louis, 1971, The C. V. Mosby Co.

Rhoads, P. S.: Management of the patient with terminal illness, J.A.M.A. **192:**661-665, 1965.

Rogers, A.: Pain and the cancer patient, Nurs. Clin. North Am. **2:**671-682, 1967.

Rosenthal, D., and Moloney, W. C.: Treating multiple myeloma, Postgrad. Med. **44:**143-148, 1968.

Ross, E. K.: What is it like to be dying? Am. J. Nurs. **71:**54-61, 1971.

Shafer, K., Sawyer, J. R., McCluskey, A. M., Beck, E., and Phipps, W. J.: Medical-Surgical nursing, ed. 5, St. Louis, 1971, The C. V. Mosby Co.

Smith, S.: Drugs and cancer, Nurs. Times **63:**283-284, 1967.

Thomas, B.: Nursing care of patients with cancer of the bone, Nurs. Clin. North Am. **2:**459-471, 1967.

Welsh, M. S.: Comfort measures during radiation therapy, Am. J. Nurs. **67:**1880-1882, 1967.

Wessels, F., Bonnet, J., and Palmer, R.: Management of metastatic lesions of bone; Part II. Chemotherapeutic aspects. Postgrad. Med. **39:**576-581, 1966.

8

Infections of bones and joints

OSTEOMYELITIS AND SEPTIC ARTHRITIS

OSTEOMYELITIS

Osteomyelitis is of three types: (1) acute infectious osteomyelitis, (2) acute localized osteomyelitis, and (3) chronic osteomyelitis.

Cause. Acute infectious osteomyelitis is usually caused by pyogenic bacteria that reach the bone through the bloodstream. Most common is the *Staphylococcus*. The *Streptococcus* is the next most common. Other organisms that may cause the disease are the pneumococcus, typhoid bacillus, colon bacillus, gas bacillus, gonococcus, tubercle bacillus, and the *Actinomyces, Coccidioides, Echinococcus,* and *Spirochaeta pallida.*

The virulence of the organism frequently determines the severity of the disease. In some instances, especially when the infective agent is the *Staphylococcus* or *Streptococcus,* the disease may be of the violent fulminating type and death may occur within 24 or 48 hours after onset of the infection. Young children are most often affected with the systemic type, and those areas of the body most subject to trauma are the ones most frequently involved.

In acute localized osteomyelitis the infection often results from compound fractures or penetrating wounds into the bone. Such infections are rarely virulent and are not usually accompanied by a general reaction in the entire affected bone, as is seen in metastatic infections.

Chronic osteomyelitis occurs in the person whose body has built up considerable resistance to the particular type of organism causing the infection. It is characterized by intermittent exacerbations of pain and inflammation—usually brought on by an attempt to throw off sequestra.

The etiology of osteomyelitis presents some factors important to nurses in their health teaching. It is, of course, a well recognized fact that compound injuries of bone may lead to osteomyelitis, but what is not always so well understood is that any lowering of the resistance or integrity of the tissue may predispose toward the disease. The body's resistance being lowered by exposure, fatigue, malnutrition, or infected tonsils and teeth seems to be a definite factor in the etiology. Bruises, blisters, deep slivers or splinters, impetigo, sties of the eyelids—all are given consideration as possible etiologic agents by writers on this subject. Any type of skin lesion deserves careful attention. When teaching the patients, the nurse should seek to make it understood that a child with extensive skin abrasions should not be allowed to resume normal athletic activities until the lesions are healed. Blisters on the heel—very common disturbances in the life of young people—should be carefully disinfected and protected from the irritating shoe by felt pads. This cannot be overemphasized. A history of boils is a common feature in osteomyelitis and these deserve medical attention. Remember that the *Staphylococcus,* chief organism in the common boil, is the same *Staphylococcus* that is a cause of the more serious osteomyelitis. It must also be remembered that persons with extensive boils carry the same phage type of *Staphylococcus* in their nose in 80% to 90% of the cases; eradication of the boils cannot be expected unless local chemotherapy is applied to the anterior nares.

Pathology. Acute osteomyelitis usually begins at the end of the long bones, where there is the greatest number of blood vessels. The disease is usually caused by the combination of two factors: (1) local selectivity resulting from trauma and (2) metastatic infection from some remote source of focal infection in the body.

After the bacteria are implanted in the bone, they grow and cause pressure and destruction of bone. The pressure serves to spread the infection (Fig. 8-1), which finally breaks through the bone surface and produces elevation of the periosteum. Most of the circulation to the bone enters through the periosteum, and the stripping effect of pus under pressure cuts off circulation to the bone. Death of the bone occurs. The periosteum maintains its circulation and under this stimulation tends to grow and lay down new bone, forming the characteristic involucrum (Fig. 8-2). This involucrum may extend part of the way along the shaft or along the entire dis-tance of the shaft. Within this involucrum of newly formed bone, the dead bone (sequestrum) becomes completely detached and must either be removed by surgery or gradually work its own way out by abscess and sinus formation.

Course. The symptoms begin with a feeling of illness, possibly headache, nausea, and a rather rapid increase in temperature. The earliest local symptom is likely to be severe sudden pain, boring in nature, near the region of a joint. Systemically, a chill followed by high fever may introduce the condition. Abruptness and severity of pain are emphasized as the two most notable features of this condition.

In the acute stages it is difficult at times to tell whether the involvement is in the joint or in the neighboring bone. The differentiation can usually be made by the fact that a certain range of painless motion is present when osteomyelitis is near a joint, but when joint involvement is present, any degree of motion is painful. The bloodstream may become infected so that positive cultures of the organism can be obtained, and the leukocyte count may rise to a very high level. Unfortunately, roentgenography is of no

1 Extracapsular metaphysis   2 Intracapsular metaphysis   3 Extra- and intracapsular metaphysis

Abscess
Metaphysis
Epiphyseal disk
Center of ossification
Capsule

4 Perforation of center of ossification   5 Dissection of capsule   6 Dissection of epiphyseal cartilage

Fig. 8-1. Illustration of the pathways for pus to decompress itself from the focal point in bone in acute osteomyelitis in the lower femur. **1,** The circle or central nidus of infection near the metaphyseal side of the epiphyseal plate can decompress into the surrounding soft tissues, producing a soft tissue abscess. **2,** The pus may burrow near the epiphyseal plate and discharge into the joint, producing a septic joint. **3,** Simultaneously the infection may erode bone and discharge into soft tissues at one point and into the joint at another. **4,** Rarely the infection can erode the epiphyseal plate cartilage and enter the epiphysis. **5 and 6,** Variations of dissection by the pus as it destroys capsule and enters the joint.

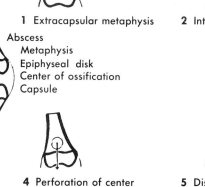

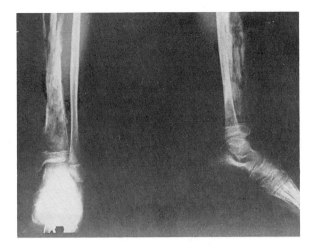

Fig. 8-2. Chronic osteomyelitis of the tibia. Note destruction of the bone, the sequestrum, and the proliferation of new bone (involucrum). (From Kenney, W. C., and Larson, C. B.: Orthopedics for the general practitioner, St. Louis, 1957, The C. V. Mosby Co.)

value in the early stage of osteomyelitis. Positive roentgenographic evidence of infection may not be found before 2 or 3 weeks. Even then the findings may be misleading when the progress of the disease has been marked by the administration of sulfonamides, penicillin, streptomycin, or other antibiotics. Localized swelling and tenderness of the involved area occur within 24 to 48 hours.

Treatment. Surgery and the use of antibiotics offer the best means of treatment. Transfusions, infusions, and supportive care must be included in the care of the patient with osteomyelitis.

In children less than 2 or 3 years of age, when the bone and periosteal tissues are flexible, it may be questionable whether surgical decompression offers any advantage. Incisions and drainage of localized abscesses may be beneficial.

In the average case of acute osteomyelitis the disease usually develops less abruptly. Although some authors have reported series of patients who seem to have been treated successfully by the use of antibiotic drugs alone, without surgery, it still seems logical that relief of pressure within the bone and periosteum by incision and drainage is an advantage. Much should depend on the local and general reaction of the patient within the immediate hours and days following onset of the disease. Immobilization in casts or in splints seems decidedly helpful in

most cases, particularly because of the effect of muscle relaxation.

The treatment of chronic osteomyelitis depends largely on the complete removal of all dead bone (sequestra) and the prolonged use of antibiotics. The use of antibiotic drugs at the first sign of bacterial activity will frequently avert the attack.

Nursing responsibilities in various methods of treatment. Perhaps it is significant that methods for treating osteomyelitis have developed during wartime. The first method was the Carrel-Dakin treatment and was used during World War I.

A second method that most nurses have read about is the Orr treatment, the closed plaster method of treating osteomyelitis. This treatment had its inception in World War I but was not used on a large scale until the Spanish Civil War. Because of the results from its use in World War II it was generally accepted as the treatment of choice for osteomyelitis.

The Orr method has been somewhat modified by chemotherapy and the antibiotic drugs, but the principles that Orr laid down are still considered sound and form the basis of modern treatment. Breifly stated, the Orr treatment consists of immediate adequate surgical drainage (saucerization), the establishment of complete rest for the involved area by the use of a plaster of paris cast that includes the joint above and the joint below the infected area, the use of petrolatum packing to maintain drainage of the affected area, and postoperative care in which rest and freedom from the interference of dressings are paramount features.

Odor from the closed plaster cast, however, may often present a real problem. Fortunately the effect of the odor on the patient is not nearly so troublesome as it is on members of the hospital staff and visitors. The nurse can give effective reassurance to the family only if she herself understands the principles underlying the closed plaster method of treating infected bone wounds and the amazing results that have been obtained by use of this method.

On the whole, attempts made to deodorize these casts have been more ingenious than successful. Commercial deodorizers are partially successful. For the most part, however, there seems to be no substitute for frequent airing of the patient's room.

Although the use of penicillin and other antibiotics has changed the treatment of osteomyelitis in some respects, provision for adequate rest of the involved area is still considered very important. In the acute stage of the disease the tendency is to institute drug therapy before resorting to surgery. However, the administration of antibiotics does not always ensure recovery and must often be accompanied by adequate drainage. There has always been controversy over surgery in the acute stage, particularly when bacteremia and general prostration are present. It is recognized that the systemic features of the disease may often be of more immediate importance than the relief of local symptoms. If surgery is performed in the acute stage, it is usually swift and conservative, consisting of a series of drill holes made through the metaphyseal portion of the bone to evacuate pus and relieve tension. More adequate drainage may need to be supplied later. Penicillin may be a lifesaving treatment in patients with the more severe forms of osteomyelitis accompanied by septicemia, provided the laboratory tests indicate that the organism isolated is sensitive to this antibiotic. In certain other cases proper choice of another antibiotic may be indicated. The patient is usually given the drug parenterally every 3 hours and, if localized abscesses occur,

the drug may be used in the wound as well. Penicillin solution is maintained in the wound by positioning of the extremity, by compression dressings, or by inserting a sterile catheter or polyethylene tube into the wound and permitting the solution to drop in slowly and continuously.

In some instances the organism causing osteomyelitis is found to be resistant to one or more of the anti-infective drugs, but penicillin will be used because it is a powerful bacteriostatic agent. It is particularly fitted to the treatment of osteomyelitis because it is not inhibited by the presence of pus or large numbers of bacteria.

General nursing care of the patient with osteomyelitis. The patient's general condition should be of as much concern as the local condition. Fluids should be given abundantly by mouth if the patient is able to retain them and intravenously if he is unable to do so. Blood transfusions are often part of the early treatment of this disease. The presence of sufficient protein and vitamin C in the diet of these patients is of the utmost importance because both of these substances are vitally necessary for wound healing. Every effort should be made to see that foods containing these are included in each meal even if the patient is receiving only a liquid diet.

A highly important fact to remember in caring for the patient with osteomyelitis is that deformity is a common sequela of the disease. The patient tends to hold the limb in a position that causes the least possible strain on the inflamed bone. Nearby joints are likely to be held in a position of flexion in order to relax muscles. In a patient with osteomyelitis of the lower end of the femur, flexion in the hip, flexion in the knee, and a tendency toward outward rotation of the whole leg may be observed. Drop foot is another feature that develops early. It is customary that as soon as drainage has been established the physician in charge will have a splint applied to the patient's extremity to hold it in an optimal position. However, if a period of days goes by, during which wet dressings are being used and no splint is in readiness, the nurse must improvise equipment to keep the foot in a normal position. A footboard or a box augmented by pillows usually causes the patient little discomfort. Many writers describe patients in whom a single focus of osteomyelitis is satisfactorily healed but the patient is nonetheless permanently crippled by flexion deformities of the knee and hip and an equinus position of the foot. Contractures of muscles alone may cause the deformity. Although edema is common in the early stages of osteomyelitis and splinting may be difficult, some attempt at maintaining optimal joint positions should be made.

Wet dressings alternated with dry dressings are sometimes ordered to be applied several times each day for the patient with an infected wound. During application of these dressings unnecessary manipulation must be avoided, and extreme gentleness is necessary when positioning the extremity. If heat is ordered to the area, this is usually accomplished by wrapping the extremity with a pad heated by an electrical unit. This assures a constant and continuous application of heat to the desired area. Controlling and checking the temperature is important, since the patient's pain may be so severe that he cannot determine when too great a degree of heat is being applied.

Laboratory findings play an important part in helping the physician prescribe treatment for this patient. Frequent blood cultures and determination of the blood level of antibiotics may be done. Urinary findings, hemoglobin studies, and white blood cell counts are a necessary part of the patient's management.

Handling of the affected area. The patient with osteomyelitis or septic arthritis is usually extremely apprehensive, and part of this apprehension is caused by his fear of being moved. He may even cry out if the bed is touched. Because it will be necessary for the nurse to move these patients to a certain extent, the manner of handling an acute inflamed joint or extremity must be brought to mind here.

Persons who have had osteomyelitis or a septic joint tell us that the pain caused by being moved is almost intolerable. The moving of an acutely inflamed joint should not be undertaken without help. All the help in the world, however, will do no good if the principles of joint immobilization are not understood and faith-fully carried out. It is not enough that the joint or the part infected is carefully immobilized; the joint above and the joint below must also be immobilized to prevent movement in the infected area. This will be readily understood when the mechanism of muscle action on joints is recalled. The muscles that act to move one joint may also serve as flexor or extensor of the one above or below it. Because this is true, moving a knee in which (or near which) a septic condition exists can be accomplished painlessly only by immobilizing the hip and ankle as well as the knee. This will require three hands. Support should be given under the hip and the knee, and another hand should support the ankle and foot steadily. Every movement of the hands in lifting must be smooth, unhurried, and infinitely careful. If he is turned to the side, the limb must stay on the same level as his body and not be allowed to sag when he is turned. His body should be supported by firm pillows, never soft ones. Gentleness in handling is imperative for another reason. Pathologic fractures have been known to occur as early as 10 days after the onset of osteomyelitis. Such fractures are frequently overlooked because the accompanying pain is often wrongly attributed to the concurrent disease.

Complications in osteomyelitis. Besides the drug reactions that may possibly occur from the use of the antibiotics or the sulfonamides, nurses should be alert to any signs that might indicate the progression of the disease to other parts of the skeleton. Any swelling, redness, or pain near a bone must be reported at once.

Amyloidosis, a waxy degeneration of the liver, spleen, and other organs, is a late and often terminal symptom. It may be mainfested by the presence of blood, pus, or albumin in the urine.

As a result of loss of bone substance there is considerable danger of pathologic fracture during and after osteomyelitis. The extremity that has been involved must be handled with great care even after the period of tenderness and pain has passed. When the patient is allowed to be out of bed, he must be guarded against falls, jerky movements, or any mishap that might threaten the integrity of the weakened bone. Sudden pain, crepitus, or deformity must be reported immediately. A sudden malposition of the limb may be the first indication that fracture has occurred in that area. Pain is sometimes disguised by the general discomfort of trying to walk after many weeks in bed.

Aftercare. In some instances long hospitalization is necessary, and careful follow-up after discharge is indispensable. The duties of the public health nurse in educating the family concerning the need for close observation and supervision of the activities of the patient are manifested. The dangers of neglect and the possibility of deformity, fracture, and stiffness of joints must be carefully pointed out, as must the possibility of recurrence. The chronicity of the condition must also be explained to avoid discouragement. Frequent return to the clinic for checkup must be stressed.

Dressings. Another important factor in the care of a patient with osteomyelitis is that of protecting other patients and personnel from the organism causing the infection. Personnel must know and understand the importance of aseptic technique. The value of and the need for proper hand washing cannot be overstressed.

Negligent technique often accompanies the dressing of draining bone wounds in hospital wards. The monotony of changing these dressings over a period of weeks or months may account for this lowering of standards. Nurses should remember that open wounds such as those encountered in patients with chronic osteomyelitis provide almost perfect culture media for bacteria. Cross infection is an ever-present danger in such wounds, and cross infection may sometimes mean the difference between recovery and chronic invalidism to the patient. Cross infection may be brought about by many agents, such as dust and lint particles in the air, soaked dressings that come in contact with contaminated bed linen or casts, upper respiratory passages, the fingers of nurses and doctors during dressing periods, and, of course, unsterile instruments and dressing equipment.

Carelessness in sterilizing instruments and in using unwashed hands to apply dressings has been the rule rather than the exception in changing septic dressings. In some instances it has been the custom to remove all dressings before ward rounds, so that the attending physi-

cian may see the wounds without unnecessary delay. This is a dangerous procedure because contamination and cross infection can so readily take place in a ward where dressings on many infected patients are opened to the air at the same time. The time a wound is exposed to the air should always be kept at a minimum.

In removing dressings from contaminated wounds it is advisable to cut the bandage and remove it in one piece. If the bandage is unwrapped, it tends to loose lint and dust into the air, and this lint may very easily hold bacteria that will infect other wounds in the area.

It is extremely important that all patients with infected wounds be housed in a separate ward. It is also desirable that patients with septic wounds be dressed in a room set aside for this purpose. Greater protection against cross infection is possible if this can be done. Cross infection with a new staphylococcal strain may not be evident unless the antibiotic sensitivities are tested or unless phage typing of the *Staphylococcus* is done.

ACUTE PYOGENIC ARTHRITIS (SEPTIC OR PURULENT ARTHRITIS)

Acute pyogenic arthritis is most frequently a disease of childhood and is caused by pyogenic organisms such as the *Staphylococcus* and *Streptococcus*. According to the virulence of the organism and the susceptibility of the host, the onset and reaction may be mild, medium, or severe. Any joint may be involved, but those most commonly involved are the joints most susceptible to trauma, such as the knee, hip, ankle, elbow, shoulder, and wrist.

Infection commonly results from the combination of trauma and focal infection and enters the joint through the bloodstream or by means of a penetrating wound into the joint.

Symptoms and signs. When the infection is mild, the joint reaction may consist of only the stimulation of synovial fluid production. This is called an effusion.

If the virulence is greater, local reaction is further stimulated and fibrinous material (coagulated white blood cells) may cover the surfaces of the joint.

If the reaction is violent, the joint may be filled with pus under considerable pressure and the symptoms are much exaggerated. The temperature may rise to 103° or 104° F.; the joint may become reddened, and a fusiform swelling may occur. Joint irritation is notoriously painful on any attempt at motion. Therefore violent muscle spasm of a protective nature usually accompanies joint irritation and exaggerates the tension and pain. There is usually a marked increase in the white blood cells.

Treatment. Early recognition and early treatment with antibiotics is the best means to prevent destruction of the joint. If response to antibiotics is not dramatic within 48 hours, surgical drainage must be considered as an emergency measure in the treatment.

Before the advent of penicillin, this type of joint infection was an extremely serious condition. The use of an antibiotic or a chemotherapeutic agent is now usually begun immediately on such patients, and surgical treatment is used only when necessary. The joint affected is immobilized by means of simple traction or a bivalved cast. Warm moist dressings will often be ordered for the joint. Fluids and blood transfusions will be given, and aspiration of the joint under aseptic conditions may be done. If the patient can be brought through the acute phase of this disease, his chances for recovery are good.

In the more severely affected patient, in whom fibrin is deposited on the joint surfaces, more extensive treatment is indicated. Joint washings may be done by using two syringes inserted on opposite sides of the joint. Quantities of physiologic saline solution are flushed through the joint until the return is clear. Then penicillin solution may be injected into the joint. Immobilization should be accomplished by splints or by Buck's extension.

If the joint reaction is severe and there is pus formation, incision and drainage are usually necessary. Drainage can be accomplished by a single or double incision adequate to allow complete exposure of the joint. All fibrinous material is picked out with forceps, and the joint is washed clean with physiologic saline solution. Penicillin solution can then be infiltrated throughout the joint, and the incision can be closed. The joint is immobilized in a splint or a plaster of paris cast, and the temperature and symptoms are watched closely.

If there should be continued elevation of temperature or continued pain, it may be necessary to bivalve the cast and inspect the joint. In a severely affected patient it may be necessary to open the wound and institute free drainage. Such technique exposes joints to secondary infection and should be avoided if possible.

General treatment should consist in the administration of proper chemotherapy combined with transfusions, infusions, and physical therapy treatments.

TUBERCULOSIS OF THE BONE AND JOINTS

The three types of tuberculosis of the bone are (1) human, (2) bovine, and (3) avian. The avian (bird type) is very rare.

Tuberculosis at the end of long bones may manifest itself in the following forms:

1. Encysted tuberculosis in which there is localized destruction of bone, surrounded by a wall of thickened bone tissue
2. Infiltrating tuberculosis that is rapid in development and frequently followed by rapid bone destruction and sequestration

3. Synovial tuberculosis with thickening of the synovial tissue and formation of rice bodies within the joint

Tuberculosis of the bone usually involves the portion that is in the vicinity of a joint. Occasionally, tuberculous infection in the bone may manifest itself in the form of an irritation of the periosteum and cortical bone, but usually it starts within a joint and extends to the medullary portion of the bone only by secondary invasion from the joint. The original involvement of the joint itself is usually through the blood-stream by means of an infarct or localization of the bacteria at the end of the arterial system. Hence, primary involvement may occur (1) at the end of long bones or (2) along the periosteum of long bones.

Clinical picture. Tuberculosis of the joint usually develops as an insidious disease. At the onset there is only occasional pain, with muscle spasm around the joint. There may be a slight elevation of temperature without leukocytosis, and a positive intradermal tuberculin test may be present. For accurate diagnosis of a tuberculous joint, material should be aspirated and injected into a guinea pig as well as cultured for tubercle bacilli. Both of these procedures should be used because one or the other may be positive. In 6 weeks the guinea pig is examined by autopsy, and the presence or absence of tuberculous organisms and exudate is determined by macroscopic and microscopic study.

Another accurate means of diagnosing tuberculosis in joints is biopsy. Material from the joint surface and synovial tissues can be removed and examined microscopically. If tuberculosis is present, it can usually be demonstrated through the presence of tubercle bacilli, tubercles, or the granulation tissue characteristic of tuberculosis.

The development of the tuberculous process in joints starts in most instances between the ages of 2 and 5 years but may begin later. The disease is not inherited and is usually acquired through association with and contamination from older persons who have active or quiescent tuberculous lesions in the lungs.

Tuberculosis of the joints is rarely transmitted to other persons except through very careless handling of dressings from draining sinuses. It must be remembered, however, that the disease is progressive when untreated and does not become checked the minute the surgeon sees it and makes the diagnosis.

Also, chest films are necessary to rule out the presence of concomitant pulmonary tuberculosis. Unnecessary exposure of other patients or nursing personnel must be avoided.

Teaching prevention. Besides the manual skill needed to treat the tuberculous patient, the nurse must realize the further challenge to educate the public regarding the causes, prevention, and necessity for prompt treatment of this disease.

One physician has stated that pulmonary tuberculosis is as contagious as measles to a child under 4 years of age. The danger in letting young children be exposed to adults with tuberculosis cannot be overemphasized. At least the exposure should not be prolonged or repeated. Recent investigations has revealed the danger that young children may receive tuberculosis from servants who have the disease in some unrecognized form. Baby-sitters coming in to relieve the parents in the evening have been shown to present a menace. Because dairy cattle have been placed so well under control, it is now known that practically all tuberculosis in children is contracted from adults.

The prophylaxis of tuberculosis, briefly stated, is the following: early diagnosis, segregation of infectious cases, and adequate treatment of discovered cases before they become clinically active.

General nursing care. Skill in the care of the patient afflicted with skeletal tuberculosis includes much more than the care given to the patient in the hospital situation. Many aspects of health care—so essential for the control of tuberculosis—must be employed to provide for case findings, early diagnosis, medical treatment, patient teaching, and the necessary follow-up care.

This disease has had its inception early in the life of the patient, perhaps in a household that included an adult relative who had tuberculosis in some contagious form. Perhaps the patient was a member of a family whose housing conditions were such that he was compelled to sleep in the same bedroom or even the same bed with that relative. Recognition must be given the important part that poor nutrition as well as poor environment may have played in his life as a child. Delay in treatment when the first mild symptoms of weight loss, fatigue, anorexia, or disinclination for his usual tasks and games became evident was perhaps engendered through ignorance on the part of parents or wrong advice given those parents by well-meaning friends.

This patient in his brace or cast will return to the same unwholesome environment, for patients with skeletal tuberculosis seldom spend their entire period of recumbency in the hospital. Therefore, the nurse sees the necessity to train the families in long-term care of these patients if they are not to return to the hospital 6 months or a year later far worse than they were when first seen.

The necessity for local rest is manifest to the nurse immediately. Frequently, concern for the spine or affected extremity is so great the one forgets that tuberculosis is a constitutional disease. Nurses do not always carry over, to the orthopedic ward and their patients with skeletal tuberculosis, their training in the care of patients with pulmonary tuberculosis. The need for rest that is general as well as local is just as great with these persons and should be borne in mind constantly.

Home care. What instructions should be given for the home care of these patients?

Families must first be taught what to observe and then be instructed in the interpretation of their observations. Second, they must be given a definite idea of the principles that underlie all details of the management of the patient at home. Last, they must be instructed carefully in the technique of carrying out these details. This third consideration will most frequently be delegated to the nurse.

The doctor will often instruct the parents of a child with tuberculosis that it is necessary to keep a daily record of temperature and to observe and estimate the amount of food intake, rest, and sunlight that the child receives. He will instruct them in the importance of recognizing any loss of weight or general strength. Signs of setback in these patients often occur so gradually that only by his impressing firmly upon the parents' minds the necessity for solicitous observation and the most painstaking care will the patient's future welfare be assured.

Where the doctor knows without question that the status of the family income will not permit proper care for this patient, social agencies will be consulted and community resources called upon. Some doctors feel quite strongly that because of the protracted character of the disease, its tedious course, and the great likelihood of complicating factors and recurrences, the patient should be cared for institutionally until solidification of the joint and quiescence of the disease are assured.

For effective instruction concerning home treatment the nurse should, if possible, employ the demonstration method. Demonstration of bath and care of cast must be given if the instructions are to have any effect at all on the parents. The nurse must have enough imagination, too, to understand how the home situation will vary from the hospital situation and to suggest means of improvising when, manifestly, equipment will be lacking. Ability to compute for the patient with tuberculosis a satisfactory diet that takes into consideration the family income is another important feature. Many little details that seem almost too small to be mentioned must be dealt with thoroughly in relation to the home treatment of the patient with tuberculosis. Rest periods tend to be curtailed in the home, and substitutions are made for essential foods because the parents think the substitute just as good.

Instructions will be individualized and vary in each case but, whatever the instructions are, they must be given kindly, with an understanding of the magnitude of the problem that confronts the confused parents, and with a genuine desire to help them solve their problems. No greater nursing service is possible than such teaching when one considers the large proportion of home care usually given such patients during the course of their disease. In addition to instructing the patient and parents, the hospital nurse will make a referral to the local visiting or public health nurse. Because most of these patients are instructed to continue with antituberculous drugs at home, it is essential that a visiting nurse make home visits, perhaps administer the drugs, and evaluate symptoms and progress. Cost of drugs must not be forgotten. Prior to discharge, inquiry into the cost of the drugs should be made, and, if necessary, appropriate arrangements made with a local authority for supplying the needed medicine.

Surgery. Surgery as an adjunct to modern drug therapy has come to be the preferred treatment in skeletal tuberculosis. Advantages of surgical treatment are as follows:

1. Biopsy may be performed for diagnostic

purposes. With the present-day use of antibiotics this procedure can be performed with little danger to the patient; since drugs used in the treatment of tuberculosis of bone and joint are more effective in the early stages of the disease, it is imperative that a diagnosis be made as soon as possible.

2. Joint motion can be obliterated by surgical interference; the operation is called an arthrodesis.

3. Evacuation or drainage of an abscess is a surgical process.

4. Decompression when an accumulation of pus has invaded parts of the body that contain vital organs, as may happen when the spinal cord is compressed by inflammatory exudates, may be accomplished.

5. Surgery may be employed to correct an existing deformtity. Osteotomies are common in this last group.

Care of the patient after spinal fusion has been described in another chapter. Joints that have undergone arthrodesis are usually well immobilized in plaster of paris before the patient is returned from the operating room, and nursing care is the same as that of any other surgical patient wearing a plaster cast. However, the systemic nature of the disease that has made the operation necessary should never be lost from the nurse's mind. Care of a patient subjected to laminectomy for decompression of the spinal cord will not vary greatly from care given the patient who has had a spinal fusion operation.

Antituberculous drugs. Streptomycin sulfate continues to be used against tuberculosis, usually in combination with isoniazid. At the initial dosage of 1 gm. per day the adverse effects on vestibular apparatus can result in hearing loss and therefore should be reduced in dosage as soon as possible.

Para-aminosalicylic acid (PAS) is a bacteriostatic drug given in conjunction with isoniazid and/or streptomycin in dosages up to 12 gms. daily in divided doses.

Isoniazid (INH) is bacteriostatic for *Mycobacterium tuberculosis* in doses of 5 mg/kg in adults, up to 300 mg. total per day. It may be used in conjunction with other drugs, but peripheral neuritis is an adverse effect, which should be kept in mind and reported whenever symptoms of numbness or paresthesias occur.

A newer drug, rifampin, is indicated for the initial treatment of pulmonary tuberculosis but is seldom needed in bone and joint tuberculosis since the other drugs such as streptomycin, para-aminosalicylic acid, and isoniazid in combination are very effective. Another drug used in conjunction with isoniazid or streptomycin is ethambutol hydrochloride given initially at 15 mg/kg in a single dose, 25 mg/kg daily for 60 days and thereafter reduced to 15 mg/kg daily. Visual fields should be tested frequently since optic neuritis has been reported with the use of this drug.

It is important, in the presence of relapse of proved tuberculosis, that sensitivity tests be carried out to determine if the organism has become resistant to the specific drug being used. It is well to remember that antituberculous drugs show their greatest value in the early treatment of the disease, before ischemia and bone necrosis have taken place, and that continuous use of the drug(s) is important in preventing development of resistant bacilli. The length of time that a drug should be taken is determined by the physician and may be a 2-year period or longer.

It must be remembered that good nutrition, immobilization, and rest are fundamental in the treatment of the patient with a tuberculous bone or joint. When good general care and surgery as indicated are combined with the use of antituberculous drugs, it is usually possible to shorten the healing period. One result of shortening the healing period is that secondary complications, such as renal calculi and joint deformity, may be prevented.

TUBERCULOSIS OF THE SPINE

Symptoms. About half of all cases of bone and joint tuberculosis occur in the spine. The first symptoms are usually stiffness, muscle spasm, and a tendency to reach things on the floor by bending the knees rather than the back.

At first symptoms may be intermittent and are relieved by comparatively short periods of rest. The intermittent characteristic may cloud the early diagnosis.

Pain may be referred to the limbs—a fact

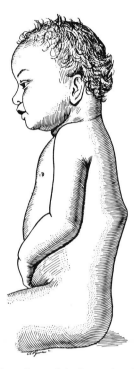

Fig. 8-3. Tuberculosis of the lower dorsal spine with angulation, or gibbus.

serving to emphasize the point that examinations should be made only after complete removal of all the patient's clothing. The area of his complaint may be remote from the actual disease.

The lower dorsal spine and the upper lumbar spine are most frequently affected, although tuberculosis of the cervical spine and the upper dorsal spine is not uncommon. The greatest deformity develops when the involvement is in the dorsal spine, and its compensatory adaptation to the neighboring uninvolved joints is less effective than in the lumbar or the cervical spine.

The characteristic deformity in tuberculosis of the spine is the development of a gibbus (Fig. 8-3), an angulation or pronounced anteroposterior curve of the spine such as is seen in the hunchback. This deformity results from destructive lesions in the spine and from fractures.

Paralysis in tuberculosis of the spine occurs occasionally. Strangely, it is rarely the result of the mechanical disturbance in the alignment of the spine but rather the effect of abscesses, granulation tissue, and other accompanying

factors in the tuberculous disease. For this reason treatment of paralysis usually consists of rest and immobilization. These agents have a tendency to diminish inflammatory factors and relieve nerve pressure. In rare instances it may become necessary to relieve bone pressure by laminectomy.

Treatment. The treatment of tuberculosis of the spine depends considerably on the advance that the disease has made at the time it is first observed and on the age of the patient.

Attempts should be made through casts and braces to maintain as nearly as possible an erect position of the spine (Fig. 8-4).

In conservative management of tuberculosis of the spine, treatment consists of immobilization and the use of drugs (streptomycin, para-aminosalicylic acid, and isoniazid). Institutional care, fresh air, sunshine, proper diet, and hygienic surroundings are important factors. Under modern treatment 6-month confinement in an institution with drug therapy, followed by continuation of the antituberculous drugs for a total of 2 years, is usually indicated.

When improvement in the patient's general condition is apparent—that is, when he has no elevation of temperature and is gaining weight, when there is a decline in the blood sedimentation rate, and when the lymphocyte-monocyte ratio is normal—surgical fusion of the spine may be indicated. Nature automatically fuses the laminae and articular facets when spinal disease has existed over a period of years. Unfortunately, nature's fusion accompanies the destruction rather than precedes it. There is a protective mechanism on her part for the area that has been involved, but no protection against advance of the disease to other vertebrae.

Ordinarily, after a spinal fusion operation the patient is protected for a time by a cast, which is followed by protective braces for an additional time. When tuberculosis exists in the cervical spine, the cast or brace must extend up to and include the chin and head.

There are many ingenious types of apparatus for obtaining and maintaining correction and immobilization in a patient with tuberculous lesions of the spine.

Abscess formation occurs in a fairly large percentage of patients with tuberculosis of the

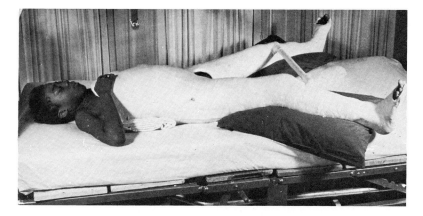

Fig. 8-4. A complete body cast has been applied to maintain immobilization and good position for this patient with tuberculosis of the spine. Note placement of pillows to support extremities.

spine. In the cervical region the abscess may develop in the pharynx, causing difficulty in breathing. In the dorsal region it may occur in the mediastinum and may rupture into the lung. In the dorsal region it may occur in the mediastinum and may rupture into the lung. In the lumbar spine an abscess may develop between the lumbar muscles or in the gluteal region, or it may follow the course of the iliopsoas muscle and point in the groin. This is the most common form (psoas abscess).

A cold abscess should be opened when pressure is great and spontaneous rupture is likely to occur. Incision may be made, through which the abscess is evacuated, and the incision is then firmly closed.

The commonest form of surgical attack on spinal tuberculosis is the anterior approach to the spine, so that infected granulation tissue, sequestra, and other necrotic tissues may be removed. Drainage of an abscess is common when the abscess is progressive and not controlled by antituberculous drugs. Approach to the abscess is usually made through costotransversectomy. If there is a great deficiency of bone at the conclusion of the operation, bone grafts can be added to bridge the gap between the vertebral bodies.

Nursing care. Because tuberculosis of the spine (sometimes called Pott's disease after Sir Percival Pott who first described the syndrome over 150 years ago) is the most frequent in occurrence of the skeletal tuberculous lesions,

care of patients having this disorder will be dealt with in full. Patients with tuberculosis of the other joints of the body need the same general care. Usually, the local care of patients who have other types of skeletal tuberculosis is somewhat simpler for the nurse because their immobilization is most commonly accomplished by circular or bivalved plaster casts.

BEDRIDDEN PATIENTS. In cases of spinal tuberculosis the nurse must employ the best techniques of cast care. This means being constantly be on the alert for abscesses that have begun to drain beneath the cast, and one's sense of smell is the best agent for discovering these. The nurse must depend upon the patient's weekly weight chart, a record of his appetite and rest habits, his general appearance of well-being, and absence of symptoms of recurrence (undue fatigue, night cries, irritability, or apathy) to be assured of his progress.

Local rest can be accomplished in a number of ways, and each orthopedist has a particular apparatus he prefers. It may be a plaster jacket applied from shoulder to hips or, sometimes, including the legs to the knees; or it may be a bivalved plaster bed of some type, extending from occiput to knees but divided into an anterior and a posterior section to permit care of the patient's skin (Figs. 8-5 and 8-6).

For the patient with tuberculosis of the spine, even in this era of early mobilization, rest is considered essential.

The care of the patient in the hospital and

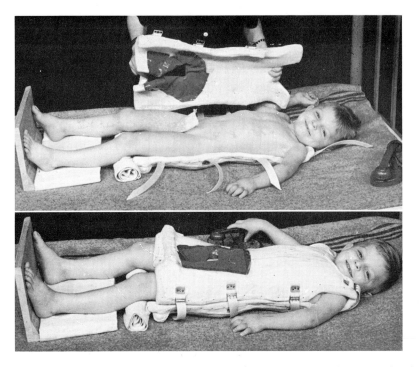

Fig. 8-5. The plaster shell or plaster bed is frequently used to immobilize the spine after fusion. Each half is lined with stockinet. The straps and buckles make it possible to remove either half for bathing and skin care. Before the patient is turned, the straps are buckled tightly. (Courtesy Iowa State Services for Crippled Children.)

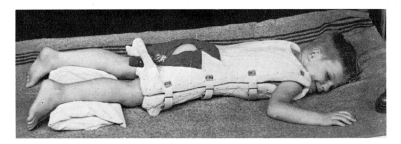

Fig. 8-6. Prone position. The anterior and posterior halves may be buckled in place to prevent the child from rising up and turning. Note the waterproof material placed about the perineum and buttocks. (Courtesy Iowa State Services for Crippled Children.)

later in the home will vary somewhat according to his type of apparatus. Extension frames have been used in the treatment of spinal tuberculosis for many years. However in recent years, with early diagnosis and the use of drugs, the orthopedic surgeon usually permits the patient to have more freedom than was prescribed previously. A straight Bradford frame may be used to restrain the child and ensure maintenance of a horizontal position. This is important, since the upright or vertical position would cause increased pressure on the diseased vertebrae. For the adult patient, recumbency on a firm mattress may be the prescribed restriction.

Care given to the patient's back is important. If he is thin and emaciated, pressure areas will demand close attention. The gibbus, or knuckling that occurs at the level of the diseased vertebra, is often the site of severe pressure. Because the patient lies on this spot over a long period, it can readily be understood why pressure necrosis occurs there. Occasionally a bursa will have formed on this gibbus, and it may be hot and indurated. Hot wet dressings are sometimes ordered.

Children with tuberculous spines should not be allowed to feed themselves because feeding oneself in so complete a state of recumbency is fatiguing. The child should be fed slowly, with careful observation of his eating habits. His diet, carefully planned for high caloric intake and for high protein and vitamin content, should be urged firmly. Between-meal nourishment should be planned to be nutritious without filling him to such an extent that he will be unable to take his next meal.

Restraints are a matter of importance in the nursing care of children afflicted with tuberculosis of the spine. They must be efficient in maintaining the position prescribed by the doctor; on the other hand, they must inflict no unnecessary restraint upon the child. Restraints to maintain position may be of the vest or jacket variety, in which a canvas garment for the upper part of the body is equipped with webbing straps and buckles.

Because the chronicity of this disease is one of its most outstanding features, early consideration must be given to the education of the child. Present educational methods have been adapted very satisfactorily to bedside teaching, so that the long treatment required by this disease does not need to interrupt the child's schooling. Most communities have arrangements wherein such children are given the advantage of a specially arranged plan of study to suit their needs. The child should not lose interests common to his age, nor must he face a future in which he is forced to return to school at a much lower level than his age justifies.

Occupational and diversional therapy are most important. Limitation of activity with these patients, of course, must be considered because the child's position makes many occupations impossible for him and also because fatigue must be avoided. However, such persons can be taught many useful crafts and be permitted to enjoy these during certain periods of the day. Many inclinations are developed and many natural gifts and talents are discovered that may play an important part in the patient's future rehabilitation. Because of the unnatural position, the possibility of eyestrain from reading and handwork should always be a matter for consideration. Lighting must be carefully supervised.

AMBULATORY PATIENTS. A new set of duties supervenes for the nurse when the patient's period of recumbency is over and healing and calcification have progressed to such an extent that the orthopedist feels he may be allowed up for short periods with some type of ambulatory support. Limitations of time designated by the doctor must be rigidly adhered to.

Periods of activity for the newly ambulatory tuberculous patient should never be prolonged or vigorous during the first weeks. Appetite must be observed lest it begin to decrease as a result of fatigue from overactivity. Weight should continue to be checked weekly. Evidences of any loss of progress should be reported to the physician. The same observations for beginning abscesses or pressure sites are as necessary now as they were during the period of recumbency.

The type of support may be an ambulatory cast, jacket, or brace. The Taylor body brace, or some modification of it, is in common use in most hospitals. It consists of two thin flexible steel bars that form a support for the vertebral column, one lying on either side of it, which fit the curves of the back perfectly. A pelvic band made of steel and leather is fastened at the bottom of these supports. Another crossbar attaches at the scapular level. Straps fastened to the vertical bars go over the shoulders, under the axillae, and back to their original attachments, making a sort of loop. In the front a canvas apron supports the chest and abdomen and is fastened to the brace by tape-webbing straps and buckles. These secure the brace tightly to the chest and abdomen. It should always be remembered by the nurse applying these braces that the pelvic band must closly encircle the pelvis slightly below the iliac crests. If this is done, the brace will be in the proper position with regard to the rest of the body. Whatever the type of body brace used, both bracemaker and physician advise that you fasten the brace around the pelvis first if the patient is lying down, and this should always be the case while fitting tuberculosis patients.

COMPLICATIONS IN TUBERCULOSIS OF THE JOINTS

The symptomatology of complications in tuberculosis of the joints should be known to the orthopedic nurse. Chronic, unreasonable irritability in the young child who has tuberculosis of a joint should be a point of observation on the part of the nurse. Symptoms of this nature may occur many weeks before evidences of lethargy, headache, neck rigidity, or convulsive states of meningitis are manifested. Rapid loss of weight in the adult, severe night sweats, temperature elevation, anorexia, and debility may indicate oncoming miliary tuberculosis.

Steindler states that tuberculosis of the kidney occurs more often with bone tuberculosis than in the pulmonary tuberculosis. Renal complications may be manifested in urinary disturbances —cystitis, hematuria, and the like. An accurate measurement of intake and output is indicated for the tuberculous patient in whom this sort of complication is suspected. Periodic urinalyses are usually ordered by the doctor. Although gastrointestinal upsets, distention, constipation, and nausea may be the result of retentive or reclination apparatus, they should be reported if they become obstinate or persist over a long period. In this connection it might be well to mention here that retropharyngeal abscess complicating tuberculosis of the cervical spine is often manifested by dysphagia or dyspnea. These symptoms have special significance and must be reported as soon as they are observed. Spasm of the muscles of the thigh and a tendency toward flexion and lateral rotation of a limb that is accompanied by great pain on motion may suggest to the doctor that a psoas abscess is in the process of formation long before a fluctuating mass may be seen in the groin.

Sudden weakness or trembling of the legs may be the first indication of further breakdown in the affected vertebrae. This is a very grave symptom, often a forerunner of paralysis, and must be reported to the physician in charge without delay.

TUBERCULOSIS OF THE HIP

Tuberculosis of the hip constitutes the second largest group of tuberculous joint involvement.

Symptoms and signs. The disease usually begins at an early age (1 to 3 years) with a limp of gradually increasing severity. The hip becomes slightly flexed, abducted, and externally rotated, and the child has a tendency to walk on the toes of the affected side. Night cries are frequently present. These are caused by a definite mechanism. The muscles relax in sleep, and the joint is unprotected. In the subconscious state body movements may occur and the joint may become irritated. There is an immediate violent spasm of the muscles that causes severe pain by bringing the irritated joint surfaces together and the child cries out as he awakens.

As the disease progresses, the destruction of the head of the femur and possibly of the acetabulum increases and the deformity changes. Adduction and internal rotation develop, whereas the flexion deformity remains.

Diagnosis. The usual methods of clinical and laboratory diagnosis of a tuberculous joint are used. In persons afflicted with the more advanced cases the characteristic destruction as shown by roentgenograms (Fig. 8-7) is in itself almost positive proof of the disease.

The symptoms are more severe than they are in Legg-Perthes disease and slipped upper femoral epiphysis and less severe than they are in acute pyogenic arthritis of the hip.

Treatment. During the early stages and in younger children, recumbent treatment is combined with the use of drugs. It is hoped that with rest (local and general), good food, and hygienic surroundings, combined with drug therapy, joint motion may be saved. Immobilization of the joint may be maintained by plaster splinting or by traction.

In patients with more severe cases fusion of the hip may be necessary. There are several methods of accomplishing fusion, but all successful methods consist of some form of bone graft between the femur and the pelvis, and growth of this graft leads to solid bone formation between these two structures and the elimination of joint function. Tuberculosis seems to lose its affinity for a joint when motion and friction are eliminated. After fusion operations a

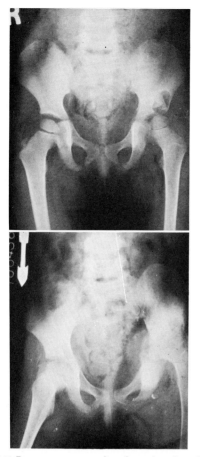

Fig. 8-7. Roentgenograms of a tuberculous hip. In the top picture the head of the left femur and the joint space are still well defined. As the infectious process continues, below, the joint cartilage is destroyed, calcium is deposited, and eventually motion in the joint is destroyed.

plaster of paris cast is applied from the chest to the toes of the affected side. The position of the hip joint is of considerable importance. There should be from 10- to 20-degree flexion and, if there has been some destruction, about 5-degree adduction to give the best weight-bearing line. Approximately 6 to 8 months are required for bone healing after hip fusion. This must be determined by roentgenography.

STUDY QUESTIONS

1. Case finding is an important factor in the prevention of tuberculosis. Why is this important in the prevention of skeletal tuberculosis? Re-view the nurse's responsibility pertaining to this aspect of patient care.
2. Discuss drug therapy as it relates to the treatment of skeletal tuberculosis.
3. Review symptoms, treatment, and nursing care of a child with an acute septic arthritis of the hip joint.
4. When dressing a draining wound, the nurse should use precautions to protect herself and to protect other patients from the organism involved. Precautions are also needed to prevent cross infection. Review technique necessary to obtain these objectives.
5. Define the following terms: Brodie's abscess, cold abscess, ankylosis, arthrodesis, fusion, gibbus, involucrum, kyphos, night cries, saucerization, and sequestrum.
6. An inflamed joint is quite painful. Describe method(s) of supporting and moving an extremity, which will cause the patient a minimum of discomfort.

REFERENCES

Bergersen, B. S.: Pharmacology in nursing, ed. 12, St. Louis, 1973, The C. V. Mosby Co.

Boland, A. L.: Acute hematogenous osteomyelitis, Orthop. Clin. North Am. **3:**225-238, 1972.

Clawson, D. K., and Dunn, W.: Management of common bacterial infections of bones and joints, J. Bone Joint Surg. **49-A:**164-182, 1967.

DiPalma, J. R.: Drugs for tuberculosis, RN **29:**53-58, 1966.

Ferguson, A.: Orthopedic surgery in infancy and childhood, ed. 3, Baltimore, 1968, The Williams & Wilkins Co.

Frenay, Sister M. A.: Drugs in tuberculosis control, Am. J. Nurs. **61:**82-85, 1961.

Hall, J. E., and Silverstein, E. A.: Acute hematogenous osteomyelitis, Pediatrics **31:**1033-1038, 1963.

Harris, N. H., and Kirkaldy-Willis, W. H.: Primary subacute pyogenic osteomyelitis, J. Bone Joint Surg. **47-B:**526-532, 1965.

Jones, W. C., and Miller, W. E.: Skeletal tuberculosis, South. Med. J. **57:**964-971, 1964.

Lawyer, R. B., and Eyring, E.: Intermittent closed suction-irrigation treatment of osteomyelitis, Clin. Orthop. **88:**80-85, 1972.

Raney, R. B., and Brashear, H. Robert: Shand's handbook of orthopaedic surgery, ed. 8, St. Louis, 1971, The C. V. Mosby Co.

Stetson, J., DePonte, R., and Southwick, W.: Acute septic arthritis of the hip in children, Clin. Orthop. **56:**105-116, 1968.

Top, F. H., and Wehrle, P. F., editors: Communicable and infectious diseases, ed. 7, St. Louis, 1972, The C. V. Mosby Co.

Williams, S. R.: Nutrition and diet therapy, ed 2, St. Louis, 1973, The C. V. Mosby Co.

Winchester, I.: Acute osteomyelitis, Nurs. Times **61:**930-931, 1965.

9

Bone metabolism

NORMAL BONE STRUCTURE AND FUNCTION

The sciences of biology, chemistry, physiology, and physics are interrelated in a molecular concept relating to function and structure. To study bone structure and function, one should examine whole bones and all structures attached to them (anatomy), the parts or types of tissue found in bone (histology), the cells that form these tissues (interrelated sciences), and the matrix material separating these cells (interrelated sciences).

Many people studying man consider the bone an inactive mechanical framework, nearly inert. This is not the case. Bone is alive and a dynamic tissue in the body; it has a unique chemical and physical construction that serves important functions. Its amazing organization—from gross shape to molecular grouping—makes for tensile strength nearly as great as that of cast iron but with relatively little weight. In many respects bone is similar to living, reinforced concrete with collagen fibers acting as tie rods and calcium salt forming the cement. Cellular components and a blood supply maintain this structure, and materials continually undergo alteration and replacement.

Long bones, such as the femur, contain four major types of connective tissue: fibrous, bone, cartilage, and blood-forming elements of of marrow.

FUNCTIONS OF BONE

1. Framework for the body
2. Storage of minerals (calcium, phosphorus, magnesium) used by all body organs

3. System of levers to help convert force generated by muscles into motion and locomotion
4. Protection of internal organs (brain, heart, and so forth)
5. Production of blood
6. Capability of growth while continuing other functions

BONE GROWTH—ANATOMIC REMODELING

Parts of a growing long bone: (Fig. 9-1).
1. Epiphysis—the secondary center of ossification of any bone (located at the ends of long bones)
2. Diaphysis—the shaft of a long bone
3. Metaphysis or epiphyseal plate—the growth zone between the epiphysis and the diaphysis

The two types of bone, intramembranous and enchondral, grow in the following manner:

Intramembranous bone formation (bone growth between membranes) generally forms flat bone such as that forming the skull. Bone forms between two layers of fibrous connective tissue or periosteum through cellular secretion of collagen matrix which then mineralizes (Fig. 9-2). Appositional growth continues as new cells continue to lay down more of the mineralized matrix. At the same time other specialized cells remodel bone by tearing it down in appropriate locations. This process allows growth yet maintains correct size and shape.

Enchondral bone formation (bone growth

Parts of a long bone

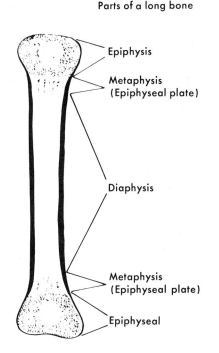

Epiphysis

Metaphysis
(Epiphyseal plate)

Diaphysis

Metaphysis
(Epiphyseal plate)

Epiphyseal

Fig. 9-1

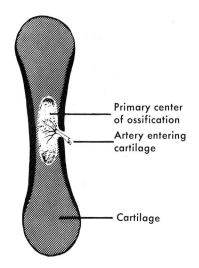

Primary center
of ossification

Artery entering
cartilage

Cartilage

Fig. 9-3. Diagram shows cartilage model of a long bone. As the blood vessels enter the shaft (diaphyseal) region, cartilage is destroyed and replaced by bone.

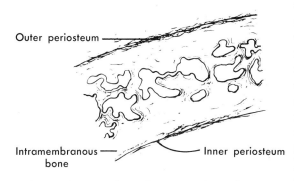

Outer periosteum

Intramembranous
bone

Inner periosteum

Fig. 9-2. Diagram shows the periosteal growth zones on the surfaces of a flat intramembranous bone. The central blood-filled cavities enlarge as the bone matures.

within cartilage) forms the long bones in the limbs, most tubular bones, and the spine. By the eighth week of embryonic life, cartilage models of most bones have formed but they have not mineralized (ossified). Three different processes of ossification occur in this cartilage model: (1) A *primary center of ossification* develops in the central shaft region of the cartilage model (Fig. 9-3). As blood vessels enter this

region, cartilage is destroyed and replaced by mineralized bone matrix. As growth proceeds, this region of ossification enlarges toward the ends of the bone, accounting for most of the increase in bone length. (2) Bone increases in diameter as it lengthens. This growth in diameter, called *periosteal bone formation,* is identical to intramembranous ossification. New bone is formed by the periosteal covering along its shaft (Fig. 9-4). (3) Many bones have *secondary centers of ossification* that develop as blood vessels enter the cartilage model in regions separate from the primary center. The epiphysis or mineralized region at the ends of the growing long bone is a secondary center of ossification (Fig. 9-4).

In a long bone the secondary center of ossification or epiphysis is separated from the primary center by the epiphyseal plate. Cartilage cells of the epiphyseal plate are highly specialized and organized in rows. A bone lengthens as ossification occurs in and along these rows of cartilage with simultaneous replacement of this cartilage by cell divisions within the epiphyseal plate. When bone reaches its adult state and growth stops, the epiphyseal plate becomes completely resorbed and replaced by bone (Fig. 9-5).

The primary and secondary centers of ossification are seen in roentgenograms of enchondral

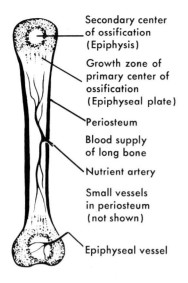

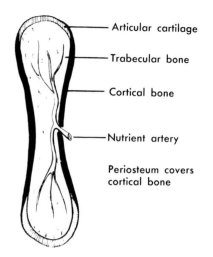

Fig. 9-4. Diagram illustrating the centers of ossification in an enchondral bone (see text). Note that each region of ossification has a well developed blood supply.

Fig. 9-5. In this diagram of an adult enchondral bone, the epiphyseal plate cartilage has been replaced by bone.

bones (Fig. 9-6). Prior to ossification, the cartilage bone model is not visible. Then, as ossification progresses, the primary center develops and enlarges, followed by development of epiphyseal centers. These centers of ossification eventually fuse in the adult.

HISTOLOGICAL REMODELING—BONE TURNOVER

Throughout life there is constant replacement of older bone elements. This takes place by the eating away (resorption) of bone in some areas together with the formation of new bone in other areas. This normally amounts to a state of constant remodeling in which the losses equal the gains, and the total amount is not changed. It is assumed that by this phenomenon the skeleton can respond to changes in strength requirements by redistribution of more bone in areas needed. It is also by alterations in the resorption and formation process that calcium can be replaced or stored according to the needs of the body.

Types of ossified connective tissue—bone. The dense region of the periphery of a bone, the cortex, is composed of very compact *cortical bone*. Bone in the central marrow space thins out to resemble a sponge and is called spongy,

trabecular, or cancellous bone. The dense cortex gives bone its major strength. The arrangement of trabecular bone along lines of stress also adds considerable strength with very little addition of weight and allows room for blood-forming elements of the marrow.

At a cellular level there are two patterns of organization, the lamellar and the woven. Woven bone is initially laid down during growth or remodeling. It is disorganized and appears woven at the microscopic level, hence the term *woven bone*. A normal mature bone is highly organized into the basic pattern diagrammed in Fig. 9-7. This architecture is described as being a *lamellar* pattern. In many pathologic conditions, and especially in fracture healing, large amounts of woven bone are produced.

Neurovascular supply. Bone, like any other living tissue, is supplied with blood and has an extensive vascular network. In fact, about 8% of the blood in each heartbeat goes to supply bone. Blood vessels in the periosteum penetrate the bone and supply the outer one-third of the cortex. Nutrient arteries course through the bone cortex to supply the bone marrow, trabecular bone, and the inner two-thirds of the cortex. Epiphyseal centers are supplied with blood via epiphyseal vessels.

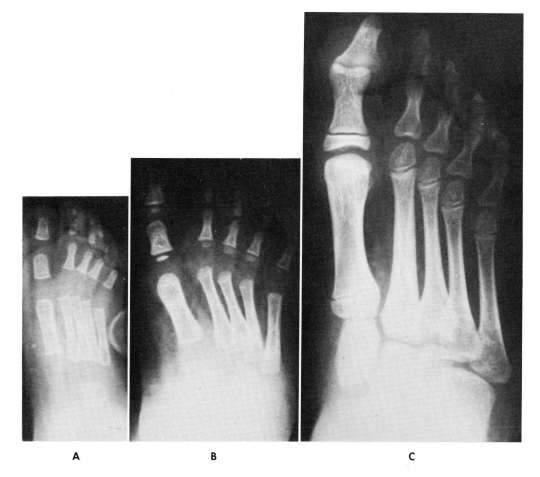

A   B   C

Fig. 9-6. Roentgenograms of a boy's foot at age **A,** 8 months, **B,** 2½ years and **C,** 13 years. At 8 months only the primary centers of ossification are visible. At 2½ years small epiphyseal centers are forming near the end of the bones. (In the foot epiphyseal centers develop only at one end of the bones.) At age 18 the epiphyseal centers are well developed and about to fuse with the diaphysis.

Nerves have been observed along the course of these vessels and even within the microscopic blood vascular canals (haversian canals) within cortical and trabecular bone. Exact function of these small nerves is not known. Studies suggest that they transmit deep bone pain, regulate blood flow, regulate growth, and control bone repair.

Structural unit of bone—the osteon. The basic structural unit of bone is called an *osteon.* An osteon includes a central neurovascular supply (the haversian canal) and the tube of cells and bone matrix surrounding this central canal (Fig. 9-7). The osteons, which are the basic structure in trabecular and cortical lamellar bone, line up along the lines of force through the bone. The diameter of any one osteon is limited by the distance bone cells can live away from their central blood supply, up to about twenty cell layers. Length is not critical, and the osteons are very often very long. It is the parallel arrangement of many osteons—like a bundle of sticks—that gives bone its great strength at the cellular level.

Bone cells. Cells of bone, like those of all living tissues, have three basic functions:

1. Reproduction—cells divide forming new cells.

2. Transformation of energy—bone cells take nutrients and oxygen supplied by the blood and convert them to substances the cell can use for energy.

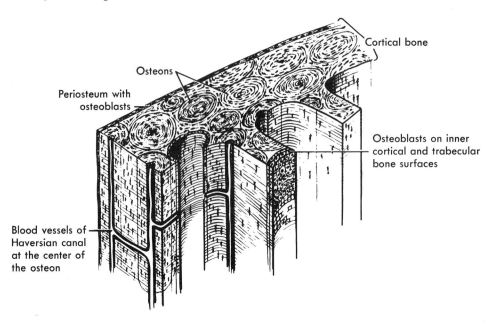

Fig. 9-7. This three-dimensional diagram illustrates both the longitudinal and cross-section of various components in the shaft (diaphysis) of a long bone. Osteons run lengthwise in the bone along lines of stress and are the basic structure of both the cortex and the central trabeculae. Osteons are formed around central canals that offer a supply of nutrients to all parts of the bone.

3. Production of new substances—the new substances are usually proteins, most significantly collagen, the tie rod of the bone matrix.

Three main types of bone cells are osteoblasts, osteocytes, and osteoclasts.

Osteoblasts are bone-forming cells that cover all growing surface of bone and initially lay down woven bone. These cells originate from undifferentiated cells located near blood vessels, then begin to form bone and eventually are surrounded by bone.

An *osteocyte* is an osteoblast that has become completely surrounded by bone matrix. Osteocytes are the mature bone cells that maintain living bone but do not form new bone.

Cells that tear down bone are called *osteoclasts.* These cells form by the fusion of osteoblasts or osteocytes into multinucleated giant cells. These giant cells usually contain about 20 nuclei, but 150 or more nuclei have been found in a single osteoclast. An osteocyte itself may be capable of bone destruction, which makes it in essence a single-celled osteoclast. The mechanisms by which these cells destroy bone are not clear.

Bone matrix and bone mineral. Matrix material surrounding osteocytes contains organic material (protein, carbohydrate, and small amounts of fat) and minerals (calcium salt crystals).

Organic bone matrix. With mineral removed, 90% of bone matrix consists of fibrous collagen proteins. Collagen is the same protein found in all fibrous connective tissue and the supporting structure on which the calcium salt crystals form. Vitamin C has an important role in collagen formation. The role of carbohydrate and fat in bone matrix is not clear, but they may play some role in the mineralization process.

Bone mineral. Blood calcium concentration remains one of the most critically regulated factors in the human body. This vitally important chemical regulates nerve impulses; muscle contractions, including heart muscle; and transport of materials into and out of all cells. The control of the blood calcium level is vital for life itself. This calcium control depends on at least three factors: (1) *bone matrix,* acting as a reservoir for calcium (Ninety-nine per cent of total body calcium is stored as bone.); (2) *hormones,* especially parathyroid hormone, which carefully controls blood calcium levels; (3)

vitamins, especially vitamins D, C, and A, which promote absorption of calcium from the intestine and help regulate bone matrix mineralization.

The higher magnification obtained with the electron microscope has added greatly to the study of bone. The structures within each cell, the formation of collagen fibers, and the laying down of needlelike calcium salt crystals around collagen fibers have been studied. Research into the integration of bone metabolism with molecular structure has just begun and will hopefully clarify more aspects of normal bone function and structure.

MINERAL METABOLISM

Metabolic bone disease describes any general disease state that stems from a disturbance of the body's normal metabolism and affects the skeleton. Affected bone often represents a response to an altered calcium metabolism. The persistent skeletal involvement seen in abnormal states of calcium balance illustrates its importance in maintaining proper amounts of this mineral in the bloodstream.

Bone contains 99% of all the body calcium. Together with structural support, its most important function is to serve as a calcium reservoir for the bloodstream. When calcium is needed to sustain life, bone and the small intestinal tract increase or decrease their supply while the kidney and the large bowel control the excretion. Calcium is also present in perspiration, but its contribution to the total excretion picture and the mechanism of its control is not yet known.

The proper supply of calcium and phosphorus is vital to every tissue in the body. Calcium is involved in most cellular systems; that is, muscle contraction, nerve conduction, blood clotting, and so forth. Phosphorus has multiple roles in metabolism; paramount is its integral role in energy producing compounds (that is, adenosine triphosphate and adenosine diphosphate). This complex system, designed to maintain a constant blood level of these divalent ions, appears to be marginally capable of passively sustaining itself as long as no outside influence attempts to upset its balance. Therefore, traffic controlling features are essential to the system (Fig. 9-8). These features are capable of opening and shutting the appropriate flood gates in a homeostatic response to its major and minor needs. The index of these features is lengthy and their execution complex and incompletely understood. We will discuss three of the more important ones.

PARATHYROID HORMONE

The glands producing this hormone are located in the neck, in and around the tissue of the thyroid gland, which is probably the main traffic controller for calcium metabolism. It monitors the calcium content of the bloodstream by constantly testing for its ionized form (free Ca^{++}). When the serum level is too low, it releases stored parathormone (PTH) and manufactures more to replace the original supply. Like most hormones, PTH is carried to different sites via the bloodstream. It operates to increase the blood calcium levels. In the intestine, parathormone interacts with vitamin D to increase the absorption of calcium by stimulating what is in effect a biologic pump mechanism.

In the bone its main affect is a release of the mineral. This is accomplished through (1) stimulation of the cells (osteoclasts and osteocytes) to eat away or dissolve the bone and (2) some similar but direct resorptive chemical effect. Interestingly, the rate of new bone formation is also moderately increased. In the kidney, PTH creates an increased excretion of phosphorus into the urine and a retention of calcium in the blood. Also reported is a conversion of vitamin D to its most active form by this hormone. This

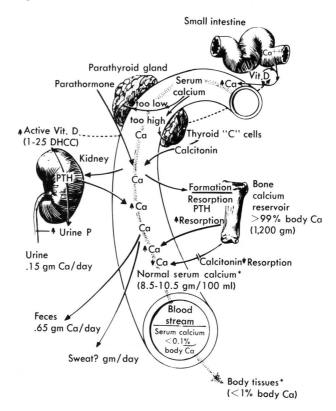

Fig. 9-8. Diagram of calcium homeostasis. The control features maintain the proper serum calcium that is needed for the body tissues. A low serum calcium stimulates absorption of calcium from the intestine, retention of calcium by the kidney, and release of it from the bone. A high serum calcium stimulates release of calcitonin, which inhibits calcium resorption from the bone.

may account for the intestinal action of PTH. In the laboratory variant factors have been found to increase or decrease the bone's response to parathormone. These include oxygen, the degree of acidity, vitamin C, vitamin D, fluoride, heparin, and so forth. However, the presence of PTH is necessary for any of these to produce an effect.

CALCITONIN

In the same general location near the thyroid gland are cells that produce another hormone, calcitonin. This hormone is released in response to high serum calcium levels (hypercalcemia). It appears to act chiefly on the bone, causing a cessation of bone resorption and an abrupt drop in the serum calcium concentration.

VITAMIN D

Vitamins are organic substances essential to the body's normal metabolism, which must be supplied by diet. Although vitamin D is called a vitamin, it behaves more like a hormone. (A hormone is a chemical substance formed by a gland or organ in one part of the body and carried through the bloodstream to another part of the body which it stimulates to functional activity.) Vitamin D is synthesized from a cholesterol compound in the skin in the presence of sunlight. It is then transported to the intestines and bone where it has a specific action. The original label *vitamin D* stemmed from the fact that most of this compound can be and is supplied through the diet, either from plant foodstuffs or meat. Initial forms either manufactured in the skin or absorbed through the intestine can be converted by the liver or kidney into metabolites significantly more potent in stimulating their target organs. The most active vitamin D metabolite (1-25 dihydrocholecalciferol or 1-25 DHCC) is produced in the kidney in the presence of parathyroid hormone. This compound is much more potent than vitamin D, which is produced by the skin. Vitamin D metabolites act principally on the intestine, and their role is one of increased calcium absorption. This appears to be by activation of a biologic "pump," which responds to: (1) a change in the resistance of the intestinal cell wall to the flow of calcium ions, and (2) the production of the calcium transport protein that actively guides the mineral across the intestinal cell into the bloodstream.

In bone, the effect of vitamin D is problematical. Certainly, in the laboratory its action is similar to PTH in that it mobilizes more mineral for the bloodstream. Since this requires the presence of PTH, it may be simply enhancement of the latter's effectiveness.

COMMON LABORATORY TESTS FOR MINERAL METABOLISM
Blood tests

1. Serum calcium. This is a standard and valuable test. Often, disease states can be placed in a broad range or category on the basis of these results alone. The range of normal values must be known for each laboratory but usually lies somewhere between 8.5 and 10.5 mg. calcium per each 100 ml. of serum. Newer methods, such as atomic absorption spectroscopy (ATM, ABS) now used in many places, offer greater precision and a smaller range of normal values. All of these values measure the *total* calcium concentration. However, about 50% of the total calcium in the blood is bound to protein molecules and not readily available for use. The parathyroid gland apparently responds to the concentration of ionized or free calcium. Presently this measurement is done in research laboratories along with the total calcium values. A low albumin concentration tends to give a false low total calcium value. Thus, the protein content should be known when a specimen is sent for calcium analysis.

Blood content values fluctuate rapidly, and repeated tests may be needed to determine normal trends. Because of the powerful homeostatic mechanisms described previously, serum calcium values can be normal despite the presence of active metabolic bone disease. For example, serum calcium may be normal in a child with bowed legs and obvious rickets caused by a diet poor in calcium or vitamin D. This situation can exist because of the sacrifice the skeleton is making to maintain the proper supply to the rest of the body. High calcium levels may be found in hyperparathyroidism, vitamin D overdose, terminal cancer patients, hyperthyroidism, and patients on prolonged bed rest. Low calcium values may be seen in rickets and hypoparathyroidism.

2. Serum phosphorus. Phosphorus values change in a predictable pattern throughout each day. Hence, blood for this test should be drawn about the same time every day. The time before breakfast is acceptable because food intake can falsely elevate this value. The normal range must be known for each hospital; but averages are 2.5 to 4.5 mg for each 100 ml. High values can occur along with low calcium levels in kidney failure and hypoparathyroidism. High phosphorus and calcium levels are seen in the normal patients on bed rest. Low values are commonly seen in rickets, salt-losing kidney conditions (renal tubular defects), and malabsorption syndromes from intestinal disease or after surgical removal of the upper intestinal tract. Hyperparathyroidism is suspected when a calcium rise accompanies a phosphorus decline.

3. Serum alkaline phosphatase. This enzyme is produced in the bone, liver, and intestine. The contribution of each can be determined if necessary. The value is usually reported as the total, and in the absence of active liver disease it is felt to represent some aspect of active new bone formation. Testing methods and resulting values used in this country are quite different. Most commonly used are Bodansky (2 to 4.5 units), King-Armstrong (5 to 10 units), and Bessey-Lowry-Brock (30 to 85 units). These values tend to become higher during fracture healing and during normal active growth periods. The maximal normal value is reached at infancy and rises again at the age of 16 or 17. High values (hyperphosphatagia) indicate that a skeletal disorder is present. The highest value is seen in Paget's Disease (200 to 3,000 I.U.), and this test can be used as a sign of disease activity. Situations causing excessive parathyroid hormone activity or osteomalacia (rickets) are also accompanied by high alkaline phosphatase levels. Active liver disease can markedly alter this test; therefore, other liver function tests should be obtained when a high value is present. Low levels are seen in a rare enzyme difficiency state named hypophosphatagia. These patients have symptoms similar to rickets but low alkaline phosphatase levels and poor ability to heal their fractures.

4. Serum parathyroid hormone. In recent years a few medical centers became equipped to directly evaluate the blood concentrations of parathormone. This is done by assay tests where antibodies are collected from laboratory animals previously injected with an extract of the human hormone. This antiparathyroid hormone serum is then labeled with an isotope for easy detection and reacted with the blood of the patient in question. This test will be used routinely as it becomes standardized and available. Presently we must rely on other more indirect tests of hormone function and on roentgenogram changes for our evaluation.

Urine tests

1. Urine calcium. Collection of urine for calcium is often used for diagnosis, imbalance studies, and as a monitor of treatment programs. It is usually collected for a 24-hour period to avoid any misleading momentary fluctuations. All else being equal, the amount of calcium released in the urine reflects the concentration in the bloodstream. Thus, changes in oral intake, vitamin D level, parathormone levels, and so forth will be reflected in this test. Renal dis-

ease will decrease the ability to excrete calcium. Therefore initial kidney function tests are necessary, for example, creatinine clearance, and so forth.

2. Urine phosphorus. Excretion of phosphorus remains a constant proportion (about 70%) of the dietary intake regardless of a disease state. It is of value to obtain this test for reflection of dietary intake and because the urine calcium is inversely related to the phosphorus content.

RADIOGRAPHIC EVALUATION

Many metabolic disease states have typical roentgenographic patterns which help to identify them. Roentgenographic changes of patients on therapy often show recognizable indications of success or failure. Quantitative density methods are also widely used for sensitively monitoring the effects of treatment.

BONE BIOPSY

Often the initial diagnosis of bone disease is best made by analysis of the bone itself. Subsequently, the success or failure of treatment in many of these diseases can be most accurately followed by repeating the biopsy after the establishment of a treatment program for 6 to 12 months. Research techniques that study bone without decalcifying it will allow quantitation of the state of bone turnover. These techniques are becoming widely used because they allow a very sensitive assessment of response to therapy.

METABOLIC BONE DISEASES

RICKETS

Rickets is a disease of childhood causing soft, deformed bones as a result of a deficiency of vitamin D. Microscopically, wide areas of unmineralized bone indicate a lack of adequate calcium content. Clinically, there is

marked bowing of the legs and arms, along with muscle weakness and bone tenderness. Roentgenograms classically display wide growth plates; long bones flare at the ends. Two basic classes of rickets can be distinguished according to their response to vitamin D replacement (Fig. 9-9).

NUTRITIONAL RICKETS

This type is a result of an actual deficiency state, either from poor diet or lack of sunlight. It is no longer common in the United States because of milk and food fortification. The minimal vitamin D requirement is about 400 I.U. daily.

RESISTANT RICKETS

This type is not corrected with replacement of a normal intake of vitamin D and may even require 50 to 1,000 times this dose for an effect. Assorted causes can produce resistant rickets; the most common include hereditary hypophosphatemic rickets, kidney salt-wasting defects, and malabsorption syndromes of childhood (Fig. 9-10).

Hereditary hypophosphatemic rickets. This inherited type has a persistently low serum phosphorus and is the most common form of

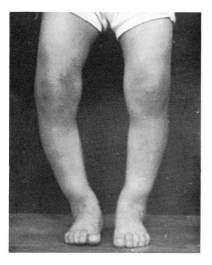

Fig. 9-9. Bowlegs (genu varum) that are the result of active rickets. If the rickets is brought under control, the bowlegs will correct themselves during further growth.

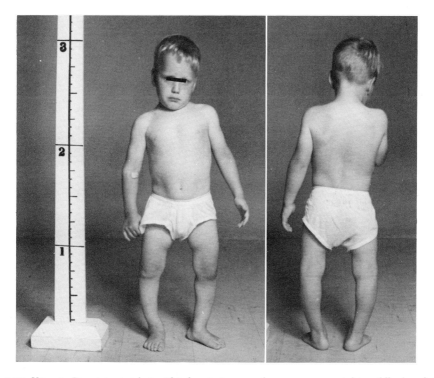

Fig. 9-10. Vitamin D resistant rickets. This boy is 5 years of age, average weight, mildly dwarfed in height, and shows the bowleg deformities that improve with proper high dosage of vitamin D intake.

rickets in this country today. Genetically, it is sex-linked dominant. Affected women transmit this trait to one-half their sons and/or daughters. Affected men transmit it to all of their daughters but none of their sons. The serum calcium is usually normal and alkaline phosphatase is high. Urine calcium and calcium balance studies are usually below normal. Urine phosphorus is often higher than normal. The actual metabolic defect is not yet known. Treatment may be successful with near-toxic levels of vitamin D.

Renal tubular rickets. Many individual salt-wasting kidney defects produce renal tubular rickets that is also "resistant" to vitamin D and mineral replacement.

Malabsorption syndromes. Studies in England of patients with rickets show that many have intestinal diseases (that is, celiac disease) where absorption of dietary vitamin D is poor.

OSTEOMALACIA

Osteomalacia is essentially the adult corollary to rickets in a child. The difference is that the mechanisms of bone growth are no longer vulnerable and only bone turnover mechanisms are affected. Thus, shortness of stature and marked bowing of extremities are not found in osteomalacia. The same factors that cause rickets are known to cause osteomalacia. Patients with colitis, postgastrectomy syndromes, cirrhosis, and so forth, as well as vegetarians and patients on anticonvulsive drugs, develop osteomalacia. Usually there is a history of bone or spine pain from crush fractures. The radiographic and clinical symptoms are often difficult to distinguish from osteoporosis. Serum calcium, urine calcium, and serum phosphorus may be slightly lower than normal.

AZOTEMIC RENAL OSTEODYSTROPHY

Most patients with uremia from chronic kidney failure also have distinct bone pathology. The skeletal changes manifest varying combinations of two pathological processes: (1) inadequate mineralization (that is, rickets or osteomalacia), and (2) hyperparathyroidism. As the renal disease progresses, the bone changes become increasingly severe and lead to more frequent orthopaedic consultations. Renal dialysis causes further deterioration, but successful renal

transplant corrects the bone problems. The serum phosphorus and urea nitrogen levels are usually very high in this category. The total calcium and ionized calcium is usually low. Parathyroid hormone levels are extremely high. Treatment modalities include correction of calcium balance, vitamin D supplements, correction of acid-base balance, and sometimes parathyroidectomy. The only absolute way to arrest and reverse the skeletal deterioration is by successful renal transplantation.

HYPERPARATHYROIDISM

Excessive production of parathyroid hormone (PTH) eventually causes predictable effects on the entire body. The high serum calcium levels cause soft tissue calcifications, alterations in muscle contractility, renal stones, and marked bone destruction. The excessive resorption of the skeleton is referred to as osteitis fibrosa. Fractures are frequent and can result in deformities. On roentgenogram there is a general decrease in bone mass with frequent cystic areas notable. Under the microscope, marked resorptive activity is obvious. There are three distinct forms of parathyroid hyperactivity.

Primary hyperparathyroidism. This state is usually associated with a tumor (adenoma) which produces PTH. Surgery is required to correct the problem.

Secondary hyperparathyroidism. A chronic state of inadequate serum calcium levels can cause an enlargement of the gland and an abnormally high production of PTH. The condition is encountered most often in patients with intestinal malabsorption and chronic renal failure. Its treatment involves correction of the low calcium levels, if possible.

Tertiary hyperparathyroidism. This term refers to the rare situation in which a patient with a long-standing secondary hyperparathyroidism develops a gland which appears to "run wild." The clinical picture is then similar to that of primary hyperparathyroidism with hypercalcemia and high levels of circulating PTH. This condition may be caused by an adenoma or an overproduction of normal-appearing glandular tissue. Again the treatment is surgical removal.

PAGET'S DISEASE (OSTEITIS DEFORMANS)

Paget's disease is a disease of the bone in which there is overactivity of osteoblasts and osteoclasts, building and destroying bone in an unaltered chemical pattern. High levels of phosphatase occur and are an index to the rapidity and amount of new bone being formed. The cause of this disease is entirely unknown, and the treatment is limited to the correction of deformities that occur. People afflicted with this disease are usually past middle age, and the bones involved may be few or many.

The bones become broader and weaker than normal and are easily fractured. The fractures heal readily. In the generalized form the patient becomes shorter and, because the skull expands, may require a larger hat. In rare instances the involved bone may show malignant changes.

OSTEOPOROSIS

Osteoporosis (porous bone) is presently defined as a clinical condition in which there is a decrease in the total amount of bone to the point that fractures occur with minor trauma. As opposed to osteomalacia, the bone in this instance appears normal under the microscope and is well mineralized, but there is simply not enough

of it. Osteoporosis is a very common end result of many different causes.

Primary osteoporosis

As the term primary indicates, in this type there is no identifiable cause. Primary osteoporosis is the most common type and the one usually understood when the general term osteoporosis is used. Many of these patients are postmenopausal women (over 50 years old) or even older men. They are usually seen because of back pain that is out of proportion to any history of trauma. If there have been old vertebral body crush fractures, loss of height and a round back posture is detected. A moderate loss of bone mass is normal with aging; however these patients have lost much more than other people their own age. As a result, they have a two-fold chance of incurring fractures of their wrist, hip, humerus, and vertebral body (usually thoracic spine). As many as 70% of the patients with hip fractures are diagnosed as having osteoporosis. Laboratory values are usually normal. Roentgenograms reveal a diffuse wash-out of bone (radiolucency) and often a loss of trabecular patterns and thin cortices. A bone biopsy reveals thin and porous but otherwise normal-appearing bone. By measurement, the osteo-

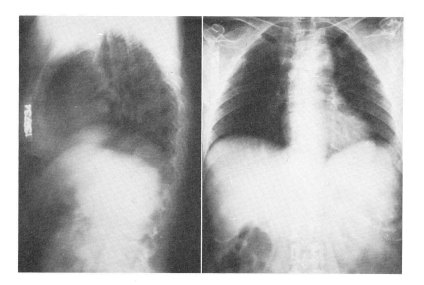

Fig. 9-11. Osteoporosis. This is a metabolic disorder of elderly persons (females especially), in which calcium in the bone is depleted and the bone matrix fails to produce replacement bone. The result is a weakening of the structure.

clastic resorption is often slightly increased. No light has yet been shed on the cause, but many factors are suspected, such as poor diet, estrogen deficiency and lack of exercise. No adequate prevention or treatment is yet proved. Presently it is common to attempt improvement in the protein, calcium, and vitamin D intake. Also, an exercise program is frequently prescribed. Estrogen replacement and high fluoride and calcium doses may have some merit. Back pain and fractures are treated as discussed in previous chapters.

Secondary osteoporosis

In this group there is an identifiable cause of the osteoporosis. The list is long and a few causes will be mentioned.

Nutritional osteoporosis. Various abnormal nutritional states are known to cause osteoporosis, such as vitamin C deficiency (scurvy), milk malabsorption syndromes (lactose intolerance and others), acid diets, and calcium deficient diets.

Endocrine osteoporosis. Abnormal function of many different endocrine glands, for example, hyperthyroidism, hyperparathyroidism (mild), Cushing's syndrome, acromegaly, and hypogonadism, will produce an osteoporosis.

Disuse osteoporosis. Bed rest and inactivity are well-known causes of osteoporosis. Lack of gravity or normal stresses and strains appears to be the main factor here since astronauts have developed the same problems despite their exercise programs while in space. On the other hand, stressing a bone by exercise is known to increase the bone mass and strengthen it.

Nursing implications

The patient who has been inactive or confined to bed rest for an extended period of time may have very fragile bones because of this demineralization process. Fractures of the long bones, vertebral bodies, or pelvis may occur with little or no trauma. Turning in bed may be sufficient stress to cause a fracture. Usually the patient experiences pain, and the "snap" may be audible. However, in some instances, because of pain already present or because of absence of normal sensation, the patient is not aware of any increased pain or discomfort. The fractures become apparent because of a deformed position of the extremity. Needless to say, extreme care and gentleness should be exercised when turning or ambulating this type of patient.

When collapse of the vertebral bodies occurs, an increase in the anterioposterior curves of the spine develop. This is particularly apparent in the thoracic region, and the result is a rounded back or kyphosis. With compression fracture of the vertebrae, the patient experiences severe back pain. The altered alignment of the spine places strain on the supporting ligaments and muscles and can cause pressure on nerve roots. The patient is uncomfortable when standing or walking and consequently is inclined to spend more time in the horizontal position, thus becoming less active. This in turn increases disuse demineralization of bone.

To overcome osteoporosis, new bone formation must exceed the process of bone resorption. Treatment consists of exercise, frequent rest periods, and avoidance of severe fatigue. For rest periods and sleep, the osteoporotic individual should have a firm supporting mattress. Exercise in the form of walking is encouraged. Wearing a spinal support such as a corset or light brace when in the upright position usually helps to decrease the back discomfort. The support serves to immobilize and protect the spine, enabling the patient to be up and about safely. It also helps the patient to use correct body mechanics—flexing knees as opposed to rounding the back when stooping. Incorrect methods of stooping or sitting cause increased pain and fatigue in the back area. In addition, the patient should be cautioned to avoid lifting or performing activities that cause twisting of the spine. Analgesics and muscle relaxants are frequently prescribed, and attention to dietary intake, to ensure adequate intake of protein, vitamin D, and calcium is an essential part of the treatment. Estrogen therapy tends to slow the process of osteoporosis.

Extensive laboratory studies are done on each of these patients. Careful instruction of nursing personnel is necessary to prevent loss of specimens, and to ensure collection of specimens at specified times.

STUDY QUESTIONS

1. List three main types of bone cells and the function of each.
2. Discuss the functions of bone.

3. List several laboratory tests for mineral metabolism, including normal values.
4. Discuss briefly several types of rickets and necessary treatment.

REFERENCES

Atkinson, P. J.: The development of osteoporosis, Clin. Orthop. **90:**217, 1973.

Dunn, A. W.: Senile osteoporosis, Geriatrics **22:**175-180, 1967.

Hass, H.: Osteoporosis, Geriatrics **22:**100-111, 1967.

Hegsted, D. M.: Osteoporosis and fluoride deficiency, Postgrad. Med. **41:**A49-A53, 1967.

Hohl, J., guest editor: Symposium on metabolic bone disease, Orthop. Clin. North Am. **3:**503, 1972.

Jowsey, J., Riggs, B. L., and Kelly, P. J.: New concepts in the treatment of osteoporosis, Postgrad. Med. **52:**62, 1972.

Lonergan, R. C.: Osteoporosis of the spine, Am. J. Nurs. **61:**79-81, 1961.

Lutwak, L.: Osteoporosis: apublic health problem, Am. Assoc. Industr. Nurses J. **14:**21-23, 1966.

Lyford, B.: Implications of osteoporosis, J. Amer. Phys. Ther. Ass. **42:**106-110, 1962.

Soika, C. V.: Combatting osteoporosis, Am. J. Nurs. **73:**1193, 1973.

Riggs, L.: Diagnosis and treatment of primary osteoporosis, Postgrad. Med. **44:**224-229, 1968.

Tapia, J., Stearns, G., and Ponseti, I. V.: Vitamin-D resistant rickets. A long-term clinical study of eleven patients, J. Bone Joint Surg. **46-A:**935, 1964.

10
Congenital deformities

Deformities that are present at birth are considered congenital. They may follow hereditary patterns or be the result of embryologic defects.

It is estimated that 2% of newborn infants have congenital malformations. It is now known that only 25% of the cases are of genetic origin, whereas 75% are the result of external factors influencing an originally healthy ovum. The importance of these external factors became evident when it was found that if a woman develops rubella in the fifth week of pregnancy she may give birth to a child with cataracts. Rubella contracted in the ninth week of pregnancy may lead to lesions of the inner ear, and if the disease is contracted between the fifth and tenth weeks of pregnancy, the child may be born with cardiac deformities. A sedative, Thalidomide, when given to pregnant women, resulted in many of their children being born with multiple congenital deformities, especially phocomelia. These malformations do not depend merely on the nature of the causative agent but more on the stage of pregnancy at which it acts on the embryo and on the vulnerability of certain cells in the embryo. Poisons or parasites, such as in toxoplasmosis, can produce ocular and/or nervous lesions. Roentgen rays or irradiation from radioactive substances can cause anencephalia, exencephalia, hydrocephalus, and ocular anomalies. Irradiation given late in pregnancy may cause spina bifida, velum palatinum fissures, and limb malformations of all types. Avitaminosis, particularly of A, E, or B_2 (pantothenic acid deficiency)—whether caused by a lack of supply, a lack of absorption, or the presence of substances that impede normal utilization—can result in malformations. Many of the progesterones (4-pregnene-3, 20-dione) can lead to virilization in female fetuses. They may cause total or partial fusion of the labia majora, hypertrophy of the clitoris, or opening of the ureter into the vagina. Over four hundred drugs are known that have teratogenic effects in animals, but only a few of these drugs can cause malformations in humans. It is important when treating a pregnant women to prescribe only those drugs that are imperative to her well-being, such as insulin, cortisone, and isoniazid.

The types and variations of deformity are almost limitless. Many deformities, however, are not disabling. Those encountered frequently will be described in this chapter.

CONGENITAL DISLOCATION OF THE HIP

The term "congenital dislocation of the hip" implies that the head of the femur is outside the confines of the acetabulum at birth. Actually, there are degrees of dislocation, from incomplete to complete, and these are identified by definite terms.

Subluxation, or predislocation, is an incomplete dislocation. This is more common than dislocation and is more difficult to detect. If they remain untreated, however, many subluxations eventually result in complete dislocations, and for this reason their early recognition assumes importance.

The exact cause is unknown, but the defect is primarily improper acetabular development. This does not cause symptoms; but when certain signs are present, the condition should be suspected and verified by a roentgenogram of the

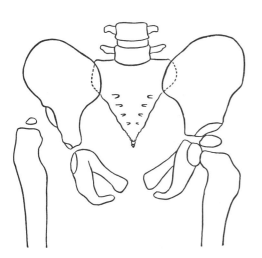

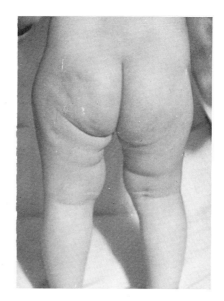

Fig. 10-1. Copy of roentgenogram of congenital dislocation of right hip. There is upward and backward displacement of the head of the femur, as well as thickening at the base of the acetabulum (prenatal).

Fig. 10-2. Congenital dislocation of the left hip. Note prominent trochanter on the affected side and asymmetry of gluteal folds.

hips (Fig. 10-1). Limited abduction of the hip in the flexed position and/or a click sign (Ortolani sign) when the hip is being abducted are the most useful objective findings. Treatment by means of a Frejka pillow splint should be instituted immediately.

Congenital dislocation refers to those cases in which there is an actual complete dislocation. This can occur during intrauterine life or result from an untreated subluxation sometime after birth. In either case it demands early recognition and treatment to obtain a satisfactory result.

The signs of congenital dislocation vary with the age of the child. Walking is often delayed, and the mother may have noted an extra gluteal fold on the affected side. Occasionally it is brought to attention by a shortness of the leg, an unusually broad perineum (especially in bilateral cases), or an unusual trochanteric prominence (Fig. 10-2). Should dislocation be unrecognized until walking begins, the most obvious sign will be a waddling limp. On examination it is usually apparent that the affected leg is shorter, the range of hip motion is freer than normal, there is lack of stability on the push test, and the trochanter is higher

than normal. In standing, the child will demonstrate a positive Trendelenburg test, which is indicative of an unstable hip joint. When the body weight is put on the normal or stable hip and the affected limb is elevated, the pelvis on the side of the dislocated hip rises (this is true with normal hip joints). However, when the body weight is taken on the dislocated hip and the normal limb is elevated, the pelvis drops on the side of the normal limb. To compensate for the pelvic drop, the body shifts to the opposite side to maintain balance (Fig. 10-3).

Treatment must be started immediately after the diagnosis is made. The aim is to reduce the dislocation to a normal position. This is ordinarily accomplished by a closed manipulation performed while the patient is under anesthesia. The reduction must then be maintained for sufficient time to allow the acetabulum to develop to a point at which it will maintain reduction. This may require months, during which time the hip will be immobilized in a plaster spica cast. The surgeon in charge will vary the position to obtain proper placement of the femoral head within the acetabulum. Various splints are available as substitutes for plaster casts and have the advantage of being remov-

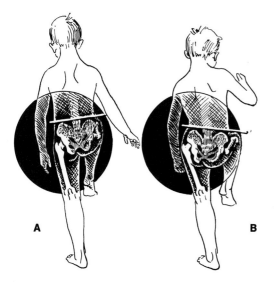

A   **B**

Fig. 10-3. A, Negative Trendelenburg sign. When the body weight is placed on the normal limb (stable hip) and the opposite limb is elevated, the pelvis rises on the side of the lifted limb. **B,** Positive Trendelenburg sign. When the body weight is placed on the unstable hip (as in congenital dislocated hip) and the opposite limb is elevated, the pelvis drops on the side of the lifted limb.

able. These are more applicable in the later stages of treatment.

Operative reduction is necessary when closed manipulation has failed to correct the dislocation. The aftertreatment is similar to closed reduction, both in time required and in type of fixation apparatus.

Late results. When treatment is begun early (within the first 18 months of life), the outcome will usually be excellent. A few patients treated early and many treated late will show degenerative changes of the hip by the time middle age has been reached. These degenerative changes cause painful disability sufficient to require further treatment. For the details of treatment at this stage as well as for unreduced dislocations found in adults, see Chapter 15.

Treatment and nursing care. The nurses's function in detecting and reporting congenital anomalies is an important one. The nurse, whether a hospital nurse working with infants in the obstetric nursery, a public health nurse giving bedside instructions to a new mother, a nurse in the pediatric ward, or a school nurse,

will have many opportunities to detect abnormalities. To do this intelligently, a clear understanding of what is normal in the structure, function, and development of the child is required. In addition to this it is necessary to know the symptoms of the common orthopedic conditions that are found at birth. Although most congenital deformities cannot be prevented, nurses should recognize the fact that certain birth injuries can sometimes be prevented by good medical supervision and care during the period of pregnancy and delivery. They should use their influence to see that all mothers are given good obstetric care.

The nurse giving a bath to the newborn infant may become aware of deviations when bathing him and watching his activities while he is unclothed. Abnormal conditions—such as limitation of joint motion, excessively free joint motion, limpness or a disinclination to move a part, a tendency to lie in one position constantly, alteration of body contours, or asymmetric folds in the skin—may rightly arouse suspicion that something is wrong.

Not all congenital anomalies, however, are detected at this early stage. The child may have reached school age before an abnormality is noted; sometimes the condition will be manifested only when the child is tired, and then a slight limp or alteration in gait will be detected.

The importance of early recognition, of course, is that it makes early treatment possible. Early treatment is paramount in the management of these patients. Delay may make any attempted treatment only palliative. The nurse should realize this factor in order to help the family accept the necessity for securing immediate medical treatment when the abnormality is recognized. Strong emotional reactions often accompany this kind of condition, and medical personnel should appreciate the feelings of the family. Parents may be afflicted by shame, pride, despair, or bewilderment, and sympathetic understanding and informed common sense are necessary to combat such feelings.

"The key that opens the door of diagnosis is suspicion," says Osgood.[*] Rather than voicing

---

[*]From Osgood, R. B.: Compression fractures of the spine, J.A.M.A. **89:**1563-1568, 1927.

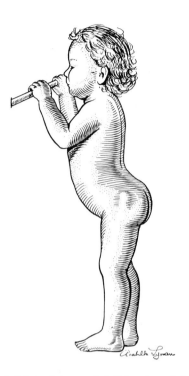

Fig. 10-4. Bilateral congenital dislocation of the hip in the older child. Note prominence in the gluteal region and swayback. The swayback position compensates for the backward displacement of the hips.

suspicions aloud, the nurse should use influence to see that the child suspected of having an abnormality is given the benefit of medical examination without delay.

It is hardly possible to overestimate the importance of early recognition of congenital dislocation of the hip. The results of the treatment are always best if it can be started early, if possible during the first 3 months of life. The possibilities of a perfect result diminish rapidly as the child grows older (Fig. 10-4).

The importance of observing the newborn infant for signs of the condition cannot be overemphasized. When bathing the infant, the nurse may note an extra fold in the buttock or thigh, or perhaps a widening of the perineum (Fig. 10-5). In flexing the baby's hips and knees with his feet flat on the table it may be observed that one knee is lower than the other. One may detect that all motion in the hip seems abnormally free except for limited abduction (Fig. 10-6). When the physician's attention has been called to these observations, the nurse may see him fix the baby's pelvis with his hand and grasp the lower end of the femur to determine if piston motion, or telescoping, is present. Roentgenograms of the hip on which these signs are noted will assist the physician in making his diagnosis if an established dislocation is present.

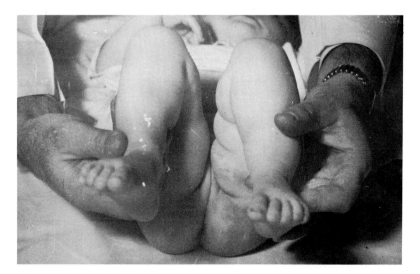

Fig. 10-5. Apparent shortening of the left thigh as the result of left hip dislocation. The left knee appears lower. Two extra skin folds are present in the left thigh.

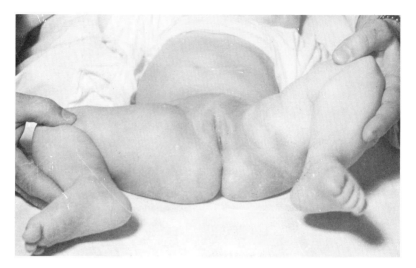

Fig. 10-6. Limitation of left hip abduction in an infant with congenital left hip dislocation.

If the anomaly of the hip is not detected in infancy or early childhood, other symptoms become apparent after weight bearing is established. Nurses should be familiar with these symptoms.

The child will walk with a lurching or a waddling gait because of the instability of the femur on the affected side. In addition to this, the buttocks may seem abnormally broad and there will be lumbar lordosis accompanied by a protuberant abdomen (Fig. 10-7). By the time the child is 10 or 11 years of age the lordosis has usually become very marked and unsightly, and scoliosis may have developed if the dislocation is unilateral. There will be shortening of the limb and often an adduction deformity of the leg. When this stage is reached, great difficulties stand in the way of treatment but much can still be done to ensure the child a fairly stable hip and to reduce the possibility of arthritis and allied conditions in later life.

Treatment of congenital dislocation of the hip will vary somewhat according to the age at which the child is seen and the kind of dislocation present. The closed reduction is probably still the preferred method if the child is seen within the first few years of life. It will usually involve the use of a spica cast, and the nursing care the child receives after this may do much to determine the success or failure of the treatment. Open reductions are sometimes nec-

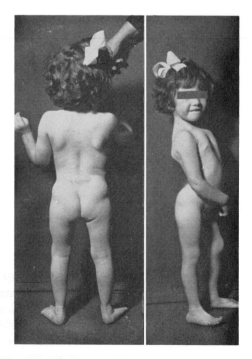

Fig. 10-7. Bilateral dislocated hips in older child. Note marked lumbar lordosis, protruding abdomen, wide perineum, and prominent trochanters.

essary to supplement the closed reduction. Palliative operations, such as shelving operations and the various types of osteotomies, may be necessary if both closed and open reductions fail. If the condition is diagnosed during what

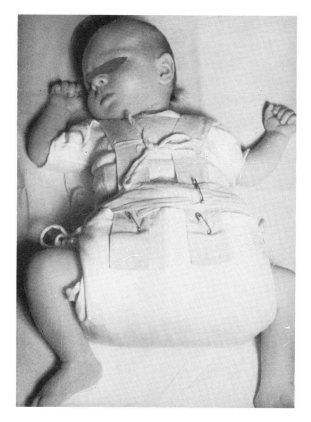

Fig. 10-8. Correct application of the Frejka pillow splint. The pillow maintains the thighs in flexion, abduction, and external rotation; it is frequently used for patients with mild hip dislocation or with tightness of the adductors.

is called the predislocation stage of the postnatal type, an abduction splint may sometimes be used.

NURSING CARE WITH THE FREJKA PILLOW SPLINT. Subluxation of the hip joint, when diagnosed during the first month of life, is usually treated with a pillow splint (Fig. 10-8). This splint, which is available in several sizes, consists of a square pillow (filled with kapok) and is held in place by a "romperlike" garment (Fig. 10-9). Usually it is not necessary for the child to be admitted to the hospital. In the outpatient clinic, while the baby is fitted with a pillow of the proper size, the mother is taught the correct application of this splint. With its correct application the baby's limbs are held in an abducted position, and in this position the head of the femur is maintained in the acetabulum. Keeping the femoral head in the acetabulum deepens the hip socket and promotes development of

a normal hip. Since the splint is applied over the diaper, it must be removed and reapplied each time the diaper is changed. Plastic pants worn by the baby can protect the pillow from wetting and soiling; however, it is advisable that the mother have a second cover for the pillow to permit change and laundry. Care of the baby wearing a pillow splint is somewhat easier than care of the child wearing a bilateral hip cast. The baby can be picked up and moved with greater ease and, generally speaking, the mother is not so apprehensive as the mother who must care for her baby while he is in a hip spica cast. The splint must be worn until roentgenograms show a normally developed hip joint, which means the baby may need to wear the splint for a period of 7 to 10 months. The splint is worn continuously at first and then use is gradually discontinued by permitting the baby to be without the splint for increasing

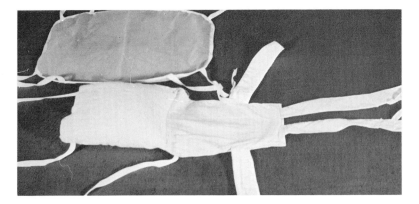

Fig. 10-9. The Frejka pillow splint ready for application. The pillow has been placed in the pocket part of the garment.

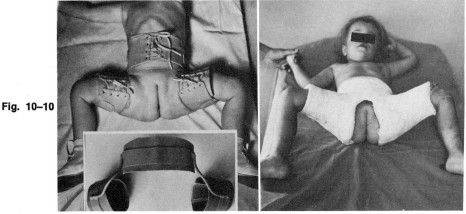

Fig. 10—10

Fig. 10—11

Fig. 10-10. Anterior and posterior views of the abduction brace used in treatment of hip subluxation and dislocation.

Fig. 10-11. Hip spica cast used in treatment of hip dislocation or subluxation.

periods of time. This should be carefully controlled by the orthopedic surgeon.

NURSING CARE WITH THE ABDUCTION BRACE. If the Ortolani test remains positive when the baby with a subluxation of the hip joint is being treated by means of a pillow splint, use of this splint will be discontinued and the baby may be fitted with an abduction brace (Fig. 10-10). This brace maintains the limbs in an abducted and flexed position. The brace is worn continuously and, with the limbs fixed in this position, the femoral head is held in the acetabulum. This tends to deepen the shallow acetabulum and to provide for the development of a well-formed femoral head. While he is wearing the brace, the baby's skin must be cleansed beneath the splint and checked for signs of irritation. Plastic material may be used to provide some protection for the leather parts of the brace; however, frequent checking and the changing of a wet or soiled diaper are very important in maintaining a clean brace. This brace is worn several months full time but, as with the pillow splint, the length of time that the abduction brace is used must be carefully controlled by the orthopedic surgeon to ensure the desired result—a normally functioning hip joint.

NURSING CARE IN THE CLOSED REDUC-

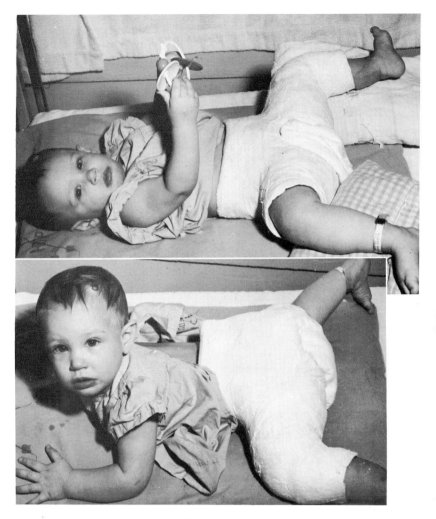

Fig. 10-12. Anterior and posterior views of a 9-month-old baby with hip spica cast applied after reduction of congenitally dislocated left hip. Her cast maintains the hips in positions of flexion and abduction. Edges of the cast have been covered with tape. Strips of protective material will be applied about the perineal and buttocks regions prior to the patient's discharge from the hospital.

TION METHOD. The closed reduction method used by Lorenz and somewhat modified in more recent years is probably the preferred method of reduction for children under 2 years of age. This reduction is performed when the patient is under anesthesia. The manipulation and manual traction used to reduce the congenital dislocated hip should be gentle and involve little force. If reducing the hip is difficult, the child may be placed in traction for several weeks. Traction can stretch the hip muscles and place the femoral head in a better position for reduc-

tion. After reduction the hip is held in a position of 90 degrees flexion and 60 to 70 degrees abduction by means of a plaster cast. Subcutaneous tenotomy of the adductor tendons is frequently done to decrease pressure on the femoral head in the reduced position. The cast is very carefully applied and well molded to maintain the reduction. With the head of the femur well centered in the acetabulum, the hip joint is considered stable, and the cast is not extended to include the knee joint on either side (Fig. 10-11). However, the cast edges need to be trimmed carefully to prevent pressure in the popliteal region. If the hip is in an unstable position, the cast is extended to below the knee on the involved side (Fig. 10-12). It is not necessary to include the feet and ankles in the plaster cast.

The small child who has had a closed reduction is usually hospitalized for 24 to 48 hours. Before the youngster is discharged, the edges of the cast are trimmed and finished with tape and plaster splints. (See Chapter 1.) If this is the first time the child has been placed in plaster, the mother will need a considerable amount of reassurance and help pertaining to his care. She should be carefully instructed in the care of both the patient and the cast. Such instruction cannot be given hurriedly if the child is to have adequate care. A discussion of many details will enter into the instruction.

The patient's mother should have an opportunity to observe the nurse while finishing the cast edges and applying Pliofilm to protect the cast from becoming wet and soiled. An additional supply of waterproof material should be sent home with the mother so that she may replace the protective membrane as needed. A perineal pad made from a folded diaper is tucked under the cast anteriorly and posteriorly. This pad also may be covered with a strip of the waterproofing, which supplies added protection for the cast. A second diaper is pinned in place to anchor the pad and to provide cover for the child. The mother should understand that making frequent checks, with prompt change of the wet or soiled diaper, is very important in maintenance of a clean and intact cast. The urine-soaked cast is not only foul smelling; it may become soft, also, and thus provide inadequate immobilization for the hip joint. A hair dryer can be used to dry the damp cast. The mother should be instructed to return the child to the hospital or clinic, if the cast is broken, and not wait until the next appointment date.

The first 24 to 48 hours following application of the cast is usually an unhappy time for the small child. Restriction of movements, which the child does not understand, is frustrating to him. He reacts by crying. This is upsetting to the mother who is already bewildered by the thoughts of caring for her baby in a cast. However, after the first several days the small child

should be quite comfortable in the cast and normal eating, sleeping, and play activities should be resumed. Nurses should bear in mind that most mothers tend to be afraid of damaging the cast. It is essential that they realize that it is possible to give the child wholly adequate care in the cast if they will take the time to do so. Methods of keeping the cast clean and dry and of caring for the skin beneath the cast should be demonstrated. The necessity of using the fingers to clean under the cast must be particularly emphasized. Many times sores near the edges of the cast, where they should be discovered without difficulty, are overlooked. The mother must be instructed to observe signs that the child is growing too large for his cast, and the freedom the child is to be allowed should be discussed. Most surgeons permit the child to stand or even walk in the crib if he so desires. Sitting astraddle a chair or some kind of kiddy-car is often permitted (Figs. 10-13 and 10-14).

Proper placement of pillows to provide correct support for the limbs and to prevent pressure from the cast edges should be explained. Placing the pillows so as to support the child's shoulders and back slightly higher than the pelvis will

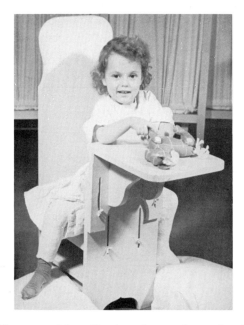

Fig. 10-13. Adjustable chair that can be used with child in hip spica cast after reduction for congenital dislocation of the hip.

help maintain a dry cast by preventing urine from running under the baby's back (Fig. 10-15). Observations to detect swelling, discoloration, or lack of motion are important. Active use of the joints not immobilized is encouraged. Normally the small child will use all joints not restricted by the cast. With the surgeon's permission simple exercises can be taught, to prevent atrophy and loss of function in the feet. Usually, dorsiflexion and inversion exercises will be prescribed.

When possible, a public health nurse should be notified of the homecoming of a child who has had a hip reduction in order to be able to assist the mother during the first daily bath and to clear up any details that have escaped the mother's memory.

After approximately 1 month, the child is returned to the clinic and roentgenograms are taken (through the cast) to check the position of the femoral head. If the position is satisfactory, the cast is worn for another 2- or 3-month period. If the knee was enclosed in plaster, the cast may be cut to allow for knee motion. Crawling and active use of the limbs, within limitation of the cast, are encouraged. An abduction brace is frequently prescribed for use after removal of the cast. This brace maintains the hip in the same position as the plaster cast and is usually worn full time until roentgenograms show good acetabular development. At that point the brace is removed for several hours daily, permitting the child free use of his limbs.

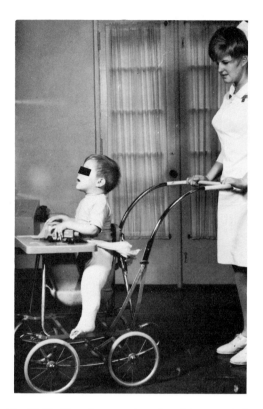

Fig. 10-14. Use of a go-cart equipped to support the child in a hip spica cast in an upright position. In addition to facilitating the care of the child, this position permits him to do many things impossible for the child who must stay in a horizontal position.

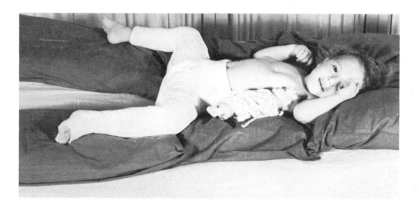

Fig. 10-15. Arrangement of rubber-covered pillows to support hip spica cast. Note space left for the bedpan and for folded diaper across the perineum. Head of bed may be elevated slightly to help prevent wetting the cast.

The time without the brace is gradually increased, and within several months the child will be able to stand and start walking. An abduction brace may be ordered to be worn at nighttime for several years to help maintain a well-developed acetabulum and to prevent a subluxation of the femoral head. As previously emphasized, this child should be examined by the orthopedic surgeon at frequent intervals to provide for early detection of undesirable changes in the hip joint.

PREPARATION FOR SURGERY. Traction may be used preparatory to open reduction or other surgery on congenital dislocation of the hip. It has been found that this procedure will shorten the time necessary for reduction while the child is under anesthesia and will often eliminate the use of undue force in placing the head of the femur in the acetabulum. The purpose of traction is to bring the head of the femur down to the level of the acetabulum. Usually, the orthopedist will maintain this traction for 10 days to 2 weeks before the operation is performed.

A small pillow may be placed under the calf of the leg to keep the heel free of the bed, thereby preventing friction.

NURSING CARE AFTER SURGERY. Open reduction of the hip may be attended by a certain degree of shock during the first 24 hours after surgery. Intravenous fluids are usually given, and shock position may be required. The child should be kept warm and observed frequently for signs of hemorrhage.

The child will usually be immobilized in a spica cast, and after his recovery from the effects of surgery, nursing care will not vary greatly from that given to the child with a closed reduction.

The treatment of neglected or recurrent dislocation of the hip in older children will usually include surgery. Nursing care after the shelving operation or after osteotomy will be similar to that given to the child with open reduction of the hip.

After removal of a hip spica cast that has been worn for several months after surgery, patients seem vulnerable to fracture of the shaft of the femur—a result of bone atrophy that takes place during long periods of immobilization. Gentle handling of the extremity is essen-

tial, and extreme care should be exercised in getting the child up in a chair or on crutches. If he is being discharged from the hospital, the parents should be instructed to guard the child's activity carefully against possible jars and falls. Fracture of the femur has been known to occur from merely turning over in bed. The fracture may often be overlooked, inasmuch as the pain associated with it is attributed to the general discomfort resulting from the removal of the cast. Nurses should be alert for any complaint that might indicate a pathologic fracture.

CONGENITAL CLUBFOOT

Congenital deformities of the foot are of many kinds and are primarily hereditary since they can frequently be traced through several generations. The typical clubfoot (Fig. 10-17) is composed of three main elements of deformity, that is, equinus, varus, and forefoot adduction (Fig. 10-16), and is known by the common term "talipes equinovarus," which was derived from the Latin (Fig. 10-17).

Intrauterine positions of the foot can easily be mistaken for true clubfoot deformity, but examinations will reveal the difference. A true clubfoot, if examined, cannot be corrected to a neutral position in all elements of deformity, whereas an apparent positional deformity corrects itself quite readily. This is important to decide because treatment should begin immediately after a true clubfoot is known to exist, whereas no special treatment is necessary for a positional clubfoot. This also holds true for other foot deformities, such as pes adductus and talipes calcaneovalgus (Fig. 10-18).

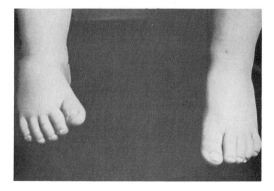

Fig. 10-16. Forefoot adduction of the right foot.

True clubfoot may be unilateral or bilateral and occurs not infrequently in association with other defects such as spina bifida and arthrogryposis. In any patient with clubfoot, therefore, other defects should be carefully looked for during examination.

Treatment of a clubfoot is quite successful in most instances. The principle of the treatment is to attain correction of all elements of deformity by manipulation and to maintain correction throughout the early growth years. This has been accomplished by various techniques, ranging from simple adhesive strapping to manipulation under anesthesia. Time and

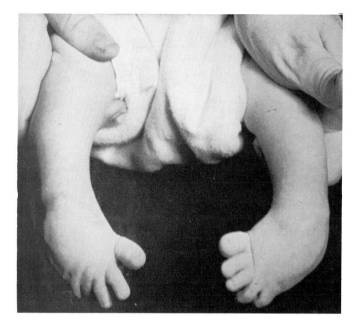

Fig. 10-17. Bilateral clubfoot (talipes equinovarus).

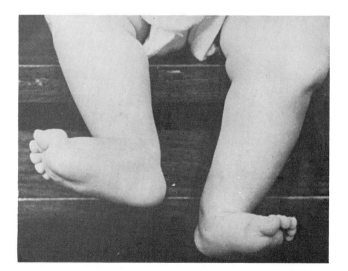

Fig. 10-18. Calcaneovalgus deformity of both feet. (From Kenney, W. C., and Larson, C. B.: Orthopedics for the general practitioner, St. Louis, 1957, The C. V. Mosby Co.)

experience have taught us that excessive force can be harmful to the growing centers. The most common technique is the use of repeated manipulations and plaster casts. By this method the foot is stretched gently into a corrected position, and a cast is applied to hold the gain. This is repeated at intervals of a few days until correction is attained. Ten or more manipulations over a period of several months may be required. Weight bearing plus some type of retentive apparatus at night will usually maintain correction.

Many variations may be made in an effort to accommodate prolonged treatment to specific needs in each case. Frequently one element of deformity, namely equinus, will be more resistant to treatment and will require special effort—even to the point of operative correction. In other instances muscular imbalance will prevent maintenance of correction so that operative transfer of tendons, such as shifting the tibialis anticus pull to a more lateral position, will be indicated.

In addition to the therapy outlined, it is important to follow these patients until growth is complete to be certain that recurrences of deformity do not occur.

Treatment and nursing care. In no other congenital orthopedic condition are early recognition and treatment more important than in clubfoot. Although severe clubfoot conditions are not likely to be overlooked at delivery, a mild involvement is sometimes not noticed for periods of weeks or months. Delivery room nurses and those in the obstetric nursery should be especially observant of exaggerated attitudes in the baby's feet. It is not abnormal for an infant to lie with the feet slightly inverted—that is, turned inward with the soles of the feet toward the midline of the body. The normal infant can easily assume and maintain the opposite position if slight manipulation is used. A child with talipes equinovarus cannot maintain the everted position. Any indication, however mild, that the baby's ability to change the position of his feet is limited should be reported.

A few years ago considerable persuasion was sometimes necessary to convince parents that the baby with a clubfoot needed immediate attention.

Public understanding is now more widespread, but the nurse will occasionally encounter parents who are extremely reluctant to begin treatment early. It will be necessary to help these parents understand the necessity for early treatment. Clubfoot is a condition of which control has been definitely established; that is, the treatment is known, its results are almost certain, and the risk attending it is very minor. The orthopedic specialist talking to parents regarding these children first and foremost insists upon early treatment, but also emphasizes continued treatment. Too often these children are given prompt early treatment, and then, when a patient has been dismissed with feet apparently satisfactory, the doctor's insistent demand that the child be seen at frequent intervals for several years afterward is ignored. The deformity, like most congenital deformities, tends to recur. The child is brought back to the clinic three or four years later with a badly deformed foot for which radical treatment is necessary. The watchword, therefore, is early treatment and prolonged observation by the specialist. One doctor made the comment that he taught a mother faithfully the care of her son with clubfoot, to be carried out over a long period of years, and then when the patient was grown he instructed the wife in the same fashion. This is a manifest exaggeration, but the idea is clear.

Treatment and nursing care may be given in the form of (1) the Kite method, (2) manipulation and casting of the clubfoot, (3) adhesive strapping of the clubfoot, (4) manipulation without casting of the clubfoot, (5) the Denis Browne splint, and (6) braces and shoe corrections.

KITE METHOD. Early treatment is always conservative. Until a few years ago it varied a great deal in manner and apparatus, and to a certain degree this is still true. The method of Kite, who believes that as many as 90% of clubfeet can be treated by the conservative method until the child is about 8 years of age, is followed to a great extent. It is a method of gradual correction that systematically deals with the different aspects of talipes equinovarus deformity. It is done by cast with a series of wedging maneuvers that seek first to correct the adduction deformity of the forefoot, then the inversion deformity, and finally the equinus deformity. From the standpoint of the nurse the case may seem simple enough. It should be kept in mind, however, that each wedging is a threat to the patient's circulation. Often the circulation of the extremity is closely observed after the application of the original cast, but the wedging may escape notice. The doctor should forewarn the nurse, and night nurses especially should be solicitous about inspecting the child's foot after such wedgings. Considerable strain is placed on tendons, blood vessels, and ligaments after the equinus correction, which forces the plantar-flexed foot into a position of dorsiflexion. Undue pain or circulatory impairment should be reported at once.

MANIPULATION AND CASTING OF CLUB-FOOT. Sometimes, with the child under anesthesia, the feet are treated by a series of corrective casts applied after forcible manipulation is carried out. Frequent changes of the cast are required in this kind of treatment.

The very young baby in the plaster cast (Fig. 10-19) should always have close attention. The danger of circulatory impairment is so important that it should never be overlooked. The

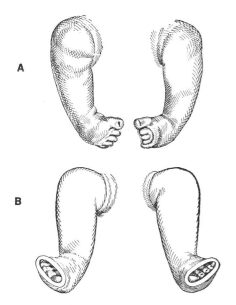

Fig. 10-19. Bilateral talipes equinovarus in the infant. **A,** Before correction. **B,** Undergoing correction in plaster casts. (From Raney, R. B., and Brashear, H. R.: Shand's handbook of orthopaedic surgery, ed. 8, St. Louis, 1973, The C. V. Mosby Co.)

foot should be inspected frequently. All the toes should be visible. This is frequently a point that must be called to the doctor's attention so that more of the cast can be cut out, for access to the two smallest toes. This cast is usually applied in a position of flexion at the knee, which will prevent its slipping downward—a complication that previously was common when the cast was applied only to the knee. In certain emergencies, when circulatory disturbance is manifest and severe and when no doctor is available, the nurse may be required to cut the cast. Bivalving the cast usually is preferred. Most doctors advise against cutting windows over the dorsum of the foot to relieve circulation, but in other clinics this is a routine measure to prevent pressure over the dorsalis pedis artery. Bandages under the cast must also be released if there is severe circulatory embarrassment. The removed portion of plaster should be taped lightly over the opening to prevent window edema.

Parents are warned about the necessity for keeping close watch on circulation when they take the infant in a clubfoot cast away from the clinic. They are advised also to watch for signs that the child is outgrowing his cast and to report to the clinic any severe chafing of the skin. Some kind of waterproofing should be applied around the thigh edge of the cast. These edges must be carefully smoothed and taped to avoid chafing the soft skin of the thigh. Failure to protect this portion of the cast lessens its life considerably; a diapered child inevitably will wet the cast each time he voids. An older child's parents must be warned that if the foot part of the cast gets soft and thin from wear much of the correction so far attained may be lost. It is not unusual, when a child returns to the clinic, to find that his cast is no thicker than a stocking and is giving about as much corrective force.

ADHESIVE STRAPPING OF CLUBFOOT. Some surgeons use adhesive plaster strapping to obtain gradual correction of the clubfoot condition in infants. They believe that plaster of paris is outgrown quickly and therefore is impracticable, whereas the adhesive tape can be changed for alteration in the corrective process as the need arises. A simple method of applying adhesive tape for this purpose is given by Sever. A single narrow strip of adhesive tape about 1 inch in width is brought around the forepart of the foot from the inner to the outer aspect and is carried up the outside of the leg. The knee is kept flexed at a 90-degree angle as this is done, and the tape is brought over it and well up on the thigh. It is necessary to exert considerable traction on the tape to secure the foot in a position of overcorrection. The danger from tape snugly applied to the baby's skin is, of course, apparent immediately. Adhesive tape and the skin of young babies, as most nurses realize, do not have an affinity for each other. It is extremely urgent that the edges of the adhesive tape be carefully watched for signs of skin erosion and that the danger of circulatory impairment to the foot be foremost in the nurse's mind.

Manipulation without casting. Mild clubfoot deformity in the very young infant is sometimes treated by frequent manipulations without the use of a corrective cast. Manipulations are usually begun immediately after birth and are carried out every 4 hours, preferably before the baby is fed. Because the manipulation is accompanied by some discomfort for the baby, it is better to perform the treatment before rather than after the feeding; if done afterward, the baby soon learns to expect unpleasantness after the feeding and will cease to take his feeding well. These manipulations may be continued until the child is 2 years of age or until the surgeon feels satisfied that reduction is complete and unremittent. Frequently this treatment is employed to lead up to later treatment by cast or splint.

There are many variations in the manner of performing manipulations, and the nurse should have demonstrations by the surgeon for each individual patient who will require such treatment. Occasionally the surgeon may feel that a complete reduction should be sought in the first manipulation and will usually perform this himself. Complete reduction is considered to be accomplished when the foot has been forcibly brought into full calcaneovalgus position to such a degree that the little toe touches the outer side of the leg. British authorities feel that this drastic early manipulation ultimately saves the child much discomfort.

The nurse must understand that when forcing the clubfoot into a position of overcorrection, by whatever method the surgeon prefers, the foot must be grasped below the tibial epiphysis. There is danger that the epiphysis may be displaced by too vigorous manipulation. This can be avoided by grasping the foot well below the malleoli with one hand while holding the ankle rigid and stable with the other hand.

Denis Browne splint. The Denis Browne splint has proved a useful device for the treatment of clubfoot in young children. The splint works on the mechanical principle that it is possible to correct the position of one foot by means of the other. In this treatment the muscles of the leg and foot may be used and strengthened while the deformity is being corrected, thereby eliminating some of the atrophy and joint stiffness that often occur when casts are used for correction. Many modifications of the original splint have been made, but the general principle remains the same. The splint is composed of a flexible horizontal bar attached to a pair of footplates. A device under the plates allows for rotation of the footplate on the horizontal bar. The apparatus is constructed so that each footplate is manipulated by means of the other (Fig. 10-20). Various means of securing the splints to the feet are used. Bandages, tape, and plaster of paris have been tried. Application with adhesive tape is probably the most commonly used method in this country at present. Sponge rubber or felt is used to cover the footplates on the surface contacting the foot.

The technique of strapping the foot to the plate varies somewhat in different clinics, but certain basic principles must be observed to assure the success of the treatment.

1. The skin of the foot must be inspected carefully to see that it is clean and free from abrasions. For the original strapping it is prepared by washing and drying and may be painted with tincture of benzoin. For subsequent strapping, however, most surgeons prefer that the skin be left as it is, and washing or cleaning of the area is not done.

2. There should be careful apposition of the foot to the footplate. The heel and sole must be firmly held to the plate; the sidepiece should contact the infant's ankle.

3. No wrinkles that might be the cause of pressure areas are allowed in the tape.

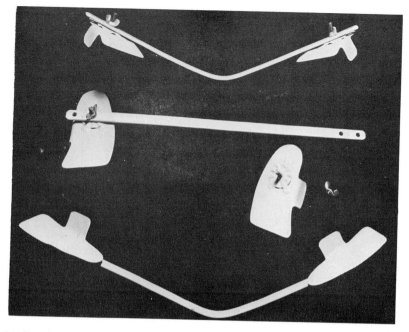

Fig. 10-20. Details of construction of Denis Browne splints. (Courtesy Dr. Arthur Steindler, Iowa City, Iowa.)

4. There should be no open spaces between the strips of tape, or window edema may occur.

Some physicians feel that is is wise to begin the treatment by attaching the feet to the plates for a short time in the position of the deformity rather than to attempt immediate correction. The bar is bent in the shape of an inverted V and applied to the footplates in such a fashion that the position of the feet is not changed. Swelling and skin irritation may sometimes be reduced and pliability of the foot encouraged by this method.

During the period of correction, which may take from 6 to 8 weeks, strapping is changed frequently, usually every 5 or 6 days. The child may be cared for in the home, if the parents can bring him to the clinic at the desired time for change of strapping. Many times, however, it is considered preferable to keep the child in the hospital during the first period of treatment —that is, until correction has been obtained.

After one or two strappings the connecting bar may be straightened to the horizontal position. The feet will follow the position of the bar, and adduction and inversion of the feet will gradually be corrected until a neutral position is obtained; that is, the feet will point straight ahead. After

that, effort is made to rotate and abduct the feet until they reach 90 degrees of outward rotation, which is the position of overcorrection essential in the treatment of clubfoot.

In order to secure a valgus position, some orthopedists prefer to angulate the bar into a true V shape at the time the foot has reached the neutral position.

As treatment proceeds, effort is made to stretch the calf muscles. This may be done by increasing the V angle of the bar when the foot is in 90 degrees of outward rotation. If the deformity is unilateral, the bar on the normal side is bent horizontally so that the normal foot is held in physiologic position at all times.

The more vigorous the baby's activity, the greater will be the correction; as the child flexes one leg and extends the other, the foot on the flexed side is forced into a valgus position, which, of course, is the corrected position, for varus deformity. Furthermore, with the foot in the valgus position, flexion of the knee will cause the foot to go into dorsiflexion, thereby stretching the posterior calf muscles. This is necessary for correcting the equinus deformity. It can readily be seen that with this treatment the baby provides his own corrective manipulation by his normal activity. As little as 5 or 6 weeks of this activity may be sufficient to obtain correction, but maintenance of correction will require a far greater length of time. The splint may be used as described for 5 or 6 months, after which shoes may be attached to the plates. Usually the shoes will be attached in reverse; that is, the left shoe will be used for the right foot and the right shoe for the left foot. This apparatus may need to be worn 6 months or longer. After the child reaches walking age, alterations are frequently applied to the walking shoe. An outside wedge or patch of leather, $^3/_{16}$ inch in thickness, may be placed on the sole. This alteration aids in overcoming any tendency the child may still have toward adduction or varus. The physician sometimes prefers that the child wear a shoe without a heel in order to continue stretching the Achilles tendon. The night splint is usually continued for a year or longer even after the child begins to walk.

Pediatricians have commented upon the increased likelihood of upper respiratory infections in children who are having clubfoot correction by the Denis Browne splint method as compared with those whose treatment is by cast. There seems to be some relationship to the fact that nurses tend to pick up babies in clubfoot casts more frequently and that babies in splints are often left in the crib for the entire day—during bathing, dressing, and even feedings. Nurses are urged to see that these babies are taken from their beds frequently and either held or placed in chairs for at least part of the day. The well-being of the baby may depend a great deal upon this simple factor.

It cannot be overemphasized that the skin of a baby upon whom adhesive tape is being used for any reason must be carefully watched for signs of swelling, excoriation, or blueness. Any abnormality of the skin around the tape should be reported to the physician immediately.

When the child is discharged from the hospital in the Denis Browne splint, some physicians instruct the parents to remove the plates from the bar once or twice daily. They feel that this will aid in preventing pressure areas. The parents are also instructed to check the position of the baby's heel at frequent intervals. If the heel is found to be slipping up, the instructions usually are to remove the foot from the plate and to return the child to the clinic at once.

Parents are sometimes asked to place a cross-bar above the baby's crib and to attach the bar of the splint to this for part of the time. It is felt that this will aid in eliminating the equinus position that results from constant resting on the bed. Instructions to parents should include advice to keep the baby in the sitting position at intervals during the day.

Braces and shoe corrections. When an over-corrected position of the clubfoot has been attained by the use of casts, the child is fitted with a splint designed to maintain the correction. This splint may be worn continuously at first and then discarded gradually as the leg and foot muscles become stronger. The Denis Browne splint may be used for this purpose (Fig. 10-21). The footplates and abduction bar are fastened to the child's shoes. The position of the feet is controlled by the abduction bar and by the mechanism used in fastening the bar to the shoes. The feet are usually held in a position of abduction, eversion, and dorsiflexion.

Exercises may be prescribed by the physician and demonstrated to the parents at this time. Experience has shown that follow-up exercises are a most neglected feature of home care. Upon return visits to the clinic, parents are questioned and frequently admit that they have omitted them for one reason or another. These exercises, however, are important. They are not difficult to perform, and parents should be urged to continue them faithfully for the welfare of the child. Failure to carry out such orders may mean that the parents have no clear concept of the importance of the exercises. A little time given to explanation will pay surprising dividends.

Shoe corrections (Fig. 10-22) may consist of an elevation to the outer border of the sole and heel. This will place the foot in a slightly everted position and aid in the maintenance of overcorrection. Here again the parents must be warned that when shoe corrections are worn down the child should be brought to the clinic. It is disheartening to observe children returning to the clinic in shoes with run-over heels and worn-down corrections, after a long and costly series of treatments by the orthopedist. Doubtless, fuller in-

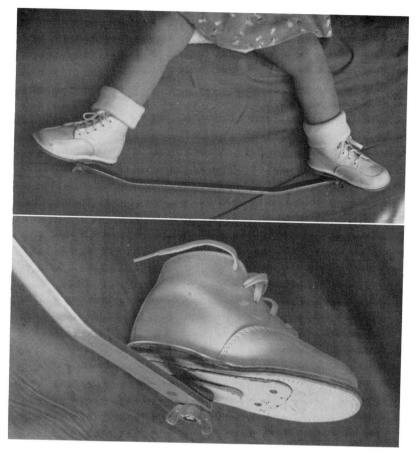

Fig. 10-21. After correction of clubfoot deformity, the modified Denis Browne splint may be prescribed to maintain correction. The splint is worn continuously at first and is gradually discarded as the child's activity increases and as muscles of the foot and leg become stronger. The desired position of the foot is controlled by positioning the abduction bar and by the screw mechanism that attaches the shoe to the bar.

structions given to the parents by doctor and nurse would obviate much of this carelessness.

Treatment of the older child. The older child with recurrent or neglected clubfoot will usually require some type of operation. It is never possible to reconstruct the foot to perfect contour and function by surgery, but a good weight-bearing foot that will minimize the deformity can usually be obtained. In order to eliminate chances of disappointment after surgery, the parents and the patient should be given a realistic understanding of what the operation will accomplish. Only a careful explanation of the expected result, given before the operation is performed, will prevent disappointment.

Soft tissue procedures, such as tendon lengthenings, stripping of the plantar fascia, or capsulotomies, are performed for neglected clubfoot. Surgery on the bone may be required for maximal correction in some patients. These operations may be wedge resections, osteotomies, or astragalectomies.

On a busy orthopedic ward where major surgery is being done daily, the problems of this patient may seem of only minor importance. The risk is not minor, however, and the danger of congestion and hemorrhage is great. The patient will usually be immobilized in a cast extending to the thigh and kept elevated with pillows or a hammock.

The nurse should be alert for seepage of blood at the site of surgery and also at the thigh where

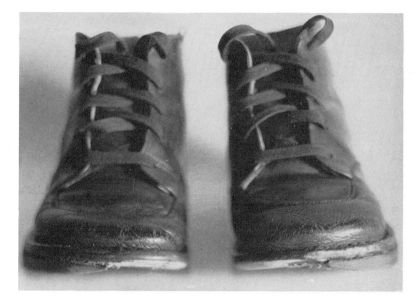

Fig. 10-22. Shoe corrections for clubfoot deformity. The elevation on the lateral aspect of the shoe sole helps prevent recurrence of the varus deformity. The importance of maintaining these shoe corrections cannot be overemphasized if recurrence of the deformity is to be prevented.

the cast ends; frequently hemorrhage may be detected there. An overhead frame with a hammock to support the cast is the preferred apparatus for support of the leg. Pillows may be used but are not so stable. Elevation is maintained usually about 48 hours but may be continued longer if congestion or pain is excessive. The nurse must heed complaints of the patient and interpret them intelligently. It is necessary to know where the line of incision is in order to be alert for any odor. Knowledge of the line of incision is necessary also in order to detect pain at other points, where pain should not be present. A complaint of pain at the heel, the patella, or the dorsum of the foot is not an expected aftermath of such surgery and should be reported at once. When the surgeon has given an order to have the cast cut over any of these points, the cutting should be done at once—not at the end of the day, when it is easier to secure an orderly. Too often casts may be marked for cutting in the morning or early afternoon but the actual process be delayed for hours if the nurse is not faithful (and persistent) in attempting to get a cast cutter to the bedside.

Dressing cart technique should be rigidly aseptic when the cast is cut and the first dressing

done. Frequently, spreading of the incision may occur if stitches are removed too soon. The surgeon will usually ask for some type of sterile adhesive strap for approximating the wound edges.

The three principal causes of failure in the treatment of clubfoot are (1) delay in beginning treatment, (2) imperfect nerve supply to muscles, as in conditions such as spina bifida, and (3) failure to obtain and maintain complete overcorrection of the deformity. Nurses will easily recognize their part in helping to eliminate at least two of these causes of failure—the delay in beginning treatment and the failure to continue medical supervision after correction has been obtained. Parents should be guided to the realization that follow-up treatment in clubfoot is as important as the active correction. They must have a clear understanding of their responsibility in this matter.

WRYNECK (TORTICOLLIS)

Signs and symptoms. At birth or shortly after, the child with wryneck may have a tendency to hold the head to one side. On palpation of the neck a mass may be felt in the sternocleidomastoid muscle. There is limitation of motion in at-

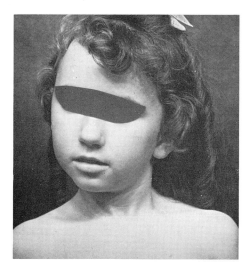

Fig. 10-23. Left torticollis before correction. Note asymmetry of the face, rotation of the head to the right, and tilt of the head toward the affected side.

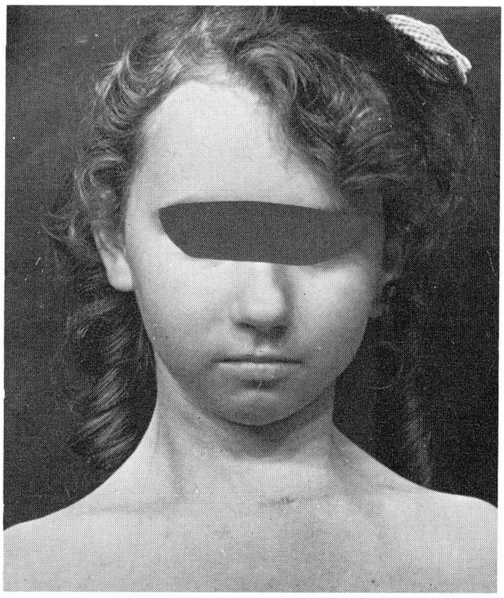

Fig. 10-24. Left torticollis after surgical correction. Same patient as in Fig. 10-23.

tempts to move the head away from the affected side.

Cause. The cause of wryneck is considered to be an engorgement of the muscle as a result of overstretching during the passage through the birth canal. Some observers hold to the theory that the affected muscle was inherently weak before birth.

Anatomy. When tearing occurs in the muscle, hemorrhage and extravasation of blood into the fibers take place. During the healing process this undergoes organization and development of scar tissue. The scar so completely involves the muscle fibers that elasticity is lost and contraction occurs. As the child grows older, this also leads to the development of a facial asymmetry (Fig. 10-23).

Treatment and nursing care. In most cases of congenital wryneck discovered shortly after birth, correction and cure can be assured within a month or two by the daily use of heat, massage, and carefully regulated stretching of the affected muscle.

In cases that have gone untreated or unrecognized, fibrosis takes place in the muscle and permanent deformity develops. Operative treatment is necessary (Fig. 10-24). This consists in the resection of the tendon of the muscle from both the sternal and the clavicular attachments (Fig. 10-25). Usually, about ¾ inch of the tendon is removed.

There are various methods recommended for maintaining correction after operation, but probably the safest is the application of a plaster of paris cast that covers the chest, neck, and head in an overcorrected position. This requires that the chin be brought high above the shoulder of the affected side.

The cast should be left on for approximately 6 weeks. After its removal a Thomas collar may be worn, and massage and stretching may be continued for several weeks.

Early recognition and treatment are essential. It is now generally recognized that much facial and postural deformity can be prevented if conservative treatment is begun early. The deformity may be so mild at birth that it is unobserved; or, being observed, it may be considered something that, with function, the child will outgrow. As time goes on, however, the ligaments on the affected side become so shortened and twisted that facial deformity becomes pronounced. Very early in the child's life an elongated swelling may be noted in the lower half of the sternocleidomastoid

Sternocleidomastoid muscle

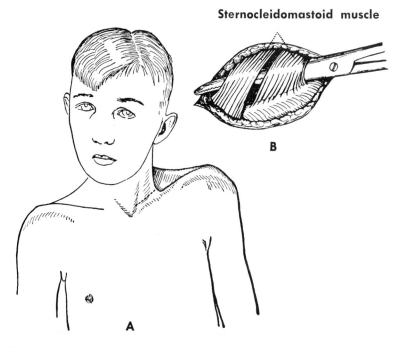

Fig. 10-25. Operation for torticollis. **A,** Line of skin incision. **B,** Clavicular and sternal attachments of sternocleidomastoid muscle withdrawn from wound and divided. (From Crenshaw, A. H., editor: Campbell's operative orthopaedics, ed. 5, St. Louis, 1973, The C. V. Mosby Co.)

muscle. It is quite tender at this time, and the child will cry if the swelling is touched or if the neck is stretched. Since the swelling and tenderness eventually disappear, the mother usually decides that there is nothing further to fear. Later, however, it can be observed that muscle tenseness exists. A band of fibrous connective tissue develops and, by contraction, pulls the head into the characteristic attitude: the ear on that side seems to be pulled downward toward the clavicle, and the face itself is turned in the opposite direction. When this condition is left without treatment, a slowly developing atrophy of the side of the face near the affected muscle will occur and become very apparent as the child grows older. This, of course, is followed by tissue changes. The soft tissues on the deformed side will become adaptively shortened; this is followed by certain definite bony deformities in accordance with Wolff's law.*

*Wolff's law: Every change in the form and the function of bones, or in their function alone, is followed by certain definite changes in their internal architecture, and equally definite changes in their external conformation, in accordance with mathematical laws. (Julius Wolff, 1868.) Briefly, the law may be remembered as "Form follows function."

The nurse caring for a young baby should be alert to detect any signs of limitations of movement in the head or neck. Frequently, when the stage of tumor and tenderness is missed, the deformity may escape notice because there are no marked symptoms except this limitation.

In mild cases, after the stage of tumor and tenderness has passed, manipulation and exercise are usually instituted; often these alone will suffice to overcome the deformity. These manipulations should be prescribed and demonstrated to the nurse by the surgeon for each patient, and progress should be checked frequently by the surgeon to ensure proper results from the treatment.

Surgery is usually indicated if the manipulative treatment fails or if the child is not seen until he is 2 years or more of age. In severe cases, surgery is sometimes performed on the young infant—in which case one of the foremost nursing problems is to care for the baby properly in the traction apparatus.

When the child with torticollis is being prepared for surgery, it is necessary to shave above the hairline on the affected side. Specific instruc-

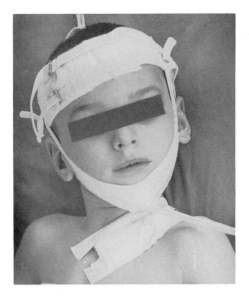

Fig. 10-26. Traction apparatus designed to maintain a position of overcorrection after surgical correction of left torticollis. Note that in the overcorrected position the chin points toward the incision and the back of the head is pulled upward.

tions should be obtained from the surgeon as to the extent of the area he wishes to have shaved. When a young girl undergoes a tenotomy of the sternocleidomastoid tendon, it is possible to part her hair low on the affected side, comb it to the opposite side, and braid it tightly. Post-operatively, the patient is especially happy to have this long hair to comb over the shaved area.

Casts are not always applied immediately after surgery. Postoperative nausea and the possibility of respiratory embarrasment make it safer to apply the cast the following day. Some type of retentive apparatus may be used in the interval (Fig. 10-26). Head traction is difficult to apply and can be dangerous if it is inefficiently done, particularly in such a young child. A flannel sling for the chin may be devised to exert head traction, but it must be inspected frequently lest it slip and impair the child's breathing or smother him by slipping upward. The amount of weight used will be ordered by the doctor, but it is usually very little. Sandbags may be used to control the position of the head.

The ordinary leather chin strap may be used, augmented by sandbags to maintain a position of overcorrection. In this type a long sandbag is placed low, forcing the chin toward the side on which the incision has been made. The second sandbag is placed on the opposite side, exerting pressure on the forehead and ear. The sandbags must be closely watched because they tend to slip.

Traction of this nature may be worn for a week or two, after which a brace is often applied. This brace is usually one that comes well down over the spine and may be a Taylor body brace with some type of corrective chin apparatus.

If the cast is applied in surgery before the patient becomes conscious, considerable care must be exercised to prevent aspiration of vomitus. Suction apparatus must be available. The area around the chin and mouth should be protected with pieces of waterproofing that may be tucked in until the cast is dry enough to finish the edges. A towel should also be tucked in around the face to further eliminate soiling.

After the cast is dry, the scalp section of the cast will usually be cut out to permit care of the head, and constant attention to this area will be necessary to prevent itching and irritation from plaster crumbs. At feeding time it will be necessary to protect the cast with a towel or napkin to prevent food from falling inside the cast. The ears must be inspected frequently to see that no plaster crumbs or pieces of food are lodged in them. Scalp and ears become sore easily when this type of cast is worn. These patients are soon ambulatory and are often left to care for themselves, but it must be remembered that careful supervision will be necessary daily to detect signs of skin irritation, pressure areas, or cracking and softening of the cast.

The cast may be kept on from 6 weeks to several months, according to the severity of the condition (Fig. 10-27). After it is removed, physical therapy will be ordered, consisting of massage, manipulation, and gymnastic exercies. These treatments may need to be continued over a considerable period, particularly in the older child. The parents should understand that torticollis cannot be completely corrected by surgery alone. A long period of follow-up care under the constant supervision of the physician will be necessary. If the child is dismissed soon after the cast is applied, the mother will need careful instruction in the details of caring for the patient and his cast.

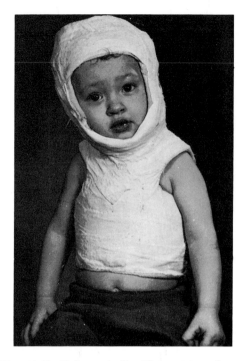

Fig. 10-27. Right torticollis. The position of over-correction is maintained 4 to 6 weeks postoperatively.

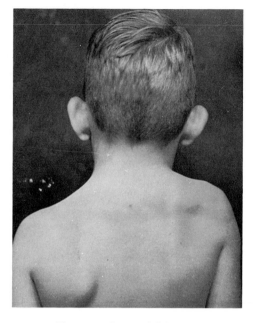

Fig. 10-28. Sprengel deformity.

CONGENITAL ELEVATION OF THE SCAPULA (SPRENGEL DEFORMITY)

Symptoms and signs. The Sprengel deformity (Fig. 10-28) is apparent in the upper part of the back of a patient with congenital elevation of the scapula. One or both shoulder blades are high. There is usually some limitation of the movement in the shoulder joints.

Anatomy. It is the opinion of most authorities that the term congenital elevation is a misnomer. The scapulae normally are high during the period of development but descend and rotate before birth. This deformity is, therefore, a failure of descent of the scapulae. It may be associated with other congenital deformities, such as abnormalities in the shape of the vertebrae, webneck or Klippel-Feil syndrome (Fig. 10-29), and possibly other deformities.

Treatment. The treatment of choice for congenital elevation of the scapulae is that recommended by Schrock. This consists in the complete subperiosteal and submuscular release of the scapulae, followed by rotation of the bone within this compartment to its normal position.

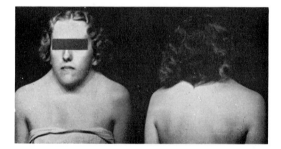

Fig. 10-29. Klippel-Feil syndrome. (From Kenney, W. C., and Larson, C. B.: Orthopedics for the general practitioner, St. Louis, 1957, The C. V. Mosby Co.)

Immobilization for a period of a few weeks follows, allowing reattachment of the periosteum. The scapulae are now in their normal position. In properly selected cases in younger children this treatment gives complete correction of the deformity.

ABSENCE OF BONES (TIBIA, FIBULA, RADIUS, FINGERS, TOES, ETC.)

Clinical picture. A child may be born with whole extremities or parts of the extremities

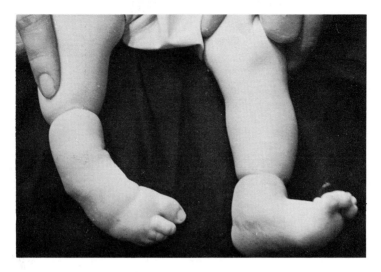

Fig. 10-30. Amnionic bands and bilateral clubfoot.

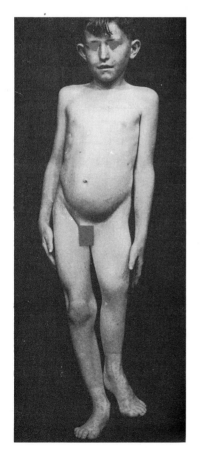

Fig. 10-31. Congenital shortening of the left femur.

missing, or with various bones missing. Extremities or digits may be partly missing, and there may be constricting bands or circular creases.

Causes. Absence of bones seems to be caused by the arrest of development during the early stages of embryonic growth. Constrictions and retarded development in the extremities in many instances are thought to be caused by amnionic bands or scars or intrauterine constrictions.

Anatomy. The deformity that develops from the absence of a bone is always characterized by loss of the propping or strutting effect of this bone. If a radius is missing, the hand is at a right angle to the forearm in a direction pointing toward the face (clubhand). It is not unusual to find associated deformities such as absence of the thumb and presence of a cervical rib (Figs. 10-30 to 10-35).

When the absence of bones occurs where there is an associated bone, such as in the forearm or in the lower part of the leg, the other bone usually becomes enlarged and frequently deformed. When there is absence of the tibia, the leg is usually shorter and the foot tends to turn inward and backward.

Congenital deformities of this type include limbs that are short and underdeveloped as a result of growth deficiencies. Occasionally, one leg or one arm will be underdeveloped so that it is

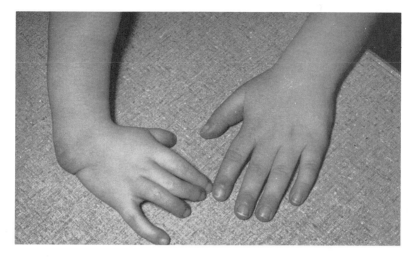

Fig. 10-32. Congenital clubhand.

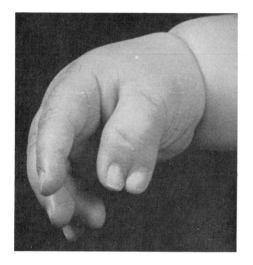

Fig. 10-33. Bifid thumb. Treatment consists of surgical removal of the accessory thumb.

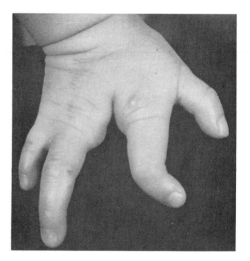

Fig. 10-34. A cleft hand. In many cases hands with this deformity are quite functional.

only about one-half the length of the opposite one.

SYNDACTYLISM

Syndactylism is a congenital anomaly characterized by the webbing of two or more fingers or toes (Fig. 10-36). The web may be formed by skin alone or by skin and subcutaneous tissue, and in severe cases there may be bony fusion between the phalanges.

The treatment consists of surgical separation of the digits and skin grafting of the denuded areas with free full-thickness skin grafts. The commissure or deepest part of the web is fashioned with a flap of skin from the palmar or dorsal aspect of the web. After skin grafting it is necessary to rigidly immobilize the digits spread apart in a plaster cast or splint for 3 weeks. The best time for surgery is during the second or third year of life.

SPINA BIFIDA

Spina bifida is a common term applied to a group of orthopedic problems that stem from an embryologic defect in the spinal canal, which is present at birth. The severity of the defect determines the amount of handicap in terms of the loss of sensation, motor paralysis, hydrocephalus

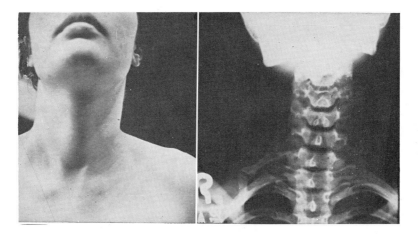

Fig. 10-35. Cervical rib. The presence of a cervical rib may produce pressure on the brachial plexus and thus cause a radiating pain in the upper extremity. This may be relieved by shoulder exercises and the use of a brace. In some instances surgical resection of the cervical rib is necessary. (From Kenney, W. C., and Larson, C. B.: Orthopedics for the general practitioner, St. Louis, 1957, The C. V. Mosby Co.)

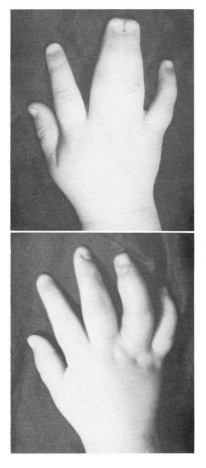

Fig. 10-36. Syndactylism (syndactylia) between middle and ring fingers. Preoperative and postoperative photographs.

and other deformities that will occur. There are various types within the general classification of spina bifida that are well recognized.

1. Spina bifida occulta is the term applied when the defect is very minor and may, in fact, have no residuals in the way of muscle paralysis, sensory loss, or other complications except for a local defect at the lower end of the spine. This is usually detected by a mild indentation of the skin over approximately the fifth lumbar segment; except for this minor cosmetic defect of indentation or a localized tuft of hair, the patient will not recognize any limitations or problems.

2. In the second type the spina bifida defect is associated with myelomeningocele (Fig. 10-37).

When the defect in the bony canal is a failure of fusion of the laminal arches posteriorly, there will be an associated outpouching of the meninges from the spinal canal. This outpouching may be large and contain only cerebrospinal fluid or may be of any size and contain elements of nerve tissue as a part of the embryologic defect. When the defect is large and the cyst is large and contains neural elements at birth, the child is ordinarily found to have very extensive paralyses and sensory losses below the level of the defect. Frequently the cyst is covered by only a thin layer of skin that easily becomes ulcerated by contact pressure; a number of these children die within a few days, from secondary infection that occurs through the ulcerated area and extends into the spinal canal.

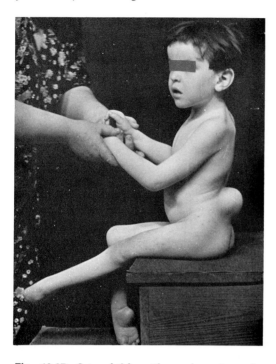

Fig. 10-37. Spina bifida with myelomeningocele. Note atrophy of the lower extremities and associated deformities of the feet. (From Kenney, W. C., and Larson, C. B.: Orthopedics for the general practitioner, St. Louis, 1957, The C. V. Mosby Co.)

The majority of children with spina bifida and myelomeningocele will have involvement that is less than actually lifetaking degree; these will survive and will do so with varying amounts of motor paralysis and sensory loss below the level of the defect. This is the group that constitutes a real problem in orthopedic surgery.

Management of myelomeningocele requires the efforts of a considerable team consisting of orthopedic surgeons, neurosurgeons, and pediatricians as well as urologists who come into the picture at a slightly later time.

From an orthopedic standpoint these children who have varying degrees of motor loss will develop distressing deformities such as dislocation of both hips, flexion deformity at the knees, and commonly bilateral clubfeet. All of these deformities are difficult to manage, since there is an associated sensory loss of the skin over the same areas, which therefore tolerates little pressure from external supports without the formation of trophic ulcers. In addition, these children frequently have loss of control of the bowels and the

bladder and frequently in the first few months of life show tendency to increasing cerebral spinal pressure that produces hydrocephalus.

The neurosurgeon has the choice of removal of the meningocele very early in life to prevent its breakdown, and there is some evidence that this procedure may even prevent an increase of paralysis in the subsequent months. The neurosurgeon has the further opportunity of providing shunts or artificial conduits from the brain ventricles into the subcutaneous tissues of the back or elsewhere to prevent the progression of hydrocephalus.

The urologist is brought into the picture with increasing frequency as techniques are being developed through which the urinary incontinence can be brought under control, either by urinary shunt operations of one kind or another or by continuous bladder drainage. This again requires very strict vigilance to guard against the possible complications, but such techniques are of value to bring the urinary flow under some type of control.

The orthopedic deformities—paralysis with resultant dislocation of the hips, flexion contracture at the knees, and clubfeet—are treated by various orthopedic means. At present there is no one standard form of therapy that is applicable in all cases, since there is great variation in the amount of deformity, paralysis, and sensory loss. For the most part the methods are similar to those discussed under the treatment for each of the individual deformities: the clubfeet, the dislocated hips, and the flexion deformity of the knees. Operative means can be utilized if conservative means are unsuccessful; in spite of the sensory loss in the skin, the healing power following operation is quite normal.

The eventual goal of the treatment is to provide these severely involved myelomeningocele patients with ability to walk even though it may require bilateral long leg braces in the instances where the paralysis is severe. Even if ambulation is accomplished, these patients must be watched continuously for the advent of pressure sores, especially on the feet. In a small number of instances, as life goes on, these pressure sores and other trophic disturbances become such that amputations are demanded. Myelomeningocele patients with deformities and loss of muscular function constitute a group of patients in which nursing techniques and vigilance by the nursing staff are perhaps more exacting than in any other of the orthopedic problems.

Nursing care. The infant with spina bifida and myelodysplasia usually is not seen first on the orthopedic service. Such conditions are considered in that early stage to be primarily pediatric and neurologic in nature. However, the congenital malformations are sometimes multiple, or, if deformity has not been present at birth, tendency toward deformity in later years is considerable. Such individuals frequently spend much time on the orthopedic services of hospitals. The patient with the milder form of spina bifida (occulta), who displays little outward manifestation of the vertebral cleft, may be admitted to the service because of clubfoot or some other deformity, but on the whole this patient does not present many problems in nursing care. It is the patient with sensory and motor involvement from some degree of cord destruction who will be discussed here.

All the problems of nursing care encountered in the patient who has destruction of the cord through disease, tumor, or trauma, accompanied by the inevitable group of symptoms engendered by this condition, are present in the paralyzed patient with spina bifida. The need to provide nursing care that will prevent or minimize the problems that confront the spina bifida patient is apparent. Urinary tract complications, trophic ulcers, and secondary contractures are perhaps the most serious of these problems. These problems not only inhibit progress in rehabilitation; they may be severe enough to pose a threat to the patient's life.

Trophic ulcers are a tremendous problem, complicated as they are by incontinence of bowel and bladder. Trophic ulcers have all the menacing features common to pressure areas, and in addition the patient lacks sensation. He is completely unaware of the condition so that there are no warning signals of pain. Furthermore, lack of nutrition to the area, which is caused by impairment of the sensory nerves supplying the muscles and blood vessels in the part, makes healing difficult or impossible. Nurses should remember that in patients with trophic ulcers the blood vessels surrounding the area have become di-

lated through failure of the nerve supply that normally regulates blood flow. The blood tends to stagnate, causing the surrounding tissues to become ischemic.

These ulcers develop in the soft tissue over bony prominences. Skin and subcutaneous tissue over the ischial tuberosities and the sacrum are areas that frequently ulcerate. Heels, lateral aspects of the feet, and skin over the malleoli are vulnerable spots. The ulcers develop in a very short period of time, are extremely slow to heal, and can lead to an osteomyelitis, which may necessitate amputation. Prevention depends primarily on relief of pressure on the involved area. This is accomplished by providing for a more even distribution of the body weight, and by frequent change of position. The alternating pressure mattress is helpful in changing pressure points, and the use of sponge rubber beneath the hips and heels provides for a more even distribution of the body weight. However, use of these "aids" does not eliminate the necessity of changing the patient's position at frequent intervals. The spina bifida patient who has difficulty ambulating is inclined to spend considerable time in the sitting position. It is desirable that this sitting time be alternated with tilt table standing, or the prone position, to relieve pressure on the sacral and ischial areas. Heel protectors made of synthetic sponge rubber may be helpful (Fig. 10-38). However, care must be exercised that they are not strapped too tightly, causing restriction of circulation; second, with their continuous use, body moisture is retained and maceration of the skin may result. When ambulation is started, careful inspection of the skin is necessary to detect beginning signs of pressure caused by the brace or shoe. The care necessary to prevent trophic ulcers is not provided by any one person, but must be the concern of all nursing personnel. In addition, as rehabilitation of the patient progresses, he must assume an ever increasing amount of responsibility for self-care, which includes skin care.

The tendency toward deformity is very great in these patients. Occasionally a child whose care has been neglected is seen in the orthopedic ward with hips and knees flexed to a right angle, back extremely rounded, and feet inverted to such an extent that the appearance is one of

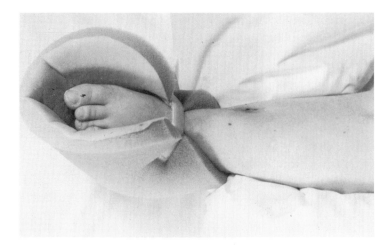

Fig. 10-38. A heel protector made from polyether urethane foam. Care must be exercised to avoid strapping the protector too tightly and thus restricting circulation. Also, because of body heat and perspiration, the protector should be used only intermittently to prevent skin maceration.

clubfeet found to have developed subsequent to birth. Dislocation of the hips is not uncommon and frequently adds to the dismaying picture.

The patient is admitted for some correction of the deformity that will enable him to walk with the aid of crutches and braces. Sometimes the immediate cause of his admission may be the grave nature of the trophic ulcers that have baffled the parents' attempts to heal.

To help prevent the types of deformity mentioned above, an exercise program similar to that designed for the paraplegic patient is needed by the spina bifida patient. This exercise program is aimed at strengthening the upper extremities and maintaining joint motion in the lower extremities. In conjunction with the exercise program, training in activities of daily living will encourage self-care and the desire to be self-sufficient.

Since past experiences have shown that these patients are prone to develop contractures and that their hips will dislocate, orthopedic surgeons have devised surgical procedures that help to prevent or minimize these complications. Various types of muscle transplant and tenotomies are done to provide for increased hip stability, to lessen muscle imbalance around the hip joint, and to help prevent or correct flexion contractures. Following any surgical procedure performed on the spina bifida patient, the nurse should solicit instruction from the surgeon in

regard to his care. The surgeon will realize how serious a problem confronts the nurse and will be able to assist in planning safe alterations of position. Frequent changes to the pronelying position must be such as will maintain the extension of the hips. The back, buttocks, and groin must have attention many times a day, certainly as often as the child becomes wet. Wrinkled, compressed, and bluish areas must be meticulously cared for. The child's skin will reflect promptly any letup in nursing care, any wrinkles or crumbs in his bed, or any neglect in changing position.

If a cast is used, the care of it is complicated. It is an extremely difficult task, particularly with female patients, to keep the cast from becoming soggy and foul smelling. Early attention to waterproofing the entire cast as well as to protecting its edges generously with a durable waterproof material is the first step.

Any apparatus must be considered a menace to the skin of these patients. Vigilant eyes, fingers, and nose cannot be emphasized too strongly here. The patient cannot tell where the pressure is; the nurse must supply this missing sensation by careful frequent inspection of the parts in the apparatus.

Soap and water cleanliness, followed by use of a dusting powder (borated), and freedom from pressure, moisture, and irritating creases in bed are essential in the care of perineum and but-

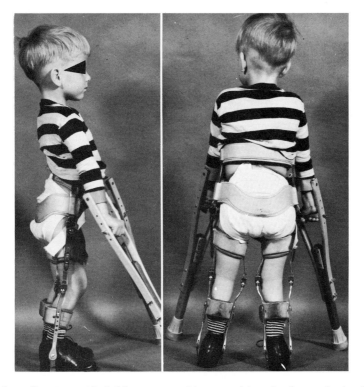

Fig. 10-39. A small patient with flail lower extremities caused by a lumbosacral spina bifida with myelodysplasia. Long leg braces attached to a body brace plus use of crutches (Canadian) make ambulation possible. Tightness of the tensor fascia lata has resulted in hip flexion contracture.

tocks. Frequently the most resistant areas of ulceration occur in the groin, as fissures, and beneath the gluteal folds, as large deep-seated sores.

Long leg braces with a pelvic band or girdle are usually prescribed when the child is ready for walking (Fig. 10-39). These, too, must be considered a threat to the integrity of the patient's skin, and the child's body must be carefully inspected for signs of irritation when they are removed. It is not usually considered advisable for a patient to remain in such braces for the entire day. Periods of bed rest without braces but in good body alignment should alternate with hours of ambulatory exercise. It is not uncommon for this patient to have a weight problem. Frequently obesity is the result of insufficient activity, and when present it becomes a major hindrance to ambulation with crutches and braces.

The parents and patient are most grateful when walking is accomplished, as it frequently is, but often they will not recognize their own parts in continuing this progress if they are not permitted to watch the meticulous nursing care that accompanies the physical rehabilitation of the child. The complications that may ensue because of brace pressure on legs must be pointed out. The necessity for preventing recurrence of deformity by watching the child's bed, chair, and walking posture, as well as by the faithful use of such night splints as have been ordered by the surgeon, should be emphasized. The care of the skin, especially around the buttocks and groin, must be demonstrated. The parents must be urged to assist the child to develop as much self-dependence as he is capable of assuming.

In addition to the development of trophic ulcers and contractures, the problem of bowel and bladder incontinency is a very real problem for the spina bifida patient. With the small youngster, it may be desirable to institute a bladder training program. This is started by placing the child on the toilet at frequent specified times throughout the day. Complete emptying of the bladder is encouraged by pressure over the suprapubic area. The mother is instructed in ways

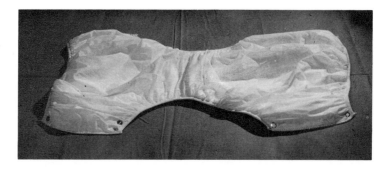

Fig. 10-40. Side-closing plastic-lined pants with grippers for easy fastening.

in which she may continue the program at home. Adequate fluid intake, plus timing of fluid intake, is important in preventing urinary tract infection and in promoting a bladder training program. With the adult patient, the problem of urinary incontinency is probably one of the most difficult problems he faces. In addition to being a continual source of embarrassment, it is a contributing factor to skin breakdown. Various methods and types of apparatus have been used in an attempt to help the patient with this problem. The male patient may be able to keep himself dry by wearing a rubber urinal, which is connected to a drainage bag attached to his leg. Protection for the woman patient may be provided by her use of a perineal pad and plastic-lined pants (Fig. 10-40). In some instances, to help prevent skin breakdown, the insertion of a Foley catheter is prescribed. This is connected to a leg bag during the day and to a drainage bottle at night. When a catheter is being worn, the possibility of urinary tract infection is always present. The patient should understand the correct care of the catheter and recognize danger signals that are indicative of need for medical care. To help the patient with an incontinency problem, surgeons are attempting to surgically redirect the urinary flow into the bowel or to the skin surface where aftercare is less troublesome. The nursing care of conduits of any type is detailed in textbooks on urology.

Fecal incontinence and the regulation of bowel movements is another nursing problem encountered in the care of the spina bifida child. The child has small, "marblelike" constipated stools, and he may constantly dribble feces. Sphincter control of the anus is not present, and there is no discomfort or special sensation in relation to the need for defecation. Measures to prevent constipation or the development of fecal impactions should be a part of his care. Good bowel hygiene may be promoted by (1) encouraging the child to eat foods with high-residue content, (2) giving bulk-producing medication, (3) maintaining adequate intake of fluid, (4) providing exercise as permitted or possible, and (5) establishing a regular time each day for bowel evacuation. It is not sufficient merely to place the child on the toilet each day at a definite time. The child must learn to press on his abdomen, to strain, and to work at having a bowel movement. The insertion of a glycerin suppository is helpful in promoting defecation and in establishing bowel habits. The patient's self-esteem can be enhanced if bowel movements can be regulated and embarrassing accidents avoided. Frequently no more pathetic individual exists on the orthopedic ward or in the crippled children's school than the patient who has this type of problem. He often feels himself to be an outcast because of his inability to take care of his toilet needs. He has, besides the motor disability that limits him in many ways, the social difficulty that becomes harder to bear as he goes into adulthood. Sometimes his hydrocephalic appearance gives him a look of subnormal intelligence that is not indicative of his actual mental capacity.

STUDY QUESTIONS

1. How will a sound knowledge and understanding of the normal infant assist the nurse in providing better care for children with congenital anomalies?
2. What routine inspection might the nurse be expected to give the newborn infant during the initial bath?

3. What nursing problems will confront the mother caring for her child in a hip spica cast? What can the nurse do to help the mother give good nursing care to the child?
4. Why is it important that the following conditions be diagnosed and treated early?
    (a) Congenital dislocation of the hip
    (b) Torticollis
    (c) Clubfoot
5. What symptoms may be observed that would indicate a congenital dislocation of the hip?
    (a) Before weight bearing
    (b) After weight bearing
6. At what sites would you be particularly alert for pressure areas after wedging of a clubfoot cast?
7. Discuss overcorrection as a means of treatment in congenital deformities.
8. List two types of spina bifida and describe each.
9. Be prepared to discuss the nursing care of the patient with spina bifida as related to the following:
    (a) Prevention and healing of trophic ulcers
    (b) Prevention of deformities and secondary contractures
    (c) Care of incontinency
    (d) Problems of the spina bifida patient with braces
    (e) Problems encountered following surgery
    (f) Psychologic, social, and economic factors
    (g) Providing adequate home instruction and follow-up care

REFERENCES

Allan, J. H.: The challenge of spina bifida cystica. In Adams, J. P., editor: Current practice in orthopaedic surgery, vol. 1, St. Louis, 1963, The C. V. Mosby Co.

Badell-Ribera, A., Swinyard, C., Greenspan, L., and Deaver, G.: Spina bifida with myelomeningocele: evaluation of rehabilitation potential, Arch. Phys. Med. **45:**343-344, 1964.

Beare, J. I.: Osteogenesia imperfecta, Nurs. Times **66:**453-455, 1970.

Bonine, G. N.: The myelodysplastic child—hospital and home care, Am. J. Nurs. **69:**541-544, 1969.

Braney, M. L.: The child with hydrocephalus, Am. J. Nurs. **73:**828-831, 1973.

Burr, C. H.: The hip in the myelomeningocele child, Clin. Orthop. **90:**11-21, 1973.

Chuinard, E. G.: Femoral osteotomy in the treatment of congenital dysplasia of the hip, Orthop. Clin. North Am. **3:**157-174, 1972.

Cowell, H. R.: Genetic aspects of orthopedic diseases, Am. J. Nurs. **70:**763-767, 1970.

D'Arcy, E.: Congenital defects 1; Some finding concerning the impact on the family, Nurs. Times **65:**1421-1422, 1969.

Deaver, G. G.: Lower limb bracing. In Licht, and Kamenetz, H. L., editors: Orthotics etcetera, New Haven, 1966, Elizabeth Licht, Publisher.

Diller, L.: Psychology of disabled children, Am. J. Nurs. **64:**131-134, July, 1964.

Ferguson, A. Jr.: Orthopaedic surgery in infancy and childhood, ed. 3, Baltimore, 1968, The Williams & Wilkins Co.

Ford, H. A.: Nursing a spina bifida child in a general hospital, Nurs. Times **66:**293-295, 1970.

Fredrickson, D. and Kinsman, D.: The child with hydrocephalus or myelomeningocele, Phys. Ther. **46:**606-615, 1966.

Funk, F. J.: Foot problems in childhood, Pediatr. Clin. North Am. **14:**571-587, 1967.

Gucker, T. III: The role of orthopedic surgeon in the long-term management of the child with spina bifida, Arch. Phys. Med. Rehabil. **45:**82-86, 1964.

Healy, H. T.: Variations in services to handicapped children, Am. J. Nurs. **68:**1725-1727, 1968.

Hill, M. L., Shurtleff, D. B., Chapman, W. H., and Ansell, J. S.: The myelodysplastic child—bowel and bladder control, Am. J. Nurs. **69:**545-550, 1969.

Kapke, K. D.: Spina bifida, mother-child relationship, Nurs. Forum **9:**310-320, 1970.

King, J. D., and Bobechko, W. P.: Osteogenesis imperfecta—an orthopaedic description and surgical review, J. Bone Joint Surg. **57-B:**72-89, 1971.

Knapp, M. E.: Physical medicine and rehabilitation in pediatrics, Part I, Postgrad. Med. **46:**173-176, 1969.

Knapp, M. E.: Physical medicine and rehabilitation in pediatrics, Part II, Postgrad. Med. **47:**219-224, 1970.

Lam, S. J.: Congenital dislocation of the hip, Nurs. Times **62:**282-287, 1966.

Lavoie, D., Liermann, C., Fletcher, A., and Corbett, D.: Spina bifida, immediate concerns—long term goals, Nursing '73 **3:**43-47, Oct. 1973.

Littlewood, J. M., Spina bifida, Nurs. Times **66:**5-8, 1970.

Lorber, J.: The child with spina bifida: medical, educational and social aspects, Physiotherapy **54:**390-397, 1968.

Lowry, M. F.: Congenital dislocation of the hip, Nurs. Times **66:**72-74, 1970.

McCarroll, H. R.: Congenital subluxation and dislocation of the hip in infancy, Postgrad. Med. **36:**102-107, 1964.

McCarroll, H. R., Coleman, S. S., Schottstaedt, E. R., and McFarland, B.: Symposium: congenital subluxation and dislocation of the hip in infancy, J. Bone Joint Surg. **47-A:**589-618, 1965.

Mihalov, Thelma R.: Bowel and bladder management of children with myelomeningocele, Nurs. Clin. North Am. **1:**459-470, 1966.

Miller, E.: Congenital clubfoot, Surg. Clin. North Am. **45:**231-237, 1965.

Morales, P.: Urinary problems in children with myelomeningocele, Arch. Phys. Med. **45:**402-409, 1967.

Murray, B. S., Elmore, J., and Sawyer, J., R.: The patient has an ileal conduit, Am. J. Nurs. **71:**1560-1565, 1971.

Murray, W.: Treatment of clubfoot, Postgrad. Med. **37:**105-112, 1965.

Peters, B.: Courage for Kim, Am. J. Nurs. **67:**1200-1203, 1967.

Ponseti, I. V., and Smoley, E. W.: Congenital clubfoot: the results of treatment, J. Bone Joint Surg. **45-A:**275, 1963.

Ponseti, I. V.: Non-surgical treatment of congenital dislocation of the hip, J. Bone Joint Surg. **48-A:**1392-1403, 1966.

Smith, E. D.: Spina bifida and the total care of spinal myelomeningocele, Springfield, Ill., 1965, Charles C Thomas, Publisher.

Steele, S.: The nurse's role in the rehabilitation of children with meningomyelocele, Nurs. Forum **6:**105-117, 1967.

Tachdjian, M.: Diagnosis and treatment of congenital deformities of the musculoskeletal system in the newborn and the infant, Pediat. Clin. North Am. **14:**307-357, 1967.

Trevor, D.: Congenital dislocation of the hip, Physiotherapy **53:**400-406, 1967.

Von Schilling, K. C.: The birth of a defective child, Nurs. Forum **7:**424-439, 1968.

Wilson M. A.: Multidisciplinary problems of myelomeningocele and hydrocephalus, Phys. Therapy **45:**1139-1147, 1965.

Winick, M.: Birth defects: what is being done about them, Nurs. Outlook **14:**43-45, 1966.

Winter, C., and Barker, M. R.: Nursing care of patients with urologic diseases, ed. 3, St. Louis, 1972, The C. V. Mosby Co.

Zimbler, S.: Practical considerations in the early treatment of congenital talipes equinovarus, Orthop. Clin. North Am. **3:**251-259, 1972.

11

Developmental diseases of bone

A number of bone and joint affections occur in middle childhood and adolescence with such regularity in age incidence that they are seemingly related to epiphyseal bone growth. Many of these conditions are self-limited within set time intervals and need treatment only to prevent deformity while the condition runs its cycle. Some are capable of inciting pain and therefore demand treatment. The more common of these conditions will be discussed in this chapter.

COXA PLANA (LEGG DISEASE, LEGG-PERTHES DISEASE, OSTEOCHONDRITIS DEFORMANS JUVENILIS)

Coxa plana at one time was frequently confused with tuberculosis of the hip because the early symptoms are almost identical. Osteochondritis of the femoral head is caused by a vascular disturbance that produces an ischemic necrosis. The reason for this disturbance is not understood. It is a self-limiting disease, usually occurring in children between 5 and 10 years of age. Boys are more frequently affected, a fact suggesting that trauma may be one of the instigating causes. Muscle spasm is rarely severe, and motions usually are restricted only in abduction and rotation, as contrasted with tuberculosis or arthritis in which all motions are restricted. In some instances the child will complain of pain in the knee rather than in the hip.

Pathology. Early roentgenograms show small vacuoles on either side or on both sides of the epiphysis. Following this, during the course of a few months to 1 to 2 years, the head of the femur undergoes degenerative changes in which segmentation first takes place (Fig. 11-1). This is combined with liquefaction over the cartilaginous surface of the joint and flattening of the upper surface of the head of the femur. In 2 or 3 years, when healing finally occurs automatically, the epiphyseal line becomes more nearly horizontal and the head of the femur becomes flattened.

This phenomenon usually does not lead to interference with joint function in early years. It may, however, lead to irritative changes around the hip joint later in life because of the discrepancies in shape between the head of the femur and the acetabulum.

Treatment. During the period of avascular necrosis the head of the femur is pliable and will heal in a deformed position if weight bearing is permitted. It is apparent that the method of treatment must provide protection for the head of the femur during this process of degeneration.

Some investigators recommend complete bed rest and traction during the developmental stages. If begun early, this type of treatment provides for restoration of the normal shape of the head. However treatment by bed rest is difficult to accomplish. Because the degenerative changes may continue for 1 to 2 years and regeneration of the head of the femur requires approximately a year, the restriction of bed rest to a child who feels well and has boundless energy requires the utmost in cooperation from parents.

Some physicians (Paul Steele, for one) recommend operation with replacement of the liquefied areas under the head with small bone graft chips from the neck of the femur; some recommend braces to relieve weight bearing, and some recommend the drilling of holes through the neck of the femur into the head of the femur to

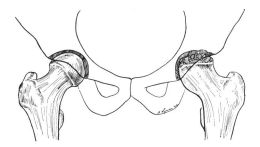

Fig. 11-1. Legg-Perthes disease. The epiphysis of the left hip (at right side in drawing) is in the middle stage, showing extensive segmentation.

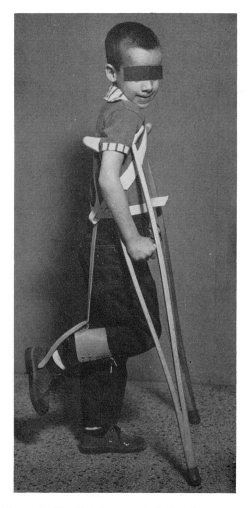

Fig. 11-2. The Fort harness is designed to prevent weight bearing on the affected extremity. The child wearing this apparatus is taught to walk with crutches, using the three-point gait.

stimulate bone growth. Some physicians prescribe that the patient be fitted with a leather harness—a Fort harness (Fig. 11-2)—that prevents bearing weight on the involved limb. The patient is required to walk with crutches. This necessarily places limitations on the child's activities but does permit his continuing school and living a somewhat normal life.

During recent years an ambulatory and weight-bearing type of treatment has been instituted. Bilateral long leg casts with an abduction bar, or long leg braces are utilized to maintain the limbs in a position of abduction (approximately 45 degrees) and slight internal rotation (20 degrees). With the limbs in this position, the femoral head is held deep in the acetabulum. As the child ambulates and bears weight on his extremities, the acetabulum serves to shape or mold the femoral head during revascularization and new bone formation. To maintain balance while ambulating, it is necessary for the child to use crutches or canes. Active range of motion exercise performed routinely will prevent hip contractures, and isometric exercises help to maintain strength in the quadriceps and gluteal muscles (Fig. 11-3).

SLIPPED FEMORAL EPIPHYSIS

Slipped femoral epiphysis (Fig. 11-4) occurs in two types of adolescents: (1) the fat overgrown adolescent (Fröhlich syndrome) and (2) the rapidly growing slender type. The condition is more prevalent in boys than in girls and is frequently bilateral. Trauma may play an important part in the precipitation of displacement and symptoms, but undoubtedly there is some underlying deficiency in calcium metabolism, and perhaps there is a deficiency in the function of the thyroid and the pituitary glands.

Pathology. The three stages to the disease are characterized as follows:

1. In the preslipped stage the condition manifests itself by the presence of a slight limp to the affected side and a slight limitation of internal rotation of the hip. Roentgenograms in the preslipped stage show little or no displacement but light rarefaction of bone on the lower femoral side of the epiphysis.

2. Through trauma or some minor injury during the earlier stages of slipping, the femoral

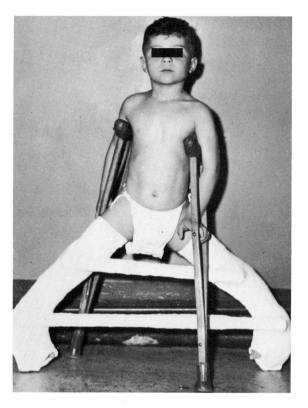

Fig. 11-3. A recent type of ambulatory treatment for coxa plana. The purpose is to hold the hips in abduction so that the major portion of the head of the femur is covered by acetabulum. In this event the acetabulum acts as a guide for shaping of the head as it goes through the repair process. (Courtesy Dr. J. G. Petrie, Montreal, Canada.)

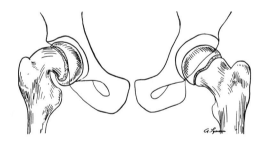

Fig. 11-4. Slipped femoral epiphysis of the right hip (shown here at the left). Note the horse-neck appearance of the neck of the femur and the erect position of the epiphyseal line.

portion of the epiphysis may slide further upward, and further eversion may occur.

3. More extensive slipping of the epiphysis upward with increased eversion of the limb occurs in the more severe or later stages. The bony changes shown by roentgenograms are accompanied by increased limitation of abduction and internal rotation. When such a degree of displacement exists, there is a rather marked limp, but pain is not a prominent symptom.

The condition usually appears during the rapid growth years—between the ages of 12 and 15.

Diagnosis. If seen in a child 7 to 10 years of age, the symptoms and signs present would be similar to those in Legg-Perthes disease. The age of the patient suggests further investigation. The roentgenographic findings are characteristic. There is an active epiphyseal line, below which the bone seems to flow into its deformity. The neck of the femur assumes a horse-neck appearance.

Treatment. The only treatment during the pre-slipped stages is immediate internal fixation to prevent possible future slipping.

When definite slipping has occurred within a

few weeks before observation, manipulation may be done by the Whitman or Leadbetter method. The leg is brought into forced abduction and internal rotation while the patient is under anesthesia. When reposition of the fragments is established, the foot will no longer evert when the heel is rested on the palm of the hand. A cast may be applied with the leg in abduction and internal rotation, or nailing with a Smith-Petersen nail is frequently recommended. Other operative procedures are also used.

When displacement has existed for months, an operation is necessary to restore alignment and improve joint function. This is accomplished by various types of osteotomy through the neck or trochanteric region of the femur.

EPIPHYSITIS OF SPINE (SCHEUERMANN DISEASE, JUVENILE KYPHOSIS, OSTEOCHONDRITIS DEFORMANS JUVENILIS)

As a result of injury that usually consists in forcible acute flexion in a young individual there may be trauma to the anterior joint margin of one of the vertebrae. The lumbar vertebrae are the most susceptible (Fig. 11-5). A small area of bone may be deprived of its normal circulation and undergo degenerative changes. Gradually, it loses its contact with the rest of the vertebral body and becomes encysted.

Symptoms. Symptoms are usually mild and consist of a slight amount of pain on certain motions and possibly an intermittent dull aching sensation in the spine. Roentgenograms show characteristic separation of the vertebral fragment, with the increased density of necrosis and a surrounding area of rarefaction.

Treatment. Immobilization in a position of extension by means of a plaster of paris body cast or a back brace for several months will usually lead either to the healing of the process or to the formation of a bridge of bone between the bodies of the adjoining involved vertebrae. Support provided by the cast or brace will help prevent deformity of the spine (kyphosis, round shoulders).

This patient should not be permitted to participate in strenuous sports, and bed rest may be necessary if pain is severe. A firm mattress with bed boards is desirable.

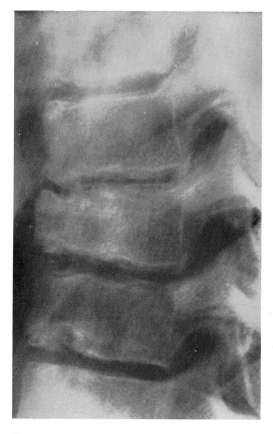

Fig. 11-5. Osteochondritis deformans juvenilis. Note wedging of the vertebral bodies and defects of the anterosuperior and anteroinferior cortical plates. (From Kenney, W. C., and Larson, C. B.: Orthopedics for the general practitioner, St. Louis, 1957, The C. V. Mosby Co.)

EPIPHYSITIS OF TIBIAL TUBERCLE (OSGOOD-SCHLATTER DISEASE, OSTEOCHONDRITIS OF TIBIAL TUBEROSITY)

Epiphysitis of the tibial tubercle (Fig. 11-6) usually occurs in rapidly growing children, most frequently in boys between 10 and 14 years of age. They complain of pain at the attachment of the patella tendon on going up and down the stairs and of acute tenderness and swelling in this region. Roentgenograms may show a small beadlike piece of degenerated bone under the epiphysis of the tibial tubercle.

Treatment. Mild cases usually respond to protection by a cast or a reinforced elastic knee support. In severe cases, operative removal of the small piece of degenerated bone may be necessary.

OSTEOCHONDRITIS OF THE KNEE JOINT

Although osteochondritis may occur in almost any joint in the body, it is comparatively common in the knee (Fig. 11-7). It usually appears under the cartilage of the outer surface of the inner condyle of the knee joint.

Cause. The cause is usually injury in which an unusual motion or strain of the joint occurs. Damage and local disturbance of the supply of circulation to a small area of bone and cartilage within the joint may result. The bone becomes separated from its blood supply and undergoes degenerative changes that separate it from the rest of the bone. This piece of dead bone may break through the covering of cartilage and enter the joint. The protective mechanism of the joint attempts to cover this loose bone (commonly referred to as a joint mouse) with cartilage until it finally becomes smooth and may slip from one point to another within the joint, causing lockage when it is caught between the joint surfaces.

Treatment. When the presence of a joint mouse is definitely established by clinical observation and by roentgenogram, it should be removed. Surgical removal is also recommended

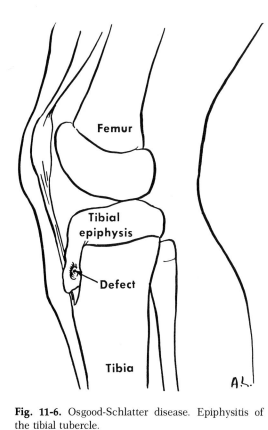

Fig. 11-6. Osgood-Schlatter disease. Epiphysitis of the tibial tubercle.

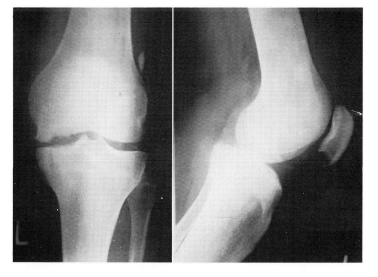

Fig. 11-7. Anteroposterior and lateral roentgenograms of the knee joint reveal a punched-out margin on the medial condyle of the femur. The "loose body" that arose from the punched-out area is visible in the quadriceps pouch along the lateral aspect of the femoral shaft.

if its presence can be determined prior to its becoming dislodged.

SCOLIOSIS

Scoliosis is a lateral curvature of the spine. It is called functional or postural scoliosis when there is no abnormality in the shape of the vertebrae and the patient can voluntarily correct the deformity. In structural scoliosis, there are changes in the shape of the vertebrae and thorax that make it impossible for the scoliotic individual to correct the deformity. The scoliosis is described as thoracic, lumbar, or thoracolumbar, according to the spinal segment involved (Figs. 11-8 and 11-9). Curvatures of the thoracic spine are frequently convex to the right, whereas curvatures of the lumbar spine are more often convex to the left. Scoliosis is usually accompanied by rotation of the vertebral bodies, toward the side of the convexity of the curve.

The rotation of the thoracic vertebrae causes the ribs on the convexity of the curve to protrude backward. The ribs on the side of the concavity are more prominent forward. In severe thoracic scoliosis the thorax is grossly misshapen. Very often the deformity consists of a right thoracic curve associated with a left lumbar curve.

Causes. Functional or postural curvatures are usually the result of faulty posture, weak musculature, and weak ligaments. Postural types of scoliosis rarely develop into structural types.

Structural scoliosis may be caused by infantile paralysis (paralytic scoliosis), congenital deformity of the vertebrae (congenital scoliosis), diseases of the lungs, certain diseases and tumors of the spinal cord and of the ribs, neurofibromatosis, hysteria, and so forth. The cause of scoliosis is unknown (idiopathic scoliosis) in a large number of cases. Poor protein intake is often observed in children with idiopathic scoliosis.

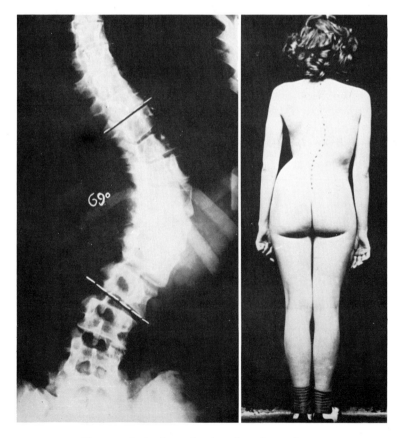

Fig. 11-8. Right thoracolumbar idiopathic scoliosis.

Symptoms. Congenital scoliosis may be detected during early childhood. Paralytic scoliosis develops several months or years after asymmetric paralysis of the trunk muscles. Idiopathic scoliosis, which is the most frequent type, occurs more frequently in girls than in boys and usually has its onset at 10 or 12 years of age.

Because scoliosis rarely causes pain until the later stages of the disease, it is frequently unrecognized until the deformity is well established. Scoliosis of the thoracic spine may be detected early by the deformity of the thorax. The ribs protrude backward on the side of the convexity of the curve, and the shoulder on the side of the convexity is higher. Scoliosis of the lumbar spine accounts for asymmetry

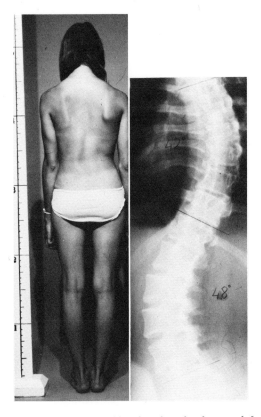

Fig. 11-9. A 17-year-old girl with right thoracic left lumbar idiopathic scoliosis. The two curves are well compensated, and the body alignment is good. This is the most common curve pattern in adolescent idiopathic scoliosis. The curves usually do not increase after skeletal maturation and remain well compensated throughout life without causing clinical symptoms.

of the hips. The hip on the side of the concavity of the curve is usually more prominent. Body alignment is often poor, and the thorax is deviated laterally in relation to the pelvis. The normal contour of the waistline is altered. It is flat on the side of the convexity of the curve and hollow on the side of the concavity.

Examination of the scoliotic patient. It is important that the patient be properly draped for the examination. The back should be completely exposed from the head to the heels. The range of motion of the spine in all directions should be noted and limitations recorded. The level of the iliac crests should be roughly estimated by pressing the hands into the flanks over them. Accurate measurement of leg length should be made, from the anterosuperior spine to the internal malleolus. Care should be taken that the position of both hips in relation to the pelvis is the same and that they bear the same relationship to an imaginary perpendicular line extending from the center of the cervical spine through the cleft of the buttocks and down between the ankles. The relative discrepancy in shoulder height should be measured, and a plumb line should be erected from between the heels to the occiput. The line should normally pass through the crease of the buttocks. The amount of lateral deviation of the spine in its various parts should be recorded and compared from time to time during observation and treatment. The range of motion of the segments of the spine should be evaluated. It will be observed that on forward flexion the rotatory deformity of the thoracic spine and the thoracic deformity are increased (Fig. 11-10, *A* and *B*). Roentgenograms of the entire spine taken with the patient in the standing position and in the recumbent position are of value in the diagnosis of the type of curve and shift of body weight. Roentgenograms taken every 3 months will show the evolution of the curve. Many curves increase little or not at all, whereas others progress rapidly. Roentgenograms taken with the patient bending as far as possible to the right and to the left will give valuable information regarding the correctability of the curve possible by fusion.

MILWAUKEE BRACE. The scoliotic patient may be treated nonoperatively by use of the Milwaukee brace, which consists of a leather or plastic

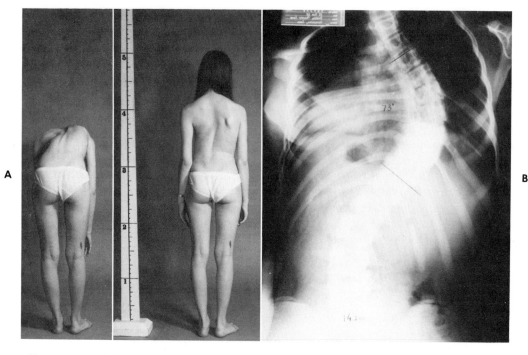

Fig. 11-10. A, Clinical photograph and **B,** spinal roentgenograms of a 14-year-old girl with a main right thoracic idiopathic scoliosis. Her thorax is shifted to the right in relation with the pelvis; therefore, her scoliosis is decompensated. Unless treated, these curves tend to increase a few degrees yearly, even after skeletal maturation, causing an increasing thoracic deformity, which may interfere with cardiorespiratory function in later life.

pelvic girdle that fits snugly and deeply over the iliac crests. This girdle serves as a foundation for the metal pelvic band and three uprights. The single anterior upright is made of aluminum to permit roentgenographic examination. The two posterior uprights are made of steel and are spaced lateral to the spine. These three uprights support the throat mold and occiput pads. The throat mold maintains the head over the occiput pads. In addition to this metal framework, which provides for passive distraction, a holding pad that is attached to the upright bars and placed below the apex of the major curve provides for lateral pressure on the spinal column (Fig. 11-11). The occiput and throat mold are adjusted to a position that permits the patient to elevate his head slightly above the head supports. These uprights may be lengthened as correction is obtained or to accomodate the child's growth. Likewise the holding pad placed over the convex side of the curve may be adjusted as necessary. The brace is designed to correct the spinal curve and to maintain the correction achieved. It should be worn almost continuously and is removed only for bathing.

In some instances it is desirable to hospitalize the scoliotic child for correct application and fitting of the brace. In severe scoliosis, head and pelvic traction may be worn for a short period of time to relieve some of the discomforts caused by the poor posture and to make wearing of the brace less difficult (Fig. 11-12). During hospitalization, prescribed exercises are taught and supervised. Exercises are of two types—those which strengthen the torso muscles, such as sit-ups used to strengthen the abdominal muscles, and corrective exercises specific for each individual patient. Also, during this time the patient has an opportunity to adjust to his brace and to gain an understanding of what he must do to attain maximum correction. The parents may feel more secure and better prepared to carry out instructions pertaining to the child's exercise, rest, and home activity if they

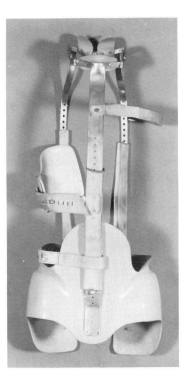

Fig. 11-11. Anterior view of Milwaukee brace. Note plastic pelvic girdle, throat mold, and occiput pads, also, provisions for adjustment of the brace to increase distraction of the vertebral column and the adjustable holding pad to provide pressure on the convex aspect of the curve.

have had an opportunity to observe and participate in the care given in the hospital situation. A better understanding of activities that should be encouraged, those which the patient may safely participate in, is helpful to the parent. Stress or emotional conflicts experienced by the teenager due to the condition itself or to the wearing of a cumbersome, seemingly unsightly brace may be dealt with. Sometimes appropriate clothing may make the brace less conspicious. Hospitalization, however, over an extended period, is not practical or desirable.

It is necessary for the child to wear the brace until bone growth is complete, which may be 1 to 3 years, or as long as there is any tendency toward increase of the curve. Before permission is given to remove the brace for short periods of time, it is important that stability of correction be demonstrated. This is accomplished by a standing X-ray film, taken after the brace has

been off for a few hours. If the major curve does not increase, permission is usually given for removal of the brace for several hours, twice a week. Roentgenograms are repeated at specified intervals, and if correction is maintained, increased amounts of time without the brace are permitted. Experience has demonstrated that removal of the brace for extended periods should be a slow process and that continued use of the brace at night may be beneficial.

For some patients, a spinal fusion will be necessary to maintain correction of the curvature. Following surgery the Milwaukee brace or a well-fitted cast is applied and worn continuously for a period of 6 to 8 months, or as prescribed. Postoperatively, when bed rest is necessary for an extended period of time, deep-breathing exercises should be encouraged and exercise of the extremities is desirable to help maintain muscle strength and to prevent the development of secondary contractures. Skin care is an important aspect of the nursing care. Pressure from the pelvic girdle may cause redness and irritation of the skin in the involved areas. If changing the child's position does not relieve the discomfort, an adjustment of the brace may be necessary. Pressure on the chin is now avoided with the throat mold.

Since this patient spends most of his time on one side or the other, the skin over the greater trochanter and the shoulder may show signs of pressure. Bathing the patient must be done with the brace in place. This takes additional time but can be accomplished much more satisfactorily than for the patient wearing a body cast.

When the patient is ready for ambulation, the brace or cast is still worn continuously. Later it is removed at night and then for graduated periods during the day; it is worn for 6 to 12 months postoperatively, depending on roentgenographic findings. Bone union at the graft site must be strong enough to maintain the correction. Follow-up care will include frequent checks by the orthopedic surgeon to provide for early detection of spinal changes. Pseudarthrosis may occur at a graft site, or the graft may fail to hold the correction.

HALO BODY CAST. The halo body cast is sometimes used in the treatment of scoliosis caused by weakness or paralysis of the neck and trunk

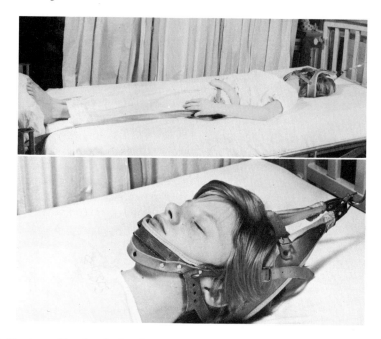

Fig. 11-12. One type of head and pelvic harness (Cotrel's) that can be used to provide for continous distraction of the spine. The doctor may prescribe that this be worn continously for several weeks prior to surgery or to the application of a scoliotic brace. By elevation of the head pulley, traction is applied primarily to the occipital bone. The patient is encouraged to actively stretch her trunk, insofar as possible, by reaching and holding to the head of the bed. The pelvic straps maintain her pelvis in a fixed position.

muscles. The halo consists of a metal head ring that is held to the outer table of the skull by means of four penetrating pins that are inserted with the patient under anesthesia. To provide for some correction of the spinal curve, a body cast may be applied and attached to the halo and suspension apparatus (Fig. 11-13). This arrangement provides for immobilization of the head and neck, and for longitudinal traction. In some instances, head traction may be applied to the halo apparatus prior to application of the body cast. To gain correction of the curve, a downward pull, in addition to the head traction, is necessary and is secured by applying skeletal traction to the lower extremities. A Steinmann pin is placed in the distal portion of each femur to facilitate traction. A body cast is applied later to hold the curve correction that has been gained by the distraction. The halo, plus the suspension apparatus, is attached to the cast by two anterior upright brackets; thus the position of the head and neck is firmly controlled. This immobilization facilitates positioning the patient and giving nursing care, prior to and following spinal fusion. The care of the patient in a halo body cast is undoubtedly a challenge to the most experienced orthopedic nurse. Care of the apprehensive patient, provision for adequate ventilation of the patient with a respiratory deficit, relief of postoperative pain, prevention of secondary contractures, plus the many aspects of nursing care necessary for the long-term patient—all are a part of the care needed by this patient.

Surgical treatment. Most of the abnormal curves of the spine are watched carefully over a period of time and measured in degrees. When conservative measures fail to prevent progression of the curve and increasing deformity cannot be prevented or when the correction gained is not stable, surgical intervention is indicated. Surgery means spinal fusion after correction has been obtained by whatever means may be chosen, and most of the fusions are done on patients at about the age of 12 to 14 years. In the moderately severe and severely progressive curves that come to fusion, it is likely over a period of

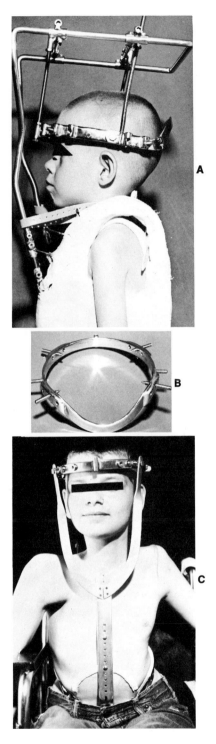

Fig. 11-13. A, Halo attached to body cast. B, The metal ring, or halo, which is attached to the skull. C, Halo attached to a Milwaukee brace. (A and B courtesy Dr. Vernon L. Nickel; from J. Bone Joint Surg. **43:**476, 1961; C courtesy Dr. Edward Miller, Chicago.)

years that the idiopathic group will retain 42% correction of the deformity. In the congenital scolioses this percentage is somewhat lower. The major problem with the surgical treatment is the failure of fusion—a condition called pseudarthrosis—and this will occur in about one-third of the patients in whom spinal fusion is attempted. When the lack is recognized, however, refusion can be obtained by further bone grafting in most instances.

There are many techniques for spinal fusion, but it has been found by experience that the most likely to succeed is one in which the facets are eradicated as a part of the technique. The correction is held by the application of bone grafts that solidify and hold the spine in the corrected position. In some cases there is difficulty in obtaining the correction desired and also in holding it by external means. An added technique, which has been introduced by Dr. Harrington, is a form of rod instrumentation. In the latter case, rods are implanted into the spine by clips that hold on the laminae. On the side of the concavity of the curve they can be utilized in a fashion to distract or correct the concavity and on the convex side they can by compression tend to correct the convexity. In experienced hands, the Harrington rods are an effective addition to this surgical treatment of scoliosis but are used in combination with, rather than as a replacement for, the external methods of support. Surgical fusion is something of a risk, since it is likely to be attended by a certain amount of blood loss and the patient with scoliosis is likely to already have a diminished pulmonary capacity.

For these reasons, the postoperative care is extremely important. Immobilization is usually continued for 6 to 12 months. In handling these patients after spinal fusion, it is well to remember that solidification is usually conceded to be present after about 4 to 6 months although this will, of course, be subject to verification by roentgenography. If a tibial graft is taken, considerable care in handling of the limb should be used for at least the first 8 weeks.

If the spinal fusion patient is to be immobilized by a brace rather than a cast, the nurse should remember that a body brace of any type should be fitted snugly around the pelvis in such

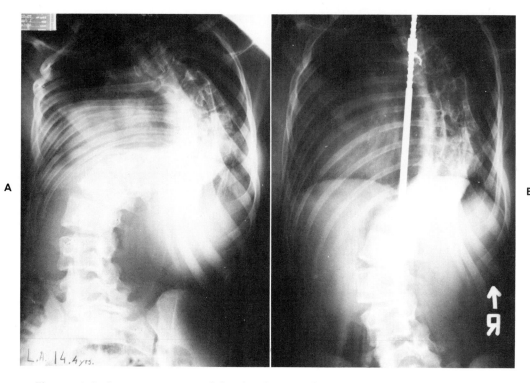

Fig. 11-14. A, Severe uncompensated dorsal scoliosis; **B,** dorsal curve considerably corrected and the correction maintained by an implanted Harrington distraction rod.

fashion that the lower band grasps the iliac crests. It should be laced or buckled from the bottom as the patient lies in bed.

If the Taylor body brace is used to immobilize the spine, the metal and leather section of the apparatus is unbuckled and lifted from the patient's body as he lies prone. The canvas apron remains under the patient. When the patient is to be turned, the brace is replaced on the back and the canvas section is buckled to the metal part before turning is done. The straps should distribute the pull evenly to avoid uneven tension. Shoulder loops are fastened to prevent the shoulders from sagging during the turning. Not all back braces are as easy to apply and remove from the patient as the Taylor. Many require forcible spreading for application. For the most part it is considered preferable to apply this back brace to the patient as he lies prone.

If a body cast is applied to provide immobilization, the nurse must realize that there is considerable strain on the patient during its application, particularly if he has been bedfast for a long period. The patient will probably be ex-

hausted upon his return from the plaster room.

The wet cast should be supported on plastic covered pillows. Cast edges should be sealed and during the time the patient is confined to bed rest, protection of the buttock area should be provided to prevent wetting or soiling of the cast. Patients in body casts are helpless, and exacting care is necessary to keep them clean. Skin care around the cast edges and frequent change of position and pressure points are essential aspects of the nursing care.

When the teenage patient becomes ambulatory, clothing becomes an important concern. Listening and encouraging the individual to express her anxieties may help to solve the clothes problem and make the adjustment and acceptance of the cast or brace a little easier.

Nursing care—general considerations for the patient's welfare. Scoliosis is often discovered in curious ways, but usually it has been present a long time before it is detected. A dressmaker's comment that she cannot get a hem to hang straight because one hip seems to be higher than the other; a teacher's observation of the

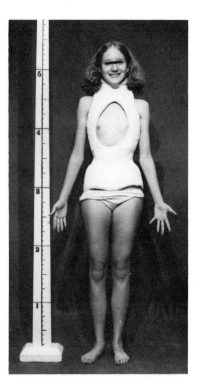

Fig. 11-15. A plaster body jacket on a girl with idiopathic scoliosis.

habitual fatigue and poor posture of a child in the classroom; a girl's complaint that one brassiere strap is always looser than the other; or a child's sleeplessness because of aching pain in the knees or in the low back—these and many similar complaints are sometimes the first hints the parents have that something is wrong with the child's spine.

Sometimes it is not until the child is in the period of rapid growth, between the ages of 12 and 16 years, that the condition becomes so evident it can no longer be overlooked. As with most crippling conditions, early recognition and treatment are vitally important.

It should be remembered that maximal improvement is obtained when the curve is small and flexible. Routine examinations of school children for the presence of curvature of the spine are very desirable. Parents and the general public should recognize the fact that it is a dangerous tendency to wait and see if the child will outgrow the condition. This attitude may keep the child from the specialist during the very time when it would be possible to minimize

the effect of the curvature. The feeling held by some individuals that scoliosis is a progressive condition and quite hopeless from the standpoint of treatment must be combated. The child with even a well-established curvature can be benefited greatly by skillful and continued treatment.

Nurses should remember that patients with scoliosis are easily fatigued. All periods of activity should be varied with periods of rest. This should be faithfully observed in the hospital as well as in the home. It is particularly advisable for such patients to assume rest positions for prescribed periods of time.

Much harm can be done if the ambulatory patient with scoliosis is allowed to slump in positions contrary to those prescribed for the maximum correction of his curvature. Encouragement from the nurse may be needed to remind the patient of this important feature of his treatment. Parents, too, will need to be reminded of this after the child has returned home. A rest position that is frequently taught is one in which the patient lies on his back with knees flexed, feet flat on the floor (or bed) with arms outstretched, shoulders rotated outward, and elbows flexed at right angles. The patient's body should be in good alignment, with head, shoulders, and pelvis in the same plane.

The health features of scoliosis should be emphasized in any article dealing with the nursing care of such patients. In the first place, a large part of the period of mobilization and wearing of corrective apparatus takes place in the home. Hospitalization over an extended period is not practical. When exercises are prescribed, the instruction is given by the physical therapist, and follow-up is usually done in the outpatient department at frequent intervals by the orthopedist. It is essential that the parents have a thorough understanding of such exercises as well as of their purpose. Written instructions, illustrated with drawings, will be helpful to the parents.

It may also take considerable ingenuity to keep the child interested in his exercises month after month.

It must be borne in mind that children with scoliotic conditions are at a time of life when appliances are often considered a cosmetic encumbrance, particularly by the child with a moderate curve that has not as yet caused him personal embarrassment. The parents, unless firmly instructed on this point, may often succumb to pleas to leave off the braces for parties and dances, and ultimately it may be found at check-up that the child is not wearing his brace half the time. Similarly the patient may often plead to omit his exercises because he is too busy or too tired. Only persistence in carrying out the doctor's orders, combined with thorough understanding of the long-term nature of treatment and the necessity for check-up at regular intervals, can be productive of permanent results in scoliosis.

It should be remembered that for his total welfare the child with scoliosis needs more than supervision of exercises and brace wearing. Fatigue is always to be avoided, and adequate nutrition is particularly important to him, as is careful supervision of his study, rest, and play habits. Tendencies toward weight loss, excessive gain in weight, or periods of rapid growth in height should be observed; in many instances, these may mean that the child should return to the orthopedic clinic earlier than had been planned. Attention to all these details may mean the difference between success and failure in the child's treatment.

STUDY QUESTIONS

1. The more severe scoliotic patient is frequently placed in some type of corrective apparatus. Review briefly the treatment and nursing care of the patient who is wearing a Milwaukee brace or a halo body cast.
2. Procedures to stabilize the spine may be done for the scoliotic patient. Explain what is meant by a spinal fusion and discuss the nursing care of this type of patient.
3. Pseudorthrosis may occur following a spinal fusion. Explain.
4. When the condition known as coxa plana occurs, there is avascular necrosis of the head of the femur. To prevent deformity during the period of necrosis, it is necessary to protect the head of the femur. Discuss methods used to accomplish this, and review nursing implications.
5. What is meant by slipped femoral epiphysis?
6. It is desirable that treatment for slipped epiphysis be started early. Explain.
7. In what age group does coxa plana occur? Slipped epiphysis?
8. Distinguish between the following terms: kyphos, gibbus, scoliosis, and lordosis.

REFERENCES

Adams, J. C.: Outline of orthopaedics, ed. 6, Baltimore, 1967, The Williams & Wilkins Co.

Baker, E. A., and Zangger, B.: School screening for idiopathic scoliosis, Am. J. Nurs. 70:766-767, 1970.

Bame, K.: Halo traction, Am. J. Nurs. 69:1933-1937, 1969.

Blount, W. P.: Bracing for scoliosis. In Licht, Sidney, and Kamenetz, H. L., editors: Orthotics etcetera, New Haven, 1966, Elizabeth Licht, Publisher.

Blount, W. P.: Use of the Milwaukee brace, Orthop. Clin. North Am. 3:3-16, 1972.

Blount, W. P., and Bolinske, J.: Physical therapy in the nonoperative treatment of scoliosis, Phys. Ther. 47:919-925, 1967.

Bobechko, W. P., McLaurin, C. A., and Motloch, W. M.: Toronto orthosis for Legg-Perthes' disease, Artif. Limbs 12:36-41, 1968.

Boegli, E. H., and Steele, M. S.: Scoliosis: spinal instrumentation and fusion, Am. J. Nurs. 68:2399-2403, 1968.

Buck, L. L.: Nursing care during the long rest period, Am. J. Nurs. 61:91-92, 1961.

Cacchiarella, A., Challenor, Y., and Katz, J. F.: Orthosis for use in Legg-Calve-Perthes' disease, Arch. Phys. Med. Rehabil. 53:286-288, 1972.

Edmonson, A. S.: Postural deformities. In Crenshaw, A. H., editor: Campbell's operative orthopaedics, ed. 5, vol. 2, St. Louis, 1973, The C. V. Mosby Co.

Ferguson, A., Jr.: Orthopaedic surgery in infancy and childhood, ed. 3, Baltimore, 1968.

Goldstein, L. A.: The surgical management of scoliosis, Clin. Orthop. 77:32-56, 1971.

Greenwald, W. F., Jr.: Scoliosis, Am. J. Nurs. 59:817-819, 1959.

Greenwish, J. F.: A new look for the youngster with scoliosis, Am. J. Nurs. 59:814-816, 1959.

Harrington, P. R.: Scoliosis in the growing spine, Pediat. Clin. North Am. 10:225-245, 1963.

Harrington, P. R.: Technical details in relation to the successful use of instrumentation in scoliosis, Orthop. Clin. North Am. 3:49-67, 1972.

Harrington, P. R.: Treatment of scoliosis, correction and internal fixation by spine instrumentation, J. Bone Joint Surg. 44-A:591-610, 1962.

James, J. I. P.: Infantile idiopathic scoliosis, Clin. Orthop. 77:57-72, 1971.

Jordan, V., Ohara, Y., Smith, M., and Townsley, J.: Halo body cast and spinal fusion, Am. J. Nurs. 63:77-80, Aug., 1963.

Keiser, R. P.: Treatment of scoliosis, Nurs. Clin. North Am. 2:409-418, 1967.

Moe, J. H.: Methods of correction and surgical techniques in scoliosis, Orthop. Clin. North Am. 3:17-48, 1972.

Moe, J. H.: The Milwaukee brace in the treatment of scoliosis, Clin. Orthop. 77:18-31, 1971.

Moe, J. H., and Gustilo, R. B.: Treatment of scoliosis, results in 196 patients treated by cast correction and fusion, J. Bone Joint Surg. 46-A:293-312, 1964.

Morton, J., and Malins, P.: The correction of spinal deformities by halo-pelvic traction, Physiotherapy **57:**576-581, 1971.

Pappas, A. M.: The osteochondroses, Pediatr. Clin. North Am. **14:**549-570, 1967.

Perry, J.: The halo in spinal abnormalities, Orthop. Clin. North Am. **3:**69-80, 1972.

Petrie, J. G., and Bitenc, I.: The abduction weight-bearing treatment in Legg-Perthes' disease, J. Bone Joint Surg. **53B:**54-62, 1971.

Ponseti, I. V., and Friedman, B.: Prognosis in idiopathic scoliosis, J. Bone Joint Surg. **32-A:**381-395, 1950.

Ralston, E. L.: Legg-Calvé-Perthes disease, Am. J. Nurs. **61:**88-91, Oct., 1961.

Raney, R. B., and Brashear, R. H.: Shands' handbook of orthopaedic surgery, ed. 8, St. Louis, 1971, The C. V. Mosby Co.

Risser, J. C. Scoliosis: past and present, J. Bone Joint Surg. **46-A:**167-199, 1964.

Roberts, J. M.: New developments in orthopedic surgery—scoliosis, Nurs. Clin. North Am. **2:**385-386, 1967.

Sells, C. J., and May, E. A.: Scoliosis screening in public schools, Am. J. Nurs. **74:**60-62, 1974.

Soren A.: Treatment of Osgood-Schlatter disease. Orthop. Surg. **10:**70-73, 1968.

Tamborini, J. M., Armbrust, E. N., and Moe, J. H.: Harrington instrumentation in correction of scoliosis; a comparison with cast correction, J. Bone Joint Surg. **46-A:**313-323, 1964.

Trott, A. W.: Orthopedic problems of the adolescent, Postgrad. Med. **49:**83-87, 1971.

Twomey, Sister M. R.: Halo pelvic traction, Nurs. Times **66:**1225-1228, 1970.

12

Cerebral palsy

Cerebral palsy is the term applied to those conditions characterized by impaired functional muscular control as a result of abnormality in cerebral areas that affect neuromuscular functions. Spasticity is a type of cerebral palsy, although frequently the terms are used erroneously in a synonymous manner.

PREDISPOSING FACTORS

Certain factors that are essentially uncontrollable increase the likelihood of a child's having cerebral palsy during the period immediately surrounding birth.

Being one of the firstborn. This factor applies until the mother's fourth or fifth pregnancy occurs. If one of these first births results in cerebral palsy, there is an increased likelihood that later children may suffer the disorder. The incidence in subsequent children, however, is not so great as in the firstborn.

Premature birth. Approximately 40% of all persons with cerebral palsy have a history of prematurity. As might be expected in premature infants, the greater the prematurity the greater the likelihood of brain damage.

Abnormalities of labor. A prolonged period of labor or an unusually rapid labor is more likely to produce cerebral palsy.

Abnormalities of delivery. Unusual fetal presentation, major manipulative procedures, or cesarean section is more prone to be productive of the disorder.

Multiple births. One of twins, usually the second delivered, has a greater likelihood of being afflicted than an infant born singly.

Heavy birth weight. Babies with heavier than average birth weights are more likely to suffer brain damage. This apparently is caused by increased probabilities of cerebral trauma resulting from increased head size.

Race. Cerebral palsy reportedly is somewhat more common in Caucasians than in persons of dark-skinned races.

Sex. Males are slightly more prone to be afflicted than females, although a great difference does not exist.

INCIDENCE

Phelps reported that the frequency of babies being born with cerebral palsy as the result of prenatal or natal causes was 7 for each 100,000 general population per year. Morbidity figures according to live births vary among observers from 1:200 to 1:568. The total number of patients with cerebral palsy of all ages has been estimated to be between 400 and 600 per 100,000 general population.

CAUSE

Conditions that produce cerebral anoxia and hemorrhage or trauma, either singly or combined, are the most common etiologic agents. These factors, if of sufficient intensity or duration, may operate during the prenatal, natal, or postnatal periods of life and produce an irreversible brain abnormality resulting in cerebral palsy.

Prenatal conditions. The more common of the prenatal conditions include infectious illnesses in the mother early in pregnancy, particularly the mild viral infections; abnormal placental attachments; toxemia in the mother; maternal hypotension; anemia; irradiation, particularly if early in gestation and if therapy is directed to the mother's pelvic organs; isoimmunization, such as Rh incompatibility between mother and fetus; and any condition in which the mother suffers intense or prolonged anoxia. The hereditary element per se is a very uncommon cause for cerebral palsy. Recent investigations have suggested that maternal nutritional deficits preceding and during pregnancy may bear an important relationship to the presence of brain abnormality and cerebral palsy in the offspring.

Natal conditions. The natal period refers to that period of pregnancy from the onset of labor to the birth of a viable child. Incidents that may produce brain damage during this time are primarily anoxia and trauma, either singly or combined. Some of the more common situations producing these damaging cerebral onslaughts are: depressing maternal anesthesia that, in turn, temporarily enfeebles the vital centers of the baby, thus delaying the onset and effectiveness of natural respirations; placenta praevia or abruptio placentae, which removes a source of oxygen to the baby before the infant's normal respiratory mechanism can operate; delaying birth unduly by force against the presenting part, pending the accomplishment of desired preparations for delivery; prolapsed cord, with delay in delivery of the head; difficult instrumental delivery; acute hypotension in the mother as a result of spinal anesthesia; precipitate birth, resulting in cerebral damage as a result of sudden change in pressure from intrauterine to extrauterine life; breech presentation with delay in delivery of the aftercoming head; and vigorous manipulative procedures.

Postnatal conditions. Most situations occurring after birth that may lead to brain abnormality are more apparent. The more important of these circumstances include: kernicterus, often the result of erythroblastosis; brain infections, such as meningitis, encephalitis, and abscesses; cerebral trauma, often resulting from falls or other accidents; intense or prolonged anoxia resulting from any cause; brain tumors; and cerebral circulatory anomalies, often leading to rupture.

Certain systemic diseases may cause brain damage as a result of secondary effects. For example, cerebral thrombosis may be a complication of nephritis, nephrosis, or other disease; cerebral embolus may result from subacute bacterial endocarditis occurring as a complication of rheumatic fever, congenital heart disease, or other conditions; and rupture of minute cerebral blood vessels may occur with severe paroxysms of coughing in an infant with pertussis.

The postencephalitic cerebral palsies, which follow some virus-induced disease that has affected the cortex of the brain, are usually severe in nature. Loss of motor function occurs, and varying degrees of impairment in speech and intelligence sometimes are so severe in nature that any return of these functions is despaired of. Until a trial is made, however, pessimistic predictions are hardly justified, for considerable return of function has been possible in a number of the most severely affected patients of this type. These children, struck down suddenly, usually from a healthy and normal childhood, present a most tragic spectacle because of the abruptness and devastation of the disease. Taking a hopeless attitude is all too easy for the nurse and parents in dealing with one of these children, and often the best treatment they can visualize is to provide complete and conscientious care of the child, with a view to his physical comfort and cleanliness. A more far-sighted attitude would be displayed in an effort to utilize the child's unaffected faculties as soon as the acute illness is over. Frequently, more is left from the wreckage than is at first apparent. One very bright boy, 14 years of age, with extremely severe involvement after encephalitis initiated by measles, was distressed immeasurably by not being able to make known his wants. A perplexed but sympathetic student nurse set herself to work out the problem with a piece of white poster paper. She divided her paper into six sections and made a crude drawing in each section: in one a bedpan, in another a urinal, in another a glass of water, and so on. When she stood at patient's bedside and pointed to the articles one after another, the boy could move his head sufficiently to let her know what he needed at the moment.

Table 1. Basic clinical types and characteristics in cerebral palsy

TYPE	BASIC CLINICAL CHARACTERISTICS
1. Spasticity	Increased resistance to manipulation; stretch reflex hyperactive deep tendon reflexes; clonus; tendency toward contracture deformities; lower extremities often more involved than upper extremities
2. Athetosis	Involuntary and uncoordinated motions without conscious control; normal reflexes when in relaxed state; upper extremities often more involved than lower extremities
3. Ataxia	Disturbance of autonomic balance; nystagmus; adiadochokinesis; difficulty in concentrating vision on a fixed field; normal tendon reflexes
4. Rigidity	"Lead pipe" resiliency of involved member; tendency to maintain position of extension; absent stretch reflex; near-normal tendon reflexes
5. Tremor	Intention-tremor contractions occur only with attempted motions; nonintention-tremor contractions are present constantly; no hyperactivity of tendon reflexes

CLASSIFICATION

The most useful classification of cerebral palsy at this time is one based on clinical findings. Autopsy material that is correlated with careful clinical observations in the same person has been insufficient to permit an authentic pathologic categorization according to types.

Table 1 lists the basic clinical types in decreasing order of frequency of occurence as recognized by most physicians particularly interested in patients with cerebral palsy (Figs. 12-1 and 12-2).

A mixture of more than one type may be present in the same person but probably is not found in more than approximately 1% of all patients.

The high spinal spastic type has been described in addition to the types as presented in Table 1. The site of damage in this type of cerebral palsy is at the level of the juncture between skull and atlas. The manifestation expected with this lesion is spasticity of the lower extremities.

The extent of involvement is variable from patient to patient. Table 2 indicates the descriptive terms used to denote parts of the body affected.

The degree of involvement is perhaps more important than the type of cerebral palsy when possibilities for physical rehabilitation are being considered. A mild degree of involvement suggests that extensive treatment measures are not necessary and can usually be accomplished by the parents in their home. One who is af-

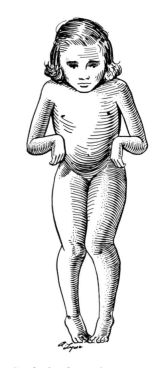

Fig. 12-1. Cerebral palsy with spastic quadriplegia. Flexion at all joints except the ankles. Adduction and internal rotation of the thighs. Scissors gait.

fected to a moderate degree needs special therapy measures that often include the use of braces and sometimes surgical procedures. One with a severe degree of involvement has only limited possibilities for physical rehabilitation even with the use of all special therapeutic measures available.

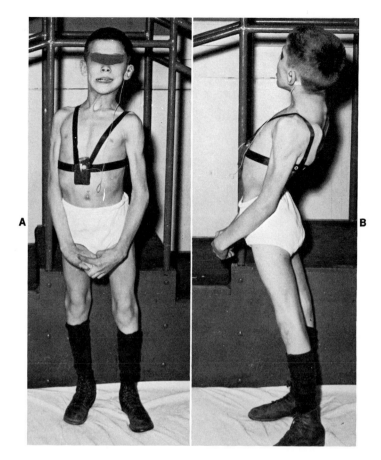

Fig. 12-2. A, Boy, 12 years of age, who has "tension athetosis" and associated hearing loss partially compensated for by a hearing aid. Note generalized hypertrophy of muscles, more involvement of the right shoulder than the left, pronated feet, and voluntary attempt to stabilize purposeless movements of the right upper extremity by clasping with the left hand. **B,** Lateral view of the same boy showing marked lordosis and genu recurvatum as a result of increased tension in an attempt to maintain standing balance as his center of gravity shifts.

Table 2. Extent of involvement

DESCRIPTIVE TERM	EXTENT OF INVOLVEMENT
Quadriplegia or tetraplegia	All four limbs
Hemiplegia	One side of body
Triplegia	Hemiplegia plus one limb of opposite side
Diplegia	Like parts of each side of body
Paraplegia	Both legs
Monoplegia	A single limb or part of body

ASSOCIATED DEFECTS

A finding of one or more associated disabilities in the person with cerebral palsy is more often present than not. These disabilities are usually the direct result of the primary brain abnormality. Table 3 enumerates the more common associated defects that are found in the cerebral palsy population.

SOCIAL INFLUENCES

Very few diseases have social factors complicating the condition as extensively as does cerebral palsy. Formerly it was considered that all persons with cerebral palsy were feebleminded; thus institutional placement was the course to

Table 3. Associated defects frequently present in persons with cerebral palsy

DEFECT	APPROXIMATE FREQUENCY OF OCCURRENCE
Mental defectiveness	25% to 40%
Educational retardation	Frequency correlated with degree of severity; very common in patients other than mildly affected
Speech involvement	70% to 80%
Hearing defects	30% to 40%
Oculomotor abnormality	30% to 40%
Convulsive disorder	40%
Perceptual defects	Frequency undetermined; more common in those with athetosis
Symbolic language disability*	Frequency undetermined; probably fairly common
Physical growth retardation	Frequency often related to the degree and extent of involvement; in part due to feeding difficulties
Emotional disturbances	Fairly common, to varying degree

*Includes dysphasia, aphasia, reading disabilities, and allied abnormalities.

follow. Unfortunately, this attitude still exists in the minds of a segment of the population, and it has been conducive to the social isolation of afflicted persons in their homes. In addition, many other factors currently exist—to the detriment of a healthful emotional state in one with cerebral palsy. Some of these are enumerated.

Parental guilt feelings and martyr complex. Studies have indicated that over two-thirds of all parents of children with cerebral palsy have feelings of personal guilt and consider that this handicapped child is theirs as a cross to bear. One would expect that such attitudes might be conveyed readily by the parents to the child in ways other than verbal expression. Parents who have these feelings to a strong degree are loathe to discuss their problems with others and tend toward voluntary introversion or extroversion and oversolicitousness as a compensatory device.

Family disagreements. Approximately one-half of the parents of children with cerebral palsy in one study admitted serious family disagreements regarding problems presented by their afflicted children.

Parental lack of information. Most parents have little or no accurate knowledge of etiologic factors, possibilities for successful rehabilitation, realistic aims, or even basic understanding of what the term "cerebral palsy" means. Perhaps, as might be expected, the majority of parents exaggerate both the severity of involvement and the mental acuity of their child, either because of lack of knowledge or because of failure to accept the facts. Approximately one-half of the parents of these children make little or no use of literature available on the subject, and most of those who have attempted self-education in this manner have found the reading to be confusing or of no help. It is not unusual to find parents who are accomplishing no rehabilitation program at home because they are uninformed as to how they should proceed.

Professional help sought. The common response of parents of children with cerebral palsy is (1) a rejection of the initial examiner and the information he gives when it is unfavorable, (2) a search for more favorable information from other sources, and finally, (3) a realistic acceptance of the child's condition. Thus, in one study of 200 parents of children with cerebral palsy having an average age near 8 years, the average amount of help sought per child was from nine medical physicians, two chiropractors, and one osteopath. Obviously, such shifting parental allegiance is detrimental to the possibility of any helpful approach to the child.

Oversolicitousness. Approximately 40% of parents admit to oversolicitousness toward their child. Experience suggests that this is a conservative estimate. Schoolteachers, playmates, and other associates of the child with cerebral palsy are prone to manifest this same attitude and thus enhance the impact of this factor.

Limitations in socialization. Socialization experiences of the handicapped child are usually curtailed proportionately according to the severity of his physical handicap or associated defects. Approximately three-fourths of all children with cerebral palsy who are not in school have few if any playmates outside their home. In addition, it is not uncommon to find a child with cerebral palsy of 5 or 6 years of age who has never been inside a supermarket or five-and-ten cent store, seen an airport, or had similar experiences that are fairly commonplace for a nonhandicapped child.

THERAPY

An effective therapeutic program may require the services of an organized group of professionals in view of (1) the physical handicap itself, (2) the associated defects, some of which are usually present in a person having cerebral palsy, and (3) the social influences encountered by the child with cerebral palsy.

The broad aims of therapy should be to establish locomotion, communication, and self-help; to work toward an appearance of normality in all motor functions; to correct associated defects as effectively as possible; and to provide educational opportunities adapted to the given child's needs.

This plan of therapy may be accomplished in the home or in a hospital, or it may require special and prolonged facilities as provided in a hospital-school. In any eventuality, continued home therapy becomes essential for those patients who may have had their therapy initiated in a hospital or hospital-school. The needs of the patient and the home facilities available become most important in deciding which approach will be most advantageous for a given patient.

Obviously, to enable one to establish more specific aims in therapy, a thorough evaluation of the entire person becomes a necessity at the beginning of his management and must be effected recurrently as his needs demand. Usually, the scope of this evaluation goes beyond the capabilities of a single person and often requires the services of a physician, psychologist, speech pathologist, social worker, nursing personnel, and other professional persons.

The services of special therapists in physical therapy, occupational therapy, and speech pathology frequently are necessary to accomplish corrective exercises in a given patient or to instruct and demonstrate to parents sufficiently so that recommended procedures may be accomplished in the home. Parents can accomplish many of these exercises if they are instructed adequately in measures to be accomplished.

Medical help is required in several ways. Of importance is one physician who may act as a coordinator of the rehabilitation program for a given patient because of his particular interest in this condition. He may be a general practitioner or specialist in any one field. It is he to whom the parents may turn for counseling when questions arise. The consultation of other medical specialists frequently is necessary for purposes of correcting associated defects as well as aiding in the basic rehabilitation program.

Appliances such as braces or splints are used frequently for purposes of correcting or preventing deformities, reducing incoordinated and purposeless movements of the limbs, or affording increased stability.

Special equipment often becomes necessary as a means of effecting therapy procedures. Kneeling benches, stand-up tables, parallel bars, relaxation chairs, and special adaptations of feeding utensils are most commonly used.

Surgical procedures on tendons, nerves, or joints become necessary in a certain number of these patients. Neurosurgery has afforded very limited benefits thus far and is seldom used therapeutically.

Medications have extremely limited usefulness. Certain products have some minor value for their relaxant properties; however, they are only adjuncts to other forms of therapy. Some medications are used to reduce salivary action and drooling. Preparations formerly advocated for improving mental acuity have now been found to have such limited value that they are unimportant. The drugs ordinarily used for control of seizures have similar usefulness in the patient with cerebral palsy.

Parent counseling is of great importance in making a program of therapy effective. The parents must be given basic information regarding cerebral palsy in general and facts pertaining to the condition as it relates to their own child. Realistic planning for rehabilitation (both physical and educational) and eventually for vocational anticipations should be accomplished. The counselor may be the physician who is coordinating the program or some other professional person if he has competent knowledge, adequate interest, and sufficient adeptness.

A person who has cerebral palsy is likely to have numerous and variable problems related directly or indirectly to his condition. Early recognition and attention to his problems, intelligent planning and accomplishment of a coordinated program of rehabilitation, and wise counseling are measures whereby satisfactory restoration may be effected in the majority of those so afflicted.

NURSING CARE

Cerebral palsy is one of the common causes of crippling in children. Yet it is not unusual for student nurses to complete their entire course of training without caring for such a patient on the hospital wards. Indeed, nurses often tell their instructors that their most impressive introduction to the patient with cerebral palsy is frequently outside the hospital entirely, on the street or in the home of some friend or neighbor.

Poliomyelitis (infantile paralysis) has received much attention in the past, and much has been done to eliminate this condition. One could hope that a similar amount of public interest might be evinced by this other comparable problem. However, cerebral palsy is a disability that does not strike spectacularly in epidemic form, and the results of it, although quite disastrous, are sometimes not appealingly dramatic. People are not instinctively drawn toward the unfortunate victim of this condition. They tend to be somewhat appalled and repelled by him, even when their sympathy for him is most manifest. Each nurse, as an individual, may sometimes make the lot of the person with cerebral palsy more bearable by interpreting his situation sensibly and realistically to friends or to the community. It can be admitted truthfully at the outset that this service may be a more important one than the relatively small amount of nursing care given these patients in the hospital.

In ward classes, student nurses discussing this condition frequently make the opinions of the public at large very graphic by their own reports of past experience. One student told how, as a child, she would cross the street to keep from passing a certain young boy. He jerked and twisted in all directions, and she was afraid of him. She knows now that the boy was an athetoid, and she remembers that he always seemed to try to smile in a friendly fashion at the people who passed him. Another student told of a girl friend of hers in high school whose younger sister "wasn't quite right." She was allowed to play only in a fenced-in backyard. One day the student saw the child in the backyard and noticed that she walked on her toes with her knees crossed and that she drooled and laughed raucously. The student remembers that she shuddered while watching the child and that she felt a great repulsion as though she were looking upon something not quite human. Now, however, she wonders why someone did not tell the parents of that child that perhaps something could be done for her.

Importance of early recognition and treatment

Early recognition is an important factor in the treatment of the condition. This is not always as easy as it might seem, particularly in the case of the mildly affected child. The more severely affected are not likely to be overlooked. When there is a history of a difficult labor, correlation between certain symptoms in the baby and his obstetric background makes the attending doctor and nurse particularly observant. Cyanosis, convulsions, dyspnea, apnea, and twitching indicate an advanced degree of involvement. Increased crying, vomiting, hiccoughs, rigidity, or tenseness may be present in less severely affected babies. All symptoms of this nature should be faithfully recorded on the infant's chart and in considerable detail. Many such babies are also intractably difficult feeders, and this may be a significant factor in diagnosis.

In the infant with very mild involvement none of the above symptoms may be present. As the infant grows older, however, certain features make their appearance which should not escape the nurse's attention. The nurse should know at least the elements of normal child development in order to recognize departures from the normal in these children.

It is not at all uncommon for this condition to escape detection until the child begins to walk, although delay in walking may be significant. Sometimes a tendency to walk on the toes (contracture of the Achilles tendon) accompanied by adduction of the thighs and knees may be the only symptoms that are noted at this time.

It has been interesting to note that babies of a year or less are frequently brought to doctors' offices for some slowness in development, such as being unable to sit up or to lift the head, and the story is told that the baby was normal until he had an attack of stomach flu or a cold, or perhaps a fall, when he was about 6 months old. These incidents in the baby's short history could be the cause of the obvious existing cerebral palsy, but in many cases doctors feel that parents have simply not noticed or admitted that symptoms existed until the child reached 6 months of age, when it was no longer possible to ignore certain retardations in development. There is a definite reluctance, even among the well-educated, to accept a diagnosis of spastic paralysis. It is still inherent in the public's understanding that these children are degenerate. There seems to be a stigma attached to them, and families tend to be ashamed, as they would never be ashamed of a child with poliomyelitis or, for that matter, one with tuberculosis, though the latter might honestly be considered to present more aspects of blame and censure for the family than cerebral palsy.

It is very important that treatment be begun early. As far as possible the training of the child with cerebral palsy should follow the development of the normal child. If the condition is not diagnosed until the child is 3 years of age or older, a great deal of valuable time will have been lost. Nurses will remember that the average child tends to sit at 6 months of age, attempts to creep at about 10 months, and tries to stand alone at 15 months. In the mildly affected child, this sequence might have been approximated with only little delay, had training been instituted early enough.

Frequently parents are tempted to follow advice secured from unreliable sources, particularly about taking the child to unqualified practitioners. This tendency is expensive and dangerous, and the nurse must marshal strong (but unhysteric) arguments against it.

Probably no parents ever need help as badly as those with a child with cerebral palsy. Nurses should know all community resource possibilities for the care and education of such children as well as those available in the state and nation. Cerebral palsy is an exceedingly complex problem, and the needs of the child for special types of treatment may be very great. Specially trained physical therapists, occupational therapists, speech therapists, and teachers may be required. The state Society for Crippled Children and Adults can usually give much valuable help on this problem and will be able to refer the nurse to other agencies for additional help. Intelligent, sympathetic information given the family by the nurse sometimes prevents a great outlay of expense and energy in traveling from one healer to another in search of a miraculous, quick recovery for the child.

The nurse and the emotional aspects of this disease

What should be the attitude of the nurse toward these children? As far as possible it should be the attitude one has with a normal child. It has been repeatedly emphasized that workers in this field must remember the patient is first of all a child and only secondarily a victim of cerebral palsy. Friendliness, interest, affection, and dependability should be manifest in the nurse's actions, for the child needs these things and they add to his feeling of security and personal importance. It should be realized that patients with cerebral palsy are quicker than many other children to detect an unsympathetic presence. They are equally sure to sense a friendly one. It is essential to secure their confidence and friendship, for upon these things much of the success in treatment may depend. Furthermore, the nurse is urged to learn everything possible about the child being cared for, concerning both background and personal history as well as the improvement that the doctor believes possible. Has the child come from a home where family life has revolved around him as though he were a pivot? Has he been shoved into the background and treated with great negligence? The nurse's attitude toward the child may need to be altered somewhat by what is learned of his background. We know that the education of the parents is a very important part of the treatment of these children. Treatment must carry on far into the future life of the child; otherwise, its value is questionable from the start. Probably the two features indispensable to successful treatment of the patient with cerebral palsy are these: (1) the patient's mental capacity to make treatment of permanent value and (2) the understanding and cooperation of the parents.

Too often the afflicted child has been utterly spoiled by the time he comes to the hospital. It may be because of a parent who has decided, with almost a religious fervor, to devote her whole life to the child to compensate him for being crippled. No responsibility of any kind has ever been given him, and he has never had to take the consequences for his misdeeds. Hospital experience will not be easy for such children, but if the situation is directed by an intelligent and understanding nurse it can be of great benefit. The child's moments of rebellion and temper will occur less frequently as he sees his unbecoming behavior duplicated in others like himself in the ward. The nurse's manner—quiet, firm, understanding, but unwavering where principle is concerned—will play a great part in the child's emotional development. This is so important that nurses should never underestimate their share in the treatment of these children. Too often a complaint is made by the nurse that the physical therapist, the occupational therapist, and the teacher are the ones who really contribute toward the rehabilitation of these children, and we as nurses have little to do with it. This attitude is quite false. The child spends more time with the nursing group than with any other while he is in the hospital. The nurse's attitude and teaching, by precept, example, and practice, can do much toward the emotional development of the child. This service to him is not to be minimized.

Intelligence in cerebral palsy is not measurable by appearance. Facial contortions, a raucous voice, emotional instability, gutteral speech, apparent inability to understand what is being said, laziness, and lack of desire to do things for himself do not always signify low mentality. Opinions about the mental capacity of persons afflicted with cerebral palsy vary considerably. Estimations of mentality based on mental tests that require some type of motor response are not considered reliable in giving an accurate measurement of the child's mental endowment. As better instruments for measurement are devised, however, and as knowledge of the various types of cerebral palsy increases, a more adequate estimation of the child's educability is becoming possible. Whereas too much optimism is always to be avoided until the child has been given the benefit of an examination by a specialist, to recommend custodial care for a badly affected child without such an examination is exceedingly unwise.

Defects of speech, hearing, sight, and sensation may be present in cerebral palsy. It can easily be seen that any of these defects might make the child seem less alert than he actually is. The athetoid is particularly likely to be slow to differentiate between sounds, and his ability to distinguish words may be greatly impaired. Defects of sight vary from lack of control of eye muscles and squinting to strabismus and nystagmus.

Clinical types of cerebral palsy are classified as spasticity, athetosis, ataxia, rigidity, tremor, and others. The list grows as the knowledge of the disease progresses. The most frequent in occurrence are the spastic and the athetoid, and discussion of nursing care will be confined largely to these.

There is considerable variation in the treatment given to the two most common types of cerebral palsy patients. The child who presents the uncomplicated cortical involvement, the true spastic, has a set of symptoms that make efforts toward muscle re-education the most important consideration. These children, confronted by a blocking of their voluntary efforts to perform an action, frequently tend to show signs of gradually developing frustration and apathy. There is reason enough to explain this, for each time the rigid spastic child attempts a movement, a sort of tug of war goes on between opposing muscles. Normal activity demands relaxation of one set of muscles while the other set contracts, but in the spastic child this does not happen. Constantly repeated blocking of his efforts may finally convince the child that the trial is not worth the effort, and he becomes harder to motivate than the person not so afflicted. Re-education of muscles forms the basis of treatment, and muscle checking to ascertain which muscles are strong, which are weak, and which are normal is essential to the program.

But the emotional manifestations that characterize these children need some concurrent attention. They are not as a rule gregarious or outgoing in their attitude toward others. They tend to be fearful of new situations and of unknown experiences. They dread sharp, unexpected noises and are very much afraid of falling. Their fear of falling is based on experience, for a fall in an unrelaxed position is indeed an unpleasant occurrence.

The athetoid patient, on the other hand, can make normal movements without the block in the antagonist muscle that confronts the spastic patient, but he is deluged by a flood of involuntary, purposeless movements that are beyond his control. He develops muscular tensions very early in life in an attempt to overcome this. Relaxation is the basis of treatment with the athetoid patient. Surgery and braces are seldom used because permanent fixed deformity does not occur in uncomplicated cases. These children are subject to spells of emotional instability approaching rages, but they are, on the whole, more outgoing and affectionate. They like people and are less self-conscious than the rigid, spastic patient.

In the third type of cerebral palsy, ataxia, the chief difficulty may be maintenance of equilibrium. Because it is hard for these patients to balance themselves, walking may be exceedingly difficult. These patients otherwise seem to be less severely involved than those with the two major types of the disease.

Certain principles apply to all types of cerebral palsy, and to avoid repetition these will be set down together. Such treatment as applies to one type or the other is usually ordered by the physician who makes the diagnosis.

Relaxation, although paramount in athetosis, is important to all types of cerebral palsy. Too much stimulation of any nature is inadvisable. Surgical wards, wards used as centers of play for a noisy group of children, and loud radio programs of syncopated music are not good for these children. The environment should be particularly quiet before meals, before the physical therapy treatments, and before retiring. The need for a controlled environment in the home is also to be emphasized. The atmosphere of the ward at all times for these children should be one of fairly even tenor. Fatigue comes quickly, even with small effort. It must be watched for and its symptoms recognized. The child tends to want to go on beyond his fatigue level. Rest periods need to be a little longer for these children because they go to sleep only after a considerable period of lying in a quiet room. In observing them after they have relaxed and gone to sleep, one will note that their exhaustion is sometimes out of all proportion to the activity they have engaged in. One of the chief lessons the patient with cerebral palsy must learn is how to relax voluntarily. In order to help the child do this, nurses should be familiar with the methods used by physical therapists in teaching relaxation. Sometimes it is possible to help the child by reference to some familiar relaxing incident, experience, or sensation. For example, the child might be asked to try to imitate a soft and cuddly kitten, or a handful of sand, or a feather or leaf floating in the wind.

Nursing responsibilities in speech training

It is now generally conceded that the ability to talk is a primary need in cerebral palsy patients and that it is much more important than, for instance, learning to walk. Speech is bound up closely with every other type of learning, and every experience might be said to have its speech component. Nurses should attempt to follow up the child's periods with the speech therapist by paralleling each experience the child has during the day with conversation appropriate to that experience—that is, talk about clothes as the child dresses and talk about food as he eats.

Speech training for the patient with cerebral palsy should be given by qualified speech therapists. To be most effective it should be begun early, preferably between 2 and 5 years of age. If this training is begun early, it will not be necessary for the child to unlearn the poor habits of communication that children with speech difficulties usually have. Parents may help prepare the child for speech training by having regular periods each day devoted to talking to the child. If the child is very young, talking should be accompanied by looking at pictures or handling the objects about which the adult is talking (Fig. 12-3). This simple beginning in speech training will aid considerably in the child's development. It is a natural tendency for the child to try to imitate and echo the sounds he hears, and the child with cerebral palsy should not be deprived of this experience.

A factor that must be remembered by both nurses and parents is that the child must be urged to ask for the things he wants. If he can get what he wants without asking for it, he will try to do so. Speech therapists emphasize the fact that it is not wise to interpret the child's speech by satisfying his wants too easily. Much of the motivation to speak more accurately may thereby be lost.

Although poor habits of speech should, of course, be discouraged on the wards when the nurse knows the patient is capable of doing better, it is unwise to constantly call attention to the child's speech, particularly in a nagging manner. An emotional block toward the whole speech problem may be induced by nagging. Encouragement and assistance rather than correction should characterize the nurse's approach to this matter.

Teaching the child to feed himself

Ability to feed himself is an important accomplishment for the child with cerebral palsy. Equipment for eating therefore should be optimal (Figs. 12-4 to 12-7). Consultation with the occupational therapist will frequently reveal to the nurse ways of adapting existing hospital equipment to fit the needs of the child for handling his own food. Spoons can be built up with sponge rubber that can be wound around the handle to make a bulky object easy for the child to grasp. If this is covered with plastic material and secured at the base with waterproof tape, it can be washed and dried with the other hospital silver. A specially constructed chair with a slight backward tilt and a table with a space hollowed out for the child's body are especially useful. If the table can be constructed with depressions to receive a bowl, a glass,

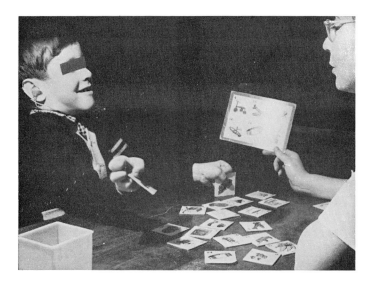

Fig. 12-3. Speech therapist using a combination of pictures and lipreading to aid speech in a deaf athetoid child. Patient's eyes covered in photograph only—not, of course, during therapy. (From Kenney, W. C., and Larson, C. B.: Orthopedics for the general practitioner, St. Louis, 1957, The C. V. Mosby Co.)

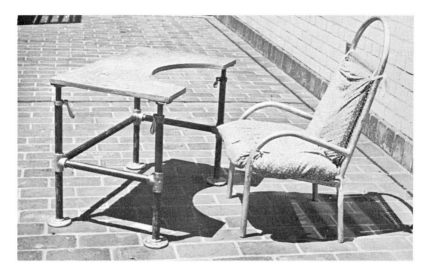

Fig. 12-4. Adjustable table and chair made by hospital carpenter for patient with cerebral palsy.

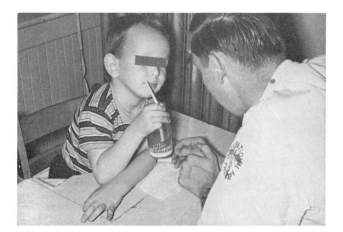

Fig. 12-5. Therapist teaching a patient with cerebral palsy to drink through a straw. (From Kenney, W. C., and Larson, C. B.: Orthopedics for the general practitioner, St. Louis, 1957, The C. V. Mosby Co.)

or cup so that things will not slide away from the child as he reaches for them, it will be particularly suitable for his use. On a table that lacks this feature, however, it has been found that small rubber mats, frequently used under tumblers, and bowls equipped with suction cups will help to keep the dishes from slipping. It is advisable to have the child's elbows supported by the table while he eats, since much greater relaxation will be obtained in that way. The feet should rest on a solid surface and not dangle in midair. A large waterproof bib will give the child freedom from fear of spilling food on his clothes. Many other details for making mealtime a more comfortable experience for the child can be worked out so that the period is less an ordeal for both the nurse and the patient than it sometimes is when no special equipment is provided.

Because much of the muscular coordination needed for chewing and swallowing is also necessary in speech, it is advisable that as soon as possible the child be given food that requires chewing. Chewing will aid considerably in developing control of the jaw and throat muscles. Some speech therapists advise that the child's training in swallowing can be aided materially by use of a lollipop. In sucking a lollipop the child will learn many of the tongue motions that are necessary in swallowing. A drinking straw is useful in teaching the child to narrow his mouth motion.

Most workers with cerebral palsy patients, however, advise that training for eating should not be done at mealtime. To avoid an emotional block, it is better for the child to learn these things at a time when his nutrition is not involved. Training in many of the details that concern eating are often incorporated in the physical and occupational therapy program. Such skills are accomplished very gradually, and the child learns to master one motion thoroughly before he is advanced to another. If he can learn to

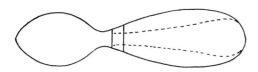

Fig. 12-6. Spoon built up with sponge rubber and covered with plastic material to make a good grasping handle for the child with cerebral palsy.

raise an empty glass to his mouth, first by being guided by the therapist's hand and then by his own effort, he has advanced considerably toward being able to feed himself. After he has mastered the empty glass, a very small amount of liquid is added to it, and this is continued until he can lift a glass containing the usual portion of liquid.

Drooling is almost always a matter of great concern to the parents of the child with cerebral palsy. Training to overcome this habit is usually begun concurrently with speech therapy because it is considered to be the result, at least in part, of an inactive tongue. Speech clinicians tell us that something can be done for drooling in almost every instance. As the child learns to chew, suck, and swallow, he will automatically develop these reflexes that will aid in the control of drooling. It is also possible to aid the child in learning to swallow by having certain periods of the day when he practices swallowing rhythmically. For instance, in one exercise the mother or nurse counts to five and the child is instructed to swallow on the fifth count. Repeated faithful efforts in this will show results in the child's gradual ability to control drooling.

The child should have the benefit of quiet

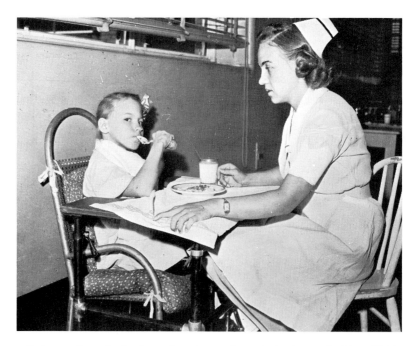

Fig. 12-7. Patient with cerebral palsy and equipment for assisting her to feed herself. Depressions in the table for holding dishes and cups are advisable for the badly affected child.

surroundings and suitable equipment when he is eating. In the hospital, where distractions are numerous, this is sometimes hard to provide without depriving the child of the companionship of his own age group. Consultation between nurse, physical therapist, and occupational therapist will frequently result in a flexible plan for the child, which can be altered as his ability to feed himself and cope with distraction develops.

It must always be remembered that the child may need help, particularly with the last part of his meal. The severely affected patient cannot be deserted and expected to accomplish even minor tasks for himself. He may need help in adjusting his equipment. When he shows obvious symptoms of fatigue, he needs assistance. If he becomes disheartened by being given too much to do or too difficult tasks to perform, he tends to lose interest and courage. The nurse should keep this in mind even when leaving him to perform a simple function of dressing or eating. Encouragement and assistance will do much to promote in the child a feeling of accomplishment without tiring or discouraging him. There is a delicate difference in the matter of creating in the child's mind the ability and desire to do things for himself and confusing him by the assignment of tasks that are beyond his capacity.

It is essential to teach the child to watch what he is doing. Once his concentration span is exceeded, he learns little by his fumbling efforts. The nurse must not be fooled, however, by the child's little tricks of feigning fatigue with a long-drawn-out sigh or a look of helplessness. He is likely to make tentative trials in this direction for the benefit of new nurses.(This is human nature and not peculiar to cerebral palsy.) Patience, understanding of the child's personality, and considerable firmness are necessary in combating these episodes. But such attitudes must be motivated by continued interest in the child's welfare, for he quickly detects when this is absent.

Nursing care for the child with cerebral palsy in the hospital

Sometimes the child with cerebral palsy is kept in the nursery wards of the orthopedic division long after his age would permit him to be moved.

This is done so that he may remain in a crib. A child 8 years of age with fairly normal intelligence does not respond well to this kind of treatment. He resents it, and it does something to his spirit. If the child can be moved into a ward with children of his own age group, some provision for this must be made.

A great effort should be put forth to speak to these children very distinctly. It is not considered wise to repeat oneself because it seems that the child has not understood. If there is some type of hearing defect, it may take him several seconds or more to understand and carry out the order or answer the question given him. Consideration must be given the problem he has with the mere task of motor response. If words are repeated, his ability to respond is interrupted by deluging him with more stimuli. Facial expression should be carefully controlled, or he will detect impatience and be discouraged at the outset. He must be spoken to clearly, simply, and directly, and sufficient time must be allowed for him to comprehend and organize his response. Repetition is in order only when he has asked for it.

It should be recognized from the outset that it is an injustice for the nurse to rush through the care of the patient with cerebral palsy. These children do not progress in the hands of a hurried, overwrought nurse. Their response to this haste is unmistakable—a tightening of all muscles, rigidity, and increased tenseness—the very things the child has been brought to the hospital to overcome. If it is at all possible, the nurse should postpone care of these patients until last in order to be able to give them more time to attempt to do things for themselves. This is sometimes impossible because of early morning assignments to physical or occupational therapy, but when it can be managed, the opportunity should not be neglected. Allowing the child to wash and dry his own face and hands or to brush his teeth may take what seems an unjustifiable amount of the nurse's time, but the reward attendant upon these efforts seems so great that no nurse should overlook it.

Toilet habits are not usually difficult to establish in the mentally unaffected patient with cerebral palsy and should be begun as early as with normal children. Specially constructed low toilet seats with armrests are desirable so that the child may be left alone. Continued use of the bedpan long after the child is progressing toward a considerable degree of independence is not wise. For the child who spends most of his time in bed, some arrangement should be made to place him securely and comfortably on the pan and leave him alone rather than to stand at his side holding him—a feature not conducive to good toilet training.

Very early in his training should come an appeal to the child to develop proper habits of cleanliness, such as clean hands, brushed teeth, and neatly combed hair. This may seem a small matter, but it will go far toward giving him a feeling of personal worth—without which no other training is of much avail.

The nurse's responsibility in teaching the patient

While the patient with cerebral palsy is in the hospital, coordination of all the services affecting him must be worked for constantly. Methods of relaxation followed by careful muscle re-education in physical therapy and hours of urging toward self-help in occupational therapy and in the schoolroom can be undone by the solicitous nurse on the ward who does not realize that the ultimate aim of treatment is to enable the patient to care for himself to the limits of his ability. It is far easier at mealtime to feed the child than to sit beside him guiding, urging, and, if need be, assisting him to eat. But if he is allowed to feed himself only on those days when the wards are not busy, he will lose the desire to do it at all; it has been observed over and over again that the child loses the will to feed himself if there are days when the nurse does it for him. He likes the presence of another person, and it is not necessary for him to put forth any effort. Another factor that leads directly to his caring. less about doing things for himself is frequently his realization that it is such a nuisance to the nurse to wait for him. These children are observant. They soon recognize signs of irritation or bother on their nurses' faces. It is not uncommon for a child with athetosis to break into fits of uncontrolled weeping in the middle of a meal for no greater reason than that he feels himself a nuisance. Probably it must be admitted from the outset that because of this necessity

to hurry, hurry, hurry on the part of busy nurses on orthopedic surgical wards, the spastic child feels that he has no business being there.

The child's own wants in the matter of attempting new activities deserve consideration. The motive is strong at this time, and attention will be directed with greater success at something he really wants to do. Guidance is necessary to prevent frustrating disappointments.

Because one of the great aims of all treatment is to give the child as great a degree of independence as is compatible with his condition, considerable attention must be given toward assisting him to care for his own physical necessities. Teaching him to manage his own clothes is a point of great importance. This may be a very slow process in the badly affected child and may start with nothing more spectacular than an attempt to fold his garments as they are taken off. The less skilled movements naturally come first, but some attempt can be made to prepare him to assume more of the task by allowing him to practice with a good sized doll that has clothes fastened by a variety of gadgets, such as hooks and eyes, buttons, and zippers, as well as drawstrings and snaps (Figs. 12-8 and 12-9).

When the child begins to walk on the ward, nurses should know exactly how he has been taught in the physical therapy department in order that consistency in instruction may be carried out. It is particularly important to note the child's habitual posture in walking and to discourage slumping attitudes or lazy methods of progression. It will help very little for the child to have 15 to 20 minutes' careful instruction in the physical therapy department once a day if he is allowed to form careless habits of walking the rest of the time on the ward.

Nurses may learn from physical therapists how mirrors can be used in the physical training of the child with cerebral palsy. It is a remarkable fact that often such a child, learning to walk by the aid of lines drawn in front of a mirror, will straighten his body almost as though by reflex when he comes within the range of vision of the mirror (Fig. 12-10). He does not like the look of the stoop-shouldered youngster he sees ahead of him, and he will do his best to alter that appearance. Physical therapists fre-

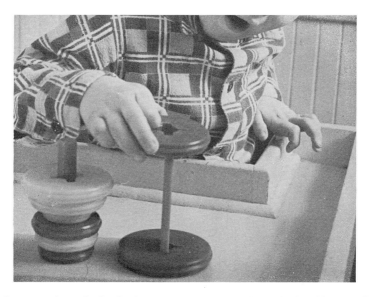

Fig. 12-8. Patient with cerebral palsy learning to grasp and release the hand by use of a large toy. Later, smaller objects will be used. Note also that the patient is in a standing table to help develop his ability to stand erect. (From Kenney, W. C., and Larson, C. B.: Orthopedics for the general practitioner, St. Louis, 1957, The C. V. Mosby Co.)

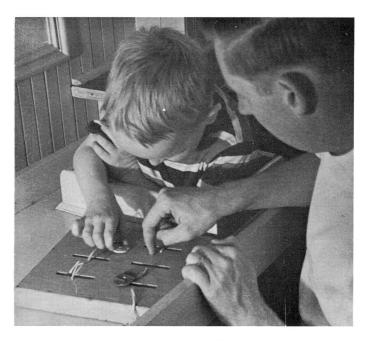

Fig. 12-9. Patient with cerebral palsy using a large model requiring, in general, the same type of movements needed to lace the shoes. (From Kenney, W. C., and Larson, C. B.: Orthopedics for the general practitioner, St. Louis, 1957, The C. V. Mosby Co.)

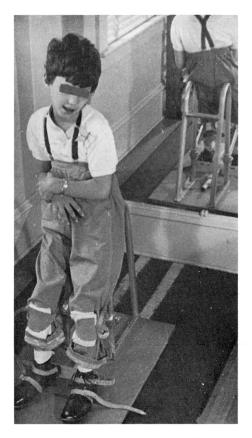

Fig. 12-10. Patient with cerebral palsy in stabilizer to achieve standing balance. (From Kenney, W. C., and Larson, C. B.: Orthopedics for the general practitioner, St. Louis, 1957, The C. V. Mosby Co.)

quently advise parents to use a weighted doll carriage in assisting the child to walk. Walkers are thought by some authorities to be inadvisable because the child, unless closely supervised, tends to push himself along without lifting his feet from the ground and thereby develops undesirable habits of progression. Parallel bars (Fig. 12-11), which furnish a sort of stabilized canelike support for the child, are considered more useful. Frequently, some type of support for the child's feet can be constructed to give a wider base for standing and walking. "Duck shoes" or "ski shoes" have been used for this purpose, and these are firmly fastened to the child's everyday shoes during his walking exercises. They are dispensed with as soon as possible, and the child is urged to attempt walking in the normal fashion.

The nurse caring for the patient with cerebral palsy over a considerable period of time will soon learn that there are certain occasions and conditions under which the child relaxes best. Soothing music, gentle rhythmic movements of the limbs, warmth, light massage, and immersion in warm pools frequently are efficacious in assisting the child to relax. Knowing that a great deal of the patient's progress depends directly upon his ability to meet new situations and environments successfully, the nurse will seek to increase the child's ability to relax in other, less favorable circumstances. This will require time and thought and will be accompanied by many setbacks, but carry-over is possible if the child's mentality is normal.

Nursing care after surgical treatment

Student nurses frequently see patients with cerebral palsy only when they are admitted to orthopedic wards for surgery. This is by no means the best time to make the child's acquaintance because he is likely to be more tense and emotional than at any other time. For this reason it would be desirable to have him admitted long enough before surgery for nurses to establish some measure of rapport with him and to assure him of their friendliness, interest, and desire to help him. Only in this way can his great burden of apprehension and insecurity be alleviated. Fortunately, most surgeons feel that it is very unwise to operate on such children until they have become adjusted to their surroundings. Their hyperexcitability is likely to lead to acidosis if surgery follows too soon upon admission to the hospital. Furthermore operations on rigid spastic patients are usually performed after a period of muscle training. If this interval devoted to muscle reeducation is spent in the hospital, the nurse can help the patient make his adjustment to the ward situation more satisfactorily than is possible if he enters immediately preceding surgery.

Many operations have been made necessary in these patients because of failure to prevent secondary contractures that come about from constant positions of creeping, crawling, and sitting. These positions are the ones maintained by the child a great portion of the time if he is unable to walk. Parents should be instructed to

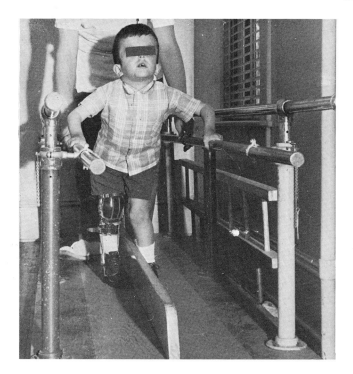

Fig. 12-11. Patient with cerebral palsy learning reciprocal gait in the parallel bars. Note the center piece to prevent scissoring. (From Kenney, W. C., and Larson, C. B.: Orthopedics for the general practitioner, St. Louis, 1957, The C. V. Mosby Co.)

have the child alternate with these some periods of prone-lying, which tends to stretch the contracted flexors of the hip and to overcome the forward position of the shoulders. Another variation can be obtained in the back-lying position with a small pillow beneath the dorsal spine. At such times elevation of the bed or crib on boxes at the head will permit the child to see what goes on around him and not leave him with a feeling of isolation from ward or home activities.

The incidence of acidosis after surgery is rather high in these children, and considerable attention is given to preoperative feeding of stick candy and orange juice. Intravenous glucose is occasionally administered to fortify the particularly excitable child against acidosis.

Postoperatively, these children sometimes display great apathy and prostration—greater than the mild surgical procedure they have been subjected to would seem to warrant. The nurse is urged to respect the child's desire to be let alone as much as is compatible with good care. If he is in casts (long leg or hip spica) after surgery on nerves or tendons, every altera-

tion of his position tends to cause agonizing muscle spasm in the extremities. Even without such movement, his face will be contorted with expressions of pain at very frequent intervals, as a result of spasm in the muscles at the site of surgery. Often, these spasms make him very resistant to any type of nursing care, and only the most skillful handling on the part of the nurse will be tolerated willingly. The patient must be turned very gently. No portion of the trunk must be allowed to change position during the turning process. Steady support along the body and cast is essential during any change of position.

The spastic child's postoperative nausea seems unduly prolonged. The intake of such children must be watched carefully. The doctor must be informed of the total 24-hour intake so that he may administer intravenous glucose when necessary.

The skin of these children tends to break down easily when subjected to constant pressure. Attention to the child's every complaint regarding a sensation of pressure is extremely important. Loss of some degree of sensation, however, is not uncommon in these children, and pressure areas may form beneath casts without any complaint from the child. Scupulous care of the patient's skin, accompanied by frequent inspection of the cast for odor, rough edges, and the like, is indispensable.

If an adductor tenotomy has been performed, the site of incision in the groin is a frequent cause of concern to the nurse, particularly if the child is very young or is one who cannot be depended upon to call for the bedpan. Sometimes collodion dressings are applied, or waterproofing may be put on over the dressings and the edges may be sealed with waterproof adhesive tape. The nurse is occasionally given permission to change these dressings when the necessity arises. Although careful aseptic technique must be carried out, it is a recognized fact that these tissues seem to be resistant to urine-induced infections.

When the order is given to bivalve the casts and to remove the child from them for certain periods during the day, it has been observed that the child may cry bitterly when the splints are put on again. Acute muscle spasm and tenseness sometimes make it almost impossible to reapply these splints, and, if force is used, the child frequently has a miserable night. It is advisable to try to bring about relaxation of the child's muscles rather than to use force in this circumstance. A prolonged bath in warm water sometimes helps to relax muscles and makes application of the splints less painful for the child. The nurse's humane urge to leave off the splints after an unsuccessful attempt to apply them must be tempered by the realization that the tendency toward recurrence of deformity in these patients is very great, and much of the improvement made by the operation may be sacrificed if splinting is not carried out faithfully.

This difficulty is not so pronounced in the application of the braces that may be ordered later for the postoperative spastic patient. By the time braces are ready, his postoperative tenderness has subsided. It has been found convenient to have the shoes that are attached to such braces cut open to the toes and have eyelets made over the dorsum of the foot, since much easier manipulation of the foot is possible in this way. Grasping the sock over the instep

and thereby guiding the foot into the shoe serves to overcome the tendency of the child's foot to go into plantar flexion as the shoe is applied.

Central nervous system operations, such as cordotomy and ramisection, are now performed much less frequently than they used to be. The nursing care for these patients is the same as combining the care of a patient who has had a laminectomy with that of a patient with hyperirritability and neuromuscular tension. Noticeable lessening of spasticity is sometimes observed, but it has been noted that this tends to be transitory. Changes in this regard must be carefully observed and recorded by the nurse throughout the postoperative period. The risk attending these operations is considerable, and the child will be seriously ill for some time.

Teaching parents home care of these children

Instruction for follow-up home care is so vital that the success of all hospital treatment may be said to be based upon it. Demonstrations of treatments and imparting information about the child are far from sufficient. If possible, the parents should spend several days in preparation for taking the child home. The mother should be allowed to see the treatments and nursing care on several occasions and to observe certain emergencies that arise in connection with the child's daily routine so that she will see how these are dealt with in the hospital. It is particularly important for the parents to realize how serious an error it is to break down or interfere with the patient's nascent sense of his own independence and worth. On the other hand, although parents should be urged to encourage the child in his activities, some warning may be needed if they seem to be overly ambitious for the child's progress. Sometimes the parents' enthusiasm and desire for the child constantly to do better serve only to increase his tension, and he may be totally unable to relax in their presence. Furthermore, parents should understand that the child will occasionally go through a period when no improvement whatever seems to occur. These plateaus are part of the natural cycle for the patient with cerebral palsy, and too much concern should not be caused by their occasional appearance.

In giving instructions for home care to the

parents of such a child, the nurse may help them see the advantages of enlarging the child's horizon by means of friendships with other handicapped children as well as with normal children. The orthopedic public health nurse may be of considerable help to the parents in finding these friends. Assisting the child to forget himself is believed by some to be the major objective of treatment, since loss of agonizing self-consciousness is one of the surest ways to improve motor skill. Developing such objectivity may be a lifelong job, but the child should be brought to understand that the human race as a whole has the same fight before it. The obstacles are greater for those with cerebral palsy, but the rewards are greater, too, in the realization of the immense obstacles overcome.

Some attempt to educate the child's friends and associates in their approach and relationship with him may be advisable. Only friends who are by nature considerate of others should be encouraged. Outright rudeness or thoughtless remarks made to the handicapped person often discourage him from further attempts of a social nature. To help the child in meeting the inescapable crises, some explanation needs to be given to him about human nature and its variable response to the handicapped person. He should be helped to realize very early that both children and grown-ups will frequently display unintelligent, ignorant attitudes toward him, which are unthinkingly cruel on some occasions and foolishly sentimental on others. Perhaps the child old enough to comprehend these things can be made to realize that he himself must develop attitudes of tolerance and forbearance toward persons of limited abilities. His own limitations, after all, are largely physical. He should therefore be able to make allowances for errors in others who are even less well equipped than himself.

There are many crafts adaptable for the home use of the child with cerebral palsy. Finger painting is excellent for the child whose hand grasp is poor. Work with clay and embroidery on burlap with yarn and large blunt needles provide training toward muscular coordination. Looms and basketry are also excellent. Occupational therapists advise us that whatever craft the cerebral palsied child undertakes should be within his mental and physical capacity.

The materials chosen for work should not be difficult to handle. In addition, the work should be the child's own, not that of the parents, nurses, or therapist. Motivation can too easily be destroyed if many alien hands interfere with the child's progress in making something that he would like to think of as entirely his own.

Community projects for the assistance of patients with cerebral palsy are numerous, and the alert public health nurse can help to interest local groups in the subject. One particularly good idea that has been worked out in a community is a so-called lending library of equipment for these patients—for example, reclining chairs, specially constructed tables with adjustable legs, dishes, and so forth. This, of course, entails having a carpenter available who can alter the equipment to suit the needs of the current borrower. As a family finishes using the particular item, it is sent back to the library, where the carpenter makes the adjustments needed for the next borrower. Another example of community cooperation is a manual training class in a high school that has taken as a special project the construction of equipment recommended by a local orthopedist for use by persons with cerebral palsy.

Public health nurses can be of inestimable help to the parents of these children in many ways. They should know definitely what instructions were given the parents before they took the child home. They are entitled to know also the treatment and success of treatment that the child had in the hospital. If these details are made available to them before the child returns home, they are fortified to assist the parents and the child in carrying out recommended treatment. It is essential that they have this information before the child goes home so that there will be no intermission or backsliding. Even a week of this can undo much of the effect of the hospital experience.

STUDY QUESTIONS

1. Study and list the possible causes of cerebral palsy.
2. What early symptoms might indicate the presence of this condition?
3. Discuss briefly the differences in treatment of the two main types of cerebral palsy.
4. Discuss the nurse's part in habit training in cerebral palsy.
5. What are some of the problems that might be

encountered in the postoperative care of the patient with cerebral palsy?

6. Does the child's physical disability influence his mental and emotional development? Explain.

7. Can you visualize the problems parents and family are confronted with when a child is born with cerebral palsy? What assitance can the nurse give the parent?

REFERENCES

Banks, H. L., and Panagakos, P.: The role of the orthopedic surgeon in cerebral palsy, Pediat. Clin. North Am. **14:**495-515, 1967.

Blockley, J., and Miller G.: Feeding techniques with cerebral-palsied children, Physiotherapy **57:**300-308, 1971.

Bobath, B.: Motor development, its effect on general development and application to the treatment of cerebral palsy, Physiotherapy **57:**526-532, 1971.

Bobath, K., and Bobath, B.: The facilitation of normal postural reactions and movements in the treatment of cerebral palsy, Physiotherapy **50:**246-262, 1964.

Bobath, K.: The normal postural reflex mechanism and its deviation in children with cerebral palsy, Physiotherapy **57:**515-525, 1971.

Cailliet, R.: Bracing for spasticity. In Licht, S., and Kamenetz, H. L., editors: Orthotics etcetera, New Haven, 1966, Elizabeth Licht, Publisher.

Cotton, E.: Integration of treatment and education in cerebral palsy, Physiotherapy **56:**143-147, 1970.

Dunn, H. G.: Physical aspects of cerebral palsy, Canad. Nurse **62:**29-32, Sept. 1966.

Ferguson, A. Jr.: Orthopaedic surgery in infancy and childhood, ed. 3, Baltimore, 1968, The Williams & Wilkins Co.

Garrett A., Lister, M., and Bresnan, J.: New concepts in bracing for cerebral palsy, Phys. Ther. **46:**728-733, 1966.

Hawke, W. A.: Impact of cerebral palsy on patient and family, Canad. Nurse **63:**29-31, 1967.

Haynes, U. H.: Nursing approaches in cerebral dysfunction, Am. J. Nurs. **68:**2170-2176, 1968.

Keats, S.: Cerebral palsy, Springfield, Ill., 1970, Charles C Thomas, Publisher.

Keats, S.: Operative orthopedics in cerebral palsy, Springfield, Ill., 1970, Charles C Thomas, Publisher.

Knapp, M. E.: Cerebral palsy I, Postgrad. Med. **47:**229-232, Feb. 1970.

Knapp, M. E.: Cerebral palsy II, Postgrad. Med. **47:**247-252, March, 1970.

Kolderie, M. L.: Behavior modification in the treatment of children with cerebral palsy, Phys. Ther. **51:**1080-1091, 1971.

Malone, P.: Danny was my patient, Am. J. Nurs. **65:**126-127, 1965.

Mercer W. and Duthie, R.: Orthopedic surgery, ed. 6, Baltimore, 1964, The Williams & Wilkins Co.

Orthopaedic surgery in cerebral palsy. In Adams, J. P., editor: Current practice in orthopáedic surgery, St. Louis, 1966, The C. V. Mosby Co.

Pendleton, T.: Trainable cerebral palsied children, Phys. Ther. Rev. **41:**582-585, 1961.

Pendleton, T., and Simonson, J.: Training children with cerebral palsy, Am. J. Nurs. **64:**126-129, 1964.

Phelps, W. M., Melcher, R. T., and Doll, E. A.: Mental deficiency due to birth injuries, New York, 1932, The MacMillan Co.

Pothier, P. C.: Therapeutic handling of the severly handicapped child, Am. J. Nurs. **71:**321-324, 1971.

Raney, R. B., and Brashear, H. R.: Shand's handbook of orthopaedic surgery, ed. 8, St. Louis, 1973, The C. V. Mosby Co.

Semans, S.: Principles of treatment in cerebral palsy, Phys. Ther. **46:**715-720, 1966.

Vennert, B. F.: A work training program for hospitalized retardates, Am. J. Nurs. **66:**2456-2460, 1966.

13
Poliomyelitis

The very fortunate trend toward the disappearance of this crippling disease has resulted from the widespread use of poliovirus vaccines (Salk and Sabin) in the United States. After the introduction of poliovirus vaccine in 1955, paralytic poliomyelitis (infantile paralysis) declined from the 18,308 cases in 1954 to a low total of 61 cases in 1965.

IPV (inactivated poliomyelitis virus) contains vaccines for types 1, 2, and 3, and is administered by subcutaneous or intramuscular injections. It is given in three doses, the second dose 2 to 6 weeks after the first, and the third 7 months later. OPV (attenuated oral live poliovirus) contains vaccines for strains 1, 2, and 3, and represents the 3 monovalent vaccines. The vaccine is liquid and may be given by dropper or teaspoon. The dosage varies depending on the potency of the pharmaceutical preparation. The oral poliovirus (OPV) trivalent is more widely used than IPV in this country because it is easier to administer and produces an immune response which, without regular booster doses, appears to be similar to immunity induced by natural poliomyelitis infection.

The three-dose immunization (OPV) should be started at 6 to 12 weeks of age. The second dose should be given no less than 6 to 8 weeks later. The third dose should be administered 8 to 12 months after the second one. The schedule, recommended by the Public Health Service Advisory Committee, will produce an immune response to all poliovirus types in well over 90% of the recipients. On entering elementary school, all children who have completed the primary oral poliovirus series should be given a single follow-up dose of trivalent oral poliovirus. All others should complete the primary series.

In spite of the decreased incidence of the illness, this chapter is being retained for the benefit of the student who may encounter poliomyelitis in other countries or need to care for patients with residual deformities and paralyses from previous epidemics here.

CAUSE

Poliomyelitis occurs most commonly in the late summer, although epidemics have occurred in the early winter months. Young children are most often affected, but there seems to be no age limit to the susceptibility to infection.

One theory is based on the probability that it is a common childhood disease but that paralysis occurs only in the severely affected persons. It is postulated that immunity against the disease is developed in many instances without the entire clinical picture being present and without knowledge that the person has had the disease. This is borne out to some extent by clinical studies in large epidemics in which it appears that only about 10% of those who are examined show some laboratory and some clinical evidence of the types that result in paralysis.

The infectious organism is known definitely to be a virus. Three strains of the poliomyelitis virus have been isolated, and an attack of poliomyelitis does not develop immunity to more than one strain of the virus.

PATHOLOGY

The destructive lesions in poliomyelitis are in the anterior horn cells of the spinal cord. The motor system of the body consists of three groups of cells: (1) those in the brain that initiate the motions, (2) those in the medulla and ganglia that coordinate the motions, and (3) those in the spinal cord (the anterior horn cells) that transmit the impulses to the muscle cells.

The anterior horn cells are distributed in groups throughout the entire spinal cord but are concentrated in the groups that supply nerve impulses to the upper and lower extremities. These groups of cells are arranged more or less in small groups supplying individual muscles, such as the deltoid, the biceps, the gluteus maximus, the quadriceps.

During an attack of poliomyelitis the following may occur: (1) There may be several areas where complete destruction of cell, either by local activity of the disease itself or by destructive effects of the toxins formed, may cause an actual degenerative process of varying size and degree. (2) Waste products and edema may endanger the vitality of a major group of cells around the destroyed area. (3) Beyond this are large inflammatory changes that temporarily incapacitate a much larger group of cells (Fig. 13-1).

Return of functional power in the muscles supplied by these cells is fairly rapid.

In the completely destroyed areas there will never be any return of muscle power. In the intermediate zone the cells may recover or may disintegrate, according to the demands placed upon them. Rest is the important factor. Only the cells damaged by relatively mild inflammatory change will recover under almost any condition.

The rapid recovery that takes place, within 1 to 3 weeks after an attack of poliomyelitis, occurs because the muscles are innervated by the cells that have been impaired temporarily by the inflammatory process.

The recovery that may or may not take place in the following weeks or months is directly related to the number of cells destroyed or not destroyed by the edema and waste products of the disease activity.

The permanent paralysis is directly related to

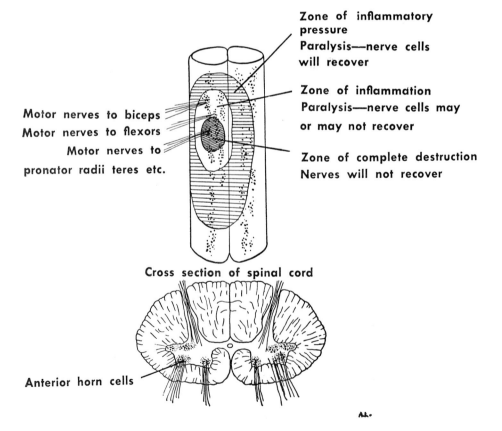

Fig. 13-1. Schematic drawing of spinal cord showing the method of attack of poliomyelitis.

the number of cells destroyed by the local activity of the disease.

Improvement continues in patients with poliomyelitis for at least several years. Any improvement after a few months, however, is not the result of any further recovery of the nerves but rather an improved functioning of the muscle fibers whose nerves of stimulation have already recovered.

There are two other types of involvement with poliomyelitis. The bulbar type consists of an involvement of the nerve cells high up in the spinal cord. If the inflammatory condition reaches the vital centers, the condition is fatal. If the damage is not sufficient to cause death, a relatively complete recovery usually occurs within a few weeks or months. These patients may require use of the respirator during the more active stage of the disease because of the paralysis of the intercoastal muscles and the diaphragm. Poliomeningitis manifests symptoms that are frequently very similar to those found in other forms of meningitis—including delirium, stiff neck, strabismus, and incontinency. Actual paralysis of the muscles is not usually present. There may be flaccidity or spasticity of the extremities.

SYMPTOMS AND SIGNS

The disease usually begins rather abruptly with a headache and an intestinal disturbance. There may be an elevation of temperature from 99° to 102° F. There is usually some evidence of spinal cord irritation that is recognized by stiffness of the neck with some resistance and pain in the back when attempts are made to raise the head from the bed. Paralysis, when it develops, usually occurs somewhere between the third and seventh day after the onset of the illness. In some cases, however, the initial symptoms are so mild that the disease is not recognized until paralysis has set in. The patient may then fall because of weakness of a limb.

In those persons in whom paralysis does not develop, all symptoms may disappear within 2 or 3 days. It is unwise, however, to make any statement regarding the severity of the disease earlier than 48 hours after the disappearance of all fever, since apparently mild cases may subsequently become severe. When paralysis develops, there may be pain on movement of the limbs and joints or on pressure upon the muscles involved. After the acute symptoms, the patient is usually quite comfortable except for this.

HOW POLIOMYELITIS IS DIAGNOSED

Diagnosis is confirmed by the spinal tap and identification of the virus (one of three strains now known). Many recently identified viruses such as the ECHO group can cause symptoms, exclusive of paralysis, that simulate the acute stage of poliomyelitis. A spinal fluid examination that reveals a slight increase in pressure, a clear appearance, and a cell count of from 10 to 300 or slightly higher is considered very significant. The cell count, if performed early enough, shows a predominance of polymorphonuclear leukocytes, but these are succeeded within 24 to 48 hours by lymphocytes. Spinal sugar is normal; nurses will remember that it should be about one-half the amount of the blood sugar. Chlorides are normal, and the Pandy test for spinal globulin may be positive, 1 to 4 plus. The total protein is usually increased, and an elevation of 45 mg. per cubic millimeter or above is thought to be significant.

If laboratory facilities are available, the poliomyelitis virus should be looked for, by the use of suitable culture techniques, in the stool of the patient or in throat washings.

CURRENT THEORIES REGARDING SPREAD OF THE DISEASE

Because it has been established that the virus may leave the body of the patient (or healthy carrier) in the discharges of the bowel or the nose and throat, it seems safe to assume that person-to-person contact must play a large part in the spread of the disease. Although the upper respiratory passages are no longer considered the primary routes of infection, nevertheless, the exact manner in which the virus enters the body is not completely understood, and care should be used in handling the discharges from the nose and throat of any patient suspected of having poliomyelitis.

It is now an accepted fact that the virus of poliomyelitis remains in the gastrointestinal tract sometimes over a period of weeks, and, therefore, considerable attention must be given to the matter of disinfecting stools.

ISOLATION OF THE PATIENT

The patient is usually isolated for approximately 2 weeks, although in some localities it may be longer. Rigid isolation precautions may be the rule in some instances, whereas group isolation may be used in others.

HEALTH TEACHING AND THE PREVENTION OF POLIOMYELITIS

At the present time, the nurse's most important responsibility pertaining to poliomyelitis lies in the area of prevention. Helping parents understand the necessity of having members of the family receive the poliomyelitis vaccine and providing them with information of immunization programs available in their community are vital if this disease is to be prevented. The oral vaccine is available at a minimal cost, and every child and adult should receive this protection against poliomyelitis. Additional teaching done by the nurse is based on a few rules of hygiene dictated by current concepts of the disease. Because in many cases it seems unquestionable that the virus is ingested, all foods should be protected from filth, flies, dirty hands, and animals. If food is to be eaten raw, it should be well washed. Hands should be carefully washed not merely before meals but before eating any food. Milk should be certified or pasteurized, and the water supply should be from approved sources. Because one of the nurse's chief duties is to prevent the spread of misinformation, it should be pointed out at this time that modern epidemiologic evidence does not seem to indicate that infected milk or water has ever been the source of an epidemic.

The necessity for having adequate rest and for avoiding strenuous exercise and chilling should be emphasized in health teaching.

TREATMENT

Treatment of poliomyelitis is discussed in reference to three stages: acute illness, convalescence, and reconstruction.

During the acute and febrile stage, rest is all-important. Use of a firm bed and relaxation of the affected extremities in a position of physiologic rest has been the treatment of choice. This consists in maintaining the shoulders in slight abduction, the elbows flexed or extended, and the wrists at slight dorsiflexion. In the lower extremities the knee and hip are flexed a few degrees, and the foot is held in a position at right angles to the leg.

Warm moist packs may be applied to the involved parts. Passive exercises performed by a physical therapist help maintain a normal range of motion. This treatment seems to have the advantage of eliminating stasis in the muscles, thereby preventing spasm and contractures, maintaining flexibility, and making the patient more comfortable; but, unquestionably, nothing can effect the recovery of the nerve cells in the anterior horn of the spinal cord.

Deformity should be prevented during the convalescent stage; but if deformity occurs or if weaknesses persist, the limbs must be protected by braces or the deformities be corrected.

Relief of muscle spasm. Methods of using heat to relieve muscle spasm vary greatly in different localities. Nurses must be guided entirely by the physician's preference in using this treatment as well as by the patient's tolerance. Parts to be packed and frequency of packing should be prescribed by the physician as any other treatment would be prescribed.

PRONE AND LAY-ON PACKING. These packs have the advantage that the patient need not be turned or manipulated during their application. Prone packing is particularly adaptable for stubborn spasm of the muscles of the back and thighs. The patient is placed in the face-lying position in good bed posture, with supports to areas where tightness exists, and the packs are applied by laying them on the parts without pinning.

Physical therapy. Early passive joint movement to all joints may also be part of the nursing duties after demonstration has been given by the physical therapist. Passive joint movement is usually done several times during the day, and it is felt that it is sometimes more convenient for nurses to do this because of their frequent contacts with the patient. Every effort is put forth to maintain complete range of joint motion in all joints from the earliest days of the disease. Warm pool treatments or hot tub baths are sometimes given several times during the week as part of the physical therapy treatment. Intensive packing of tight or contracted muscles, followed by forcible stretching, may be done after the acute period of pain and spasm is over.

Bulbar involvement. Both medical treatment and nursing care in bulbar poliomyelitis are based on four considerations: preventing asphyxia, averting exhaustion, maintaining adequate nutrition, and checking secondary infections. Restlessness, wakefulness, an increase of mucus in the throat, difficulty in swallowing, drawing the head back, rigidity, and an expression of apprehension are significant and should be reported without delay.

Involvement of muscles of respiration. In the spinal type of poliomyelitis or in the combined spinal and bulbar type, weakness of shoulders and arms is sometimes an early sign that impairment of some muscles of the chest (pectorals) and those of respiration (intercostals and diaphragm) may take place. The nurse must be alert for signs of approaching respiratory embarrassment when caring for a patient with obvious involvement of the upper extremities.

PRINCIPLES UNDERLYING USE OF THE RESPIRATOR. Some review of the mechanics of respiration is necessary in order to adequately understand the operation of the respirator. The respiratory function is accomplished by inspiration and expiration. When the individual breathes in, the thoracic cavity enlarges by contraction of the muscles of inspiration—the diaphragm and intercoastal muscles. The contraction of the intercostal muscles lifts the rib cage, and contraction of the diaphragm depresses the floor of the chest, both thereby increasing the chest capacity. This enlarged chest cavity returns to normal more or less passively. Expiration is considered to be by some physiologists almost entirely passive. It is a result of the relaxing of the intercostal muscles and the diaphragm, as well as the returning upward pressure of the abdominal walls, now free from the pressure of the contracted diaphragm. When paralysis of the diaphragm and intercostal muscles is present, all this is obviously impossible, and it is in these patients that the respirator has made its greatest contribution.

The patient's body is placed in the airtight chamber of the respirator, but with his head out-side. The respirator bellows upon expansion will cause the air pressure in the tank to become lower. Because it is a physical fact that air pressures tend to equalize themselves, air from the outside will rush into the lungs through the nose and throat, expanding the lungs and thereby lessening the pressure in the chest; equilibrium of air pressure will thus be restored. The contracting bellows immediately increase air pressure on the body in the tube, the chest cavity is compressed, and the patient exhales. This constant rhythmic procedure aerates the lungs in the manner of natural respiration but with no effort on the part of the patient.

ROCKING BED. A rocking bed has been used by some physicians to assist the patient in gaining independence from the machine. The mechanism of this bed provides a seesaw motion, and inhalation occurs more or less passively as the head is elevated and the abdominal viscera are shifted downward. Then, with the feet up and the head down, the viscera move upward against the diaphragm and assist in exhalation (Figs. 13-2 and 13-3). These oscillations are regulated so that they are at the rate of normal breathing.

CHEST RESPIRATOR. In some instances it is possible to use a chest respirator (Fig. 13-4) to replace the tank respirator. This respirator gives the patient more freedom and greatly facilitates nursing care. Various kinds of material may be used for the chest covering. The edges, which must fit snugly against the chest wall, are made of rubber. The shell is held in place with tape-webbing straps. Considerable care must be given to the skin that comes in contact with the rubber, since it tends to break down easily.

Rehabilitative aspects for poliomyelitis residuals

The student will find that much of the following discussion pertaining to "rehabilitative aspects," is also applicable to individuals physically disabled from other causes.

Poliomyelitis is said to have reached the chronic stage after the muscles have made their maximum recovery, usually from 18 months to 2 years. A great deal of the progress, however, that has been made during the convalescent stage can be lost if careful medical and nursing supervision is not provided thereafter. Weight bearing

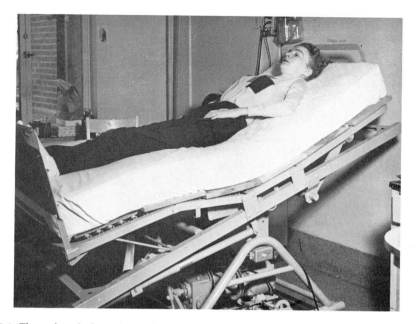

Fig. 13-2. The rocking bed may be used to promote early weaning of the patient from the respirator. Each day, or several times daily, the patient is placed on the bed for increasingly longer periods. The length of time tolerated is determined by the patient's facial expression, pulse rate, and color. Nursing activities can be performed with the bed in motion. Liquid or food is given when the head of the bed is highest. During this phase the abdominal viscera tend to move downward, favoring movement of the diaphragm and inhalation of air.

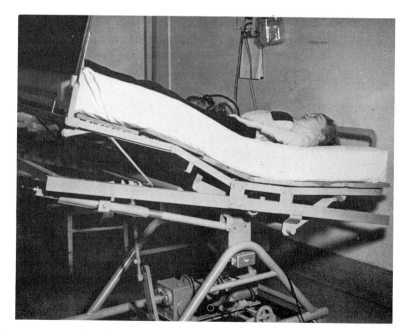

Fig. 13-3. As the head of the bed lowers, the viscera shift upward against the diaphragm and air is exhaled. At this time, when air is going out through the larynx, it is easier for the patient to speak. The patient learns to inhale as the head of the bed rises and exhale as the head of the bed lowers.

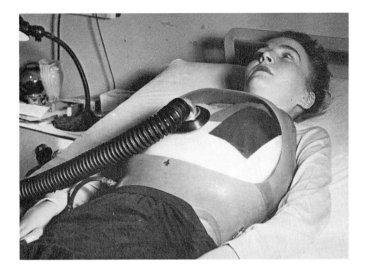

Fig. 13-4. The chest respirator is placed over the chest and held in place by straps that encircle the patient's body. The rubber edges must fit snugly about the chest wall if the person is to receive benefit from the respirator.

and similar activities place considerable strain on muscles, and even patients who have had very minor involvement may develop unsuspected weaknesses at this time unless a close check is kept on their progress.

EMOTIONAL ASPECTS

The treatment of poliomyelitis in the early weeks is dramatic enough that the full import of the patient's disability does not always become apparent to him for some time afterward. Progress during the first weeks tends to be more rapid than it will be after 6 months' time has elapsed. A gradual awareness of the permanent nature of his handicap may in some instances, particularly with the adolescent and the young adult, be the cause of major depressions and personality changes. Indifference, apathy, or self-pity may replace the patient's original attitude of hope, courage, and determination to recover.

Nurses should be forewarned that these things are likely to happen and that this is a rough spot over which they must be expected to guide the patient, with considerable permanent involvement. They should be able to warn parents and relatives that such an occurrence is a natural reaction. To limit this period and to cut it down to its minimum by sympathetic, intelligent advice should be part of the nurse's skill.

Management of these situations demands early recognition of their likelihood. Although the nurse's attitude—like that of the patient—must be based on faith and optimism, statements must be guarded. The patient should very gradually be brought to accept his handicap from the first days of his paralysis and to plan his life in terms of that, rather than in terms of a complete functional recovery. This is the only honest course for any of his associates to take. It is kinder than unguarded optimism and cheeriness that break down under the strain of long-deferred hope. It goes without saying that the principles of mental hygiene that the nurse applies when working with the patient must be given to the family of the patient to guide them in their understanding of the patient's problems. That this takes ingenuity is an understatement. The nurse may be instrumental in helping the parents of a child patient plan, in relation to the patient's homecoming, such alterations of environment and living that will make relative independence possible for him. The importance of friendship and relationship with young people of his own age must be pointed out so that the parents may make special efforts to see that friendships he enjoyed in school are continued while he is homebound.

The patient's problem is a very real one. Faced in the cold light of day and robbed of the mitigating factors that attend the early illness and the dramatic fight for survival, the outlook may be very black indeed. It is a situation that the newly crippled person realizes, however dimly, he has to face alone. The pattern of his life is smashed. He must collect the fragments and make what he can of them; and the task may look hopeless, the effort not worth the while.

It is impossible to lay down a schedule of treatment for this situation. To meet it adequately, the nurse's preparation must be broad. Besides courses in orthopedics, sociology, community health, and mental hygiene, a deep-seated interest in people and their problems is necessary. It is also important to be aware of what community resources for education and rehabilitation may be available to help this person. He will not know of them, for 3 months ago he was a healthy person with no knowledge or need of such services. If ever there was an urgent necessity for broad information on these points, it is at this time when the nurse earnestly accepts the challenge to assist a young newly crippled individual attacked by all the forces of pessimism and personal disintegration.

The student nurse should know the ways in which the physical therapist and the occupational therapist keep the patient interested in making further effort toward physical reclamation. These team members must do this day after day in their work, and there is more skill involved than the student often realizes. Facile encouragement, more or less mechanical, will not accomplish much. The patient soon learns to detect patent signs of insincerity in the nurse.

Nurses can do much to provide diversional activity for young people in the hospital if they will remember the things they liked to do at that age and find some means of encouraging the patients to develop like interests. To encourage hobbies in their patients, nurses should have a few of their own that they can offer to explain to the patient. Many nurses initiate such hobbies by contributions of their own. Stamp collecting, postmark collecting, and matchfolder collecting are cheap and interesting and might provide a beginning for activity by a disabled child.

Where it is possible, a ward-governing body may be developed. Such groups can have more functions than might be apparent at the outset, and they often do much to improve ward spirit and morale. Complaints, requests, plans for activities and parties, and welcoming committees for new patients are functions that can be worked out of the original self-governing group. Great pride in this matter has been observed in areas where such a democratic system of regulation is carried out over a period of time.

General health supervision. Nurses who supervise the care of patients after poliomyelitis should aim to assist their patients in the daily requirements of living in the home, such as bathing, dressing, getting out of a chair, going to the toilet, and other, similar activities. It will often take considerable planning and ingenuity to make it possible for the severely affected patient to do some of these things, but certainly no service can be more important. To achieve these ends, adaptation in home equipment may often be necessary. Nurses will frequently be able to secure help and advice from members of the family who have an aptitude for mechanical construction and carpentry. Consultation with a physical therapist or an occupational therapist will often give the nurse valuable hints needed for attaining some of the objectives.

Frequent inspection to detect habitual faulty positions in sitting, walking, or standing should be made during the period when functional activity is being resumed. The public health nurse should be alert for incomplete extension of hips, for tendencies to stand in the back-knee position, and for deviation of the spine as a result of poor habits of sitting and standing. She should observe unequal growth of the legs or feet that might indicate overuse of one extremity because of a disguised weakness in the other. The parents should be instructed to observe signs that the unaffected parts of the patient's body are becoming weakened because of overuse and fatigue. No matter how mild the involvement from poliomyelitis, patients must be taught to avoid fatigue for a long time after their recovery. Periods of rather strenuous activity will often reveal weaknesses in muscles that were not originally thought to be affected. Periods of bed rest should always follow periods of prolonged or strenuous activity. The after-lunch nap for an hour should be part of the patient's daily program. It should be taken in a darkened, ventilated room, free from the distraction of radio or toys.

The child with only a short leg brace or splint often tends to sit or lie for long periods with the leg rolled outward because of the weight of the apparatus. The mother's attention should be called to this position, which is often the cause of troublesome deformity at the hip level when the child begins to walk.

The danger of eyestrain should be borne in mind, particularly in the older patient, who spends so much of his time reading or doing handwork that requires close attention. Attitudes denoting eyestrain—squinting, frequent headaches, reddened lids, or holding the work too close to the eye—should be reported to the physician. Glasses can sometimes relieve much of this strain.

The child's eating habits should have close attention. Because of his relative inactivity, combined with normal appetite, the patient often tends to gain weight easily. The diet may need to be limited sensibly, but it should not be limited in features essential for a growing person. The child's functional disability will be greatly exaggerated by a substantial gain in weight, and weakened muscles will undergo further strain from having to support it.

Consideration of the patient as an individual is necessary, and his individual problem, which is bound to be a little different from that of the child in the next bed, must be given consideration. If he seems unruly and twists and turns in bed despite all pleas, perhaps the nurse can arrange his bed so that he is able to see different parts of the ward at different times of the day.

On the whole, the younger child tends to adjust to his condition much more easily than the older one, which is not difficult to understand. The older patient will be affected by periodic spells of gloom and depression, accompanied in some cases by definite refusal of cooperation. Such a patient needs some definite assurance of advancement. It is the long period of confinement, the inactivity, and the limitation of body motion that bring on these periodic spells of depression.

SURGERY IN POLIOMYELITIS

The entire plan of reconstructive surgery in poliomyelitis is based on the fact that joints are controlled by groups of coordinating but opposing muscles. In the ankle, for example, plantar flexion results from the action of the gastrocnemius (calf muscle group) and flexors of the toes. This is opposed and balanced by the extensor group of muscles—the tibialis anticus, the peroneus brevis, and the extensors of the toes. Inversion of the ankle is accomplished by action of the tibialis anticus and the tibialis posticus, assisted by the flexors of the toes.

If the extensors of the toes are paralyzed, the foot will turn inward and there will be a drop-foot deformity. Likewise, weaknesses of various types will develop with paralysis of other groups of muscles.

Reconstructive surgery is based on the elimination of the joint actions that allow the deformity to occur—by operative fixation, by transplantation of certain selected tendons to replace the action of paralyzed ones, or by a combination of joint fixation and tendon transplantation.

There are a number of mechanical tricks learned through experience in operative surgery that may in some instances save part or all of the motion in certain joints and still eliminate the ability of the stronger group of muscles to create deformity.

Many operations are designed to correct various deformities and contractures that developed before the patient was first observed. These consist frequently in detaching the contracted muscle from its origin and allowing it to reattach to bone in a position that will accomplish straightening of the joint or limb.

Some special operations. When there is a permanent paralysis of the deltoid muscle with a frail and useless shoulder, the shoulder may be stiffened in a position of abduction (60 degrees for children and 65 degrees for adults), provided there is good power in the muscles around the shoulder blade and reasonably good power in the hand. Following the operation, the entire upper extremity and the upper half of the body (shoulder spica) are placed in a cast until bony union within the joint is present. Joint fusions are usually accomplished by the complete removal of all cartilage from the component surfaces. Frequently, a bone graft is used to transfix the joint, stabilize it, and speed the fusion time. Complete fusion usually takes place in from 3 to 6 months.

HAND. One of the commonest deformities in the hand consists in a paralysis of the opposing muscles of the thumb. This causes the loss of grasping and holding power. The condition may be improved or corrected by tendon transplantation. One method (Steindler) consists in transplanting one half of the long extensor tendon of the thumb to the posterior surface of the proximal phalanx of the thumb near its articulation with the metacarpal bone. The method of Bunnell utilizes the flexor carpi ulnaris or the palmaris longus tendons, attaching them by a transplantation to the flexor tendon of the thumb through a loop around the carpal bones of the outer side of the hand.

SPINE. Many of the worst cases of curvature of the spine are the result of spinal or abdominal muscle paralysis. These curvatures should be prevented as much as possible during convalescence, but when they do occur they must be corrected.

The first step in the correction of paralytic curvature of the spine is through the use of corrective casts, such as the Risser cast. When the spine has been straightened, it is fused by surgery on the affected area and becomes rigid where the curve is most severe. The operation is frequently performed through a window that is cut in the back of the cast. The cast usually includes the head, the body, and one leg. It is worn for 4 to 6 months. This cast is replaced by another cast extending from the armpits, down to and including the pelvis, thereby allowing the patient to become ambulatory.

When curvature of the spine is the result of abdominal weakness, transplants of the strong ligamentous material from the other side of the thigh (fascia lata) are made, replacing the paralyzed muscles (Lowman and Mayer). These bands are usually stitched to the brim of the pelvis and to the ribs to form inelastic stabilizing sinews beneath the skin, which prevent rotation of the body and curvature. There are a number of applications of this method of stabilization.

HIP. When there is a flexion contracture of the hip, the muscle attachments, including a shell of bone, can be freed from the anterior and lateral portions of the iliac crest (Speed), thereby releasing the contracted muscles and giving correction of the deformity. A plaster hip spica is used to maintain correction for 6 to 10 weeks.

KNEE. There are a number of operations designed to stabilize the knee. If both the knee and the ankle are severely paralyzed, however, a long leg brace that extends from the ischium to the shoe frequently constitutes the best form of treatment. If stabilization of the knee is desired, it may be done by a bone block operation to limit flexion of the knee joint, by a bone block operation to prevent hyperextension of the knee joint (backknee), or by a complete ankylosis or fusion of the joint in the position of greatest usefulness as far as the occupation of the particular person is concerned.

Before operative fusion is performed, it is good to test the probability of success and satisfaction to the patient by applying a plaster of paris cast over the thigh and leg and allowing him to get about for a few weeks with the leg in a fixed position.

Knock-knee and outward rotation of the tibia and foot are common deformities in patients with poliomyelitis. They can be corrected by an ostectomy of the bone just below the knee with inward rotation of the tibia. Immobilization in plaster for 8 to 10 weeks is required for healing.

ANKLE. At the ankle, operations are designed to correct the most common deformities. Drop foot with inversion of the ankle and foot (equinovarus) is best treated by a modified Hoke operation that consists in the removal of a wedge-shaped portion of bone from the undersurface of the astragalus. The base of the wedge is forward and outward so that both deformities are corrected at the same time. The bone surface is freshened on both sides, and all cartilage is removed so that prompt ankylosis takes place. A plaster of paris cast from the toes to the groin maintains the corrected position during healing. The portion of the cast above the knee may be removed about 2 months after operation, but complete ankylosis rarely occurs in less than 4 to 6 months.

When the drop foot is uncomplicated by associated deformities, a posterior bone block in the astragalus will hold the foot at a right angle. When the arch is abnormally high as a result of a contracture of the plantar muscles, the detachment of these muscles from the os calcis (Steindler) followed by manipulation and stretching will give correction in the more mildly affected patients. In the more severely affected patients the removal of a wedge-shaped piece of bone from the tarsal region (dorsal surface) may be necessary to supplement this procedure.

There are comparatively few tendon transplantations that are permanently successful in the lower extremities, but there is one that gives quite satisfactory results. In patients with claw-foot (retraction of the toes), successful results are obtained by the transplantation of the extensors of the toes into the metatarsal bones near the heads. It is usually necessary to fasten these tendons through drill holes in the metatarsal bones so that anchorage will be secure.

EPIPHYSEAL ARREST. Unequal growth of the legs may be an aftermath of poliomyelitis contracted in early childhood. To correct this condition by equalizing the length of the legs is an important consideration in orthopedic surgery.

Phemister and others a number of years ago showed that arrest of epiphyseal growth could be effected by forms of localized epiphyseal destruction or disturbance. Their plan was based on the fact that equalization of leg length could be obtained by such disturbance, and retardation of growth at the epiphyseal line could be accomplished by a block osteotomy over the line with a 90-degree rotation of fragment (a square plug). When this is rotated, it causes a fusion or elimination of the growth line, resulting in the stoppage of growth of the limb. The state of the epiphysis as shown by roentgenography and a family history of height statistics give a clue as to the time that epiphyseal growth should be stopped.

Walter Blount has shown clinically that the principle of epiphyseal arrest can be applied to many more problems. By the use of stainless steel staples, it can be applied not only to the equalization of leg length but also to the calculated control of knock-knees and bowlegs. Moreover, this process may be stopped and controlled by the timely removal of the staples. Blount has found that one staple on each side may break as a result of epiphyseal growth strain. About three staples are necessary to stop the growth. Strangely enough, however, if the staples are removed before complete closure of the epiphyses, growth is restored. These findings open up a new field of leg equalization as well as the correction of bowleg and knock-knee deformities at a calculated time before puberty or the closure of the epiphyseal lines.

In addition, deformities such as a flexed knee

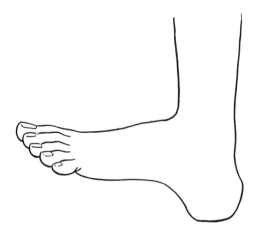

Fig. 13-5. Paralytic calcaneovalgus deformity.

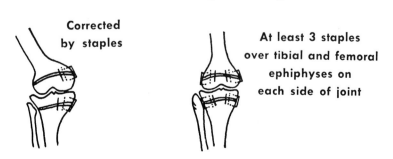

Knock-knee

Corrected
by staples

Leg shortening

At least 3 staples
over tibial and femoral
ephiphyses on
each side of joint

Fig. 13-6. Drawings showing epiphyseal arrest used in knock-knee and for leg shortening.

or a hyperextended knee can be corrected by staple fixation. Use of the staples can be discontinued at the proper time (Fig. 13-6).

Nursing care. As has been stated, surgery may be performed after poliomyelitis to correct deformities, to secure stability of the joints, and to improve function. Sometimes surgery is necessary because of neglect in early treatment or because of carelessness in following the instructions given for home treatment. Nurses, therefore, should be very earnest in their attempts to see that instructions for home care are followed to the letter.

Surgery for stabilization of the joints may frequently be performed to permit the patient to walk without braces or crutches. Even though it may accomplish this purpose satisfactorily, some disappointment is often felt by the patient or his parents because the cosmetic effect has not been all that they had expected. Time should always be taken before surgery to explain all the factors involved in the surgery and its probable outcome in order that disappointment may be avoided. Stories in newspapers and magazines during the past years have spoken so lavishly of miracle surgery that many persons expect an almost impossible result from orthopedic surgery and are disappointed when the outcome falls short of their anticipations.

The immediate aftercare is the same as that given to any orthopedic surgical patient, and it is an extremely important factor in the eventual outcome. Because most operations performed on patients with poliomyelitis are classified as clean surgery, the greatest care should be taken to eliminate the possibility of wound infection during dressings. Casts or other immobilizing apparatus must receive continued intelligent care both in the hospital and at home in order to accomplish the purpose for which they are intended. A great deal of the ultimate success of muscle transplants will depend upon prolonged and skillful physical therapy treatments, and nurses should make every effort to see that follow-up treatments are continued until the maximum recovery of function has been obtained.

STUDY QUESTIONS

1. Discuss the nurse's duties pertaining to prevention of poliomyelitis.
2. Explain the sequence of giving the Sabin oral vaccine (OPV).
3. Review the treatment and nursing care of the patient with chronic poliomyelitis in relation to (1) prevention of deformity, (2) maintenance of muscle strength, (3) types of surgical procedure that may be done to prevent or correct deformity, stabilize joints, and improve muscle balance.

REFERENCES

Ager, E. A.: Current concepts in immunization, Am. J. Nurs. **66:**2004-2011, 1966.

Bergersen, B. S.: Pharmacology in nursing, ed. 12, St. Louis, 1973, The C. V. Mosby Co.

Dail, C. W.: Respirators. In Licht, S., and Kamenetz, H. L., editors, Orthotics etcetera New Haven, 1966, Elizabeth Licht, Publisher.

Ferguson, A., Jr.: Orthopaedic surgery in infancy and childhood, ed. 3, Baltimore, 1968, The Williams & Wilkins Co.

Gregg, M. B.: Communicable disease trends in the United States, Am. J. Nurs. **68:**88-93, 1968.

Holguin, A. H., Reeves, J. S., and Gelfand, H. M.: Immunization of infants with the Sabin oral poliovirus vaccine, Am. J. Public Health **52:**600-610, 1962.

Huckstep, R. L.: Poliomyelitis in Uganda, Physiotherapy **56:**347-353, 1970.

Krugman, S., and Ward, R.: Infectious diseases of children, ed. 7, St. Louis, 1968, The C. V. Mosby Co.

National Communicable Disease Center: Morbidity and Mortality Weekly Report, **16:**[33], Aug., 1967.

Peach, A. M.: Poliomyelitis—a Conquered fear?, Nurs. Times **66:**107-109, 1970.

Raney, R. B., and Braschear, H. R.: Shand's handbook of orthopaedic surgery, ed. 8, St. Louis, 1971, The C. V. Mosby Co.

Riley, H. D.: Current concepts in immunization, Pediat. Clin. North Am. **13:**93-102, 1966.

Sideman, S.: Surgery of poliomyelitis of the lower extremity, Surg. Clin. North Am. **45:**175-200, 1965.

Top, Franklin H., Sr., and Wehrle, P. F., eds. Communicable and Infectious Diseases, ed. 7, St. Louis, 1972, The C. V. Mosby Co.

14
Neuromuscular affections

PROGRESSIVE MUSCULAR DYSTROPHY

Types. A number of neuromuscular disorders are included under the term "progressive muscular dystrophy." The most common type is that of the pseudohypertrophic muscular dystrophy. With this type, symptoms (Fig. 14-1) may be noted by the time the child is 2 or 3 years of age. The mother becomes aware that the child stumbles and falls more readily than do other children. He may not be able to run, and he tends to walk on his toes with a slightly waddling gait. The calf muscles become enlarged; as the disease advances, intermittently, the waddling nature of the gait increases and an exaggerated hollow in the back develops (Fig. 14-2). The muscles around the thighs, hips, and shoulders atrophy. The fibers of the enlarged calf muscles become displaced by fat and fibrous tissue. It is characteristic that when these children are placed in a sitting position on the floor they arise first to their knees and hands, awkwardly bring each leg up separately to a flexed, weight-bearing position, and then with their hands against the knees and thighs gradually force themselves up into an erect position (Gowers' sign, Fig. 14-3). Even then they have great instability, and a small blow against their knees or other parts of their bodies may throw them off balance and cause them to collapse to the floor.

In later stages extensive wasting of the muscles occurs, and the limbs and spine may assume grotesque deformities. Respiratory infections become more difficult to control, and frequently are the cause of death. A second cause of death is involvement of the heart muscle. In recent years the use of antibiotics has helped to prolong the life of the child with muscular dystrophy.

Facioscapulohumeral muscular dystrophy is a second type that involves both sexes. Symptoms of this type may appear during the early teens or sometimes later in life. It is not so incapacitating as pseudohypertrophic muscular dystrophy, and most of these patients may live a relatively long and useful life.

Limb-girdle muscular dystrophy, a third type, has its onset usually in the second or third decade of life. It develops more rapidly and may incapacitate the individual within a few years.

Cause. The cause of pseudohypertrophic muscular dystrophy is unknown. There is a definite hereditary factor, and it is transmitted in the same manner as hemophilia—through an unaffected mother to the male children. A test that determines the blood level of creatine phosphokinase (CPK), an enzyme, may be used as an aid in identifying muscular dystrophy carriers as well as early detection of the disease. At the present time no cure is known, and the prognosis is poor. Much research has been and is being done, however, in an attempt to find the cause and thus a method of treatment.

Care. Even though the prognosis is poor, much can be done to help these children live useful and happy lives. Education for the child with muscular dystrophy should not be neglected. Attendance at a regular school is desirable as long as his physical condition permits.

417

When this is no longer possible, his education should be continued in a school for handicapped children. As the disease progresses and the physical activities that he can participate in lessen, reading may become his chief means of entertainment.

Muscular dystrophy children should be encouraged and taught to help themselves as much as possible and for as long as possible. They may

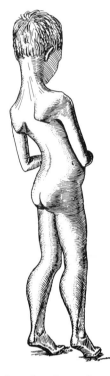

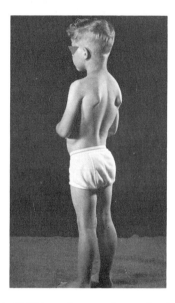

Fig. 14-1. Child in early stage of muscular dystrophy. Note winging of scapulae, lumbar lordosis, and enlarged calf muscles.

Fig. 14-2. Moderately advanced case of infantile pseudohypertrophic progressive muscular dystrophy. Note enlarged calves, contracted heel cords, swayback, and winged shoulders.

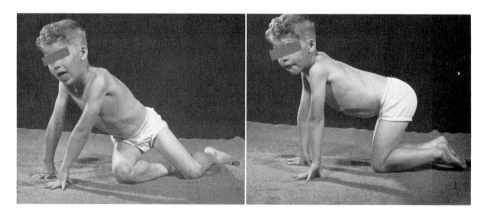

Fig. 14-3. Child with pseudohypertrophic progressive muscular dystrophy arising from the floor in a typical fashion. After getting on his hands and knees he braces his hands against his thighs and pushes himself to an upright position (Gowers' sign).

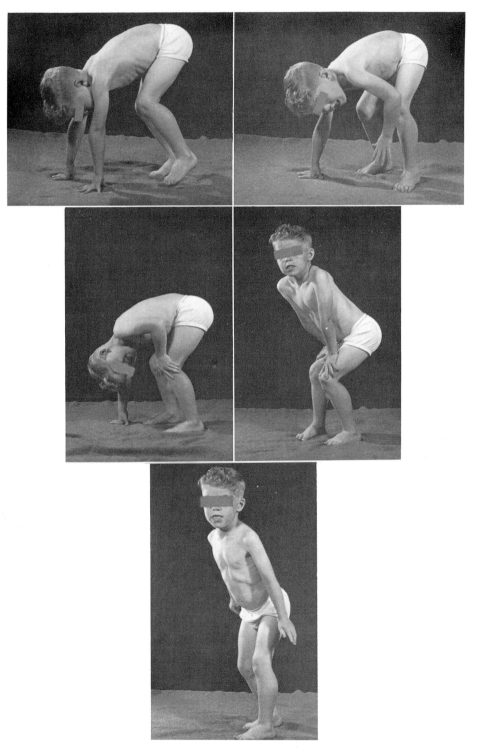

Fig. 14-3, cont'd. For legend see opposite page.

be slow and clumsy, but active use of their muscles helps maintain strength, which, when lost, is never regained. Parents need help in understanding this, and because muscular dystrophy is a slowly progressive disease, the parents or other family members must assume most of the responsibility for the child's care. Preventing joint contractures is of the utmost importance. It is necessary that the family be taught the value of a foot support, to prevent development of drop foot, and proper bed positions to prevent knee and hip flexion contractures or other deformaties.

Excessive weight frequently becomes a problem as the child grows older and is less active. Overeating is to be guarded against.

The nurse should remember that the family of a child having muscular dystrophy needs guidance and assistance in securing equipment that facilitates care and at the same time lessens the demands on the mother's physical strength. Rehabilitation aids, such as a trapeze for the bed or a lift for moving the patient from bed to wheelchair, should be made available.

Many muscular dystrophy patients have received assistance through the Muscular Dystrophy Association of America. This organization was founded in 1950 by the parents and families of muscular dystrophy victims, and through local and state agencies it assists the needy muscular dystrophy patient by providing school facilities, physical therapy, braces, wheelchairs, and other items needed for his care. It has also made provision for grants to finance research pertaining to this disease.

BIRTH PALSY (ERB'S PARALYSIS)

Cause. Birth palsy consists in a paralysis of the arm caused by damage to the brachial plexus during the process of birth. It may occur spontaneously during a relatively difficult labor, or it may result from the use of instruments or traction on the arm in abnormal labor.

Types. There are two types (both becoming less frequent with improved obstetric methods): (1) the milder type in which only the muscles around the shoulder are paralyzed (Erb's paralysis) and (2) a more severe form in which the lower arm is paralyzed (Klumpke's paralysis). In both types the arm is rotated inwardly by the unparalyzed pectoral and scapular muscles. These muscles become contracted if the condition remains untreated for any great length of time, and the deformity becomes fixed.

The prognosis in Erb's paralysis is good. It is poor in paralysis of the whole arm or the lower arm (Klumpke's).

Treatment and nursing care. Early recognition of birth paralysis is not difficult. It is frequently suspected by the obstetrician when he delivers the child. The causative factor is a forcible separation of head and shoulder during delivery. This produces a tearing injury of the nerves of the brachial plexus. The nurse giving the initial bath will note the characteristic position of the arm as it hangs flaccidly with the elbow in extension, the shoulder adducted and rotated inwardly (often accompanied by a cupping appearance of the shoulder), and the hand pronated, palm facing the back (Fig. 14-4). The infant does not use the arm and will object to its being moved for him during the first days of life. This reaction gradually subsides, and the arm can be moved without pain to the child.

Difficult, prolonged labor seems to play a definite part in the etiology of this condition, since anesthesia is employed in these cases, and considerable muscular relaxation is present during birth.

In the milder form of birth palsy the nerves are injured and the paralysis is usually caused by stretching of the brachial nerve trunks. As recovery takes place, treatment is directed at the prevention of contractures. This is accomplished by providing for active or passive motion of the joints involved. Sometimes a "Statue of Liberty" position, which consists of abduction and external rotation of the shoulder, flexion of the elbow, and supination of the forearm is prescribed for short periods, several times daily. This position may be maintained by means of a splint (Fig. 14-5), or by careful positioning of the baby's body and arm. Freedom of the arm is permitted at other times. This is important, since no one position should be maintained continuously.

In the more severe lower or whole arm paralysis, there is usually formidable damage or complete severance of some of the roots of the brachial plexus. Inspection by operation and suturing of these nerve roots is seldom justified. Again, early care and management must provide for passive range of motion and changes of position for the involved extremity. This treatment is directed at the prevention of contractures. Later, muscle transplants or other surgical procedures may be performed to correct any existing deformity and to improve function.

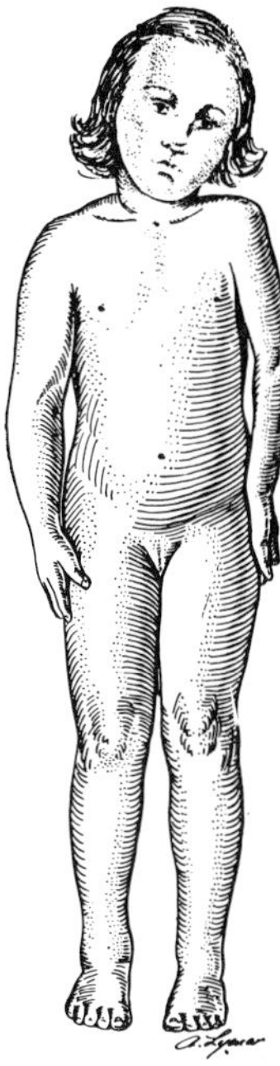

Fig. 14-4. Birth palsy (Erb's) of the left arm in a child 6 years of age. Inward rotation, adduction, and atrophy are shown.

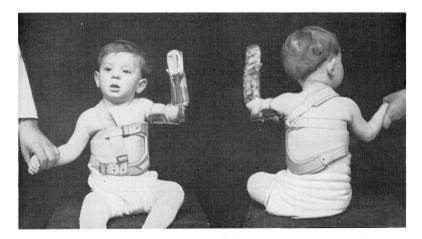

Fig. 14-5. Abduction arm brace. The arm is maintained in abduction and external rotation. The thoracic and iliac portions ensure stability of the brace, and a part of the weight of the apparatus is distributed to the normal shoulder.

CHARCOT JOINTS AND OTHER NEUROMUSCULAR AFFECTIONS (NEUROPATHIES)

Charcot joints are not truly neuromuscular affections but are allied enough to be included in this chapter.

It has been established—clinically and roentgenographically—that bone, cartilage, and ligaments can at times literally melt away, leaving a very misshapen, unstable, unserviceable, and yet quite painless joint. This is known as a neuropathy and occurs particularly in association with certain nervous tissue disorders such as neurosyphilis, diabetic neuritis, syringomyelia, and occasionally paraplegia. The name Charcot has been applied to such joints (Fig. 14-6).

There is no specific treatment except to treat the underlying cause: penicillin for neurosyphilis, diet and insulin for control of diabetes, and radiation therapy for syringomyelia. The unstable joint does not heal, but occasionally the progression of the process can be checked. Attempts at fusion or application of braces will benefit the affected joints.

STUDY QUESTIONS

1. Briefly review the types of muscular dystrophy, symptoms and treatment.

2. As a rule, the youngster with muscular dystrophy is cared for in the home. What can the nurse do to help the family provide proper care for this type of patient?

REFERENCES

Alder, J., and Patterson, R.: Erb's palsy, J. Bone Joint Surg. **49-A:**1052-1064, 1967.
Bresnan, M. J.: Neurologic birth injuries, Post grad. Med. **49:**202-206, 1971.
Cohen, J.: Laboratory diagnostic measures in generalized muscular disease, Pediat. Clin. North Am. **14:**461-477, 1967.
Elementary rehabilitation nursing care, Public Health Service Publication no. 1436, Washington, D. C., 1966, U. S. Department of Health, Education, and Welfare.
Golub, S.: Muscular dystrophy, R. N. **31:**34-37, 1968.
Gucker, T.: The orthopedic management of progressive muscular dystrophy, J. Am. Phys. Ther. Ass. **44:**243-246, 1964.
Johnson, E. W., and Kennedy, J. H.: Comprehensive management of Duchenne muscular dystrophy, Arch. Phys. Med. Rehabil. **52:**110-114, 1971.
Kenrick, M. M.: Certain aspects of managing patient with muscular dystrophy, Southern Med. J. **58:**996-1000, 1965.
MacGinniss, O.: Muscular dystrophy, Nurs. Outlook **10:**588-591, 1962.

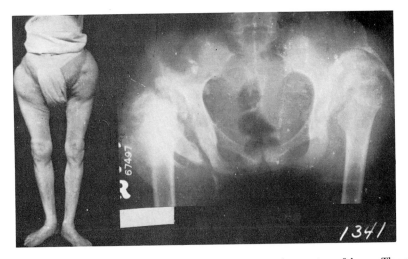

Fig. 14-6. Charcot joints. Roentgenogram illustrates extensive destruction of bone. The patient experiences little or no pain, but such joints are quite unstable and weight bearing is difficult.

Miller, J.: Management of muscular dystrophy, J. Bone Joint Surg. **49-A:**1205-1211, 1967.

Morris, A. G., and Vignos, P. J.: A self-care program for the child with progressive muscular dystrophy, Am. J. Occup. Ther. **14:**301-305, 1960.

Siegel, I. M.: Pathomechanics of stance in Duchenne muscular dystrophy, Arch. Phys. Med. Rehabil. **53:** 403-406, 1972.

Spencer, G. E.: Orthopaedic care of progressive muscular dystrophy, J. Bone Joint Surg. **49-A:**1201-1204, 1967.

Summary of progress in neuromuscular disorders, Research profile number 7, Public Health Service Publication no. 1159, Washington, D. C., 1966, U. S. Department of Health, Education, and Welfare.

Walton, J. N.: Progressive muscular dystrophy, Postgrad. Med. **35:**102-110, 1964.

Wershow, H. J.: Muscular dystrophy: a positive approach to care, Nurs. Outlook **14:**49-53, 1966.

Zundel, W. S., and Tyler, F. H.: The muscular dystrophies, New Eng. J. Med. **273:**537-543, 596-601, 1965.

15
Special operative procedures

TYPES OF OPERATIVE PROCEDURE

This chapter has been included to acquaint the student with the types of operative procedures carried out for disabilities of bones and joints. It is not meant to include all varieties of operation but rather to point out broad categories and to discuss a few in detail.

ARTHRODESIS (FUSION)

A number of operative techniques have been designed to fuse various joints that are disabling. The main purpose of any fusion is to eliminate motion from the joint. This is helpful in healing disease such as tuberculosis of the hip, knee (Fig. 15-1), or spine. Fusion may also serve to eliminate instability of a paralyzed foot, or it may be useful to correct deformity such as might occur in the ankle after a severe injury.

Triple arthrodesis. Triple arthrodesis is a surgical procedure performed on the foot to increase stability (Fig. 15-2). The poliomyelitic patient with a flail extremity or the older child with an untreated clubfoot may have this procedure performed to eliminate motion and to maintain a better position of the foot. It consists in fusing three joints of the foot: the subastragalar joint, the astragaloscaphoid joint, and the calcaneocuboid joint. The fusion of these joints eliminates the movements of inversion and eversion of the foot and lessens the amount of abduction and adduction of the forefoot. Ankle motion is not changed. Fusion is accomplished by removing the articular cartilage of the joints involved.

After this surgical procedure a short leg plaster cast is applied. The foot is immobilized in plaster

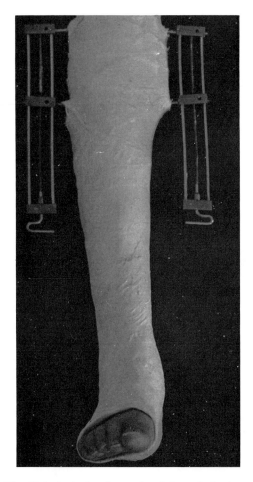

Fig. 15-1. A pin has been placed through the lower end of the femur and the upper end of the tibia to maintain compression apposition during the healing stage after an arthrodesis of the knee. The two hand screws allow for daily adjustment to bring the two bone wires closer together to maintain compression at the site of the fusion.

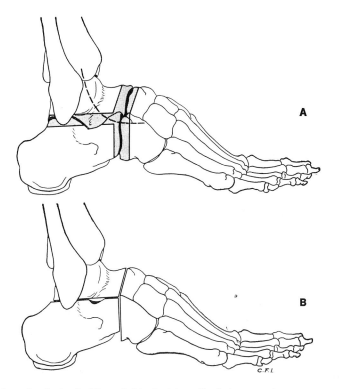

Fig. 15-2. Triple arthrodesis. **A,** Line of skin incision. Shaded area indicates amount of bone removed. **B,** Completion of operation. (From Speed, J. S., and Knight, R. A.: Campbell's operative orthopaedics, ed. 3, St. Louis, 1956, The C. V. Mosby Co.)

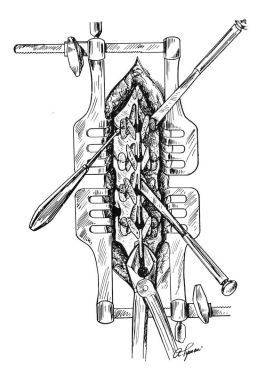

until healing and fusion have taken place, approximately 8 to 12 weeks. Weight bearing is not permitted during this time. Postoperatively, a considerable amount of bleeding may be expected. The limb should be elevated for 3 to 5 days after surgery to minimize swelling and thus lessen the pain. Even so, narcotics usually must be given to provide comfort for this patient. Careful and frequent check of the circulation in the toes must be made. Often it is necessary that the cast be split and spread.

Fig. 15-3. Fusion of the spine—Hibbs method. Upper chisel for obtaining bone chips from superficial surfaces of articular facets. Curette for removing cartilage from articular facets. Lower chisel for producing bone flaps from spinous processes in four directions. Bone-cutting forceps for cutting chips from remaining portion of spinous processes, to be laid down center. Muscles and ligamentous structure hold chips in place when wound is closed.

Spinal fusion. Spinal fusion warrants detailed discussion because it is so common and involves considerable nursing care. Fusion of the spine is accomplished by obtaining solidity between the posterior segments of the vertebrae. Usually, the solidity is achieved by the use of bone grafts placed on the lamina of the area to be fused.

Refinements of technique are diverse and are determined by the type of graft, placement of the graft, and preparation of the graft bed. In addition, most surgeons fuse the facets at the proper levels to assure solidity of fusion (Fig. 15-3).

It has been implied that spinal fusions are performed to relieve backache, which is true, but there are other equally important indications. Scoliosis can be corrected in part, and the correction can be maintained by fusing the spine in the corrected position. Here as a rule many levels are fused, and the aftercare to ensure fusion must be closely supervised. The same is true when fusion has been performed to control active tuberculosis of the spine. The patient must remain for some months in recumbency with immobilization, and thereafter ambulation must be begun gradually with continued support to prevent motion of the spine.

Halo pelvis apparatus. When fusion is carried out to provide stability for the cervical spine, the halo traction is useful as a means of immobilization. Occasionally in severe deformities the additional fixation of the pelvis by means of skeletal pins fixed to the brace will provide more support. The halo apparatus, originally devised for patients with severe scoliosis, is a versatile fixation apparatus that secures the head at four points instead of two. It is easy to apply and maintain. This apparatus has been used in scoliosis with femoral pins for traction and with a cast or Milwaukee brace for cervical or high thoracic curves. The halo, used with a pelvic hoop attached to two rods piercing the iliac crest, achieves the maximum possible exterior skeletal fixation of the spine. Presently this is used for spine procedures in which rigid fixation is needed but a cast is not advisable (for example, emphysema patients). The ease of maintenance and the rigid fixation make this useful also for unstable spine injuries. It allows most patients to become ambulatory. The care of the pins in-

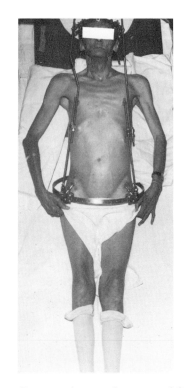

Fig. 15-4. Patient with cervical spine instability. Halo pelvic apparatus.

volves daily cleansing, and replacement of the skull pins can be performed without disturbing the rest of the apparatus.

ARTHROPLASTY

An arthroplasty is an operative procedure that attempts to re-create a joint as nearly like the original as possible. It has been applied to the elbow, hip, knee, shoulder, and small joints of the hand with varying degrees of success in the order listed.

The creation of a new joint is a reconstructive operation and requires skill by the surgeon as well as strong will by the patient to achieve a good result. At best a surgically constructed joint will not equal a normal joint; but if the operation is well done technically, the results can approximate the normal if the patient will faithfully carry out a long program of exercises to maintain motion and to build muscle strength (Fig. 15-5).

Hip arthroplasty. In arthroplasty of any joint some material must be superimposed between

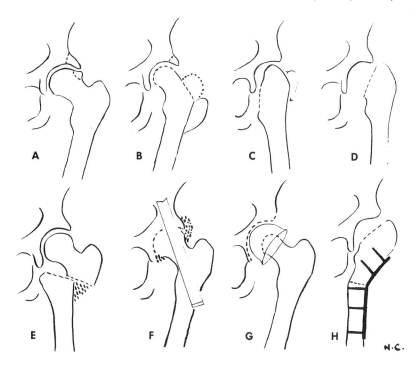

Fig. 15-5. Diagrammatic sketch to illustrate principles of the technique of various types of hip reconstruction: **A,** acetabuloplasty; **B,** trochanteric transfer; **C,** Colonna procedure; **D,** Girdlestone method; **E,** osteotomy, subtrochanteric; **F,** arthrodesis with metallic fixation; **G,** mold arthroplasty; **H,** Bachelor technique. There are others, such as use of the prosthesis shown in Fig. 5-54. Each reconstruction has its own indication, and the choice in each case must rest with the surgeon.

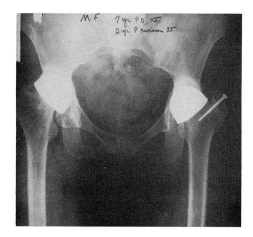

Fig. 15-6. Roentgenogram showing position of Smith-Petersen Vitallium cup after bilateral arthroplasty of the hip.

the newly shaped joint surfaces to prevent ankylosis of the joint. In the elbow, fascia lata has been found to be satisfactory interposition material. In the hip, where weight bearing is necessary, fascia lata is not so satisfactory;

therefore, stronger material has been used, namely Vitallium, which is a metal that the body tolerates well. Vitallium cup arthroplasty (Fig. 15-6) has so far been used mainly for the hip in adults and for the following conditions:

Indications for cup arthroplasty of the hip:
1. Malum coxae senilis (painful osteoarthritis of the aged)
2. Traumatic arthritis (secondary arthritis that follows surgery)
3. Rheumatoid arthritis (arthroplasty indicated to relieve pain, correct deformity, and improve function)
4. Unreduced congenital dislocation of the hip
5. Old septic arthritis
6. Complications following fracture of neck of the femur
   (a) Aseptic necrosis of head of the femur
   (b) Nonunion (calls for various types of reconstruction using the arthroplasty principle with Vitallium cup; reconstruction dependent on what remains of the original joint that can be utilized)

To illustrate what has already been mentioned regarding the importance of supervised con-

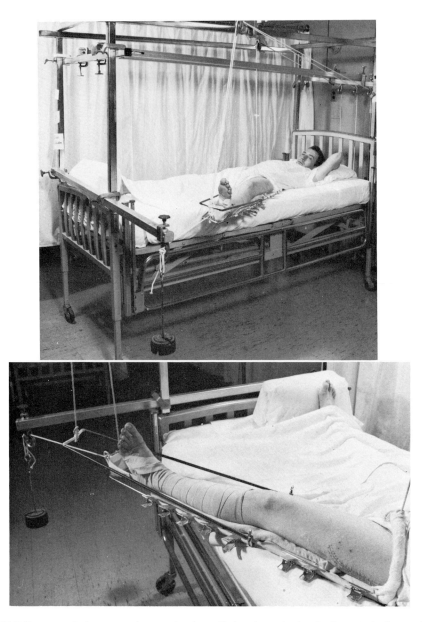

Fig. 15-7. Postoperatively, suspension traction is applied, to keep the involved extremity in a position of abduction. This position helps maintain the cup and head of the femur in the acetabulum. The half-ring Thomas splint with Pearson attachment provides support for the limb. To maintain his position, the patient must learn to keep the crests of the ilia level, his chest and shoulders in the center of the bed, and his uninvolved limb near the edge of the bed (position of abduction). Sandbags placed along the inner aspect of the uninvolved limb and along the lateral aspect of the chest wall (uninvolved side) may be used to help him maintain the correct position. When the patient lies diagonally across the bed, abduction of the extremity is lost. In addition to the position of abduction, it is usually desirable that the limb be maintained in a neutral position or in one of slight internal rotation.

valescence, the following routine is frequently employed after cup arthroplasty.

Postoperatively this patient is placed in suspension traction (Figs. 15-7 and 15-8). The purposes of using such traction then are (1) to provide support for the limb, (2) to maintain the extremity in a position of abduction, (3) to provide increased comfort for the patient, and (4) to facilitate nursing care. Bed position and posture are extremely important for the patient with cup arthroplasty. The affected limb is maintained in a position of abduction and internal rotation. To help the patient maintain this position, the nurse will not only need to teach him what constitutes good position but also help him attain it in many instances. A sandbag placed against the medial aspect of the unaffected limb will remind the patient that he must not recline so that his body lies diagonally on the bed. If this position is permitted, abduction of the extremity is lost. A sandbag placed against the chest wall on the unaffected side will help him

to keep the iliac crests level. A footboard or bolster for the unaffected extremity will help maintain good position, and when the backrest is elevated, there will be flexion of the hip joints and not flexion of the lumbar spine. A small pad placed beneath the lumbar region will add greatly to the patient's comfort. It must be remembered, however, that extension of the hip joint without increased lumbar lordosis is desirable. Several days after surgery the patient should be doing things for himself. He may need to be encouraged to use the trapeze for shifting his position and to assist with nursing care procedures. Exercise and use of the unaffected extremity will help maintain muscle strength and prevent generalized weakness.

The exercises that promote flexion and extension of the hip joint and that increase muscular strength are illustrated. These exercises are a very important part of the treatment and care of the patient with a cup arthroplasty, and they are ordered specifically by the surgeon for the indi-

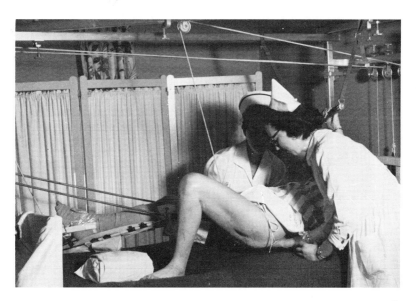

Fig. 15-8. Method of giving back care to the patient in suspension traction. By grasping the trapeze and pushing with the normal extremity, with knee and hip flexed, the patient is able to lift the buttocks off the bed. Because of the balanced weights, the splint supporting the affected extremity elevates as the patient's body is lifted. When linen beneath a patient is being changed, the soiled linen is loosened on the patient's uninvolved side and moved toward the center of the bed. The clean sheet is then placed on this portion of the bed beneath the uninvolved foot. As illustrated above, the patient raises his shoulders and hips off the bed, and both the soiled and the clean linen are pushed beneath him toward the involved side. The nurse then goes to the opposite side of the bed and completes the bedmaking process.

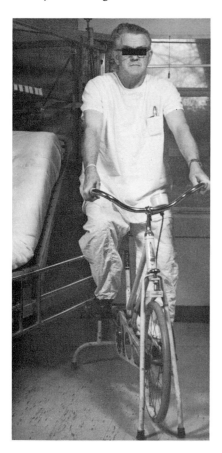

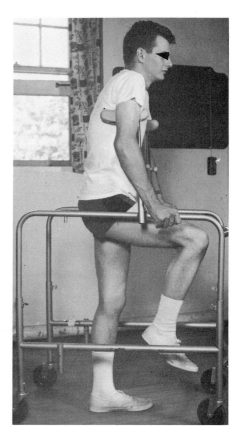

Fig. 15-9. The stationary bicycle provides flexion and extension exercises of the hip and knee joints. The patient must sit well back on the bicycle seat, with his foot placed squarely on the pedal. The first time he may not be able to make a complete turn with the pedal. The nurse must remember, however, that in the beginning all of these exercises are for short periods and are gradually increased to periods of 10 minutes or more and are performed several times daily. To promote development of the hip muscles, resistance may be applied against the bicycle wheel. To increase flexion of the hip joint, the bicycle seat may be lowered.

Fig. 15-10. Walking in the walker. Note extreme flexion of the affected extremity. When using the walker or crutches, the patient should be encouraged to use this type of step rather than a shuffling gait. With unilateral cup arthroplasty the patient is taught the three-point crutch gait. Both crutches are advanced with the affected extremity, and the patient takes approximately half his body weight on the affected extremity. With bilateral cup arthroplasty, the four-point gait is taught: left crutch, right foot, right crutch, left foot. The patient is also taught stair climbing. This is the same for the patient with a cup arthroplasty as for any patient with crutches. When he goes down the stairs, the crutches and affected extremity are placed on the lower step, preceding the normal leg. When going up the stairs, the patient's normal leg is placed on the next step and then followed by the crutches and the affected extremity.

vidual patient. The patient undertakes gradually one exercise after another to keep motion and to build muscle until further gain cannot be made. After a year or so, the new joint will have reached its optimal function, although small gains may still be made year after year.

TOTAL HIP REPLACEMENT

Total hip replacement is a relatively new operation used in the treatment of most types of hip disease in the adult. The operation consists of replacing the acetabulum with an artificial acetabulum, usually made of plastic, and an artificial femoral head, usually made of metal (Fig. 15-13, *A* and *B*). These prosthetic components are cemented to the bone with another plastic, methyl methacrylate (Fig. 15-13, *C* and *D*). A roentgenogram of the components in place is shown in Fig. 15-13, *E*. The procedure is applicable in all forms of adult hip disease other than infection. If the expected postoperative condition of the patient is considered to be sufficiently better than his preoperative state to warrant the risks involved, then the procedure is indicated. It is not yet known how long the artificial joint will last beyond 10 years. The younger the patient, the greater the risks that the joint will wear out and, therefore, the procedure is more commonly done in older people. Degenerative arthritis is the most common diagnosis, but rheumatoid arthritis and the residuals

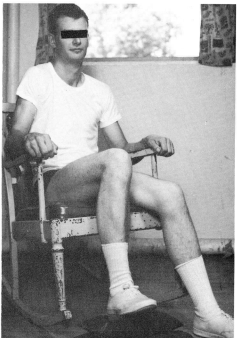

Fig. 15-11. Rocking chair exercise. Note that the patient sits with hips well back in the seat of the chair and that the foot of the affected extremity is placed on sandbags. This increases the amount of flexion at the hip joint as he rocks forward.

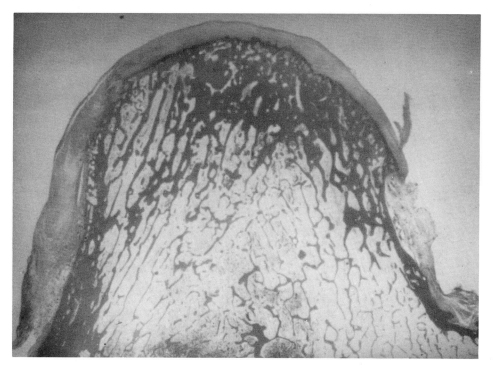

Fig. 15-12. Microscopic slide to show the repair of fibrocartilage and dense subchondral bone that occurs on the head of the newly constructed femoral head 1½ years after cup arthroplasty. These have maintained good repair for 25 years after operation.

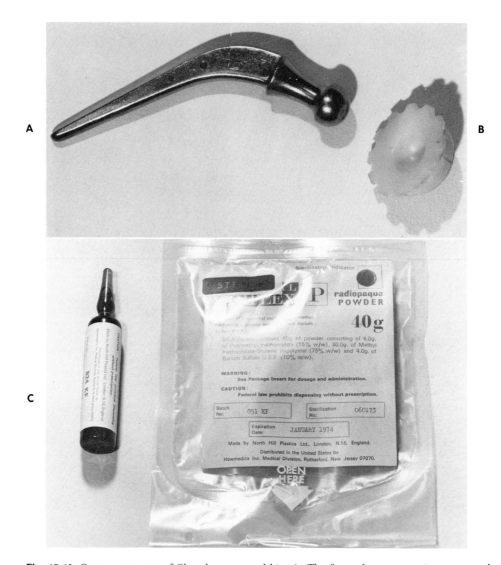

Fig. 15-13. Component parts of Charnley type total hip. **A,** The femoral component is constructed of surgical stainless steel, and various lengths are available. The diameter of the head is small to reduce frictional wear. Other types such as the Meuller utilize a larger size head to spread the weight bearing load over a larger surface area. **B,** Acetabular component is constructed of high density polyethylene to reduce friction and better withstand impact loading with each step. **C,** Bone cement consisting of a powder (polymer) and a liquid (monomer), mixed as needed during the operation by the scrub nurse. **D,** After 6 to 10 minutes the mixture at a "dough" stage is ready to be placed in the bone bed. The component part is immediately inserted into the dough, which then sets and firmly fixes the component part to the bone in 3 to 5 minutes. **E,** The roentgenogram shows the intrapelvic protrusion of the hip preoperatively and the total hip replacement in the postoperative roentgenogram. Both the amount and distribution of the bone cement can be seen since a radiopaque material is present in the mixture.

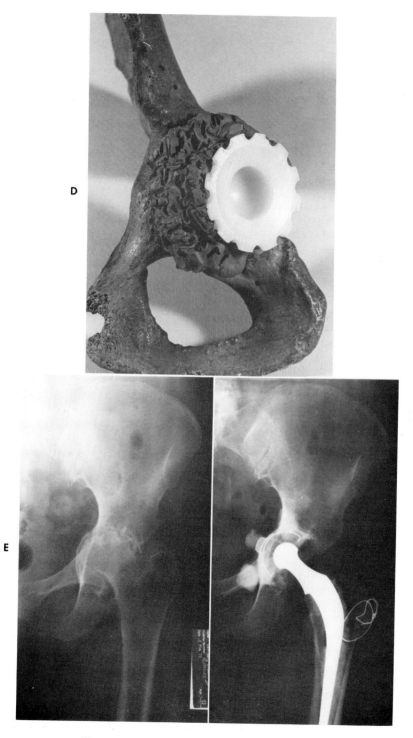

Fig. 15-13, cont'd. For legend see opposite page.

of trauma or congenital problems are frequent diagnoses.

The operation is a relatively major one, and the blood loss, because of the exposed vascular bone, can be rather large. Much of the blood loss may occur during the early postoperative period. Blood replacement can vary from none to 10 units, but usually 3 units of blood are required. Much of the blood loss can go unnoticed because it takes place in the deep soft tissues in the upper thigh and buttock.

Postoperatively the patient usually remains in bed for 4 days to a week with his operated extremity kept in abduction by either splints or traction. The length of the hospitalization postoperatively is usually between 2 and 3 weeks. The patient will walk with crutches for several weeks after the operation and then with a cane for several months.

By 6 months after the operation the patient has a 95% chance of having minimal or no pain, walking with minimal or no limp, and having enough motion to sit and stand normally and probably to bend down to tie his shoes. He should be able to do almost anything he wants to do. Many patients are working at their usual occupations full time after the operation.

Preoperative teaching. Preoperative teaching is essential for the total-hip-replacement patient. Preparation of the patient and his family for this procedure includes an explanation of the surgical procedure and information concerning the care necessary postoperatively. Helping the patient understand what to expect, such as type of apparatus to be used, positions maintained, and exercises he will need to perform, will help prevent some of the anxiety and fear the patient and family must experience when confronted with this operative procedure.

Nursing care. Coughing and deep breathing should be encouraged at least every hour while the patient is awake. However, this in itself is not always enough to prevent complications of bed rest. The patient must be encouraged to remain active while in bed. A trapeze is helpful in having the patient lift from the bed, position himself correctly in bed, and assist in the daily nursing care activities. It is important that the patient and the nurse understand that remaining active may "hurt" his new hip but not "harm" it.

Leg exercises should be stressed frequently. These are important in maintaining muscle strength, range of motion, and in preventing phlebitis. Commonly used exercises are (1) quadriceps-setting, (2) plantar and dorsiflexion of the foot, (3) internal and external rotation of the hip, and (4) gluteal setting.

The hips should remain abducted during bed rest and while the patient sits in a chair. Patients must be discouraged from crossing their legs during this early postoperative period.

If the patient remains active, serious skin problems usually do not occur. Those areas needing frequent observation and massage are the coccyx, heels, and elbows.

The nurse should be alert for symptoms of complications that are common after any major operation. These include shock, pulmonary emboli, pneumonia, phlebitis, paralytic ileus, bladder retention, wound infection, and bowel impaction.

Dislocation of the prosthetic parts can occur after total hip replacement. Symptoms of a dislocation include inability to rotate the hip internally or externally, inability to bear weight, shortening of the affected leg, and increased pain. The nurse should also realize that the patient will not necessarily experience severe pain when his hip dislocates. The physician should be notified immediately.

Temporary discouragement is common after the patient begins to get out of bed and learn to walk and take care of himself. Frequent reassurance and encouragement are essential to help the patient remain motivated and cooperative. Learning to walk with crutches can be difficult at first. If the patient believes that there will be improvement and gets daily encouragement, this phase will progress more quickly. The patient should be encouraged to use his hip as normally as possible and not to be overprotective of it. He should be helped, not just told, to do everything for himself. A positive attitude by all concerned is very important.

It is the nurse's responsibility to see that the patient and his family are prepared for the posthospital phase. The surgeon should explain his regimen to the patient. A list of important activities, restrictions, and exercises can be a helpful guide for the patient. Reviewing such a list with the family can more fully prepare them for the weeks and months ahead. It can also serve as a reference for the patient if a question arises after he is home.

TOTAL KNEE JOINT REPLACEMENT

The advent of the total hip replacement has introduced a new concept in joint surgery. Wherever a joint has been irreparably damaged by disease, a replacement of the entire joint by mechanical implants is available today. The knee joint, which in the past has been difficult to repair by arthroplasty, has become the most recent priority in efforts to design a proper mechanical replacement. At present there are a number of designs available, but none has been tried sufficiently to become a routinely acceptable standard. As engineers and orthopedic surgeons working together continue to study the complicated mechanics of the knee joint, there is reason to believe that a standard design will be forthcoming. The same may be said for many other joints that have heretofore received less attention.

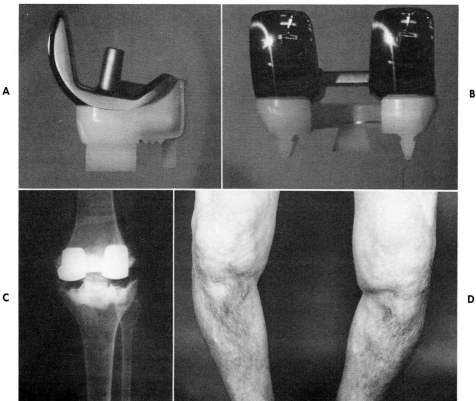

Fig. 15-14. A, Side view of the component parts of the geomedic design for total knee replacement. The upper metallic portion substitutes for the femoral condyles, while the lower high polymer plastic portion substitutes for the tibial joint surfaces. **B,** Front view of the component parts of the geomedic total knee replacement implants. Each of the upper components are convex to fit a similar concave groove in the tibial component. Bone cement (methyl methacrylate) is used to fix both components to bone. **C,** This shows a marked varus deformity of both knees, which could be corrected by osteotomy if a good joint surface is present on the tibia. In this case no cartilage remained in the joint, and bone had already eroded on the medial tibial plateau. **D,** Component parts of the total knee replacement inserted and aligned to correct the deformity and provide a joint surface for motion and weight bearing. Note that the tibial component is radiolucent and has markers present to aid in interpretation of position.

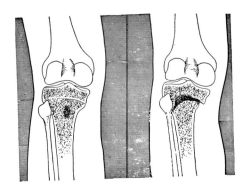

Fig. 15-15. Line drawing illustrating osteotomy of the tibia used in correction of genu valgum deformity.

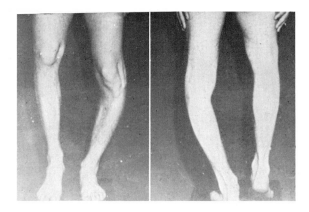

Fig. 15-16. Anterior and posterior views illustrating extreme bowing of left tibia.

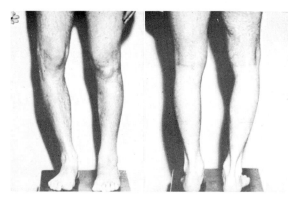

Fig. 15-17. Postoperative photographs of patient in Fig. 15-16, showing correction gained by osteotomy of the proximal end of the tibia.

OSTEOTOMY

The shaft of any long bone may be malaligned as a result of congenital deformity, disease such as osteogenesis imperfecta, or a fracture that healed in malposition. Any such deformity may be corrected by operative means; this constitutes an osteotomy.

When it is feasible, the osteotomy will be fixed by internal means, such as wire, metal screws and plates, bone grafts, or specially designed fixation material. The aftercare will be similar to the treatment of a fracture at a comparable site, for in essence an osteotomy is a controlled fracture.

Osteotomy of the femur for a painful hip is a recognized and acceptable operation. In selected early cases of degenerative arthritis an osteotomy will relieve a good deal of pain in 80% of the cases operated upon. A new joint space is created by nature's repair as shown in the example (Fig. 15-18).

TENDON TRANSPLANTATION

Several principles of tendon transplantation might be of interest to nurses. It is good to know the reason in a given case for the tendon transplant.

Substitution. In patients with poliomyelitis there is frequently residual paralysis of certain muscle groups that can be easily determined. In any such circumstance if strong muscles exist in the same extremity, the strong muscle may be transplanted (1) to gain certain function, as in opponens pollicis transplantation to the thumb, or (2) to eliminate bracing, as in anterior tibial substitution.

Replacement. In crushing hand injuries certain tendons may be damaged beyond repair. In such instances a tendon from a less important area may be surgically grafted to replace the damaged tendon, and this is known as a free graft.

Realignment. Uncorrected deformities are

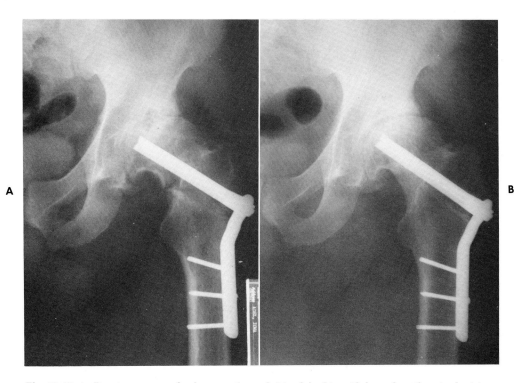

Fig. 15-18. A, Roentgenogram of a degenerative arthritis of the hip with loss of cartilage in the joint space and early subchondral cyst formation. The osteotomy at the base of the neck of the femur has been fixed with a nail and side plate. **B,** Roentgenogram of the osteotomy 1 year later. Note that the osteotomy is well healed, and a new joint space has regenerated. The patient is pain-free.

sometimes increased by the pull of normal muscles in an abnormal direction. Such muscle pull can be redirected by surgical transfer so that it tends to correct the deformity. An example is a shift of the anterior tibial tendon to a more lateral position in a patient with clubfoot.

ARTHROTOMY FOR INTERNAL DERANGEMENT OF THE KNEE

The knee, the elbow, and the phalangeal joints are the only true hinge joints in the body. The knee, being a weight-bearing joint, is the most susceptible to strain and ligamentous injury. Such injuries commonly occur in athletes and industrial workers and usually are the result of twisting motions or lateral strain. When the knee is in complete extension, stabilization is accomplished by the internal and external lateral ligaments. These become taut in the extended position but relax somewhat in flexion (Fig. 15-19). The anterior cruciate ligament also is tightened in extension and tends to stabilize the joint in complete extension.

The posterior cruciate ligament prevents forward displacement of the tibia on the femur when the knee is in flexion.

Types of injury. Rupture of the anterior cruciate ligament may occur when the knee is forced into a backknee position. Rupture of the posterior cruciate ligament may occur when the force is exerted on the lower leg from behind with the knee in flexion.

The most common athletic injury is tearing of the internal lateral ligament. It is caused by exerting pressure against the other side of the knee when the foot is anchored against the ground. This is often called football knee and requires a period of 3 to 6 weeks to heal. The first 3 to 4 weeks are spent in a walking cast that extends from the groin to above the ankle. To prevent the cast from sliding down by gravity, adhesive tape is usually applied over a coat of compound tincture of benzoin (to prevent skin irritation) and is turned upward at the lower end of the cast. After this, a knee support is frequently used for a period of several weeks. The reinforced, laced, elastic type seems to be the most efficient. The knee-cage brace with a steel reinforcement and joint may be preferable in some cases.

Rupture of the cruciate ligaments is usually caused by rather severe knee injuries. Fortunately, most of these ruptures will heal if cast immobilization is used for sufficient periods of time. If not, operations for the replacement of the ligaments with tendons or strips of fascia become necessary.

Rupture of the internal and external semilunar cartilages occur frequently. Rupture of the internal cartilage is the most common. It occurs

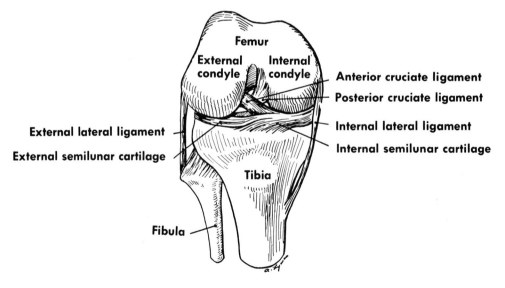

Fig. 15-19. Ligaments of the knee joint and semilunar cartilages shown with the knee in flexion.

as a result of a twisting motion. The foot is anchored on the ground, and the body and thigh twist when the knee is flexed, in a way that causes rotation of the condyles of the tibia on the condyles of the femur. Rupture of the external semilunar cartilage occurs as a result of a reversal of this motion.

The rupture may occur as a detachment of the anterior attachment of the cartilage or the posterior attachment of the cartilage, or it may be the bucket handle type in which the cartilage is split, part of it entering the central compartment of the knee joint and part of it remaining in the normal position along the outer margin of the joint. Repeated locking is indicative of this type.

Treatment. Immediate operation is not always necessary in semilunar cartilage injury. Many patients will recover if closed reduction is accomplished with or without anesthesia and a walking leg cast is applied for a period of 3 to 4 weeks. If there is recurrence, then removal of the cartilage is usually indicated. Removal produces a mild rotatory instability of the knee that can usually be overcome by maintaining strong stabilizing muscles to the knee and does not usually lead to any interference with the function of the joint. There are many active athletes who have had a cartilage removed.

After surgery no cast is used, but a compression bandage helps prevent postoperative hemorrhage. Quadriceps setting and straight leg raising exercise as well as protected weight bearing are begun after 24 to 36 hours. About 3 months are required for full recovery.

AMPUTATION SURGERY AND REHABILITATION

Although amputation surgery is as old as surgery itself, the past 25 years has brought enormous progress to the field. With the help of antibiotics, vascular surgery, and effective control of diabetes, many limbs are now being saved that would have required amputation in the past. Since World War II intensive research in the development of artificial limbs, or prostheses, and an excellent education program have been sponsored by several federal agencies. Greatly improved care for the patient with a threatened or doomed limb is now generally available. The outlook for returning to a nearly normal life is much brighter today for the amputee, as a result of these developments.

Amputation is far more common in civilians than in members of the Armed Services, even during wartime. Nurses will encounter patients with amputations on the general surgical wards as well as on the orthopedic wards. The ultimate goal in the care of each patient is maximum restoration of physical, economic, emotional, and social capacity. This means the amputee must learn to walk, using his artificial limb, learn to care for his own toilet and dressing, and sometimes learn a new job in keeping with his new abilities. To accomplish this goal requires effective teamwork and meticulous nursing care. Nurses must have a fund of knowledge that will enable them to offer advice or asistance when the occasion arises. Besides the knowledge of the care required immediately after surgery, they must teach stump hygiene and know something of prosthesis construction, fit, and function.

The major causes for amputations are as follows:

1. Injury. Amputation sometimes becomes necessary as a result of severe crushing or extensive lacerations of arteries and nerves.

2. Disease. Vascular disease, especially arteriosclerosis, may result in gangrene of a limb because of inadequate blood supply to the tissues. The elderly patient with an above-knee amputation as a result of arteriosclerosis is by far the most common amputee. Diabetes is often

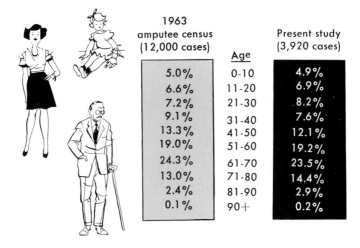

Fig. 15-20. Distribution of amputees by age ("new" cases). (From Davies, E., Friz, B., and Clippinger, F.: Amputees and their prostheses, Artif. Limbs **14:**19-48, 1970.)

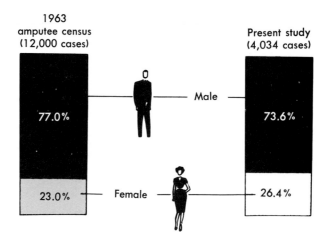

Fig. 15-21. Distribution of amputees by sex ("new" amputations). (From Davies, E., Friz, B., and Clippinger, F.: Amputees and their prostheses, Artif. Limbs **14:**19-48, 1970.)

accompanied by severe vascular disease as well as loss of the skin sensation and marked susceptibility to infections. Extensive osteomyelitis may so damage a limb that the patient prefers amputation and a prosthesis.

3. Tumors. Malignant bone tumors are most common in the second decade of life and in many cases are best treated by amputation.

4. Congenital disorders. Absence of limbs (phocomelia) or severe malformations of a limb present at birth are the result of faulty embryonic development. Thalidomide, a sedative, has caused multiple severe limb malformations in the infants born of mothers who had taken the drug. Amputation may be necessary if a malformed limb will not respond to other, corrective treatments.

Figs. 15-20 through 15-24 illustrate comparative data of the Glattly study made in 1963 and a study reported in 1970. Findings of the recent study closely parallel the findings of the Glattly study in relation to sex and age of new amputees and the cause and level of amputations.

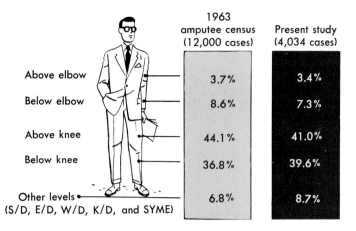

Fig. 15-22. Distribution* by site of amputation ("new" cases). (From Davies, E., Friz, B., and Clippinger, F.: Amputees and their prostheses, Artif. Limbs **14:**19-48, 1970.)

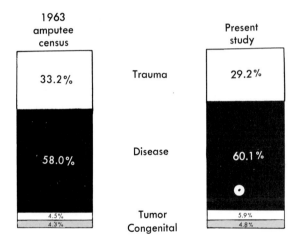

Fig. 15-23. Distribution by cause of amputation ("new" amputations). (From Davies, E., Friz, B., and Clippinger, F.: Amputees and their prostheses, Artif. Limbs **14:**19-48, 1970.)

AMPUTATION SURGERY

As much as possible the surgeon attempts to perform the amputation with standard techniques at standard sites, saving as much of the limb as feasible. Each level of amputation, therefore, has certain characteristic features and problems with which the nurse should be familiar. For example, the Syme amputation is a removal of the foot at the ankle joint (disarticulation), and it is done in younger patients with good circulation. It provides an excellent weight-bearing stump that allows the patient to walk with or without a prosthesis. Below-the-knee (BK), knee-bearing (KB), above-the-knee (AK), hip disarticulation (HD), and hemipelvectomy (HP) are other standard levels in the lower extremity. Wrist disarticulation, below-elbow (BE), elbow disarticulation, above-elbow (AE), and shoulder disarticulation (SD) are standard upper extremity amputation levels.

The surgeon designs neat skin flaps to cover the new stump. Each tissue is handled carefully and in its own prescribed way to avoid unnecessary damage. The major vessels are

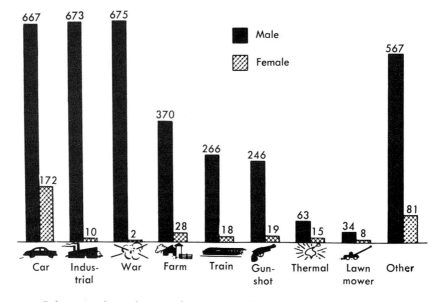

Fig. 15-24. Relative incidence, by sex, of amputations due to trauma. (From Davies, E., Friz, B., and Clippinger, F.: Amputees and their prostheses, Artif. Limbs **14:**19-48, 1970.)

doubly secured with suture ligatures before being divided. In closure of the wound only enough sutures are used to bring the tissues into approximation without undue tension. Drains placed deeply within the wound may be brought out through the skin incision line to allow escape of fluid and blood from beneath the skin flaps. Suction tubes to serve the same purpose may be brought out from the skin adjacent to the incision line.

Occasionally, a guillotine amputation is necessary because of uncontrolled infection. In this type of amputation the tissues and bone are severed at the same level without skin flaps being made. The wound is not closed but usually can be approximated by use of skin traction postoperatively, or it may require secondary closure in the operating room some days later. A snug compression dressing is applied in the operating room. Some surgeons prefer skin traction that can be applied in the operating room or immediately after the patient is conscious. This is necessary in some cases to ensure proper conditions for healing. Methods of applying traction may vary somewhat. Stockinet and skin glue, moleskin straps, and rubber surface traction are in common usage (Fig. 15-26).

If stockinet is used, the material is rolled doughnut fashion and applied over the dressing. The top of the stockinet is secured to the skin of the leg above the dressing by some kind of skin adherent.

The most commonly used type of traction is made by four strips of adhesive tape, one applied on each of the four aspects of the thigh above the dressing—medial, lateral, posterior, and anterior. Either a circle of heavy wire, stabilized by two crosspieces of wire, or a wooden hexagon may be used as a spreader for the adhesive. Rope extends from this spreader to a pulley attached to the end of the bed. A 5-pound weight attached to the traction is usually considered adequate.

Rubber surface traction differs in having the adhesive tape strips previously described also lined with thin strips of sponge rubber. These strips are then bandaged to the skin above the stump, and the weights are applied as in most skin adhesive traction. The suction of the rubber on the skin maintains it in place. The advantage of this kind of traction is that it can be removed entirely for physical therapy treatments. Occasionally, a protective wire cage or plaster cast is applied to keep the fresh wound undisturbed, to keep the limb in the desired position, or to prevent contractures.

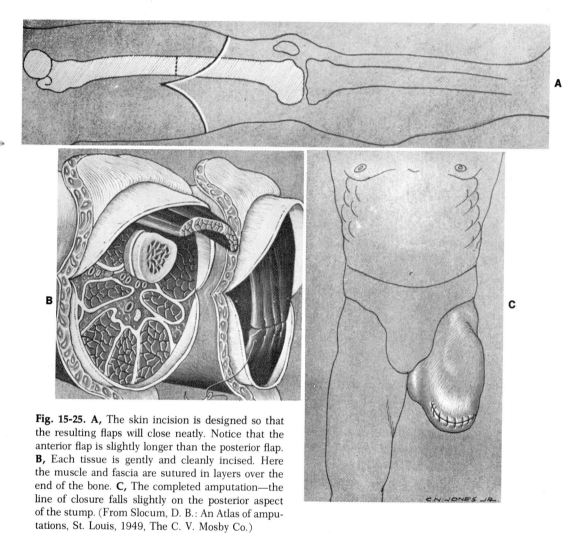

Fig. 15-25. A, The skin incision is designed so that the resulting flaps will close neatly. Notice that the anterior flap is slightly longer than the posterior flap. **B,** Each tissue is gently and cleanly incised. Here the muscle and fascia are sutured in layers over the end of the bone. **C,** The completed amputation—the line of closure falls slightly on the posterior aspect of the stump. (From Slocum, D. B.: An Atlas of amputations, St. Louis, 1949, The C. V. Mosby Co.)

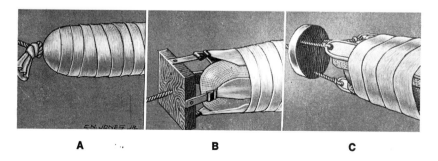

A **B** **C**

Fig. 15-26. Skin traction. **A,** Stockinet and skin glue. **B,** Adhesive tape. **C,** Rubber pad. (From Slocum, D. B.: An atlas of amputations, St. Louis, 1949, The C. V. Mosby Co.)

CARE OF THE PATIENT AFTER AMPUTATION

Immediately after surgery, the patient who has had an amputation is subject to complications inherent in the administration of any anesthetic and major surgical procedure. Close observation in a recovery room or another facility where suction apparatus, oxygen, infusion packs, and other emergency equipment are at the bedside must be maintained for several hours after surgery. It is not enough to have these facilities in the next room—they must be at the bedside for immediate use. This is the sole responsibility of the nurse who is in charge of the recovery area. Nothing whatsoever must distract attention from the postoperative patient, because this time is nearly as critical for the welfare of the patient as is the actual operation. Frequent observations and recordings of the vital signs are necessary. Restraints may be necessary until the patient is fully alert to prevent disturbing the dressing, the intravenous infusions, and suction tube apparatus. The patient is encouraged to cough and take deep breaths every 15 minutes. The doctors may have him placed temporarily in the side-lying position to prevent aspiration of vomitus into the airway. If elevation of the extremity is necessary because of shock or hemorrhage, it is wiser to raise the end of the bed than to place pillows under the stump. Extensive bleeding from a loosened ligature on a major vessel is fortunately very rare. When it does occur, it is an emergency of the gravest degree. To avert a possible catastrophe, many surgeons order a tourniquet routinely kept at the bedside during the postoperative period.

Curiously enough, the pain after amputation is almost always quite mild. Mild analgesics usually suffice, and often no analgesic at all is necessary after the first 24 hours. Pain of great severity may indicate a wound complication, and the doctor should be notified at once of the patient's discomfort.

The doctor will usually permit sips of fluids as soon as the patient is fully awake and free of nausea. The following day, a light diet is usually well tolerated. The insulin requirements of diabetic patients undergoing amputation may fluctuate in the postoperative period. This is especially true when infection is a complicating factor. When control is difficult, the doctor may order frequent small doses of regular insulin and may request frequent fractional urine determinations for urinary glucose.

Amputation is usually accompanied by a more or less profound degree of psychologic shock, which, of course, can be readily understood. This reaction is seen less frequently in patients who have been psychologically well prepared for their surgery. It is most profound in the patient who has an amputation as a result of an injury and has not had time to adjust to the loss. The nurse may note evidence of this psychologic shock in the patients through their manifestations of depression, hostility, denial, and occasionally, feelings of futility. The elderly patient often demonstrates extreme confusion during the postoperative period, and young patients may have feelings of mutilation or emasculation. These reactions in general are seen less often in the patient with a well-balanced, stable personality. The patient will need reassurance—starting even before surgery and continuing during the first few difficult days after surgery. Nurses are in an excellent position to supply reassurance that he is not to become a cripple, unable to walk or look after his own needs. Because they are fully aware of the advances made in the past few years in regard to walking with artificial limbs, nurses can be a source of great encouragement to the patient at this time. They should supply continual firm, affirmative support and constant reassurance. This type of assistance should be continued throughout the rehabilitation period.

Nurses should be alert from the outset to detect signs of flexion and abduction contractures at the hip. A position of flexion and abduction is a natural one for the patient to assume in bed, partly because he feels he is protecting the fresh wound from any disturbance. The hip then may become contracted quite insidiously. Strenuous measures must be taken to avoid this complication because it makes efficient walking with a prosthesis difficult, if not impossible (Fig. 15-27). Even a slightly sagging bed can contribute to contractures, and bed boards may be necessary to provide a firm support. Pillows under the thigh are almost certain to result in some degree of flexion at the hip level. To prevent these complications, the above-knee amputee should lie prone for half-hour intervals several times during the day (Fig. 15-28). If the patient uses the backrest or a wheelchair for long periods during the day, he should be encouraged to spend comparable periods in a position of full extension to prevent contracture of the hip flexors. Bed exercises will be started after a day or two, not only to prevent contracture but also to start building needed muscle strength.

A great deal of the patient's future ability to walk will depend on the remaining limb, and

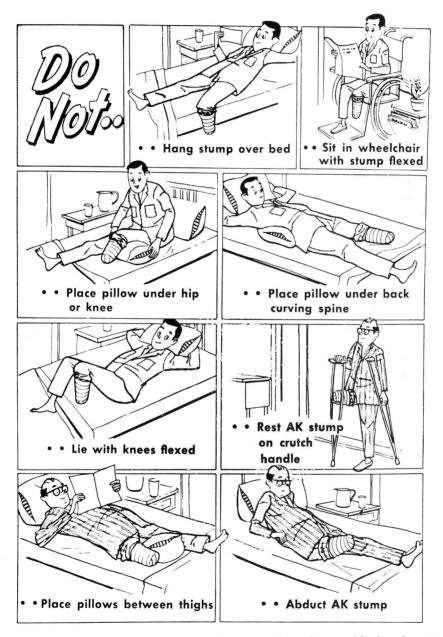

Fig. 15-27. To avoid contractures and to assure the best conditions for wound healing the patient should be cautioned to avoid the activities shown. (From Wilson, A. Bennett, Jr.: Artif. Limbs 7:1-42, 1963.)

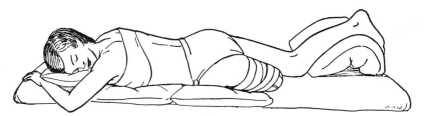

Fig. 15-28. Prone position. The pillow under the patient's lower trunk protects the wound from pressure on the bed and maintains the hip in extension. (From Moskopp, M., and Sloan, J.: Am. J. Nurs. **50:**550-555, 1950.)

care should be taken to keep it in normal muscle tone. Supports should be provided to encourage good anatomic position in bed. A sensitive heel sometimes develops in the remaining foot because of the patient's inclination to push himself up in bed by digging his heel into the mattress. An overhead trapeze will help the patient to pull himself up in bed without using his heel.

The patient may be allowed out of bed as early as the day after amputation, to reduce the danger of embolism. He should be fitted with a good shoe when he begins to bear any weight on the foot.

These things will not be difficult to encourage in the healthy adult, but the debilitated, elderly patient will need to be encouraged by frequent explanations about the necessity of what he is doing. Otherwise, it seems too much trouble to him to warrant the effort he must put forth.

PHYSICAL THERAPY

Two forms of treatment that are almost universally followed after amputation are bandaging and exercise. It is desirable, although sometimes not possible, that these be given under the direction of a physical therapist. If such service is not available, nurses must request demonstration from the physician. It is not enough in these circumstances that the demonstration be given to the patient alone, since the nurse will need to encourage and guide the patient in the doctor's absence.

Bed exercises may be started on the first or second postoperative day. These help greatly in the prevention of contractures as well as in preserving and increasing muscle power for the training to come. While lying in the prone posi-

tion, the patient is instructed to bring the stump close to the normal leg, to lift it, and to contract the gluteal muscles as he does so. Nurses supervising this bed exercise should see to it that the patient lies with his foot over the edge of the mattress, keeping the normal leg on the mattress while he is extending the stump. Another exercise the surgeon may sometimes suggest is that of squeezing a pillow between the thighs. If the patient has a below-knee amputation, considerable attention may be given to strengthening the quadriceps muscle as well. One commonly used exercise is to tighten the kneecap, using the quadriceps muscle, for 10 seconds and then to relax for 10 seconds. The exercise is repeated four or more times, several times each day. Patients understand more quickly if they do this in unison with the normal leg and are taught to feel the medial portion contract during the final 10 degrees of full extension.

Heat and massage may also contribute a great deal toward preparing the stump for efficient weight bearing. These treatments should be done in accordance with the doctor's prescription and by a person trained in physical therapy if at all possible. Otherwise, the nurse entrusted with the treatments should seek explicit instructions and demonstrations from the doctor.

Radiant heat may be provided by sunlight or by an electric ultraviolet lamp. Infrared lamps may be helpful in improving local circulation and promoting scar healing but carry the danger of burning the stump. The stump should be kept dry at all times until healed, and it is not permissible to use hot packs or the whirlpool bath. Heat should be used with extreme care, particularly in patients with diabetes or diseases of the vascular system. For such patients the doctor may order a foot cradle and a lamp sus-

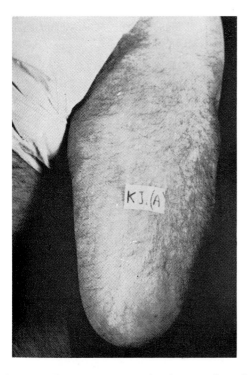

Fig. 15-29. Proper compression bandaging will result in a well-molded stump that is ready for prosthetic fitting. (From Wilson, A. Bennett, Jr.: Artif. Limbs **7:**1-42, 1963.)

pended over the limb area. This type of heat will increase the circulation of the limb without endangering the stump area itself.

When the patient can be out of bed, it is essential that he learn to balance himself properly as he stands on his remaining foot. Parallel bars or crutches will assist him in attaining this balance. In the patient with poor vision, poor balance, or tremors, a walker may be of great benefit. The body should be held straight and the stump should hang straight without flexion or abduction. There should be no distortion of the body because of the missing limb. Drawing in of the abdominal muscles and pinching the gluteal muscles together will give the patient a girdle sense that will help him to avoid shifting his weight to the side of the normal leg.

COMPRESSION OR SHRINKER BANDAGING OF STUMP

As soon as the wound is healing well, the doctor may order some type of shrinker or compression bandage to be applied to the stump. The preferred material for this bandage is usually cotton elastic. Bandages are worn at all times except during physical therapy treatments and until the patient is fitted with a prosthesis. With careful bandaging, the stump can be molded into the desired shape for fitting with a prosthesis. With careful bandaging, the stump can be molded into the desired shape for fitting with a prosthesis (Fig. 15-29). Without bandaging, the stump tends to remain boggy, swollen, and flabby—and in this condition a prosthesis cannot be satisfactorily fitted. The chief cause of delay in the fitting of the prosthesis and rehabilitation of the patient is an improperly molded stump as a result of inadequate or incorrect compression bandaging. A poorly applied bandage is probably worse than no bandage at all. If it is properly applied, however, a shrinker bandage may play a most important part in the ultimate rehabilitation of the amputee.

Because the bandage needs to be reapplied several times during the day to be most effective, nurses should be familiar with the correct application. Too often nurses are satisfied to leave this task to the physical therapist, but this is hardly a wise procedure, since the bandage will frequently need to be reapplied when no physical therapist is available. Occasionally, in busy seasons, it has been necessary to permit patients to apply their own bandages. Results from this, for the most part, have not proved satisfactory.

For the thigh of an average adult two or three 4- to 6-inch all-cotton elastic bandages will be necessary. For convenience and security they are sewed together end-to-end. The bandage is started on the front of the thigh at the groin level (Fig. 15-30). It may be anchored in place by having the patient hold it with his thumbs, one on either side of the thigh. The bandage is then carried down the center front of the thigh, over the end of the stump, and up the back of the thigh to the gluteal fold, where the patient may secure it with his index fingers. (Unless the patient is very large, his hands should be able to encircle his thigh in this fashion.) Now the bandage is carried down the back of the thigh, going somewhat obliquely this time, over the end of the stump, back up to the groin level, and then down obliquely again, this time over the inner aspect of the stump. Each time the recurrent loop is held by the patient's fingers and thumbs and each time the end of the stump

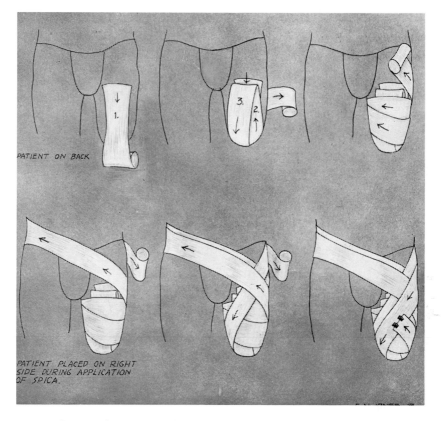

Fig. 15-30. Application of compression bandage. (From Slocum, D. B.: An atlas of amputations, St. Louis, 1949, The C. V. Mosby Co.)

must be compressed securely. The maximum force of the bandage should always be at the stump end and should diminish as the bandage ascends. These recurrent loops (three) are then secured by one or two circular turns of bandage around the thigh at the groin level.

Two spiral turns of the bandage downward to the end of the stump are now made, and the patient is turned on his normal side. The bandage is then carried spirally upward around the thigh, compressing the soft tissues on the side of the stump in an upward and outward direction, and then over the outside of the buttock near the iliac crest. It crosses the abdomen and then passes around the hip of the normal side, across the back, and around the amputated leg at the groin level. A spiral to the end of the stump is made and a second spiral is made as before, always working from within outward and always using the bandage to compress soft tissues at the stump end. The bandage is finally brought back to the stump and completed by a few spiral turns as the length of the bandage allows. It may se secured by safety pins or by bandage clips.

The finished bandage should be observed to see that the spiral crossings to make the hip spica bandage do not lie on the front of the thigh, a condition that encourages hip flexion. Also, the bandage must cover the inner surface of the thigh as high as possible on the groin. If this is not done, a fleshy roll will be likely to occur at the top of the bandage, which will be uncomfortable to the patient and will also cause the bandage to slip downward from that level. An unhealed stump must not be bandaged too snugly, and bandages for healed stumps should not be applied so snugly that actual discomfort occurs.

The below-knee bandage is applied in much the same manner as the one for the thigh stump, omitting, of course, the technique for the hip spica. If the bandage extends above the knee, the patella should remain uncovered and the leg should be held in extension. The popliteal area must not be compressed by too snug a bandage.

Because compression bandages must be reapplied several times during the day, it is advisable to have several sets on hand. They should be carefully washed after each wearing, with mild soap and warm water, and be very thoroughly rinsed. They should be squeezed out and laid on a flat surface to dry because they tend to lose their elasticity if hung. When dry, they should be rolled snugly but without stretching.

As soon as the wound is well healed and the patient understands stump wrapping, exercises, and positioning, he will be discharged from the hospital. He is seen at frequent intervals by the doctor to supervise these activities. As soon as his stump is well molded and firm, he is ready for prescription of an artificial limb and rehabilitation.

PROSTHESIS PRESCRIPTION

When the stump is well healed and firmly molded (ordinarily 2 to 3 months after operation), the patient is ready for consideration of a prosthesis. In well-run amputee clinics, experience has shown that the prescription and training in the use of the limb are best carried out jointly by a doctor familiar with amputees and prostheses, the prosthetist who will construct and fit the limb, and the physical therapist or occupational therapist who will train the patient in its use. Rehabilitation counselors and social workers usually are also involved. Interested nurses are in an excellent position to contribute to this team through their familiarity with the patient. Many factors must be considered in selecting the proper type of prosthesis and prosthetic component. Some of the more important considerations are the following:

1. Age. Special problems exist at the extremes of life. Children need simpler mechanical devices than adults, and their limited attention span makes special training techniques necessary. They outgrow the prosthesis every 2 to 3 years. The elderly amputee may need extra stability to prevent falls.

2. Occupation. Obviously, an active laborer will require heavy-duty components and construction, whereas a weak, elderly nursing home patient will desire a lighter prosthesis.

3. Agility and intelligence. A feebleminded patient cannot be expected to master a complicated upper extremity prosthesis, and an obese clumsy patient will require more safeguards and stability than the average patient.

4. Other health problems. Cardiac reserve is seldom an absolute limiting factor in training because the exertion required to walk with an artificial limb is less than that required for crutch walking. Poor vision, poor balance, paralysis, diminished skin sensation, and tolerance are other health considerations.

5. Finances. Artificial limbs are very expensive. Recently developed components—for example, the commercially available hydraulic knee unit—add greatly to this expense. Charitable or governmental agencies furnish 70% to 80% of all prostheses today. Therefore cost must be kept as low as possible. Luxury components can rarely be used.

6. Motivation. The most important consideration of all is motivation, for without it the patient will not use the prosthesis and all rehabilitation efforts are doomed. The nurse, with knowledge of the patient, can contribute greatly in this evaluation. In general, it is uncommon for a prosthetic prescription team to decide that the patient is not a candidate for an artificial limb of any sort.

After a prescription has been made, the prosthetist takes a mold and certain measurements of the stump to use in construction of the prosthesis. When the mold has been taken, shrinker bandaging should be discontinued because further shrinkage of the stump will result in an ill-fitting prosthetic socket. The construction of artificial limbs requires the highest standards of craftsmanship and technical skill. The prosthetist must have a thorough understanding of the intricate mechanics of body motion that he is attempting to replace. Construction of the socket is critical for the proper fit and distribution of weight. Sometimes the unit is hand carved in basswood or willow wood; otherwise a plastic laminate socket is constructed from a plaster mold. Only certain definite areas on the stump and buttocks are capable of withstanding the pressures of body weight, and the socket must distribute the weight accordingly. Alignment is equally critical, since the position of the prosthesis at all times must closely match that of a normal limb. The prosthetist must finish the prosthesis so that it will be pleasing to the eye, carefully matching the patient's own coloring and contour, or else the patient may not wear the limb at all. The prosthetist must be exacting in each detail of construction. This is no mail-order procedure.

PROSTHESIS COMPONENTS
Lower extremity

Familiarity with prostheses can be gained only be seeing several of each type. The nurse should examine the workings and fit of each artificial

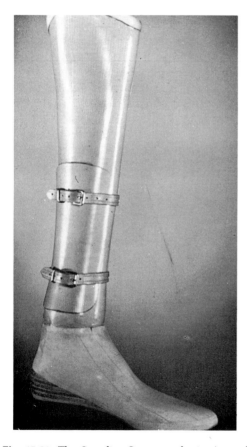

Fig. 15-31. The Canadian Syme prosthesis. A panel on the medial side permits the bulbous stump to enter the prosthesis. A SACH foot is used in this prosthesis. (Courtesy Prosthetic and Sensory Aids Service of the Veterans Administration, Washington, D. C.)

limb encountered. For the interested nurse whose duty requires working with large numbers of amputees, attendance at one of the three large prosthesis schools (Northwestern University, New York University, or University of California at Los Angeles) would be invaluable. The following brief account of the commonest prosthesis components can best be understood if actual prostheses can also be seen and investigated.

The Syme prosthesis is constructed to permit direct weight bearing on the end of the tibia (Fig. 15-31). A small side or rear opening panel in the shank allows the bulbous stump to enter the prosthesis. The socket is made entirely of plastic laminate. A SACH (Solid Ankle, Cushion Heel) foot is provided, and this has no actual moving ankle joint. Sponge rubber in the heel simulates the ankle function of absorbing the impact of heel strike with each step. With no moving parts, this foot combines a pleasing appearance with trouble-free wear.

For the below-knee amputee, the patellar tendon bearing (PTB) socket has become widely

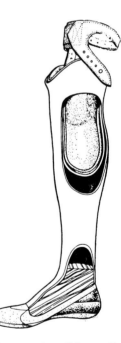

Fig. 15-32. Cutaway view of the patellar tendon bearing prosthesis for below-knee amputees. Usually, only a light strap above the knee is necessary for suspension. (From Wilson, A. Bennett, Jr.: Artif. Limbs **7:**1-42, 1963.)

popular (Fig. 15-32). This socket is constructed of plastic laminate with a thin leather and sponge rubber liner. The bulk of the weight in this instance is distributed to the patellar tendon, which is admirably suited for the job. Usually a single cuff around the thigh just above the kneecap is sufficient for suspension. The SACH foot is generally used in combination with the PTB socket prosthesis. The older hand-carved wooden socket, or so-called soft socket, depends on hinged upright thigh bands and leather lacers to carry much of the weight. The lower end of the socket is left open and it is combined either with a SACH foot or with single axis ankle-foot components. Although for years it has proved to be a satisfactory prosthesis, it has a few disadvantages and is being gradually replaced by the PTB socket.

The above-knee amputee faces additional problems because the prosthesis must have a knee articulation (Fig. 15-33). Many types of knee units are in current use, but nearly all incorporate a design that promotes friction during the swing phase of walking. This is necessary to

limit the height of the rise of the heel from the floor and to prevent a jarring impact as the knee is again extended just prior to the time the heel strikes the floor. The knee is so aligned that in standing, with knee fully extended, it is balanced against sudden flexion—a disaster that would send the wearer sprawling on the floor. An automatic knee brake (the Bock safety knee) is useful for elderly or infirm patients because it prevents the knee from buckling whenever weight is borne on the prosthesis, whether the knee is safely extended or not. For the especially active wearer, there are new hydraulic (Hydra-Cadence) knee units available that produce a marvelously smooth gait. These are expensive and occasionally troublesome.

The quadrilateral socket, or Berkley socket, has virtually replaced the older, round socket or plug socket for the above-knee amputee. As the name implies, its rectangular shape does not conform to the shape of the stump, but it does make use of the remaining muscles of the stump. Weight is distributed principally on the ischial

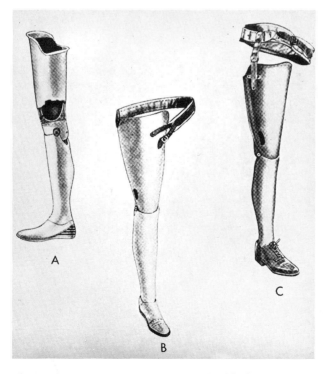

Fig. 15-33. Three means of suspension in above knee artificial limbs. **A,** Cutaway view of suction socket. Note again the SACH foot. **B,** Silesian bandage. Note the single axis ankle-foot component. **C,** Pelvic belt suspension. (From Wilson, A. Bennett, Jr.: Artif. Limbs **7:**1-42, 1963.)

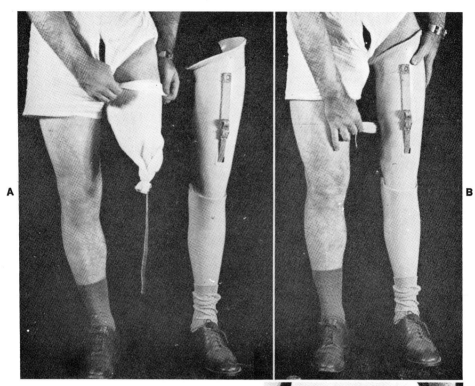

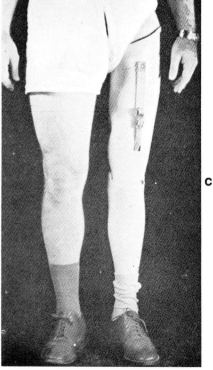

Fig. 15-34. Application of the suction socket above-knee prosthesis. **A,** A thin cotton sock is placed on the stump. Note that a string is attached to the bottom of the sock. When the stump is placed in the limb, this is threaded out through the valve to facilitate drawing the sock from the stump. **B,** The stump is placed in the limb, and the sock is pulled out through the open valve. **C,** Weight is placed firmly on the limb to evacuate any possible air; the suction valve is closed. The limb is now ready for use and is maintained on the stump through negative pressure and muscle action. No stump sock is worn with this type of suspension. (From Slocum, Donald B.: An atlas of amputations, St. Louis, 1949, The C. V. Mosby Co.)

tuberosity and the tough origins of the hamstring muscles. The socket is carved from wood or molded in plastic. In some cases a total-contact socket is used to alleviate or prevent certain stump skin problems. As the name implies, all portions of the stump are in contact with the socket wall. The suction socket has definite advantages for the active above-knee amputee. It not only reduces the need for harnessing, but also gives improved perception of the movement and location of the prosthesis. The wearer feels that the prosthesis is more a part of his body. When once applied, the stump is pumped up and down to expel all air from the bottom of the socket. A valve is then closed that permits no air to enter, and a suction effect is created.

The Canadian hip disarticulation prosthesis is the current standard prescription for patients who have had a hemipelvectomy or hip disarticu-

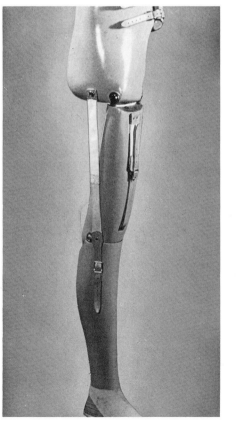

Fig. 15-35. The Canadian hip disarticulation prosthesis. (Courtesy Prosthetic and Sensory Aids Service of the Veterans Administration, Washington, D. C.)

lation (Fig. 15-35). The socket is a plastic laminate mold designed to distribute weight on the ischium or other available structures. The hip joint hinge is located toward the front of the socket in a position ahead of the thigh. This alignment eliminates the need for a lock at the hip joint because it cannot buckle suddenly during standing or normal walking. This arrangement also facilitates sitting while wearing the prosthesis. The remaining components consist of a constant-friction knee and a SACH foot.

Immediate postsurgical fitting of the lower extremity prosthesis. Fig. 15-36 illustrates the type of prosthesis that is applied to a below-knee amputee, when ambulation and weight bearing are advocated within 24 to 48 hours after surgery. Immediately after surgery, a sterile stump sock is applied over the fluffed gauze dressing. This protects the stump from the plaster of paris dressing. In addition, felt pads are placed in position to protect bony prominences from pressure caused by weight bearing. An elastic plaster of paris bandage is then applied to the stump in a specified manner. This dressing is reinforced with the conventional plaster of paris bandage. A suspension strap, as illustrated, is incorporated into the plaster. Later, this suspension belt is fastened to the waist belt. When the cast is dry, additional layers of plaster of paris are used to attach and hold the adjustable portion of the prosthetic unit in the correct position. This cast is worn for 8 to 14 days postoperatively, unless there are indications for removing it, such as an elevated temperature, discomfort, or a loose-fitting bandage. If the cast is removed or accidentally comes off, it is important that another stump cast be applied very soon to prevent edema of the stump. The first postoperative day, active assistive exercise of the hip joint and weight bearing on the prosthesis are encouraged as tolerated by the patient. During the next 3 to 4 weeks, ambulation, with three-point partial weight bearing, is increased as determined by the surgeon and as tolerated by the patient. With some patients, the mold for a permanent prosthesis may be made approximately 3 weeks following amputation. The rigid dressing tends to prevent severe pain when weight bearing is instituted soon after amputation and phantom pain has not been a problem. When early ambulation

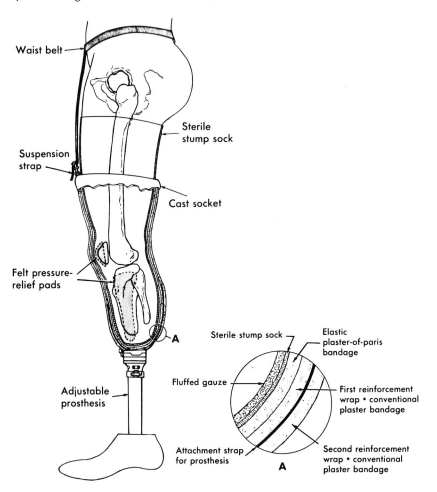

Fig. 15-36. Schematic cross section showing most of the elements in application of a prosthesis to a below-knee amputee immediately after surgery. For the sake of clarity, the suture line, silk dressing, and drain are not shown. View **A** is an enlarged schematic section of the cast socket, prosthetic unit attachment strap, stump sock, and fluffed gauze at the distal portion of the stump. The fluffed gauze does not extend beyond the area indicated. (From Immediate postsurgical prosthetics, Washington, D. C., 1967, Veterans Administration.)

is accomplished, the patient feels encouraged, and the complications frequently caused by inactivity may be avoided. With this regime for the amputee, the rigid bandage and early ambulation with weight bearing, it appears that the process of stump shrinking and shaping begins much earlier than in treatment by the conventional method.

Upper extremity

For the upper extremity amputee, prosthesis function and fitting present some quite different problems. Replacing the prehensile human hand is clearly an impossibility, and prostheses can make available only a rough approximation of the hand's function. In most cases the prosthetic hand provides only holding and assistive functions for the intact hand. Placing the hand at a desired position in space away from the body and holding it there becomes an intricate problem in levers, cables, and locks. Cosmetic appearance is of far more concern to the average upper extremity amputee. These many problems lead to a lower rate of success in the number of amputees who successfully wear upper extremity prostheses as compared to those with lower extremity prostheses.

For the wrist disarticulation or below-elbow

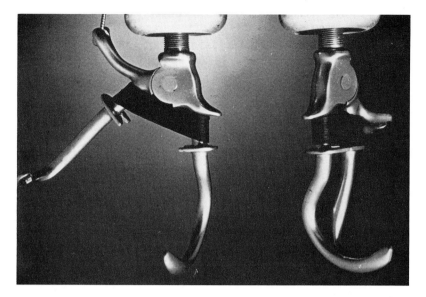

Fig. 15-37. A common type of voluntary opening hook. Opening is achieved when the wearer applies pull to the cable. Closure is powered by stout bands of elastic rubber. (Courtesy Prosthetic and Sensory Aids Service of the Veterans Administration, Washington, D. C.)

(BE) amputee, the replacement consists of some type of terminal device that is powered by a cable arrangement from the shoulder. Many types of terminal devices are available, but these divide naturally into hooks (Fig. 15-37) and mechanical hands. The term hook is a misnomer that conjures ugly visions of pirate captains, but it is so entrenched in common usage that we are left little alternative except to refer to it nonspecifically as a terminal device. Actually, it is seldom used as a hook, and it would make a clumsy weapon in combat. Most hooks are of the voluntary opening variety, which means that the wearer actively opens the hook to grasp objects, but that closure is powered by stout bands of elastic rubber. Voluntary closing hooks remain open until the wearer activates the mechanism to close or pinch an object. This provides more delicate function, but it is inclined to malfunction more frequently. A simple voluntary opening hook is the more efficient, functional, and trouble-free terminal device. It is the logical choice for the new amputee.

Mechanical hands are complex pieces of apparatus that are made in answer to the demand for better cosmetic appearance. In this they do quite well, for they do simulate the form of the hand and a flesh-colored rubber glove adds a reasonable approximation to human skin. They operate on a voluntary closing principle. The dexterity they afford is less than that of the hook, and because they are intricate devices, they are subject to more frequent malfunction. Many amputees prefer the hook for everyday use and the mechanical hand for dress-up occasions.

Just as prosthesis design is more complex for the above-knee amputee than the below-knee amputee, so is it for the above-elbow amputee than for the below-elbow amputee (Fig. 15-38). Elbow joint function must be replaced in order to place the hand at a desired position in space. This requires some kind of cable control to provide elbow flexion (forearm lift) and the elbow lock. Often the forearm lift is controlled by the same cable and shoulder harness as that which operates the terminal device. The elbow lock control unit is usually operated by a separate control cable.

The shoulder disarticulation prosthesis (Fig. 15-39) varies from the above-elbow prosthesis in only two ways. A friction joint is provided in the shoulder region, which allows the wearer to preposition the shoulder joint for special uses. There is no mechanical device that activates the shoulder joint, and most of the time the shoulder remains by the side. The second difference is that

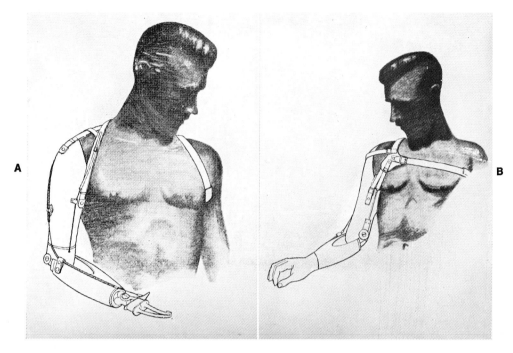

Fig. 15-38. A, Typical prosthesis for an above-elbow amputee. The voluntary opening hook is powered by a cable arrangement from the shoulder harness. Two cables are required for use of this prosthesis. **B,** The elbow disarticulation amputee requires a slightly different elbow joint. Note the mechanical hand and the harness. (From Wilson, A. Bennett, Jr.: Artif. Limbs **7:**1-42, 1963.)

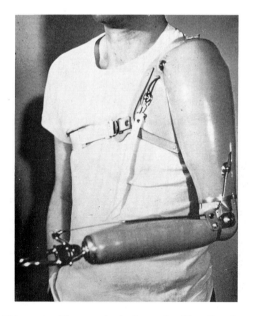

Fig. 15-39. The prosthesis for a shoulder disarticulation amputee has a larger, wider socket to receive the remaining shoulder. A hinge joint in the shoulder provides some passive motion. (Courtesy Prosthetic and Sensory Aids Service of the Veterans Administration, Washington, D. C.)

an excellent power source for operation of control cables (humeral flexion) has been lost. Consequently, less convenient movements at a greater distance from the shoulder must be harnessed to operate the terminal device, the forearm lift, and the elbow lock.

The sockets for all upper extremity prostheses are usually made from plastic laminates that are individually constructed to fit each patient. Terminal devices, elbow joints, and other hardware are available in a variety of sizes. The harness is made of leather and heavy cotton-web belting. The axillary loop is coated with impervious, smooth plastic because of the constant smooth moisture and friction in the axilla. The control cables are mounted upon the harness in such a way that they derive power from the relative motion between two parts of the body.

PROSTHETIC USE TRAINING

Immediately after receiving his prosthesis, the patient should again be seen by the prescription team. The prosthesis should be checked to see that it is satisfactory in every way. The stump should be checked for edema, joint contracture, and muscle strength. If faults exist, the appropriate therapy is instituted. As soon as it is determined that the prosthesis fits properly and consists of the components prescribed, training can begin. The amputee must not be allowed to attempt to put on the limb and begin using it without guidance—faulty habits and pressure sores cannot easily be undone.

The therapist's first job is to teach the amputee to care for the prosthesis and how to put on and to remove the aid himself. The patient should be instructed in the mechanisms of the prosthesis; every effort should be made to give him confidence that it will not collapse. To apply the typical above-knee prosthesis, the amputee places the wool stump sock over his stump. The stump is placed in the limb socket and the wearer settles his weight into it until he feels proper weight distribution on the proper place. The pelvic belt or harness is then buckled securely.

The patient is usually given instructions by the limb maker in caring for his prosthesis or, if he is an elderly person, some member of the family may be provided with these instructions. With reasonable care the length of useful wear is greatly increased beyond that of a prosthesis carelessly worn and cared for. The patient is instructed never to allow the limb to become excessively wet because this will do irreparable damage to the appliance.

Most limb makers recommend that the prosthesis be cleaned at frequent intervals. The socket, at least, should be cleaned daily with mild soap and water. It is especially important that the socket be dried thoroughly after each use. The patient may be allowed to lubricate and to adjust the friction of certain hinges. The shoe worn on the prosthetic foot should not become excessively worn. The patient should not varnish the wooden socket himself because varnish may prove to be an irritating substance. Stockings may be held up by adhesive tape or by garters; the use of thumb tacks is discouraged. Hooks should not be used as tools to pry or hammer. Anything other than the most minor repairs should be performed by the prosthetist and should be done without delay. Preventive maintenance will greatly prolong wear.

The patient will need a period of intensive practice and learning to balance himself in this new limb before he attempts to walk with it. When he has mastered balance in standing with the new limb, he will be ready to take a few steps using the parallel bars. From this he graduates to crutches or to two canes that will later be discarded, one at a time. In crutch walking, a three-point crutch gait is advised; a four-point crutch gait is rarely prescribed. The patient should not be allowed to consider crutches or canes indispensable. The artificial limb is strong enough to support the patient if he learns to use it properly.

Since a fall may occur, the patient is taught how to fall as gracefully as possible and how to rise from the floor. When level walking has been mastered, ascending and descending stairs can be taught. Throughout the period of gait training, three essential points must be emphasized in teaching the patient to use the artificial limb. He must learn (1) to balance his body in good posture, (2) to use steps of equal length, and (3) to attain normal speed in walking.

One of the commonest errors observed in people who use artificial limbs is the rolling gait caused by abduction of the stump and prosthesis in taking a step. It is extremely difficult to overcome once it is acquired, and nurses should be alert to a tendency to walk in this fashion. The patient should not raise or hike his hip and shoulder on the amputated side as he walks.

Use training for the upper extremity amputee starts with operation of the terminal device. It may be necessary to strengthen the groups of muscles that power the terminal device. This is followed in the above-elbow amputee by learning to manage the elbow lock and forearm lift. One by one, such skills as using a knife and fork, tying shoelaces, and managing a billfold are mastered. Training emphasizes two-handed activities or those that require special techniques.

The patient sometimes becomes discouraged and frustrated during the period of training. The nurse should make every effort at this time to give special encouragement and commendation for his achievements. The major single cause for failure is lack of motivation.

Care of the stump

Good care of the amputated stump is essential to continued successful use of prosthesis. Skin problems of many sorts arise unless positive action is taken to avoid them. Enclosing the stump in an airtight container (the socket) inevitably leads to the accumulation of perspiration, skin waste products, and skin bacteria. Incubation of this mixture at normal body heat all day long produces a noxious brew. The slightest abrasion or ingrown hair quickly becomes a boil.

The stump should be washed thoroughly each night at bedtime with warm water and a mild soap containing hexachlorophene. Thorough rinsing and drying are also essential. The stump should be kept free of irritating substances such as oil, alcohol, and medicated talcum powders. Iodine and strong disinfectants are never allowed. A high-quality, nonmedicated talcum may be used occasionally. During initial use training especially, the stump should be inspected frequently for red spots, blisters, and boils. The patient should be specifically asked whether he has any pinched or painful areas. If the slightest skin irritation is in evidence, wearing of the prosthesis should be discontinued until the stump and the socket are checked by the doctor. Neglect of these apparently innocent friction spots can lead to serious problems that may make the fit of any future prosthesis difficult.

A stump sock, which is worn with the lower extremity prosthesis, should be made of pure virgin wool. The patient will need two or three of these because they must be changed at least once daily. In hot weather more changes will be needed. Socks should never be used if they are torn, patched, or roughened, and they should fit snugly except at the end. Wrinkles in the sock will inevitably lead to irritation and discomfort. These socks need special washing care. They should be washed with mild soap in lukewarm water and rinsed several times. Woolite used in cold water is quite satisfactory. The wool sock should be squeezed dry, not wrung, then spread flat or placed on a sock stretcher to dry. A rubber ball of proper size will help maintain shape of the distal end. Three measurements are needed when ordering stump socks. These are the circumference of the upper rim of the socket, the circumference of the distal end of the stump, and the length of the stump (distal end of stump to the place where the upper rim of the prosthesis strikes the leg, plus a couple of inches to turn back over the socket of the prosthesis).

Some shrinkage may continue in the stump over a period of years, and it is not unusual to find patients attempting to fill the space between the stump and the socket by wearing more and more stump socks. If it is discovered that the patient is wearing three or four of these to raise the stump, he should be advised to contact the limb maker at once because a new socket liner or even a new socket may be necessary. The maximum number of stump socks worn at one time should not exceed two.

Phantom limb sensations are experienced by some adult amputees after removal of the limb. These are usually not distressing to the patient, and upon direct questioning he is likely to regard them as a curiosity. Over a period of years the feelings from the absent limb seem to shrink into the stump gradually until the phantom sensation is gone altogether. Distressing phantom limb pains are fortunately a rather rare occurrence—1% to 2% of all amputations. When present, the amputee often feels that the absent toes are being pinched and squeezed or being burned. The phantom limb pains may not make their appearance until years after the amputation. Invariably there is a heavy emotional overlay, and these patients can think and talk of nothing else. The cause of the phantom limb pain is not clear. Many types of operative procedures have been devised, but little seems to benefit the wretched condition of patients suffering from this sensation.

On the other hand, true neuroma formation is a fairly frequent condition. Actually, this is the natural reparative reaction (attempted regrowth) of any periphheral nerve that has been cut. If the neuroma is in a location subject to pressure or trauma, it may become quite sensitive. It is characterized by electric or lightning-like pains that are triggered at one well-localized spot. Surgical removal of the offending neuroma is usually very beneficial.

In children with amputations bony overgrowth

of the amputated limb is a common complication. The explanation for this phenomenon is not clear, but the bone simply outstrips the surrounding soft tissue in its growth. Again, resection of the excessive bone is usually necessary, and this may have to be repeated several times until the growth of the skeleton ceases.

The public health nurse inspecting a prosthesis on a home visit should observe the apparatus for loose or worn joints, for signs of deterioration in rubber, leather, or other fabrics, and for signs of wearing or cracking in the wood or plastic. Any of these are indications that the prosthesis should be seen by the limb maker at the earliest possible moment. The nurse should also observe the number and condition of the stump socks that the patient is using. The skin of the stump should be inspected for swelling or irritation, and the nurse should inquire about the stump hygiene routine. The patient should be reminded that any abnormality or discomfort—such as swelling, redness, blisters, irritation, or induration—is a danger signal that needs immediate attention. When these things occur, he must stop weight bearing until suitable adjustment can be made in the socket of his prosthesis.

The nurse may also observe the patient's walking habits to see that he is making the best mechanical use of the prosthesis. Poor walking habits that are acquired early by the wearer of an artificial limb are extremely hard to overcome, but considerable improvement is often possible if the patient understands what is expected of him and if he is given practical suggestions for increasing his ability to use the limb more effectively.

REHABILITATION OF THE AMPUTEE

Rehabilitation ideally should start before the patient enters the hospital for his amputation. As previously stated, psychologic problems in the well-prepared patient are minimal. The average patient of today is likely to be much more cooperative and less subject to emotional shock if he is provided in advance with a reasonable expectation of what he is to experience. Often the surgeon will give the patient a general explanation of this, including a rough timetable not only of events during hospitalization but also of postoperative office visits up to the time when the stump is ready for limb prescription. The doctor will also tell the patient in a general way what activities he can reasonably expect to do after training with his new limb. It is not within the scope of nurses' training or responsibility to provide this information. They should be prepared, however, to answer the patient's direct questions as honestly as possible. If any doubt exists, the questions should be referred to the doctor, but cheerful reassurance can be a source of great comfort to the patient at this time. On the other hand, unfounded optimism can be extremely cruel.

The young person who has had a single-limb amputation and who has been fitted with a prosthesis and trained in its proper use should be able to carry on an active self-supporting life. His family and friends should recognize that the greatest help they can give him is to treat him as normally as possible. The problem of the person with two amputations is manifestly more complex. It is absolutely necessary that such persons be given the benefit of the specialized therapy—physical, diversional, and vocational—that will enable them to attain the maximum degree of independence.

When amputation has resulted from some systemic disease, vitality is usually lowered and habits of invalidism are easily acquired. The patient may tend to prefer a wheelchair rather than to struggle with the problems associated with the use of an artificial limb. As his general health improves, however, the patient should be encouraged to resume his normal activities insofar as possible. Sensible goals set for him to work toward, accompanied by encouragement and an attitude of hopefulness on the part of the public health nurse, will often pay dividends in the patient's increased capacity and willingness to care for his own needs.

Amputees as a group offer better results in terms of returning to social and economic independence than do patient with many other major maladies—for example, blindness and paraplegia. The chief cause for failure in rehabilitation of the amputee is lack of motivation. In this regard the nurse can be of enormous benefit to the patient.

STUDY QUESTIONS

1. Care of the patient after an amputation includes prevention of contractures in adjacent joints. Describe types of contractures most likely to develop following (a) below-knee amputation, (b) above-knee amputation. Discuss care necessary to prevent each of these contractures.
2. Describe method of applying a compression bandage following a mid-thigh amputation.
3. Early application of a prosthesis and early ambulation are being advocated for the lower limb amputee. Discuss advantages the patient may gain from the activity.
4. Following an arthroplasty of the hip joint, the involved limb is usually maintained in a position of abduction and of neutral or internal rotation. Explain why this position is necessary and the method(s) by which it may be attained.
5. Suspension traction is usually applied after an arthroplasty of the hip joint. Explain the purpose of the traction and equipment needed.
6. Quadriceps-setting and gluteal muscle–setting exercises are usually prescribed following an arthroplasty of the hip joint, as well as dorsiflexion and plantar flexion of the ankle joint. Describe these exercises and explain why they are necessary.
7. Flexion contracture of the hip joint may develop after an arthroplasty. Explain why this is a possibility and discuss care necessary to prevent.
8. It is not desirable for the cup arthroplasty patient to turn for back care. Describe method of giving back care and changing bed linen for this patient.
9. Define the following terms: arthrotomy, arthrodesis, arthroplasty, ankylosis, tenotomy, osteotomy, and fusion.

REFERENCES

Adams, J.: Modern management of traumatic amputation, Nursing '72 **2**:46, 1972.
Amputations, Physiotherapy **52**:180-203, 1966.
Amstutz, H. C.: Complications of total hip replacement, Clin. Orthop. **72**:123-137, 1970.
Anderson, A. D., Levine, S. A., and Colmer, M.: The temporary walking device for the mobilization of the elderly amputee, Geriatrics **21**:186-188, 1966.
Anderson, M. H.: Upper extremity orthotics, Springfield, Ill., 1965, Charles C Thomas, Publisher.
Arnold, H. M.: Elderly diabetic amputees, Amer. J. Nurs. **69**:2646-2649, 1969.
Aufranc, O.: Constructive surgery of the hip, St. Louis, 1962, The C. V. Mosby Co.
Bain, A. M.: Surgical treatment of osteoarthrosis, Physiotherapy **59**:47-52, 1973.
Bechtol, C.: The fitting of a lower-extremity prosthesis in the immediate postamputation period, Arch. Phys. Med. **48**:145-146, 1967.
Bosanko, L. A.: Immediate postoperative prosthesis, Am. J. Nurs. **71**:280-283, 1971.
Brady, E.: Grief and amputation; ANA clinical sessions, New York, 1968, Appelton-Century-Crofts.
Brooks, M. B., Beal, L., Ogg, L., and Blakeslee, B.: The child with deformed or missing limbs, his problems and prostheses, Am. J. Nurs. **62**:88-92, Nov., 1962.
Burgess, E., Traub, J., and Wilson, A. B.: Immediate postsurgical prosthetics in the management of lower extremity amputees, Washington, D. C., 1967, U. S. Government Printing Office.
Clayton, M. L.: Care of the rheumatoid hip, Clin. Orthop. **90**:70-76, 1973.
Compere, C.: Early fitting of prostheses following amputation, Surg. Clin. of North Amer. **48**:215-226, 1968.
Cummings, G. S.: A clinical assessment of immediate postoperative fitting of prosthesis for amputee rehabilitation, Phys. Ther. **51**:1007-1011, 1971.
Davies, E. J., Friz, B. R., and Clipinger, F. W.: Amputees and their Prostheses, Artif. Limbs **14**:19-48, 1970.
Demopoulos, J. T., and Selman, L.: Rehabilitation following total hip replacement, Arch. Phys. Med. Rehabil. **53**:51-59, 1972.
Drain, C. B.: The athletic knee injury, Am. J. Nurs. **71**:536-537, 1971.
Evarts, C. M., editor: Symposium on interposition and implant arthoplasty, Orthop. Clin. North Am. vol. 4, 1973.
Eyre, M. K.: Total hip replacement, Am. J. Nurs. **71**:1384-1387, 1971.
Fliegel, O., and Feuer, S. G.: Historical development of lower extremity prostheses, Arch. Phys. Med. **47**:275-285, 1966.
Gerhardt, J. J., King, P. S., Peirson, G. A., Fowlks, E. W., and Altman, D. C.: Immediate post-surgical prosthetics: rehabilitation aspects, Amer. J. Phys. Med. **49**:3-105, 1970.
Glattly, H. W.: A preliminary report on the amputee census, Artif. Limbs **7**:5-10, Spring, 1963.
Golbranson, F. L., Asbelle, C., and Strand, D.: Immediate postsurgical fitting and early ambulation, a new concept in amputee rehabilitation, Clin. Orthop. **56**:119-131, 1968.
Graves, S., and Vincent, S.: Total hip replacement is a family affair, RN **34**:35-41, 1971.
Guy, F. M.: Implants used in orthopaedic surgery part I, Nurs. Times **68**:463-466, 1972.
Guy, F. M.: Implants used in orthopaedic surgery, part II, Nurs. Times **68**:500-503, 1972.
Harrold, A. J.: Internal derangements of the knee, Nurs. Times **67**:1575-1577, 1971.
Holt, P. J.: Upper-limb endoprostheses, Physiotherapy **59**:112-115, 1973.
Jackson, J. P.: Internal derangement of the kneejoint, Physiotherapy **52**:229-232, 1966.
Jeglijewski, J. M.: Target: outside world, Am. J. Nurs. **73**:1024-1027, 1973.
Johnston, R. C., and Larson, C.: Surgical management of osteoarthritis of the hip. In Cooper, P.: The craft of surgery, ed. 2, Boston, 1971, Little Brown and Co.
Kessler, H. H., and Kiessling, E.: The pneumatic arm prosthesis, Am. J. Nurs. **65**:114-117, June, 1965.
Kirkpatrick, S.: Battle casualty, amputee, Am. J. Nurs. **68**:998-1005, 1968.

Kluge, L. B.: The Walldius prosthesis; a total treatment program, Phys. Ther. **52:**26-33, 1972.

Knapp, M.: Lower-extremity amputations and prosthetics, Postgrad. Med. **44:**259-264, Nov., 1968.

Knapp, M.: Lower-extremity amputations and prosthetics, Postgrad. Med. **44:**259-264, Dec., 1968.

Knapp, M.: Lower-extremity amputations and prosthetics, Postgrad. Med. **44:**170-172, 1968.

Lineberger, M. I.: Habilitation of child amputees, J. Am. Phys. Ther. Ass. **42:**397-401, 1962.

Longton, E. B.: Orthopaedic surgery in arthritic lower-limb joints, Physiotherapy **59:**116-119, 1973.

Marquardt, E.: The Heidelberg pneumatic arm prosthesis, J. Bone Joint Surg. **47-B:**425-434, 1965.

Martin, N.: Rehabilitation of the upper extremity amputee, Nurs. Outlook **18:**50-51, 1970.

Marx, H. W.: Some experience in hemipelvectomy prosthetics, Orthotics and Prosthetics. **21:** 1967.

May, B. J.: Stump bandaging of the lower-extremity amputee, J. Am. Phys. Ther. Ass. **44:**808-814, 1964.

McKee, G. K.: Development of total prosthetic replacement of the hip, Clin. Orthop. **72:**85-103, 1970.

McKee, G. K., and Watson-Farrar, J.: Replacement of arthritic hips by the McKee-Farrar prosthesis, J. Bone Joint Surg. **48-B:**245-259, 1966.

Muller, M. E.: Total hip prostheses, Clin. Orthop. **72:**46-68, 1970.

Patterson, T., Loche, M., and Flournoy, M.: Traumatic amputation, Nursing '72 **2:**40-45, 1972.

Plaisted, L. M., and Friz, B. R.: The nurse on the amputee clinic team, Nurs. Outlook **16:**34-37, Oct., 1968.

Rockwell, S. M.: Total hip replacement: the OR nurse's role, RN **34:**1-9, 1971.

Rosenberg, E. F.: Total hip replacement—viewpoint of a rheumatologist, Postgrad. Med. **51:**124-127, 1972.

Sarmiento, A.: Recent trends in lower extremity amputation, Nurs. Clin. North Am. **2:**399-408, 1967.

Sarmiento, A., editor: Symposium on amputation surgery and prosthetics, Orthop. Clin. North Am. **3:**265-494, 1972.

Soules, B. J.: Thalidomide victims in a rehabilitation center, Am. J. Nurs. **66:**2023-2026, Sept., 1966.

Staros, A., and Gardner, H. F.: Direct forming of below knee PTB sockets with a thermoplastic material, Artif. Limbs **14:**57-64, 1970.

Stinchfield, F. E., and Chamberlin, A. C.: Arthroplasty of the hip, J. Bone Joint Surg. **48-A:**564-581, 1966.

Stolov, W. C., Burgess, E. M., and Romano, R. L.: Progression of weight bearing after immediate prosthesis fitting following below-knee amputation, Arch. Phys. Med. Rehabil. **52:**491-502, 1971.

Thompson, A.: An early walking aid for geriatric amputees, Physiotherapy **57:**585-588, 1971.

Tooms, R. E.: Amputations. In Crenshaw, A. H., editor: Campbell's operative orthopedics, vol. 1, ed. 5, St. Louis, 1971, The C. V. Mosby Co.

Warren, R.: Early rehabilitation of the elderly lower extremity amputee, Surg. Clin. North Am. **48:**807-816, 1968.

Wesseling, E.: The adolescent facing amputation, Amer. J. Nurs. **65:**90-94, Jan., 1965.

Wilson, A. B., Jr.: Limb prosthetics—1970, Artif. Limbs **14:**1-52, 1970.

Wilson, A. B., Jr.: A material for direct forming of prosthetic sockets, Artif. Limbs **14:**53-56, 1970.

Wilson, K.: Hand and foot prostheses, Practioner **201:**759-766, 1968.

Zalewski, N., Geronemus, D., Siegal, H.: Hemipelvectomy—the triumph of Ms. A., Am. J. Nurs. **73:**2,073-2,079, Dec., 1973.

16

Legal liability of nurses

JOHN W. LARSON, B.A., J.D.

The purpose of this chapter is to convey a basic general understanding of the legal liability of the nurse. It is limited to a survey of the most general points; attention is directed to the list of references at the end of the chapter, provided for the reader who desires to explore the subject in greater depth. If any trend is ascertainable in this area of the law, it is the courts' ever-increasing recognition of nursing as a true profession with a corresponding increase of responsibilities and accompanying legal obligations. However, there is considerable disagreement among the courts as to the treatment of specific legal issues and, consequently, there is often an inconsistency in result between the decisions in the various states.

Any discussion of the legal aspects of nursing is necessarily interwoven with the relationship of the nurse to the physician and to the hospital and with the complex series of legal obligations and duties between them and with respect to the patient. The basic inquiry will be to ascertain the standards applied to determine if the nurse has been negligent in the performance of professional functions and then to determine who else may also be liable for that negligence.

LEGAL DEFINITION OF A NURSE

There is no agreed legal definition of nursing, and each state has attempted to establish the meaning through statute. From a composite of the various statutes, the following may be suggested as the definition of a nurse. A nurse is one who engages and is considered to be qualified in the application of biologic, physical, or social sciences for the observation of symptoms and reactions of patients, the accurate recording of fact, and the carrying out of treatments and medications or other lawful orders under the direction or supervision of a physician. In addition, the typical statute specifies the basic educational and training requirements, distinguishes between the various subclasses of nurses—for example, registered, practical, and student—and provides an exception for those performing similar services in the home without claim of nursing qualifications.

To establish a common basis for discussion of the legal consequences of various nursing acts, it is necessary to deal with the various functions of a nurse, which historically have been classified as follows:

1. Independent nursing functions—the functions and duties a nurse can properly perform without the direction, supervision, or control of a physician, such as the following:
   (a) Accurate observation and recognition of symptoms and reactions of the patient
   (b) Accurate recording of fact and maintenance of various required hospital records
   (c) Application of general nursing procedures concerned with hygiene of the patient, such as bathing patients, making beds, and answering the requests of patients
   (d) Supervision of the safety and security of the patient, such as properly situating

the patient in his bed or chair and locking the windows

2. Dependent nursing functions—the functions that can be performed by a nurse only under the direction and supervision of a physician, including acts normally considered as falling within the definition of the practice of medicine.

LIABILITY OF THE NURSE FOR NEGLIGENCE

One of the basic concepts of our legal system is that every person must govern his conduct so as to minimize the possibility of injury to others to the extent that a reasonably prudent man would do under the circumstances. This is known as the standard of due care, and violation of this standard is considered negligence. Where such negligence is the proximate cause of injury to another person, the negligent person may be held legally liable to the injured person for compensatory damages. Negligence is one form of a class of civil wrongs which the law refers to as a tort.

As essential element of the standard of due care is the ability to foresee harm to another. Perhaps one of the best statements of the standard of due care is found in the opinion of the English Court of Appeals in the landmark case of *Heaven v. Pender*, decided in 1883. Said the court:

[W]henever one person is by circumstances placed in such a position with regard to another that every one of ordinary sense who did think would at once recognise that if he did not use ordinary care and skill in his own conduct with regard to those circumstances he would cause danger or injury to the person or property of the other, a duty arises to use ordinary care and skill to avoid such danger. 11 Q.B.D. 503, 509.

Professional nurses, however, have had the benefit of special training and experience, and are considered as possessing professional skill and competency. It is expected, therefore, that they will exercise the degree of care which reasonably prudent nurses, practicing their profession in the community, would exercise under the same or similar circumstances. Accordingly, nurses, in their professional activities, are not measured against the standard of care expected of a prudent layman, but against the standard of care expected of a prudent nurse.

If they fail to exercise that degree of care and as a result of that failure a patient suffers harm, they are considered negligent and are subject to civil liability for money damages in an amount sufficient to compensate the patient for any injuries caused by the nurse's negligence. In this regard, it may be of interest to the student nurse that the courts have held student nurses to the standard of care expected of graduate nurses in the community, rather than of other student nurses, apparently on the rationale that a patient has the right to expect his nursing care will be performed with the same degree of skill and competency whether it is entrusted to a registered nurse or to a student nurse. See, *e.g., Nickley v. Skemp*, 239 N.W. 426, 427 (Wisc. 1931); *cf. Christensen v. Des Moines Still College of Osteopathy*, 82 N.W.2d 741, 746 (Iowa 1957) (intern held to standard of knowledge, skill, and care of osteopathic profession). The lesson would seem to be that student nurses assigned to perform a task, who realize that they are inadequately prepared or will be inadequately supervised, should bring such fact to the attention of the supervisor or perhaps altogether refuse to perform the task. The line between due care and insubordination is obviously a delicate one, and the student nurse would be well advised to anticipate as many situations as possible so that she may seek the advice of a qualified supervisor before an emergency arises.

On the other hand, it is not possible to provide the nurse with an exhaustive list of the various possible situations and the appropriate responses necessary to avoid liability. This question has evoked considerable litigation, each concerning a specific and somewhat different fact-situation; however, it is not the purpose of this chapter to analyze the numerous court decisions involving the tort liability of nurses, but rather to suggest a few of the broad patterns into which many of the cases fall.

It is important to note that the law does not require the nurse or physician to be an absolute insurer of the patient's welfare throughout the course of care and treatment. If the nurse practices due care in accordance with established nursing practices in the community and injury to the patient nevertheless results, that nurse will not be liable for such damages. By analogy to the field of medical malpractice, which uses the same standard to determine whether or not the physician was negligent, the recent case of *Thompson v. Lillehei*, 273 F.2d 376 (8th Cir. 1959), is illustrative of this point. An attempted surgical repair of a ventricular septal defect in an 8-year-old girl by using the mother as a donor under the technique of cross control circulation resulted in an air embolism in the donor, which in turn resulted in permanent brain damage and corresponding mental deficiency. After carefully reviewing the evidence and expressing sympathy for the plight of the donor-plaintiff, the court held the doctors not liable, since they had taken every precaution then known to medical science and the injury occurred nevertheless, but without negligence on their part.

To illustrate the application of the standard of due care as it pertains to nursing, it may be useful to review briefly a few of the professional functions normally performed by nurses, which have led to litigation and liability for negligence.

1. Nurses are often required to recognize and record symptoms in patients. Although not required to perform this function to the extent and with the skill of a physician, failure of the nurse to recognize abnormal reactions to prescribed treatment or drugs or the improper administration of treatment or drugs has resulted in personal liability.

2. An error in the recording of fact can obviously have serious consequences for the patient, and such errors, as well as illegible notations, have led to liability.

3. Even the more menial nursing skills, such as bathing the patient, assisting him into a wheelchair, or administering ice or hot packs, have frequently led to liability for injury. For example, placing the patient in bath water that results in a burn or failing to support a patient properly during his transfer to a wheelchair has resulted in liability for negligence.

4. One of the most difficult areas is found in the so-called dependent nursing functions that require the direction and supervision of a physician. Performance of such functions without the required direction or supervision is in itself a negligent and improper nursing activity. Even though properly supervised and directed, such functions may still be improperly performed, resulting in the nurse's liability for negligence.

A major cause of the difficulty in this area is that the nurse normally has some independent diagnostic and remedial functions that do not require any direction or supervision by the physician. For example, the nurse, in checking the pulse of a patient or in administering a simple medication and noting the patient's reaction, is making a diagnosis that is in the realm of her legitimate functions. Just where the line must be drawn between this type of diagnosis and treatment and that which requires the training and skills of a physician is a subtle question that has caused disagreement between courts. On the other hand, the courts have rather uniformly held that such acts as suturing, changing dressings, and administering anesthetics do require the direction and supervision of a physician.

Another problem in this regard is that as a practical matter physicians do not and cannot exercise direct physical control and supervision over some dependent nursing functions. The only guide available to the nurse is the advice that, if it is generally accepted practice in the immediate medical community, a particular function can be performed by an experienced nurse without direct supervision of the physician. Under such circumstances, it is unlikely the nurse will incur liability for negligence merely by performing such function. For example, in many areas it is common practice for the nurse to administer intravenous and hypodermic injections upon the request of a physician but without any supervision by him. In such areas, accordingly, the nurse is not considered negligent simply because of administering such injections rather than having the physician do so. However, the nurse may still be liable if the injections are performed in a careless manner.

5. The nurse has the unpleasant legal duty of questioning a physician's obviously incorrect order that will result in injury to the patient if the instructions are carried out. At the risk of becoming unpopular, the only safe course of

conduct for the nurse, when in doubt, is to inquire.

6. The scope of the nurse's normal functions may be extended in an emergency situation, which is defined as one in which there is immediate danger of death or serious injury to the patient if prompt remedial action is not taken and no physician is available to do so. In this situation nurses may properly perform functions normally beyond the scope of authorized nursing activities, with one important limitation —they may never perform acts for which they were not trained, such as surgery. They could, for example, clean a wound and suture it if immediately necessary. One consolation for nurses is that under the pressure of the moment the law does not expect cool detached reflection such as will produce 100% accuracy in diagnosing the actual existence of an emergency condition as defined but requires only that under the circumstances a reasonably prudent nurse might have reached the same conclusion.

In the final analysis, the application of the standard of due care to the alleged negligent act of the nurse will turn upon the judgment of the particular community, as expressed through the members of the jury, with regard to what is just, sensible, and proper under the circumstances. Inability to predict the results of this process makes any positive guide for the nurse inadequate.

LIABILITY OF OTHERS FOR THE NURSE'S NEGLIGENT ACTS

Once the liability of the nurse for negligent acts has been established, the next step is to determine if the hospital, physician, or both are also liable. This depends upon the classification of the nurse, either as an employee or as an independent contractor within the basic concepts of agency law. At the risk of oversimplification, it may be said that if the nurse was an employee of the physician or hospital and the injury to the patient occurred within the course of that employment, the physician or hospital, as the case may be, is also liable. If the nurse was not employed by either the hospital or the doctor, however, but was hired directly by the patient, the nurse alone is liable

for negligence. Perhaps the only example of the independent contractor nurse is the private duty nurse who is usually furnished by a listing service and is hired and paid directly by the patient.

The usual problem is to determine whose employee the nurse was at the time of injury— that of the physician or hospital. Obviously, the physician is liable for an injury caused by his own office nurse. It is also rather clear that the hospital is liable for injury caused by a nurse who is employed by the hospital as a member of the regular nursing force, at least for those injuries resulting from the nurse's performance of her *independent* nursing functions.

The real problem exists in the area of the *dependent* nursing functions, which must be performed under the direction and supervision of a physician. The majority, and historic, rule of law is that, since the physician has the power to control and supervise the acts of the nurse in the dependent functions, he should be held liable for any injury caused by the nurse in the performance of such functions. Several other theories also are advanced in support of this view. One theory is based upon the borrowed servant doctrine in the field of agency law. As applied here, this rationale provides that although nurses are primarily the hospital's employees, they temporarily become the physician's employees at the time he takes over the direction and control of their actions in performing a certain act. Another theory is that the physician cannot delegate his responsibility for the performance of these dependent nursing functions and therefore he remains liable despite the fact such functions are actually performed by the nurse. The most persuasive theory, and perhaps the real basis for the majority rule, is that our society desires to place the responsibility on the physician because this is the person who is selected by and relied upon by the patient and who usually has the financial ability to pay for the damages.

As a result of the majority view, the surgeon is held responsible for all of the actions of the nurses in the operating room, since he is deemed to be in complete control of all personnel during the operation. Therefore, if the nurse fails to count the sponges correctly and one is inadvertently left in the patient, the surgeon as well as the nurse is liable for the injuries caused.

Increasingly, however, courts are coming around to the view that the physician should not be held liable in such situations unless he exercises *actual* supervision over the nurse or unless delegating to the nurse the responsibility for performing such function was in itself negligent. The rationale in support of this view is that often the physician does not in fact have the opportunity to exercise actual supervision over the nurse and that he should be free to concentrate upon his primary functions rather than these secondary duties. In addition, it is contended that the physician should be able to rely upon the hospital for providing qualified and competent nurses. In the final analysis, the confusion arises because of the elasticity of the distinction between medical and nursing duties, caused in part by the medical profession's willingness to recognize the increasingly professional characteristic of nursing while continuing to pay lip service to more traditional notions with respect to what functions constitute the practice of medicine and, thus, are reserved exclusively to the physician's dominion.

THE NURSE'S LIABILITY FOR INTENTIONAL ACTS

The nurse will usually encounter the area of personal liability for intentional torts (as distinguished from unintentional torts such as negligence) in only two situations: assault and battery and false imprisonment. It should be noted that such acts subject the nurse to civil liability for both compensable or actual damages and punitive damages.

Assault is the act of putting another in immediate *fear* of personal injury, whereas battery is the act of harmful or offensive *physical contact* against another. Both acts must be intentional as contrasted to accidental and must be without legal justification. The nurse may have occasion to restrain a patient from an act that is harmful to the latter's condition even though the patient may think otherwise. Certainly, when the patient is mentally ill, restraint is required; and when no more force than necessary is applied, there can be no action for assault and battery. The same result occurs when restraint is necessary to prevent the pain-racked patient from injuring himself. If the physical contact is not justifiable in terms of necessary medical treatment to which the patient has expressly or impliedly consented, the nurse may be liable to the patient for damages. It is essential that the patient consent to the treatment involved, inasmuch as the mentally competent patient can refuse to accept any treatment offered. When such a refusal occurs, the remedy is to require that the patient either consent to the treatment or leave the hospital. The patient must comply with hospital rules and must limit himself to areas of the hospital in which those rules permit his presence. If the patient violates the rules, physical restraint to enforce them should be no more violent than necessary and in no event should include such force as would be likely to produce great bodily injury. If the patient persists in violating hospital rules, he should be requested to leave the hospital. The nurse has the right to prevent the patient from injuring other patients, hospital personnel, and guests so long as only a reasonable amount of force is used, and of course one has the right of self-defense in the event of a physical attack by a patient.

False imprisonment is total restraint against a person's will by violence or the threat of violence. To be actionable, the restraint must be intended and the victim must be aware of the restraint. A nurse who refuses to permit a patient to leave the hospital and uses violence or the threat of violence to enforce the restraint, will be subject to civil liability for false imprisonment. Again, however, restraint based upon justifiable medical treatment to which the patient has expressly or implicitly consented will not create liability. If a patient is told under threat of violence that he cannot leave the hospital until his bill is paid, on the other hand, false imprisonment occurs, and the nurse who has so advised the patient may be subject to liability.

REFERENCES

Cady, E. L., Jr.: Law and contemporary nursing, Paterson, N. J., 1961, Littlefield, Adams & Co.

The doctor and the law, vols. 2 and 3, Fort Wayne,

Ind., 1959, Law Department of The Medical Protective Co.

Harrison, G.: Nurse and the law, Philadelphia, 1948, F. A. Davis Co.

Hayt, E., and Hayt, L.: Legal guide for American hospitals, New York, 1950, Hospital Textbook Co.

Hershey, N.: The law and the nurse, a regular column in American Journal of Nursing.

Lesnik, M. J., and Anderson, B. E.: Nursing practice and the law, Philadelphia, 1955, J. B. Lippincott Co.

Lott, J., and Gray, R.: Law in medical and dental practice, Chicago, 1942, Foundation Press.

Morris, R. C., and Moritz, A. R.: Doctor and patient and the law, ed. 5, St. Louis, 1965, The C. V. Mosby Co.

Scheffel, C.: Jurisprudence for nurses, New York, 1945, Lakeside Publishing Co.

Glossary

achondroplasia a form of dwarfism in which the trunk and head are almost normal size but the limbs are short and sometimes distorted; caused by a disturbance in epiphyseal growth that originates in intrauterine life; definitely congenital and frequently inherited.

acromegaly (gigantism) overgrowth of stature, enlargement of the jaw, shoulder girdle, pelvis, hands, and feet; usually develops during periods of rapid growth in adolescents but may occur in adult life.

actinomycosis (blastomycosis lumpy jaw) infection usually first manifested in the bones of the jaw; in a small proportion of patients, the spine is affected; destructive areas, of interest to orthopedists, found in spine, and usually some abscess formation; diagnosis made by the ray-fungus obtained by aspiration of abscess; treatment by drainage, evacuation of abscessed area, or radiation therapy that usually leads to cure within 6 months or a year.

adactylism absence of the fingers or toes.

amputation neuroma enlargement at the end of a cut nerve usually composed of jumbled scar and regenerating nerve tissue and often painful.

amyotonia congenita inherited weakness of the muscles; may persist through adult life or may respond to antirachitic therapy in earlier life.

ankylosis stiffening of a joint; caused by scar tissue or bone growth between the two surfaces of a joint; occurs as result of infection or irritation.

arthrodesis surgical fusion of a joint.

arthrogryposis flexion contractures of the limbs; congenital.

arthroplasty operative creation of a new joint to replace a stiff or ankylosed joint.

arthrotomy operative exploration of a joint.

brachydactylism congenital shortening of the fingers or toes.

Brodie's abscess localized circumscribed osteomyelitic abcess, usually of the long bones; virulence of organism low; treatment by drainage and curettage and infiltration with powdered sulfanilamide; prolonged sulfonamide therapy may be required.

calcaneovalgus sometimes called congenital flatfoot; consists in a deformity in which the tibialis anticus is contracted and the gastrocnemius (heel cord group) is weak; a deformity in which, at birth, toes and top of foot may lie against anterior surface of leg.

cartilaginous exostoses (multiple) see dyschondroplasia.

cavus hollow foot; contracture of the plantar fascia.

cervical rib a congenital anomaly; consists of a supernumerary rib attached to one of the cervical vertebrae; because of pressure, the rib may produce sensory, motor, and vasomotor symptoms in upper extremity.

Charcot joint degenerative proliferative joint lesion of tertiary syphilis causing instability and enlargement but lacking in pain.

Charcot-Marie-Tooth disease characterized by atrophy and paralysis of muscles as a result of degenerative changes in the peripheral nerves; peroneal muscles usually affected first; progresses slowly, has familial tendency, and occurs more frequently in males than in females.

chondritis inflammation of a cartilage.

chondrodystrophy (hypertrophic) see dyschondroplasia.

cineplasty a type of operation in which a skin tunnel is constructed through muscle belly in an arm amputation; by a pulley arrangement the tunneled muscle is made to activate the artificial hand.

Clutton's joints bilateral synovitis of the knees and elbows as a result of congenital syphilis.

congenital absence of the clavicle (sternocleido-dysostosis) absence of the clavicles associated with delay in closure of frontal sutures of skull; causes box-head deformity of skull and groove down center of forehead.

coxa hip.

coxa plana flattened head of the femur.

coxa valga increase of the angle between the neck and shaft of femur.

coxa vara decrease of the angle between the neck and shaft of femur.

cretinism representing type of dwarfism caused by insufficient function of thyroid gland; persons affected have large tongues, thick lips, flattened noses, and puffy eyelids, and should be treated by the administration of thyroid extract.

cubitus elbow.

Dupuytren's contracture scar formation in superficial skin tissues of palm as a result of trauma and focal infection; one or more fingers flexed toward palm; treatment by elimination of foci and complete operative removal of scar.

dyschondroplasia (Ollier's disease) an overgrowth of bone or bony prominences (exostoses) near epiphysis caused by congenital misplacement or abnormal distribution of growth cells; characterized by multiple overgrowth of bones near joints; more common in males than females; if bony projections interfere with joint function or are subject to local irritation, they should be removed.

echinococcus cyst destructive bone lesions infected by the *Taenia echinococcus* when the parasite lodges within bone tissue.

epiphysitis (acute) disease of epiphyseal region near joints; characterized by pain and tenderness near joint; motion usually normal; treatment by immobilization in plaster cast for mild cases and incision and drainage for more active ones.

equinus (like the foot of a horse) consists in contracture of Achilles tendon to extend that ball of foot in walking makes contact with ground but heel cannot touch.

fibrositis rheumatoid involvement of superficial tissues of bony surfaces and of intramuscular and periarticular tissues of bony surfaces; "muscular rheumatism, periarthritis"; pain usually referred to joint but motions not much limited; fibrous nodules found in hands, back, and hips; patient feels stiff and has many spots of tenderness; treatment by removal of focal infection with physical therapy treatments and probably use of vaccines.

flatfeet (rigid) in certain young persons, pain and stiffness of ankles without apparent cause; characterized by progressive knock-ankle deformity and limitation of motion in joints of foot; result of an inherent congenital weakness or reaction to inflammatory changes resulting from focal infection; treated by manipulation (under anesthesia) with correction of deformity and application of plaster cast; corrective procedure combined with removal of any detectable focal infection; for fixed deformity reconstructive operation to restore arch may be required.

Friedreich's ataxia characterized by weakness of leg muscles and caused by degenerative changes in nerve fibers in dorsal and lateral tracts of spinal cord; a progressive condition; familial; treatment by bracing and muscle re-education; stabilization operations may be helpful.

Gaucher's disease generalized bone disease associated with pathology of spleen; bone lesions similar to hyperparathyroidism.

genu knee.

genu valgum knock-knees.

genu varum bowlegs.

genu recurvatum hyperextended position of the knee (backknee position).

gigantism disease of youth as a result of overactivity of anterior portion of pituitary gland; bony growth usually symmetric, and person may attain height of 7 to 9 feet.

"glass" arm athlete's arm weakened by presence of subdeltoid bursitis or epicondylar bursitis.

glioma malignant tumor of brain or nerve cells.

goniometer special protractor used to measure joint motion.

gout disease usually seen in acute attacks that may involve various joints but most commonly the first metatarsophalangeal joint; acute attacks accompanied by extreme pain, redness, and swelling; treatment, elimination of foods high in purines and administration of colchicine.

Gowers' sign "climbing up the legs" to attain an erect position in progressive muscular dystrophy.

Guillain-Barré syndrome (polyneuritis) symmetric paralysis that develops slowly; frequently follows some mild infection; often confused with poliomyelitis; respiratory embarrassment may develop and necessitate a tracheotomy and use of respirator; prognosis good for return of normal muscle power.

hallux great toe.

hallux valgus angulation of great toe away from the midline of the body.

Heberden's nodes enlargements around finger joints accompanying chronic arthritis; enlargements composed of partly bony and partly gelatinous material.

hemophiliac joints occur frequently when disease is present; joints assume a fusiform swelling; areas of subcutaneous hemorrhage; tend to subside with administration of cold packs and vitamin K; immobilization and blood transfusions important factors in preventing further bleeding; joints, after repeated attacks become ankylosed; any surgery distinctly contraindicated.

intermittent hydrarthrosis usually occurs between 30 and 40 years of age; occurs most frequently in knee or both knees and is transient; swelling characteristically painless, lasts a few days, and then disappears only to recur in a month or two; absence of pain or tenderness or of any abnormality in roentgenographic findings in joints; thought that disturbance of allergic or endocrine nature responsible; spontaneous disappearance of disease may occur in pregnancy, but as a rule synovectomy offers best prospect of cure.

involucrum new bone that grows around the sequestrated shaft of an old bone, such as in osteomyelitis.

Kümmel's disease delayed collapse of an injured vertebra in which a minor fracture or no fracture was demonstrated roentgenographically immediately after injury; collapse may occur as late as 5 or 6 months after injury.

kyphosis increase in posterior curve of thoracic vertebrae (hunchback).

Little's disease congenital cerebral palsy or spastic paralysis.

lordosis anterior flexion of lower part of back causing hollow back deformity.

macrodactylia congenital enlargement of one or several digits of hand or foot; may be hereditary.

Madelung's deformity deformity of wrist in which distal end of radius displaced anteriorly; causes dorsal prominence of distal end of ulna and limitations in dorsiflexion of wrist.

Marfan's syndrome (arachnodactyly) characterized by weakness of muscles, hypermobility of joints, marked scoliosis, long thin extremities, including bones of hands and feet (spider fingers and toes).

melorheostosis (flowing bones) extremely rare condition in which cortical portion of bone is overgrown and gives a flowing appearance; usually confined to a single extremity.

meningococcus arthritis joint infection following meningitis; surrounding tissues more involved than joints; prognosis good when immobilization and sulfonamide injection used; anklyosis not infrequent.

Morquio's disease syndrome of mild dwarfism that is hereditary and involves body asymmetrically as compared to achondroplasia.

myleomas, multiple cancerlike type of generalized bone destruction; always fatal.

myositis inflammation of a muscle.

myositis ossificans (progressiva) rare disease of unknown origin in which the muscles and fascia are converted into bone; childhood disease involving first the spinal muscles and gradually spreading to other parts of the body.

Nélaton's line extends from the anterosuperior iliac spine to ischial tuberosity.

osteitis deformans (Paget's disease) disease of unknown origin that affects persons of middle age and manifests itself by gradual thickening and bowing of shafts of long bones and thickening of skull; cystic areas in bone that are filled with gelatinous and fibrous material with great increase in vascularity; trunk may gradually become shortened and chest barrel-shaped; legs and arms may become bowed; roentgenograms show characteristic bone changes; patient usually complains of aching pains in spine and extremities; treatment directed toward support or correction of deformities.

osteitis fibrosa cystica (von Recklinghausen's disease) decalcification of bone caused by hypersecretion of parathormone from parathyroid glands; excretion of calcium and phosphorous markedly increased; formation of renal calculi is not uncommon; bone fractures may result from decalcification process.

osteitis of Garré (chronic diffuse sclerosing) usually occurs in shafts of long bones in late childhood; thickening of bone and cortex; may be redness, tenderness, and a dull ache; treatment by excision of thickened bone cortex or drilling holes through it.

osteochondromatosis formation of multiple loose cartilaginous bodies within joints.

osteoclasis fracturing a bone surgically by means of an osteoclast.

osteogenesis imperfecta (fragilitas osseum, brittle bones) congenital or inherited disease in which calcium content and size of bones is far below normal; numerous fractures usually result from even mildest types of trauma; represent a difficult nursing problem on this account; healing of fractures normal; dwarfism common; eyes have peculiar bluish discoloration of sclera; condition has a tendency to disappear after puberty but is distinctly hereditary in character; prevention of deformities and later correction of deformities are orthopedic problems.

osteomalacia deficiency disease of bone in which decalcification takes place and bones may collapse; characterized by heart-shaped pelvic ring.

osteopetrosis (marble bones) thickening of bone cortex throughout bones of body including the pelvis, vertebrae, and skull; blindness frequently associated with the disease.

osteopoikilosis (spotted bones) a rare condition in which there is scattered spotting in ends of long bones usually discovered accidentally by roentgenography; usually no symptoms.

osteoporosis decalcification of the bone.

osteosclerosis group of diseases characterized by abnormal increase in calcium content of bone as shown in roentgenograms; thickening of cortex and narrowing of medullary canal; cause unknown.

osteotomy cutting of bone.

plantar wart ordinary wart that occurs on weightbearing surface of foot and is usually extremely painful on pressure.

pneumococcus arthritis usually follows pneumonia in about 2 weeks with an active and painful joint infection; plus formation; poor prognosis held for joint; treatment by drainage, splinting, and the administration of sulfonamides.

polydactylism excessive number of fingers or toes.

podagra gouty inflammation of great toe.

Raynaud's disease vasomotor constrictor disturbance that may affect upper or lower extremities or both.

renal rickets dwarfism; rare disease of childhood in which there is replacement of red bone marrow by fat; seen in combination with chronic interstitial nephritis.

Schüller-Christian disease (xanthomatosis) childhood disease characterized by deposit of fat in bone as result of disturbed fat metabolism; roentgenographic findings of multiple cystic areas characteristic.

scorbutus scurvy.

scurvy caused by dietary deficiency of vitamin C (antiscorbutic vitamin); characterized by subperiosteal and submucous hemorrhages.

sequestrum usually refers to dead bone that acts as medius for continuing drainage, as in osteomyelitis.

spasmodic wryneck characterized by jerking motions

of head and neck as a result of chronic nerve irritation; treatment by long immobilization in plaster cast that includes head, shoulders, and chest.

spondylitis inflammation of vertebra.

Still's disease generalized rheumatoid arthritis in children.

subluxation incomplete dislocation.

synostosis when two contiguous bones become united as variant from normal; congenital synostosis of the radius and ulna is example; trauma can be productive of synostosis.

synovitis inflammation of the synovial membrane lining joint capsule.

talipes refers to ankle.

tenodesis securing tendon to bone.

tenotomy cutting of tendon.

tuberculous dactylitis tuberculous infection of bones of fingers and toes; develops in early childhood; areas of destruction in phalanges and metacarpals, usually accompanied by pus formation and bone sequestration; responds to conservative treatment with rest and sunshine.

typhoid spine typhoid bacillus infection of vertebra coincidental with typhoid fever; characterized by extreme pain in back and extremities and elevation of temperature; roentgenograms show localized destruction and proliferation of bone in low dorsal or lumbar region; treatment usually by immobilization in plaster casts; recovery usually takes place, but there may be permanent but localized stiffness.

Index